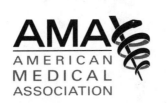

# Principles of CPT® Coding

*Fifth edition*

**American Medical Association**
**Executive Vice President, Chief Executive Officer:** Michael D. Maves, MD, MBA
**Chief Operating Officer:** Bernard L. Hengesbaugh
**Senior Vice President, Publishing and Business Services:** Robert A. Musacchio, PhD
**Vice President, Business Products:** Anthony J. Frankos
**Director, Editorial and Operations:** Mary Lou White
**Senior Acquisitions Editor:** Elise Schumacher
**Director, CPT:** Michael Beebe
**Director, CPT Education and Information Services:** Danielle Pavloski
**Director, CPT Editorial Research and Development:** Marie Mindeman
**Former Director, CPT Editorial and Research Development:** Grace Kotowicz
**Director, CPT Product Development:** Dan Reyes
**Director, Production and Manufacturing:** Jean Roberts
**Director, Business Marketing and Communication:** Pam Palmersheim
**Director, Sales and Strategic Partnerships:** J. D. Kinney
**Developmental Editor:** Elizabeth Dudek
**Senior Production Specialist:** Rosalyn Carlton
**Senior Production Specialist:** Boon Ai Tan
**Senior Print Production Specialist:** Ronnie Summers
**Marketing Manager:** Amy Burgess

Internet address: www.ama-assn.org

For information regarding the reprinting or licensing of *Principles of CPT® Coding, Fifth Edition,* please contact:

American Medical Association CPT Intellectual Property Services
515 N State St
Chicago, Ill 60610
312 464-5022

Additional copies of this book may be ordered by calling 800 621-8335 or from the secure AMA Web site at www.amabookstore.com. Refer to product number OP501007.

ISBN 978-1-57947-967-1
AC24:07-P-026:10/07

# Table of Contents

## Chapter 6  Anesthesia   315

## Chapter 7  Radiology   327

## Chapter 8  Pathology and Laboratory   367

## Chapter 9

# Medicine
# 405

# Foreword

Since 1966 the American Medical Association (AMA), working with the CPT Editorial Panel, has maintained Current Procedural Terminology (CPT®) as a code set that clearly and comprehensively describes the clinically recognized and generally accepted services provided by health care professionals to individual patients and populations. The CPT code set is designed to communicate uniform information about medical services and procedures and to accurately describe medical, surgical, and diagnostic services among physicians, coders, patients, accreditation organizations, and payers for administrative, financial, and analytical purposes. Given the diverse uses and users of the CPT code set, the consistent and accurate application of CPT coding rules and guidelines is important for everyone in the health care system.

The CPT Editorial Panel and the CPT Advisory Committee consider CPT section guidelines, specific code level instructions and definitions, and the application of modifiers at the same time the language for CPT code descriptors is developed. Thus, proper use of CPT codes must be based on all the associated material within the CPT codebook. For example, "simple, intermediate, and complex repair" are defined in the CPT codebook prior to the actual repair codes so that users understand the circumstances for reporting. Also, coding conventions, such as add-on codes, are explained in the guidelines. The use of codes and descriptions apart from this information limit the functionality of CPT coding and uniform application that contribute to improper coding interpretations, which is counter to the purpose of having national standard code sets. The AMA believes that the consistent and accurate application of CPT coding rules and guidelines is an important aspect of controlling health care costs by reducing administrative complexity.

The purpose of *Principles of CPT Coding* is to serve as an in-depth exploration of the rules and guidelines for applying the CPT code set. In this sense, *Principles of CPT Coding* is a textbook to help educate users of the CPT code set. Insights are shared on CPT coding rules that have been developed and refined over the course of the AMA's involvement in the development of the CPT codebook. By building on the work and collective experience of the CPT Editorial Panel, the CPT Advisory Committee, and AMA CPT staff, this text conveys information on the CPT code set that has been gained from more than 40 years of work with medical terminology and its functional integration with health care clinical and administrative processes.

But *Principles of CPT Coding* is more than a textbook; it is an invitation to participate in the future of the CPT code set. Because the CPT code set is a working terminology that continually incorporates the practical wisdom of physicians, health care professionals, administrators, and coders, you are part of the CPT community and a participant in its growth and enhancement. As you study this text and answer the questions following many of the chapters, I encourage you to consider how the rules and guidelines should be applied in practice and then how to improve the CPT code set for the benefit of patients and all CPT users.

Michael Beebe
Director, CPT
American Medical Association

# Preface

When we were developing *Principles of CPT Coding*, we decided that the text would be designed to serve as a guide for learning and using the CPT nomenclature, and not as a substitute for the CPT codebook. With this in mind, we have intentionally excluded long listings of code descriptions. In addition, as you work your way through the book, you will notice that it follows the same basic format as the CPT codebook. So for those of you familiar with the CPT code set, you will find this makes the book easy to follow. For others, you will probably want to familiarize yourself with the basic layout of the CPT nomenclature before reading *Principles of CPT Coding*.

In some of the chapters, we include brief anatomy and physiology reviews. They are included simply to help orient you to the subjects being discussed in the chapters, and not as a substitute for your medical reference books (some of which are listed in our appendix of resources) or more formal education in anatomy and physiology.

Finally, when reading the *Principles of CPT Coding*, you must always bear in mind that the information presented is from the CPT coding perspective, and conveys the intent of the CPT Editorial Panel. Payment policies are determined by third-party payers, and not by the American Medical Association. Therefore, any specific payment-related questions or issues should be directed to the respective third-party payers.

# Acknowledgments

We wish to acknowledge the efforts of AMA CPT Coding Specialists Martha Espronceda, DeHandro Hayden, Grace Kotowicz, Anita Majerowicz, Janette Meggs, Susan Tracy, Peggy Thompson, and Ada Walker; Senior Coding Specialists Karen O'Hara, Mary O'Heron, Lianne Stancik, and Desiree Rozell; also Staff Assistants Rejina Glenn, Desiree Evans, and Joyce A. Dalton, for managing the development and production of the book. Finally, we want to thank the CPT Editorial Panel and the CPT/HCPAC Advisory Committee for their contributions and review of the material presented in *Principles of CPT Coding, Fifth Edition.*

For information about all the coding and reimbursement references and resources available from the American Medical Association, call 800 621-8335 or visit www.amabookstore.com.

## Additional Study Material Available on AMA Web Site

**www.amabookstore.com**

As a special interactive feature, the AMA developed a Web page to give book purchasers the opportunity to test their knowledge after reading the book. Log onto www.amabookstore.com and type in "Principles of CPT Coding" in the Search box for additional study materials and also the opportunity to earn up to three continuing education units (CEUs), by successfully completing our on-line quizzes.

# CHAPTER 1

# Introduction to CPT® Nomenclature

In this chapter, the history behind the development and maintenance of the American Medical Association's (AMA) Current Procedural Terminology (CPT®) nomenclature is discussed.

# What Is the CPT® Nomenclature?

CPT nomenclature is a listing of descriptive terms, guidelines, and identifying codes for reporting medical services and procedures. The purpose of CPT nomenclature is to provide a uniform language that accurately describes medical, surgical, and diagnostic services—serving as an effective means for reliable nationwide communication among physicians, patients, and third parties.

Inclusion of a Category I CPT code descriptor and its associated specific five-digit identifying code number in CPT coding is generally based on the procedure being consistent with contemporary medical practice and performed by many physicians in clinical practice in multiple locations. Inclusion of a procedure or service in CPT coding does not represent endorsement by the AMA of any particular diagnostic or therapeutic procedure, nor does it imply any health insurance coverage or reimbursement policy.

# How Is CPT Nomenclature Used?

CPT codes and descriptive terms currently serve a wide variety of important functions in the field of medical nomenclature. CPT coding is the most widely accepted medical nomenclature used to report medical procedures and services under government and private health insurance programs.

CPT coding is also used for administrative management purposes such as claims processing and developing guidelines for medical review. The uniform language is also applicable to medical education and research by providing a useful basis for local, regional, and national utilization comparisons.

# How Was CPT Nomenclature Developed?

The AMA first developed and published CPT nomenclature in 1966. The first edition helped encourage the use of standard terms and descriptors to document procedures in the medical record, helped communicate accurate information on procedures and services to agencies concerned with insurance claims, provided the basis for a computer-oriented system to evaluate operative procedures, and contributed basic information for actuarial and statistical purposes.

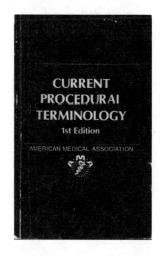

The first edition of *Current Procedural Terminology®*, published in 1966, contained primarily surgical procedures, with limited sections on medicine, radiology, and laboratory procedures. When first published, CPT coding used a four-digit system. The second edition, published in 1970, presented an expanded system of terms and codes to designate diagnostic and therapeutic procedures in surgery, medicine, and the specialties. It was at that time that the five-digit codes were introduced, replacing the former four-digit system. Another significant change to the book was to list procedures related to internal medicine.

In the mid to late 1970s, the third and fourth editions of CPT nomenclature were introduced. The fourth edition, published in 1977, represented significant updates in medical technology, and a system of periodic updating was introduced to keep pace with the rapidly changing medical environment.

In 1983, CPT nomenclature was adopted as part of the Healthcare Common Procedure Coding System (HCPCS) developed by the Centers for Medicare and Medicaid Services (CMS) (formerly the Health Care Financing Administration [HCFA]). (Refer to discussions later in this chapter for more detail on HCPCS.) With this adoption, the CMS mandated the use of HCPCS to report services for Part B of the Medicare program. In October 1986, CMS also required state Medicaid agencies to use HCPCS in the Medicaid Management Information System. In July 1987, as part of the Omnibus Budget Reconciliation Act, CMS mandated the use of CPT codes for reporting outpatient hospital surgical procedures.

Today, in addition to use in federal programs (Medicare and Medicaid), CPT nomenclature is used extensively throughout the United States as the preferred system of coding to describe health care services. In August 2000, the CPT code set was named as a national standard under the Health Insurance Portability and Accountability Act of 1996 (HIPAA).

## Who Maintains CPT Nomenclature?

The AMA's CPT Editorial Panel is responsible for maintaining the CPT nomenclature. This panel is authorized to revise, update, and modify CPT codes. The panel is made up of 17 members as follows:
- Eleven are nominated by the AMA.
- One member is a representative of the Performance Measures development organizations.
- Two members are nonphysicians, representing the Health Care Professionals Advisory Committee (HCPAC).
- One is nominated by the Blue Cross and Blue Shield Association.
- One is nominated by the Health Insurance Plans.
- One is nominated by CMS.
- One is nominated by the American Hospital Association.

The AMA's Board of Trustees appoints the panel members. Of the 11 AMA seats on the panel, 7 are regular seats, having a maximum tenure of two four-year terms, or a total of eight years for any one individual. One of these seats is designated for a physician who can represent the performance measures development organizations. The four remaining seats, called rotating seats, each have one four-year term. These rotating seats allow for diverse specialty input.

Five members of the Editorial Panel serve as the panel's Executive Committee. The Executive Committee includes the chairman, the vice chairman, and three panel members-at-large, as elected by the entire panel. One of the three members-at-large of the executive committee must be a third-party payer representative.

The AMA provides staff support for the CPT Editorial Panel and appoints a staff secretary who records the minutes of the meetings and keeps records.

## The CPT Advisory Committee

In addition to the CPT Editorial Panel, there is a larger body of CPT advisers that supports the CPT Editorial Panel in its work. The CPT Advisory Committee members are primarily physicians nominated by the national medical specialty societies represented in the AMA House of Delegates. Currently, the Advisory Committee is limited to national medical specialty societies seated in the AMA House of Delegates and to the AMA HCPAC organizations representing limited-license practitioners and other allied health professionals. Additionally, a group of individuals, the Performance Measures Advisory Committee (PMAC), who represent various organizations concerned with performance measures, also provide expertise.

The Advisory Committee's primary objectives are as follows:
- To serve as a resource to the CPT Editorial Panel by giving advice on procedure coding and appropriate nomenclature as relevant to the member's specialty or practice.
- To provide documentation to AMA staff and the CPT Editorial Panel regarding the appropriateness of various medical and surgical procedures under consideration as CPT codes.
- To suggest revisions to the CPT nomenclature. (The Advisory Committee meets annually to discuss items of mutual concern and keep informed on current issues in coding and nomenclature.)
- To assist in the review and further development of relevant coding issues and in the preparation of technical education material and articles pertaining to CPT coding.
- To promote and educate its membership on the use and benefits of CPT coding.

## AMA Health Care Professionals Advisory Committee

Current CPT nomenclature contains many codes that are used by both doctors of medicine (MDs)/doctors of osteopathy (DOs) and non-MD/DOs. In some instances, use of CPT codes by non-MD/DOs is required by legislation and regulation. In other instances, third-party payers have retained limiting policies governing how non-MD/DOs report their services by means of CPT codes. In 1992, the AMA Board of Trustees concluded that an HCPAC should be established for the CPT Editorial Panel and the Relative Value Scale Update Committee (RUC) to open up these processes to all the groups legally required to use CPT codes to report their services.

Responding to this recommendation, organizations representing physician assistants, nurses, occupational and physical therapists, optometrists, podiatrists, psychologists, social workers, audiologists, speech pathologists, chiropractors, dietitians, and, most recently, respiratory therapists, naturopaths, and genetic counselors were invited to nominate representatives to the HCPAC.

The HCPAC allows for participation of organizations representing limited-license practitioners and allied health professionals in the CPT and RUC processes. The co-chairman and one member of the HCPAC are also voting members of the CPT Editorial Panel. (Refer to the Appendix of Resources regarding where to obtain information about the RUC and the RUC process.)

## Who Can Submit Suggestions for Changes to CPT Nomenclature?

Anyone can request a change to CPT coding. The effectiveness of the CPT nomenclature depends on constant updating to reflect changes in medical practice. Suggestions of physicians, medical specialty societies, state medical associations, and those who deal regularly with health care information are the only way to ensure that CPT nomenclature reflects current practice.

The AMA welcomes correspondence, inquiries, and suggestions concerning old and new procedures. Specific procedures exist for addressing suggestions to revise CPT coding, add or delete codes, or modify existing nomenclature. Coding change request forms are available through the AMA and are required to initiate a review of a proposed coding change by the CPT Advisory Committee. These forms play a vital role in maintaining and increasing the efficiency of the CPT process. One can visit the CPT Web site at www.ama-assn.org for information regarding submitting suggestions for changes to CPT nomenclature.

## How Are Suggestions for Changes to CPT Nomenclature Reviewed?

Before submitting suggestions for changes to CPT nomenclature, the requester should consider the following questions:
* Is the suggestion a fragmentation of an existing procedure/service?
* Can the suggested procedure/service be reported by using one or more existing codes?
* Is the suggested procedure/service performed by many physicians/practitioners across the United States, or is it highly regionalized?
* Does the suggested procedure/service represent a distinct physician's service?
* Is the suggested procedure/service merely a means to report extraordinary circumstances related to the performance of a procedure/service already having a specific CPT code?
* Why are the existing CPT codes inadequate?

As indicated in the CPT Process flow chart on page 8, this is a multistep process. Being a multistep process naturally means that deadlines are very important. The deadlines for coding change requests and Advisory Committee's comments are based on a schedule that allows at least three months of preparation and processing time before the issue is ready to be reviewed by the CPT Editorial Panel.

The CPT Editorial Panel meets three times each year to address the complexities associated with new and emerging technologies and to manage outdated procedures.

When a suggestion to revise CPT nomenclature is received, AMA staff reviews the proposal to evaluate the coding suggestion. If the AMA staff determines that the panel has already addressed the question, the requester is informed of the panel's prior interpretation. If the staff determines that the request is a new issue or significant new information is received on an item that the panel previously reviewed, the request is referred to the appropriate members of the CPT Advisory Committee. The requester must have completed and submitted a coding change request form.

If the advisers determine that no new code or revision is needed, the AMA staff provides information to the requestor on how to use existing codes to report the procedure or service. If all the advisers agree that a change should be made or if two or more advisers disagree or give conflicting information, the issue is referred to the CPT Editorial Panel for resolution.

This first step, which includes staff and specialty adviser review, is complete (1) when all appropriate advisers have been contacted and have responded and (2) when all information requested of a specialty society or an individual requestor has been provided to the AMA staff.

The next step involves AMA staff preparing materials for the CPT Editorial Panel meeting agenda. The topics for the agenda are gathered from several sources. Medical specialty or other professional societies, individual physicians, hospitals, third-party payers, and other interested parties may submit materials for consideration by the Editorial Panel. Each agenda item includes a ballot for the request to be acted upon by the panel.

The panel actions can result in one of the following three outcomes:
- Add a new code or revise existing nomenclature, in which case the change would appear in a forthcoming edition of the CPT codebook.
- Postpone/table an item to obtain further information.
- Reject an item.

Once the panel has taken an action and approved the minutes of the meeting, the AMA staff informs the requester of the outcome. If the requester wishes to appeal the panel's decision, there is an appeal process to follow.

To appeal a decision, AMA staff must receive a written request for reconsideration. The request must contain the reason the requester believes that the panel's actions are incorrect and should respond to the panel's stated rationale. Once this information is received, the issue is referred to the CPT Executive Committee for a decision to reconsider. A proposal whose appeal is rejected by the Executive Committee and/or panel cannot be reconsidered for one year from the date of that meeting.

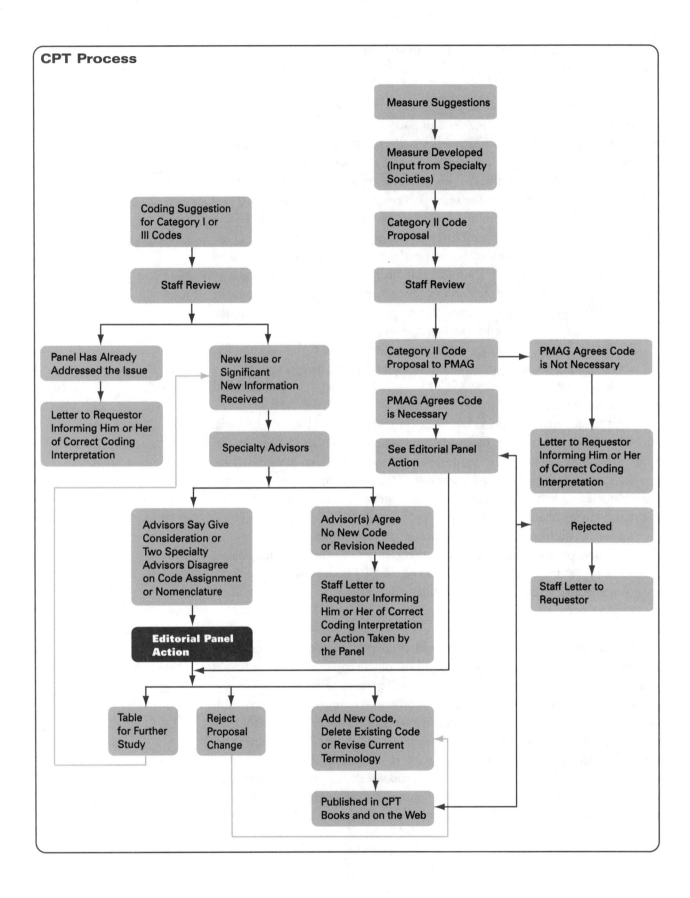

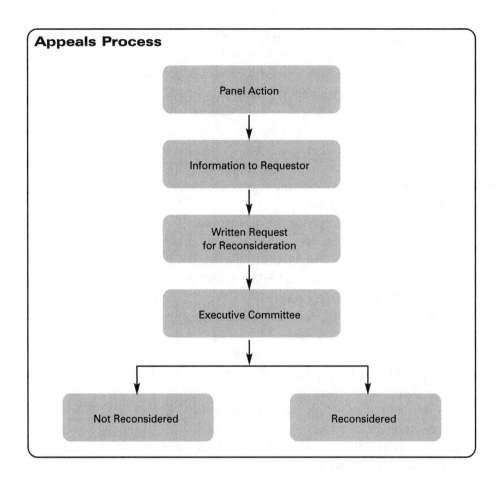

**Appeals Process**

- Panel Action
- Information to Requestor
- Written Request for Reconsideration
- Executive Committee
- Not Reconsidered
- Reconsidered

## Categories of CPT Codes

In order to adapt CPT to allow maximum participation of users and key stake-holders, the AMA began a project that used the workgroup process to assess the ability of CPT to address issues of clinical practice, data management, government, organized medicine, and coding. This project, CPT-5, examined issues such as coding for nonphysician professionals, coding to facilitate the collection of data for quality health services and public health research, the elimination of ambiguity and enhanced specificity, the development of uniform coding rules, and changes to the editorial process to allow greater participation and efficient development of new descriptions of service. New ways to maintain CPT nomenclature were also examined, including enhanced databases and other new technologies.

The final recommendations of the CPT-5 workgroup were that CPT processes should (1) enhance the existing functionality of the CPT nomenclature, (2) correct problem areas, and (3) expand the codes and descriptors to accommodate emerging demands in the provision of health care. The recommendations of the CPT-5 workgroup have been introduced to CPT in an incremental fashion since the conclusion of the workgroup. The changes resulting from these recommendations preserve the core elements that define CPT nomenclature as the language to communicate clinical information for administrative and financial purposes. These core elements include the following:

- Descriptions of clinically recognized and generally accepted health care services
- A five-character core with concept extenders (modifiers)
- Professional responsibility for a mechanism for periodic review and updating

On the basis of the activities of the workgroup, CPT nomenclature attributes that have been developed or continue to evolve include the following:

- Codes for new technology
- Standardized codes for performance measures
- Codes to capture preventive medicine/screening services
- Codes to capture education/counseling services
- Development of nonphysician health professional evaluation services
- Expanded Editorial Panel process
- Decrease of the time frame involved in obtaining a CPT code through Web and Internet communications
- Expansion of the CPT Advisory Committee
- Improvement of CPT nomenclature instructions/guidelines to be more comprehensive, user-friendly, and specific
- Development of a CPT glossary to standardize definitions and differentiate use of synonymous terms
- Maintenance of the CPT code set through a database that incorporates data modeling tools and vocabulary structures to formalize the hierarchical relationships within the CPT code set
- Computer management of intellectual content data and transition into various print publication processes
- Development of CPT educational material and training for postgraduate medical education, health care professional societies, and others who use CPT terminology

As a part of the drive to extend the functionality of CPT nomenclature, in which CPT nomenclature would meet the needs of data reporting in the areas of enrollment, encounter, outcomes, and quality data, and to enhance data collection with CPT codes without significantly altering the current structure and payment focus of CPT nomenclature, the workgroups involved in the CPT-5 project recommended that CPT codes be tiered to accommodate inclusion of codes to report performance measures and codes for emerging technology, services, and procedures.

With the implementation of the workgroup recommendations, CPT codes have been introduced to facilitate collection of data for performance measures (Category II codes) and to report emerging technology, services, and procedures (Category III codes). These codes appear after the Medicine section of *CPT* and before Appendix A. All five-character codes other than these are considered to be CPT Category I codes.

# Category I CPT Codes

Category I CPT codes describe a procedure or service identified with a five-digit numeric CPT code and descriptor nomenclature. The inclusion of a descriptor and its associated five-digit identifying code number in this category of CPT codes is generally based on the procedure being consistent with contemporary medical practice and being performed by many physicians in clinical practice in multiple locations.

# Category II CPT Codes

Category II CPT codes are a set of optional codes developed principally to support performance measurement. These codes are intended to facilitate data collection by encoding specific services and/or test results that have an evidence base for contributing to positive health outcomes and quality patient care. These codes describe performance of clinical components that are typically included in an evaluation and management (E/M) service or other component part of a service. Consequently, Category II codes do not have a relative value associated with them. The use of these codes is optional and not required for correct coding.

The decision to develop Category II codes for performance measurement was based on a desire to standardize the collection of data for performance measurement, a response that agrees with current Health Insurance Portability and Accountability Act (HIPPA) guidelines. Among many other provisions, the HIPAA guidelines designate that providers "use the same . . . code sets, and identifiers" (Centers for Medicare and Medicaid Services [CMS] Web site, Transactions and Code Set Standards: Overview, www.cms.hhs.gov/TransactionCodeSetsStands). This process has been engaged to promote better communication between providers, payers, and patients through the use of a designated set of codes to identify services, procedures, and other information related to the delivery of health care. For more information regarding HIPAA, visit the CMS Web site.

Former methods of capturing performance data were based on detailed chart review, data abstraction, or site surveys—processes that are costly for physicians and health plans. Measurement based upon claims data used for payment was limited to process measures with specific Category I or HCPCS Level II codes. Coding data elements of performance measures on a claim provide an opportunity for the administrative data system to allow physicians to supply information on performance measures directly to health plans.

Category II codes are ideally developed from measures that are evidence-based—that is, the element being measured has published evidence that it is associated with improved clinical outcomes, eg, a better hemoglobin A1c (HbA1c) being associated with reduction in end organ complications of diabetes as published in the Diabetes Control and Complications Trial (DCCT) trials. Some measures are based upon consensus panels and Category II codes may facilitate collecting the data that will determine if the process is or is not associated with improved outcomes.

The first step involved in development of quality measures is to identify those activities that are nationally recognized and have an evidence base that demonstrates contribution to quality patient care. In other words, the measure has to be shown to be well known throughout the country as a practice that contributes to positive patient outcomes when done and has been tested/surveyed (or "vetted") to prove this to be true. Performance measurement of attributes of care not widely recognized to be valid components of high-quality care is unlikely to improve care.

The CPT Editorial Panel does develop CPT codes (including Category II codes), however it does not develop measures. Instead, Category II codes that are released via the efforts of the CPT Editorial Panel and the Performance Measures Advisory Group (PMAG) are codes based on specific measures that are developed by certain designated national organizations. These groups include the following:

- The National Committee for Quality Assurance (NCQA),
- The Agency for Healthcare Research and Quality (AHRQ),
- The Joint Commission on Accreditation of Healthcare Organizations (JCAHO),
- The American Medical Association-convened Physician Consortium for Performance Improvement® (Consortium [PCPI]).

These organizations develop broadly accepted measures that are currently used in health care performance improvement. Each group has its own requirements and established method for developing quality measures. As a result, individuals/parties seeking to develop new measures through one of these organizations should contact the organization directly to identify its specific requirements regarding the development of performance measures.

The measures have also typically been further accepted by the National Quality Forum (www.qualityforum.org/) and the Ambulatory Quality Alliance (AQA) (www.ambulatoryqualityalliance.org). These two organizations work to prioritize the implementation of quality improvement activities focusing on public reporting and to create consistency in measures. Measures endorsed by these organizations are also eligible for development into CPT Category II codes.

## Measure Requests

Details for measure requests developed by the AHRQ, JCAHO, and/or NCQA should be obtained directly from those organizations. Web site information is as follows:

- Agency for Healthcare Research and Quality (AHRQ), www.ahrq.gov
- Joint Commission on Accreditation of Healthcare Organizations (JCAHO), ORYX Initiative Performance Measures, www.jcaho.org/pms
- National Committee on Quality Assurance (NCQA), Health Employer Data Information Set (HEDIS®), www.ncqa.org
- The AMA-convened Physician Consortium for Performance Improvement® (Consortium), www.physicianconsortium.org

The AMA-convened Physician Consortium for Performance Improvement is committed to enhancing quality of care and patient safety by taking the lead in the development, testing, and maintenance of evidence-based clinical performance measures and measurement resources for physicians. The Consortium is comprised of over 100 national medical specialty and state medical societies, the Council of Medical Specialty Societies, the American Board of Medical Specialties and its member-boards, experts in methodology and data collection, the AHRQ, and CMS. The Consortium's mission is to improve patient health and safety by

- identifying and developing evidence-based clinical performance measures that enhance quality of patient care and that foster accountability,
- promoting the implementation of effective and relevant clinical performance improvement activities, and
- advancing the science of clinical performance measurement and improvement.

## Category II Code Release Schedule

Code release for Category II codes will generally follow the quarterly dates for implmentation of HCPCS changes. Due to the dynamic nature of the Category II code set, the best method for identifying the latest changes, release, and implementation dates for these codes is to visit the AMA Web site. In addition, information regarding CPT Category II codes, instructions for preparing a code proposal, and a template form are available under the Code Education and Information section within the AMA CPT Web site at www.ama-assn.org/go/cpt.

## Performance Measures Advisory Group

The PMAG, appointed by the AMA Board of Trustees, is composed of physician representatives from: AHRQ, CMS, JACHO, NCQA, and the Consortium. The PMAG, charged with the review of requests for the development of new Category II codes, forwards recommendations to the CPT Editorial Panel (which may include comments from the CPT Advisory Committee). Proposals for Category II codes must be validated by the PMAG before they are passed onto the CPT Editorial Panel. Once approved by the CPT Editorial Panel, the information is posted on the AMA Web site for release and implementation. Implementation of Category II codes typically occurs three months after code release onto the Web, but exceptions do occur for certain code updates. Information regarding release and implementation for specific codes can be obtained by visiting the Category II codes section of the AMA Web site at www.ama-assn.org/ama/pub/category/10616.html.

## CPT Category II Code Format

A Category II code consists of five characters with the letter **F** as the last character (eg, **1234F**) to distinguish it from Category I and Category III CPT codes. Category II codes are located immediately following the final Category I codebook subsection (Medicine). Introductory language in the section explains the purpose of these codes. Similar to codes contained in the Category I section of the CPT codebook, Category II codes are defined by specific code numbers with corresponding descriptor language and include parenthetical notes to guide coders in the use of these codes. When codes are deleted, cross-reference may be added to identify replacement codes when they exist.

In some instances, certain codes may be deleted without replacement, usually due to changes in the measure. Parenthetic notes in the Category II Code Section and reporting instructions in Appendix H are included to instruct users in the appropriate reporting for services whose descriptions have been deleted or revised.

Consistent with the arrangement of codes in other sections of the book and to facilitate flexible code number assignment for future codes, Category II codes are grouped into predefined categories based on established subjective-objective-assessment-plan (SOAP) guidelines for clinical documentation. In addition, Appendix H is included in the CPT codebook to assist users in identifying all measures related to a given clinical condition or topic. The description for each measure also describes the organization that developed the measure(s), the associated Category II code(s), and a synopsis of the use of Category II codes for a given measure. Readers are directed to the aforementioned Web sites for the measure development organizations for more technical specifications and details related to the measure.

Category II codes are grouped according to the following eight predefined categories (definitions for each category are included in the codebook):

- **Composite Measures—0001F:** Facilitate reporting of a group of services when all components are met.
- **Patient Management—0500F:** Utilization measures or measures of patient care provided for specific clinical purposes (eg, prenatal care, presurgical and postsurgical care, referrals).
- **Patient History—1000F:** Aspects of patient history and review of systems.
- **Physical Examination—2000F:** Aspects of physical examination.
- **Diagnostic Screening Processes or Results—3000F:** Results of clinical laboratory tests, radiological, or other procedural examination.
- **Therapeutic, Preventive, or Other Interventions—4000F:** Pharmacologic, procedural, or behavioral therapies, including preventive services such as patient education and counseling.
- **Follow-Up or Other Outcomes—5000F:** Review and communication of test results to patients, patient satisfaction or experience with care, patient functional status.
- **Patient Safety—6000F:** Patient safety practices.

Each code descriptor also includes a *suffix* or an abbreviated clinical topic listing at the end of the descriptor that reminds users of the specific clinical topics and measures in which that code is included. The translations for these suffix listings can be found in the Appendix H listing in alphabetical order next to the full name for that abbreviation.

**EXAMPLE:** 3120F 12-lead ECG performed (**EM**)[5]—the "EM" suffix abbreviation can be located alphabetically in Appendix H, next to the full name for that topic, Emergency Medicine (EM).

More information regarding this topic can be found in the discussion for Appendix H and in Diagrams A and B located in this chapter.

CPT Category II code descriptors include a superscripted number that references the footnote. This footnote provides the name of the organization that developed the measure upon which the code is based and the URL for the measure developer's Web site to facilitate user location of additional data specifications for each measure. Diagram A lists the different components of the Category II Code Section listing.

Diagram A has been included to identify each of the specific parts of the Category II Code Section document and how each part is used to assist in determining the appropriate code for the procedures and measures that are being identified. Since the document included in the CPT codebook and the document included on the AMA Web site have similarities and differences, both have been noted to inform users of the distinctions between each document as both are necessary to obtain a complete listing of all Category II codes available for use.

## Diagram A – Category II Code Section – Web Document and Codebook document

**Category II Code Section Heading –** This title divides the Category II Code Section into groups according to standard clinical documenation format.

**Heading definition –** Gives the user a brief synopsis of the types of codes (and therefore the types of measures) that are included as part of that section of the Category II codes.

**Superscripts & Footers –** The superscripted number shown after the descriptor language and suffix acronym refers users to the footnotes that display the specific developer for the measure. The information noted in the footnote includes the URL for the developer's Web site where a complete listing of the measure langauge can be found.

**Disease Condition/Suffix Acronym** Provides an abbreviation of the clinical conditions or topics at the end of the code descriptor. This is added to the code to help the user identify each clinical condition or topic in which the code is associated. The suffix acts as a "cross reference" to the Appendix H Clinical topic, allowing users a quick method to find *where* the code can be found in the Appendix H listing. The full translated title for each suffix may be found alphabetically in the Appendix H listing.

# Physical Examination

Physical examination codes describe aspects of physical examination or clinical assessment.

▲ 2001F    Weight recorded (CHF, PAG)[1]

Released: July 1, 2006

Implemented: October 1, 2006

First appearance of change in CPT Coding Manual: **CPT 2008**

▶ (Code 2003F has been deleted. For performance measurement coding information regarding heart failure, see the Heart Failure Clinical Topic listing in Appendix H) ◀

Released: March 17, 2006

Implemented: July 1, 2006

First appearance of change in CPT Coding Manual: **CPT 2007**

▲ 2010F    Vital signs (temperature, pulse, respiratory rate, and blood pressure) documented and reviewed (CAP)[2], (EM)[5]

Released: December 1, 2006

Implemented: January 1, 2007

First appearance of change in CPT Coding Manual: **CPT 2008**

Footnotes
[1] Physician Consortium for Performance Improvement, www.physicianconsortium.org
[2] National Committee on Quality Assurance (NCQA), Health Employer Data Information Set (HEDIS®), www.ncqa.org
[3] Joint Commission on Accreditation of Healthcare Organizations (JCAHO), ORYX Initiative Performance Measures, www.jcaho.org/pms
[4] National Diabetes Quality Improvement Alliance (NDQIA), www.nationaldiabetesalliance.org
[5] Joint measure from The Physician Consortium for Performance Improvement, www.physicianconsortium.org and National Committee on Quality Assurance (NCQA), www.ncqa.org
[6] The Society of Thoracic Surgeons, http://www.sts.org, National Quality Forum, http://www.qualityforum.org

Copyright © 2007 American Medical Association

**Date Information – Release, Implementation, & Appearance Dates (WEB DOCUMENTS ONLY):** These dates note 1) the code's first appearance on the Web, and 2) when the code will be ready to use for reporting purposes (implementation), as well as the next CPT codebook in which the new codes will appear. The time between these dates is allowed to provide users a chance to incorporate the new codes and changes into their billing systems. **Note:** Codes that appear in the codebook are already implemented. As a result, release/implementation/codebook appearance dates are not included as part of the hardcopy manual.

## Category II Performance Measurement Exclusion Modifiers

Three modifiers are available for reporting in addition to Category II codes when certain reasons may exist that warrant exclusion of a certain group of patients from a given measure. These modifiers report circumstances identified in a performance measure for services that were considered but not provided because of medical, patient, or system reasons documented in the medical record. These reasons are identified as *exclusions,* meaning that they identify a population of patients for whom the ordinary measure requirements do not apply. For the services being measured for these patients, one of three exclusion modifiers is appended to the Category II code to note the special circumstance for the service/procedure/criteria being measured.

> **Modifier 1P identifies exclusions for medical reasons.** This includes any restrictions from meeting the measure parameters because of medically related issues, such as nonprescription of medication noted in the measure due to patient allergies or absence of the organ or limb identified by the measure.

> **Modifier 2P identifies exclusions for patient reasons.** This modifier has been included to identify certain circumstances that allow for patient decisions to influence the provision of the service(s). This includes reasons such as patient exclusions due to patient refusal of services, religious reasons, or economic reasons.

> **Modifier 3P identifies system exclusions.** These exclusions include lack of availability of resources for the procedures/services, lack of insurance coverage, or payer-related issues.

Note that exclusion modifiers should be appended only to Category II codes and should not be used with Category I codes. In addition, these modifiers are not intended to be used for all Category II codes. Instead, reporting instructions are included to provide users information that identifies the specific exclusions that are appropriate for the codes listed in the measure. References to circumstances regarding the exclusions are included in the detailed specifications of the measure itself. The user should review the full measure (by visiting the developer's Web site) to identify more specific information regarding the intent of the measure.

> **8P Modifier added as a reporting modifier.** Modifier 8P is used to report circumstances when an action described in a measure's numerator is not performed and the reason is not otherwise specified. This can include reasons or circumstances such as provision of services to a patient that are unrelated to the measure (for example, treatment of a broken leg for a patient with diabetes where the diabetes is being managed by another physician). This includes *any* non-medical, patient, or system reasons for not meeting measure requirements. This is the only Category II modifier that is not used as an exclusion modifier.

## Appendix H

Appendix H in the CPT codebook is an index arranged in alphabetical order according to clinical condition or topic (Asthma, Chronic Obstructive Pulmonary Disease, etc., with one or more measures per condition or topic). Each measure within the condition listing contains information related to the measure developer, the performance measure, and the associated descriptor and code(s). Appendix H allows the user the ability to identify and locate codes according to the disease conditions or topics that each code is associated with. In addition, it includes a "snapshot" of the associated measure information. This includes:

- The title of the measure
- The measure statement, which tells what the measure is intended to identify
- The numerator, which identifies the population of patients for which the physician/health professional met the measure requirements (ie, the patients for whom the doctor/practitioner has performed the noted services/ procedures)
- The denominator, which identifies the total population of patients for which the measured service was available provided
- The percentage statement, which verbally combines the numerator and denominator into a single statement that notes the population of patients that is being measured
- The Reporting Instructions, which provide valuable information about how the codes are intended to be used. These are statements that are similar to guidelines and parenthetical notes in the Category I and III sections, since they note usage information such as appropriate replacement codes, codes that should be reported in addition, codes that exclude use of another code, and the appropriate use of exclusion modifiers.

A labeled diagram is included on the next page.

## Diagram B: Appendix H

The following diagram has been included to identify the specific components of Appendix H to assist in the selection of the appropriate performance measure and CPT code(s) used with each measure.

**Superscript** – The superscripted number at the end of the Measure Title refers users to the developer for the measure in the footnotes. This information includes the URL for the developer's Web site where a complete listing of the measure language can be found.

**Performance Measure Title** – Displays the title of the specific performance measure consistent with the language of the measure developer's Web site.

**Clinical Topic/Condition** – Displays the specific measure group. All Clinical Topics listed in Appendix H are in alphabetical order and include corresponding abbreviations (in parenthesis).

**Code Number Listing**. This column lists all CPT codes that address compliance with the measure, including Category I, II, and III codes.

### Asthma

| Brief Description of Performance Measure, Source and Reporting Instructions | CPT Code(s) | Code Descriptor |
|---|---|---|
| **Asthma Assessment**[1]<br>Whether or not patient was evaluated during at least one office visit during the reporting year for the frequency (numeric) of daytime and nocturnal asthma symptoms.<br><br>**Numerator:** Patients who were evaluated during at least one office visit during the reporting year for the frequency (numeric) of daytime and nocturnal asthma symptoms.<br>**Denominator:** All patients aged 5–40 years with asthma.<br><br>**Percentage** of patients aged 5–40 years with asthma who were evaluated during at least one office visit during the reporting year for the frequency (numeric) of daytime and nocturnal asthma symptoms.<br><br>**REPORTING INSTRUCTIONS:**<br>To be counted in calculations of this measure, symptom frequency must be numerically quantified. Measure may also be met by physician documentation or patient completion of an asthma assessment tool/survey/questionnaire. Assessment tool may include the Quality Metric Asthma Control Test™, National Asthma Education & Prevention Program (NAEPP) Asthma Symptoms, and Peak Flow Diary. | 1005F | Asthma symptoms evaluated (includes physician documentation of numeric frequency of symptoms or patient completion of an asthma assessment tool/survey/questionnaire) |

**Measure Statement** – Provides a "snapshot" of measure.

**Numerator Statement** – Identifies the patient population for whom the measure requirements were met.

**Denominator Statement** – Denotes the total population eligible for inclusion.

**Percentage Statement** – Percentage of patient population measured compared to eligible population.

**Code Descriptor** – Displays the complete full descriptor for all Category II codes and many Category I codes.

**Reporting Instructions** – Provides specific information including appropriate exclusion criteria, modifier usage, and documentation requirements.

**Footnotes**
[1] Physician Consortium for Performance Improvement, www.physicianconsortium.org
[2] National Committee on Quality Assurance (NCQA), Health Employer Data Information Set (HEDIS®), www.ncqa.org
[3] Joint Commission on Accreditation of Healthcare Organizations (JCAHO), ORYX Initiative Performance Measures, www.jcaho.org/pms
[4] National Diabetes Quality Improvement Alliance (NDQIA), www.nationaldiabetesalliance.org
[5] Joint measure from The Physician Consortium for Performance Improvement, www.physicianconsortium.org and National Committee on Quality Assurance (NCQA), www.ncqa.org
[6] The Society of Thoracic Surgeons, www.sts.org, National Quality Forum, www.qualityforum.org

**Footnotes** – Direct the user to 1) the appropriate developer for each measure, and 2) a link to the developer's Web site. There, users will find the specific performance measure referenced in Appendix H.

Remember that the Appendix H listing is only a snapshot of the measure information. The complete measure parameters should still be accessed to identify all specifications as explanations regarding the intended use of the measure, including details regarding what the measure is for (ie, what it is intended to help), the population that is being measured for quality performance, and any other important details regarding the condition/topic being addressed by the measure will be found there. This information can be found on the source organization's (or measure developer's) Web site.

Because some of the measure codes apply to more than one condition, a code may appear more than once within Appendix H. For example, code **2000F**, *Blood pressure measured*, is a code that identifies a measure that is included as part of both the coronary artery disease clinical topic and the heart failure clinical topic. A listing of Appendix H can be found in the latest edition of the CPT codebook as well as on the AMA Web site at www.ama-assn.org/go/cpt.

## Category II Code Section, Appendix H, and the Web

Users of the Category II code set should note that Category II codes exist both in the CPT codebook and on the AMA Web site. The Appendix H section on the AMA Web site includes a complete listing of all codes. The codes are listed within the Appendix in disease conditions that are provided in alphabetic order. The Web version of Appendix H is regularly updated to reflect the latest codes developed. Therefore, the Web version of Appendix H should be reviewed regularly to identify the latest changes (a posting date is included as part of the listing to identify the date of the latest update to the listing).

The Category II Code Section included on the Web lists only those Category II codes that have been added to the code set since the latest printing of the CPT codebook. Therefore, use both the book and the Web site to identify the complete code set listing for the Category II Code Section.

In addition, each code included on the Category II Code Section notes dates that identify 1) when the code was released (that is, when the code was first posted for viewing and inclusion into user databases), 2) when the code will be implemented (that is, when the codes will be ready for use), and 3) when the code will appear in the hardcopy of the CPT codebook. An implementation period (usually three months) is included between the dates when the code is posted and the date when the code can be used (implemented). This period is included to give users a chance to incorporate the newest codes into their systems. As was stated earlier, codes listed on the Web in the Category II Code Section will remain on the Web until the next publication of the CPT codebook.

# Category III CPT Codes

Category III (Emerging Technology) CPT codes are a set of temporary codes for emerging technology, services, and procedures. Category III CPT codes allow data collection for these services/procedures. These codes are intended to be used for data collection purposes to substantiate widespread usage or in the

Food and Drug Administration (FDA) approval process. Since Category III CPT codes are intended to be used for data collection purposes, they are not intended for services/procedures that are not accepted by the CPT Editorial Panel because the proposal was incomplete, more information is needed, or the Advisory Committee did not support the proposal.

Category III codes were developed to provide an alternative for addition of codes because of the length of time required to develop a CPT code and the requirements for approval of a CPT code. These factors in the development of a Category I code in the CPT process conflicted with the needs of researchers for coded data to track emerging technology services throughout the research process. For a procedure to be approved as a Category I code, the CPT Editorial Panel at a minimum requires that

- services/procedures be performed by many health care professionals across the country;
- FDA approval be documented or be imminent within a given CPT cycle; and
- the service/procedure has proven clinical efficacy.

As such, the Category III CPT codes may not conform to these usual CPT code requirements. For services/procedures to be eligible for Category III codes, the service/procedure must have relevance for research, either ongoing or planned.

Category I CPT codes are restricted to clinically recognized and generally accepted services, not emerging technologies, services, and procedures. Another important consideration in the development of Category III codes was the elimination of local codes under HIPAA. The August 17, 2000, Final Rule supported the elimination of local codes and the transition to national standard code sets. Many of the local codes were temporary codes used by payers until services/procedures were more fully substantiated through research and received a CPT code. On December 31, 2003, CMS eliminated the local codes for reporting. Thus, Category III codes can take the place of temporary local codes used for this purpose.

As with Category I CPT codes, inclusion of a descriptor and its associated code number in CPT nomenclature does not represent endorsement by the AMA of any particular diagnostic or therapeutic procedure/service. Inclusion or exclusion of a procedure/service does not imply any health insurance coverage or reimbursement policy.

Category III codes contain an alphanumeric identifier with **T** in the last field (eg, **1234T**). These codes are located in a separate section of the CPT codebook, after the Category II Code Section. Introductory language in this Code Section explains the purpose of these codes.

To get new CPT Category III codes into the field as soon as possible, once they have been approved by the CPT Editorial Panel, the newly added Category III codes are made available on a semiannual basis via electronic distribution on the AMA CPT Web site (www.ama-assn.org/go/cpt). The full set of Category III codes are then included in the next published edition for that CPT cycle. Such an early release is possible for Category III codes because payment is based on the policies of payers and not on a yearly fee schedule. The AMA's CPT Web site features updates of the CPT Editorial Panel actions and early release of the Category III codes in July and January in a given CPT nomenclature cycle.

The dates for early release correspond with the CPT Editorial Panel meetings for each CPT cycle (February, June, and October).

Category III CPT codes are not referred to the AMA/Specialty RUC for evaluation because no relative value units are assigned to these codes. Payment for these services/procedures is based on the policies of payers and not on a yearly fee schedule.

These codes are archived after five years if the code has not been accepted for placement in the Category I section of the CPT codebook, unless it is demonstrated that a Category III code is still needed. These archived codes are not reused.

# When Are CPT Codes Implemented?

For federal programs, January 1 of each year is generally the effective date for using the new CPT Category I codes. The AMA prepares each annual update so that the new CPT codebooks are available in late fall of each year preceding their implementation. However, other third-party payers might not implement the new codes on the same date. It is important to be familiar with individual payer policies for implementation schedules of new codes each year.

Category II codes are typically released one month after the CPT Editorial Panel meeting at which they were accepted, and implemented three months later. Category III CPT codes and Category I vaccine codes are typically "early-released" for reporting on either January 1 or July 1 of a given CPT cycle.

# The HCPCS Coding System

HCPCS is CMS's Healthcare Common Procedure Coding System. This system was developed in 1983 by HCFA (now CMS) to standardize the coding systems used to process Medicare claims on a national basis. The HCPCS coding system is structured in two levels. Each of the two HCPCS levels is its own unique coding system.

## Level I—CPT Nomenclature

Level I is the AMA's CPT nomenclature, which makes up the majority of the HCPCS coding system. Most of the procedures and services performed by physicians and other health care professionals, even with respect to Medicare patients, are reported with CPT codes. Highlights of the CPT nomenclature are as follows:
- Each procedure or service is identified with a five-digit numeric code or a five-character alphanumeric code.
- Two-digit modifiers are used (refer to Chapter 10 for further discussion).
- Codes are revised and updated on an annual basis.
- Updates and revisions become effective in January.
- Revisions, additions, and deletions are prepared by the AMA's CPT Editorial Panel.

## Level II—National Codes

Level II national codes are assigned, updated, and maintained by CMS. These codes describe services and supplies not found in the CPT code set. Some examples of the procedures and services described by Level II national codes include durable medical equipment, ambulance services, medical/surgical supplies, drugs, orthotics and prosthetics, dental procedures, and vision services. Highlights of the Level II national codes are as follows:

- Five-character alphanumeric codes are used; the first character is a letter (**A** through **V**, except **I** and **S**), followed by four numeric digits.
- Alpha (eg, **LT**) and alphanumeric (eg, **E1**) modifiers are used.
- The codes are updated annually by CMS.
- The codes are required for reporting most medical services and supplies provided to Medicare and Medicaid patients.

The **I** codes are reserved for use by the Health Insurance Association of America to fulfill their member companies' unique coding needs. The **S** codes are created and maintained by the Blue Cross and Blue Shield Association for their needs.

**CHAPTER 1**

# EXERCISES

1 Who developed and maintains the CPT nomenclature?

2 What are the two levels of the HCPCS codes?

3 Who maintains the HCPCS Level II codes?

4 When are Category I, II, and III CPT codes implemented?

5 Which CPT codes are five-digit numeric codes?

6 True or False: Inclusion of a procedure descriptor and its associated code number in the CPT code set indicates health insurance coverage.

7 True or False: The first character of HCPCS Level II codes is numeric.

8 Where is information regarding changes to HCPCS Level II codes obtained?

9 What is the CPT nomenclature?

10 True or False: Category II codes may be used as a substitute for Category I codes.

11 True or False: Appendix H lists the Category II codes in alphabetical order to allow the user to easily find each performance measurement code according to the measure being identified.

12 Fill in the blank: _____ combine several measures within a single code descriptor to facilitate reporting for a particular clinical condition when all components are met.

13 Fill in the blank: Newly added Category II codes are made available on a _____ basis via electronic distribution on the AMA Web site: www.ama-assn.org/go/cpt.

## CHAPTER 2

# CPT® Nomenclature Basics

The prospect of learning Current Procedural Terminology (CPT®) coding can be overwhelming. That is why it is crucial that you have a solid foundation on which to build knowledge. This chapter guides the reader through the basics of the CPT codebook. Go ahead, pick up the book and get a general feel for its layout. Become familiar with the section numbers and their sequences. Take a look at the various code symbols that appear throughout the book. Learn about the format of the terminology in CPT coding. Taking the time to review these basic concepts will help develop the solid foundation needed for CPT coding.

# Section Numbers and Their Sequences

There are eight sections in the CPT codebook. The first six sections pertain to Category I CPT codes. See the following table:

| Section Names and Code Sequences | |
| --- | --- |
| **Section Name** | **Code Sequence** |
| Evaluation and Management | 99201–99499 |
| Anesthesia | 00100–01999, 99100–99140 |
| Surgery | 10021–69990 |
| Radiology | 70010–79999 |
| Pathology and Laboratory | 80048–89356 |
| Medicine | 90281–99199, 99500–99602 |

The seventh and eighth sections pertain to the Category II performance measure CPT codes and the Category III new or emerging technology/devices codes, respectively. The section names and sequences for the Category II and Category III codes are as follows:

| Section Names and Code Sequences for Categories II and III | |
| --- | --- |
| Category II Performance Measurement codes | 0001F–6020F |
| Category III New/Emerging Technology codes | 0016T–0183T |

The procedures and services listed in the CPT nomenclature are presented in numeric order with one exception: the Evaluation and Management (E/M) section appears at the beginning of the book. Since these codes are used by most physicians in reporting a significant portion of their services, they were placed at the front of the book for ease of reference.

# Instructions for Using CPT Nomenclature

When CPT codes are used to report procedures and services, the name of the procedure or service that most accurately identifies the service performed should be selected. Any service or procedure reported should be adequately documented in the medical record to support the specific code(s) reported.

For example, when coding for tumor antigen testing, select the most specific code for the testing procedure performed. Prostate-specific antigen (PSA) testing is reported with codes **84153** and **84154**. These codes are analyte-specific for PSA testing. Carcinoembryonic antigen (CEA) testing is reported with code **82378**.

CPT code **86316**, Immunoassay for tumor antigen; other antigen, quantitative (eg, cancer antigen 50, 72–4, 549), also describes tumor antigen testing but would not be appropriately reported when testing is specifically for PSA or CEA. Code **86316** describes tumor antigen testing by the methodology (ie, immunoassay). This code is used to report tumor antigen testing when an analyte-specific listing (eg, PSA, CEA) is not available in the CPT code set. As indicated in the code descriptor, one example of the use of code **86316** would be for the reporting of cancer antigen 50 testing.

# Placement of a Code in the CPT Code Set: Nomenclature vs Classification

When procedures are evaluated for reimbursement or other purposes, it is important to consider each procedure on its own merits and not simply on the placement of the code in CPT nomenclature. It should be recognized that the listing of a service or procedure in a specific section of the CPT codebook does not restrict its use to a specific specialty group. Any procedure or service in any section of the book may be used to designate the services rendered by any qualified physician or other health care professional.

Questions are often raised regarding the CPT classification of procedures as "surgery." In other classification and definitional systems, such as the Uniform Hospital Discharge Data Set, a definition of a significant procedure has been adopted that includes surgery. As defined in this data set, surgery is incision, excision, amputation, introduction, endoscopy, repair, destruction, suture, and manipulation. Although many of these terms are familiar and included in CPT coding, neither this nor any other definition of surgery has been used to place items in any particular section of the CPT codebook.

Because the CPT nomenclature is not a strict classification system, there may be some procedures that appear in sections other than in those where they might ordinarily be classified. From a historical perspective, CPT coding has always placed procedures in general sections according to where physicians will most conveniently find them.

For example, the code for a diagnostic colonoscopy, although not involving an incision, is located in the Digestive System Surgery section. Keeping the endoscopies involving a biopsy, tumor removal, or other operative interventions in proximity to the diagnostic procedure was an important consideration. Similarly, cast applications are listed in the Musculoskeletal Surgery section in proximity to the fracture and dislocation treatments, but clearly, cast application is not a surgical procedure.

The semantic differences have led to difficulties for physicians and patients in receiving reimbursement for procedures that have been performed. Some patient insurance contracts strictly limit the definition of a surgical procedure and do not cover other "surgical" procedures. Other patient insurance contracts may not cover "surgery" of any type, and the inclusion of a procedure in CPT coding under the Surgery section may lead payers to deny benefits. The issue is sometimes further complicated by "type of service" indicators, which third-party payers often require on their claim forms. Although these indicators are often similar to or the same as the section names of CPT coding, they may be defined differently by payers, and the definitions may vary between payers.

# Format of the Terminology

Without developing a basic understanding of the format of the terminology in CPT coding, appropriate use of the CPT codebook would be almost impossible. Understanding how to read the full description of the CPT codes is a necessary fundamental concept to learn and will assist the reader in appropriate use of the CPT codebook.

The format of the terminology was originally developed as stand-alone descriptions of medical procedures. However, to conserve space and avoid having to repeat common terminology, some of the procedure descriptors in CPT coding are not printed in their entirety but rather refer back to a common portion of the procedure descriptor listed in a preceding entry. Within any indented series of codes, the reader must refer back to the first left-justified code (parent code) within that series to determine the full procedure descriptor of the indented code(s) following.

| | |
|---|---|
| **97010** | Application of a modality to one or more areas; hot or cold packs |
| **97012** | traction, mechanical |
| **97014** | electrical stimulation (unattended) |
| **97016** | vasopneumatic devices |
| **97018** | paraffin bath |
| **97022** | whirlpool |
| **97024** | diathermy (eg, microwave) |
| **97026** | infrared |
| **97028** | ultraviolet |

The common part of the parent code **97010** (that part of the description to the left of the semicolon—"Application of a modality to one or more areas;") should be considered part of each of the following indented codes in that series (**97012–97028**).

For example, the full procedure descriptor represented by code **97012** is as follows:

| | |
|---|---|
| **97012** | Application of a modality to one or more areas; traction, mechanical |

Simply because a code is indented within a series does not mean that one code from a series cannot be reported with another code within the same indented series. If two distinct procedures are performed, both procedures can be coded. However, in such a case, the use of CPT modifiers becomes necessary. (Refer to Chapter 10 for further discussion of modifiers.)

# Code Symbols

To make CPT nomenclature more user-friendly, over the years a number of code symbols have been incorporated into the book. Following are the various code symbols that appear throughout the CPT codebook:

●      Whenever new procedure codes are added to the CPT code set, they are identified throughout the manual with the bullet symbol preceding the code number. Note that this symbol appears for only one year, the year that the code is added.

▲      The triangle is used to designate codes with substantially altered descriptions. Once again, this symbol appears for only one year, the year that the code is revised.

►◄      These sideways triangles are used throughout CPT coding to indicate new and revised text, such as new parenthetical notes and language added to guidelines. They do not apply to code descriptors (see ▲). These symbols appear for only one year, the year that the new and revised text is added. Before these symbols were added in 1998, the only way to determine changed text was to compare books from year to year.

✚      Add-on codes (a special category of CPT codes) are identified with the plus symbol preceding the codes. This symbol was introduced in 1999. Add-on codes can also be identified by specific language in the code descriptor, such as "each additional" or "(List separately in addition to primary procedure)." A complete list of all add-on codes in the CPT code set can be found in Appendix D of the CPT codebook. (Add-on codes are discussed in greater detail in Chapter 4.)

⊘      This symbol designates codes that are exempt from the use of **modifier 51** but have not been designated as CPT add-on procedures/services. As an added reference, Appendix E in the CPT codebook also contains a complete list of the codes exempt from **modifier 51** usage. (Refer to Chapter 4 for further discussion of these codes.)

⊙      This symbol designates codes that include conscious sedation as an inherent part of providing the procedure. As an added reference, Appendix G in the CPT codebook also contains a complete list of the codes that include conscious sedation.

✗      This symbol designates codes for vaccines that are pending approval from the Food and Drug Administration (FDA). Appendix K in the CPT codebook lists all of the codes that are pending FDA approval.

⊃ A green arrow symbol identifies CPT Assistant feature articles and educational instruction related to new, revised, and deleted codes published annually in CPT *Changes: An Insider's View*. For example, an entry that reads CPT Assistant Feb 96:4 and appears after a specific code descriptor indicates that information regarding that code can be found in the February 1996 issue of the newsletter, on page 4.

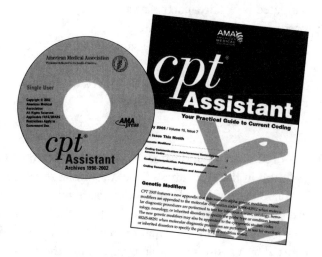

A red arrow symbol identifies *Clinical Examples in Radiology*, a collaborative quarterly publication between the AMA and the American College of Radiology. *Clinical Examples in Radiology* moves coders from theory to practice by providing several carefully selected procedure reports that are dissected and annotated by nationally recognized experts in radiology coding. For example, an entry that reads ⊃ *Clinical Examples in Radiology* Winter 04:7 and appears after a specific code descriptor indicates that information regarding that code can be found in the Winter 2004 issue on page 7.

Contact the AMA's Customer Service department at (800) 621-8335 for pricing and purchasing information for either of these publications. (CPT Assistant is also available on CD-ROM.)

# Guidelines

Specific guidelines can be found at the beginning of each of the six sections of the CPT codebook. The guidelines provide information that is necessary to appropriately interpret and report the procedures and services found in that section.

In addition to the guidelines that appear at the beginning of each section, several of the subheadings or subsections have special instructions unique to that section, resulting in guidelines and instructional notes appearing throughout the CPT codebook (eg, at the beginning of a category or subcategory of codes and in parenthetical notes either preceding or following a code).

All of the guidelines and notes in the book are there to assist users of the CPT nomenclature in appropriate interpretation and application of the codes throughout the book. These guidelines and notes are critical to using CPT coding correctly.

# Modifiers

CPT nomenclature uses modifiers as an integral part of its structure. Modifiers are used to indicate that a performed service or procedure has been altered by some specific circumstance but not changed in its definition.

Modifiers may be used in many instances. Following are some examples:
- To report only the professional component of a procedure or service
- To report a service mandated by a third-party payer
- To indicate that a procedure was performed bilaterally
- To report multiple procedures performed at the same session by the same provider
- To report that a portion of a service or procedure is reduced or eliminated at the physician's discretion
- To report assistant surgeon services

CPT modifiers are two-digit numeric indicators, with the exception of the Physical Status modifiers found in the guidelines of the Anesthesia section and Appendix A of the CPT codebook. Physical Status modifiers are represented by the initial letter **P** followed by a single digit from **1** to **6**. (Refer to the Anesthesia guidelines in the CPT codebook for more information regarding these modifiers.) The modifier is reported by a two-digit number placed after the five-digit CPT code, like this:

**49500 50**

The code and modifier are reported as a one-line entry on the claim form. Further discussion and specific examples of the use of modifiers can be found in Chapter 10, modifiers.

# Unlisted Procedure or Service

Because of advances in the field of medicine, there may be services or procedures performed by physicians or other health care professionals that have not yet been designated with a specific CPT code. To report unlisted procedures or services, a number of specific code numbers have been designated. Each of these unlisted procedure code numbers relates to a specific section of the CPT codebook and is referenced in the guidelines of that section. Unlisted codes provide the means of reporting and tracking services and procedures until a more specific code is established in the CPT code set.

It is very important that the CPT code accurately describe the service that was performed. For that reason, it is equally important that a code that is close to the procedure performed not be selected in lieu of an unlisted procedure.

Some people maintain that they are not allowed to use unlisted procedures or that the use of the codes is undesirable. Although the use of an unlisted procedure code will require a special report or documentation to describe the service, correct coding demands that a square peg not be fit into a round hole.

# Appendixes

In the CPT codebook, there are appendixes located in the back. Each contains helpful information as indicated in the following sections.

## Appendix A—Modifiers

This appendix contains a complete list of the CPT modifiers and their definitions. Also, to provide a more complete reference for the hospital outpatient users of CPT coding, the Healthcare Common Procedure Coding System (HCPCS) Level II national modifiers that have been approved by the National Uniform Billing Committee for hospital outpatient reporting are included in this appendix. (Chapter 10 features a comprehensive discussion of modifiers.)

## Appendix B—Summary of Additions, Deletions, and Revisions

This appendix summarizes the additions, deletions, and revisions applicable to the current edition of the CPT nomenclature.

## Appendix C—Clinical Examples

This appendix contains the clinical examples of the CPT codes for E/M services. These clinical examples were developed in conjunction with the implementation of the new codes for E/M services, which were introduced in *CPT 1992.*

The explanatory paragraphs preceding the actual clinical examples provided contain very important information regarding the use of these clinical examples. The clinical examples, when used with the E/M code descriptors found in the full text of the CPT codebook, are intended to be used as a tool for reporting services provided to patients. Coders should take the time to read and understand the intent of these clinical examples, because the examples can lead to a deeper understanding of the services encompassed in the E/M codes.

## Appendix D—Summary of CPT Add-on Codes

In this appendix, users will find a summary of the codes designated as CPT add-on codes for the current edition of the CPT codebook. These codes are also identified throughout the text of the CPT codebook with the symbol placed before the code. (Refer to Chapter 4 for further discussion of add-on codes.)

## Appendix E—Summary of CPT Codes Exempt From Modifier 51

The codes in the listing that appears in this appendix are exempt from the use of modifier 51 but have not been designated as CPT add-on codes. These codes are identified throughout the text of the CPT codebook with the ⊘ symbol placed before the code. (Refer to Chapter 4 for further discussion of CPT codes exempt from modifier 51.)

## Appendix F—Summary of CPT Codes Exempt From Modifier 63

The codes in the listing that appears in this appendix are exempt from the use of modifier 63. These codes are identified through the text of the CPT codebook with the parenthetical instruction, "(Do not report modifier 63 in conjunction with . . . )."

## Appendix G—Summary of CPT Codes That Include Moderate (Conscious) Sedation

The procedure codes listed in this appendix include conscious sedation as an inherent part of providing the procedure. These codes are identified throughout the text of the CPT codebook with a ⊙ symbol placed before the code.

## Appendix H—Alphabetic Index of Performance Measures by Clinical Condition or Topic

This appendix provides an alphabetical index of performance measures categorized by clinical condition or topic. Prior to reporting a code, the user must review the complete description of the code in the Category II section of the CPT codebook and the complete description of its associated measure by accessing the measure developer's Web site provided in the footnoted reference of the table.

## Appendix I—Genetic Testing Code Modifiers

The modifiers in the listing that appear in this appendix are intended for reporting with molecular laboratory procedures related to genetic testing. Genetic test modifiers should be used in conjunction with CPT and HCPCS codes to provide diagnostic granularity of service to enable providers to submit complete and precise genetic testing information without altering test descriptors.

## Appendix J—Electrodiagnostic Medicine Listing of Sensory, Motor, and Mixed Nerves

This appendix contains a summary that assigns each sensory, motor, and mixed nerve with its appropriate nerve conduction study code in order to enhance accurate reporting of codes **95900**, **95903**, and **95904**. Each nerve constitutes one unit of service.

## Appendix K—Product Pending FDA Approval

This appendix contains a list of vaccine product codes pending approval from the FDA. These codes are indicated with the symbol ⁄ and will be tracked by the AMA to monitor FDA approval status.

## Appendix L—Vascular Family Listing

This appendix provides an assignment of first-, second-, and third-order branches in a vascular family. This table makes the assumption that the starting point is catheterization of the aorta. This categorization would not be accurate, for example, if a femoral or carotid artery were catheterized directly in an ante-grade direction. Arteries highlighted in bold are those more commonly reported during arteriographic procedures.

## Appendix M—Crosswalk to Deleted CPT Codes

This listing is a summary of the deleted *CPT 2007* codes and descriptors that have been crosswalked to *CPT 2008* codes to more easily follow the large number of changes to the codes. Substantial revisions include deletion and renumbering of many codes and adding new subhead titles to provide more appropriate Code Sections for more meaningful, logical location of the codes in the CPT codebook.

# Alphabetic Index

The alphabetic index is located after the appendixes in the CPT codebook. It cannot be stressed enough that the alphabetic index is not a substitute for the main text of the CPT nomenclature. Even if only one code appears in the index, the user must refer to the main text of the CPT codebook to ensure that the code selection is accurate.

The index is organized by main terms. Following are the four primary classes of main index entries:
- Procedure or service, eg, Allergen Immunotherapy, Arthroscopy, Biopsy, Cardiac Catheterization, Debridement, E/M Laparoscopy, Osteopathic Manipulation, Physical Medicine/Therapy/Occupational Therapy, Vaccines
- Organ or other anatomical site, eg, Abdomen, Bladder, Esophagus, Hip, Intestines, Malar Area, Olecranon Process, Prostate
- Condition, eg, Abscess, Blepharoptosis, Dislocation, Esophageal Varices, Hemorrhage, Omphalocele, Varicose Vein
- Synonyms, eponyms, and abbreviations, eg, Anderson Tibial Lengthening, CBC, Clagett Procedure, ECG, Patterson's Test

A main term may be followed by a series of up to three indented terms that modify the main term. These modifying terms should be reviewed, as these sub-terms have an effect on appropriate code selection.

Cross-references provide additional instructions to the user. Following are the two types of cross-references in the index:
- "see": This type of reference is used primarily for synonyms, eponyms, and abbreviations. As an added reference, a list of common abbreviations can be found on the back cover of the professional edition of the CPT codebook.
- "See Also": This directs the user to look under another main term if the procedure is not listed under the first main index entry.

CHAPTER 2

# EXERCISES

1   The CPT codebook is divided into how many sections? Name the sections.

2   Which section of Category I CPT codes appears first in the CPT codebook, and why?

3   In which section of Category I CPT codes are the following codes located?

**71060**

**49060**

**99241**

**01440**

**99058**

**84443**

**64831**

4   Write the full Category I CPT code descriptor for the following codes:

**31625**

**73202**

**42415**

**28805**

**64704**

5   Identify the parent code for each of the following indented Category I CPT codes:

**97028**

**87530**

**59515**

**40844**

**99292**

6   True or False: If a Category III code is available, this code must be reported instead of a Category I unlisted code.

7   True or False: With the exception of the anesthesia physical status modifiers, all CPT modifiers are two-digit numeric.

**8** Match the appendix listed in column 1 with the contents in column 2.

| Appendix | Contents |
|----------|----------|
| A | 1. Summary of CPT Add-on Codes |
| B | 2. Modifiers |
| C | 3. Summary of CPT Codes Exempt From Modifier 51 |
| D | 4. Summary of Additions, Deletions, and Revisions |
| E | 5. Clinical Examples |
| F | 6. Electrodiagnostic Medicine Listing of Sensory, Motor, and Mixed Nerves |
| G | 7. Vascular Family Listing |
| H | 8. Summary of CPT Codes That Include Moderate (Conscious) Sedation |
| I | 9. Alphabetic Index of Performance Measures by Clinical Condition or Topic |
| J | 10. Product Pending FDA Approval |
| K | 11. Summary of CPT Codes Exempt From Modifier 63 |
| L | 12. Genetic Testing Code Modifiers |
| M | 13. Crosswalk to Deleted CPT Codes |

**9** True or False: The Category I CPT codes in the Radiology section of the CPT nomenclature can be reported only by a qualified radiologist.

**10** Which code symbol is used to identify new procedure Category I, II, and III CPT codes?

**11** The alphabetic index of the CPT codebook located after the appendices is organized by main terms. List the four primary classes of main index entries.

# CHAPTER 3

# Evaluation and Management Services

The Evaluation and Management (E/M) Services codes were introduced into Current Procedural Terminology (CPT®) nomenclature in 1992. These codes describe services provided by physicians to evaluate patients and manage their care. The E/M codes replaced "visit" codes that described services generally as a "brief visit," intermediate, or comprehensive, for example. These codes are widely used by physicians of all specialties and describe a large portion of the medical care provided to patients.

The levels of evaluation and management (E/M) services include examinations, evaluations, consultations, treatments, conferences, counseling with patients and/or family, preventive pediatric and adult health supervision, adult and pediatric critical and intensive care, emergency department, home care, nursing home care, and similar medical services, such as the determination of the need and/or location for appropriate care.

This chapter focuses on the E/M services guidelines, including such topics as the categories and subcategories of E/M service, definitions of commonly used terms, and the instructions for selecting a level of E/M service. Guidelines from some of the categories and subcategories of E/M service are then highlighted. Finally, there is discussion about procedures or services included when E/M services are reported.

Although specific codes are addressed throughout this chapter, code descriptors have not been printed in this text. This text should be used in conjunction with the current edition of the CPT codebook to reference the entire code descriptor for the specific codes discussed.

The basic format of the E/M codes follows. (See the schematic diagram that follows.)

- A unique code number is listed.
- The place or type of service is specified (eg, office or other outpatient setting).
- The content of the service is defined (eg, a problem-focused history, a problem-focused examination, straightforward medical decision making).
- Counseling and/or coordination of care with other providers or agencies is/are included when an E/M service is reported, if appropriate.
- The nature of the presenting problem(s) usually associated with a given level is/are described.
- The time typically required to provide the service is specified in many codes.

**99201** **Office or other outpatient visit** for the evaluation and management of a new patient, which requires these three key components:

— unique code number

— place or type of service

- A problem-focused history

- A problem-focused examination

- Straightforward medical decision making

— content of service defined

Counseling and/or coordination of care with other providers or agencies are provided consistent with the nature of the problem(s) and the patient's and/or family's needs.

— counseling and/or coordination of care

Usually, the presenting problems are self-limited or minor. Physicians typically spend 10 minutes face-to-face with the patient and/or family.

— nature of presenting problem

— typical time

# Classification of E/M Services

As noted in the following table, the E/M section is divided into broad categories of services such as office visits, hospital visits, and consultations. Most of the categories are further divided into two or more subcategories of services, such as new patient, established patient, initial hospital care, subsequent hospital care, initial inpatient pediatric critical care, subsequent inpatient pediatric critical care, initial neonatal critical care, and subsequent neonatal critical care.

The subcategories are further classified into levels of E/M services that are identified by specific codes. This classification of E/M services is important because the nature of physician activity and practice resource costs vary by the type of service, place of service, and patient's status and age.

## Categories and Subcategories of Service

Following is an inclusive numeric listing of the categories and subcategories of E/M services to familiarize readers with the range and scope of these services.

### Categories/Subcategories of E/M Services

| Category/Subcategory | CPT Code Numbers |
|---|---|
| **Office or Other Outpatient Services** | |
| New Patient | 99201-99205 |
| Established Patient | 99211-99215 |
| **Hospital Observation Services** | |
| Observation Care Discharge Services | 99217 |
| Initial Observation Care | 99218-99220 |
| **Hospital Inpatient Services** | |
| Initial Hospital Care | 99221-99223 |
| Subsequent Hospital Care | 99231-99233 |
| Hospital Discharge Services | 99238-99239 |
| **Observation or Inpatient Care Services (Including Admission and Discharge Services)** | **99234-99236** |
| **Consultations** | |
| Office or Other Outpatient | 99241-99245 |
| Inpatient | 99251-99255 |
| **Emergency Department Services** | **99281-99285** |
| **Pediatric Critical Care Patient Transport Services** | **99289, 99290** |
| **Critical Care Services** | |
| Hourly Critical Care | 99291, 99292 |
| Inpatient Pediatric (29 days to 24 months of age) | 99293, 99294 |
| Inpatient Neonatal (birth through 28 days) | 99295, 99296 |
| Continuing Intensive Care Services for Infants | 99298-99300 |

| Category/Subcategory | CPT Code Numbers |
|---|---|

**Nursing Facility Services**
Initial Nursing Facility Care . . . . . . . . . . . . . . . . . . . . . . . . . . . . . . 99304-99306
Subsequent Nursing Facility Care . . . . . . . . . . . . . . . . . . . . . . . . 99307-99310
Nursing Facility Discharge Services. . . . . . . . . . . . . . . . . . . . . . . 99315, 99316
Other Nursing Facility Services . . . . . . . . . . . . . . . . . . . . . . . . . . 99318

**Domiciliary, Rest Home (eg, Boarding Home),**
**or Custodial Care Services**
New Patient . . . . . . . . . . . . . . . . . . . . . . . . . . . . . . . . . . . . . . . . . . 99324-99328
Established Patient. . . . . . . . . . . . . . . . . . . . . . . . . . . . . . . . . . . . . 99334-99337
Domiciliary, Rest Home (eg, Assisted Living Facility),
or Home Care Plan Oversight Services . . . . . . . . . . . . . . . . . . . . 99339-99340

**Domiciliary, Rest Home (eg, Assisted Living**
**Facility), or Home Care Plan Oversight Services**    **99339-99340**

**Home Services**
New Patient . . . . . . . . . . . . . . . . . . . . . . . . . . . . . . . . . . . . . . . . . . 99341-99345
Established Patient . . . . . . . . . . . . . . . . . . . . . . . . . . . . . . . . . . . . 99347-99350

**Prolonged Services**
With Direct (Face-to-Face) Patient Contact . . . . . . . . . . . . . . . . 99354-99357
Without Direct (Face-to-Face) Patient Contact. . . . . . . . . . . . . . 99358, 99359
Physician Standby Services. . . . . . . . . . . . . . . . . . . . . . . . . . . . . . 99360

**Case Management Services**    **99363-99368**
Anticoagulant Management . . . . . . . . . . . . . . . . . . . . . . . . . . . . . 99363-99364
Medical Team Conference, Direct (Face-to-Face) Contact
With Patient and/or Family . . . . . . . . . . . . . . . . . . . . . . . . . . . . . . 99366
Medical Team Conference, Without Direct (Face-to-Face) Contact
With Patient and/or Family . . . . . . . . . . . . . . . . . . . . . . . . . . . . . . 99367, 99368

**Care Plan Oversight Services**    **99374-99380**

**Preventive Medicine Services**
New Patient . . . . . . . . . . . . . . . . . . . . . . . . . . . . . . . . . . . . . . . . . . 99381-99387
Established Patient . . . . . . . . . . . . . . . . . . . . . . . . . . . . . . . . . . . . 99391-99397
Individual Counseling . . . . . . . . . . . . . . . . . . . . . . . . . . . . . . . . . . 99401-99404
Behavior Change Interventions, Individual. . . . . . . . . . . . . . . . . . 99406-99408
Group Counseling. . . . . . . . . . . . . . . . . . . . . . . . . . . . . . . . . . . . . 99411, 99412
Other Services . . . . . . . . . . . . . . . . . . . . . . . . . . . . . . . . . . . . . . . 99420-99429

**Newborn Care**    **99431-99440**

**Non-Face to Face Physician Services**
Telephone Services. . . . . . . . . . . . . . . . . . . . . . . . . . . . . . . . . . . . 99441-99443
On-line Medical Evaluation . . . . . . . . . . . . . . . . . . . . . . . . . . . . . . 99444

**Special Evaluation and Management Services**
Basic Life and/or Disability Evaluation Services. . . . . . . . . . . . . . 99450
Work-Related or Medical Disability Evaluation Services. . . . . . . . 99455, 99456
Other Evaluation and Management Services. . . . . . . . . . . . . . . . . 99477, 99499

## Levels of E/M Services

Within each category or subcategory of E/M service, there are three to five levels of E/M services available for reporting purposes. The number of levels within a category varies and is dependent on the scope or types of services that might be provided in a given setting. The various levels of E/M services describe the wide variations in skill, effort, time, responsibility, and medical knowledge required for the prevention or diagnosis and treatment of illness or injury and the promotion of optimal health.

The code descriptors for the levels of E/M services identify seven components, six of which are used in defining the levels of E/M services. The seven components of E/M services are as follows:

- History
- Examination
- Medical decision making
- Counseling
- Coordination of care
- Nature of presenting problem
- Time

The six components used in defining the levels of E/M services are history, examination, medical decision making, counseling, coordination of care, and the nature of presenting problem.

The seventh component, time, was implied before the introduction of the E/M section of the CPT codebook. When the E/M section was introduced in 1992, typical times were included, where appropriate, as a distinct component to assist physicians in selecting the most appropriate level of E/M service.

When counseling and/or coordination of care constitute more than 50% of the physician-patient and/or family encounter, time may be considered the key or controlling factor to qualify for a particular level of E/M service.

### Key Components

History, examination, and medical decision making are considered the key components in selecting a level of E/M services. As a general rule, these are the first components considered when determining the level of E/M service to report. But as with most rules, there are exceptions, eg, in the case of visits that consist primarily of counseling or coordination of care (see the discussion of time).

### Contributory Factors

Counseling, coordination of care, and nature of presenting problem are considered contributory factors in the majority of physician-patient encounters. It is not required that these services be provided at every or any patient encounter.

### Time

Typical times have been included in many of the code descriptors of the E/M codes. The specific times in the visit code descriptors are averages and therefore represent a range of times that may be higher or lower depending on the actual clinical circumstances. The times included in the CPT nomenclature are more reflective of the actual face-to-face time (or intraservice time) involved in an

E/M service. Other components of the service, such as review of X rays, telephone calls, review of other laboratory tests (or preservice and postservice work) involve additional time not reflected in the time stated but are included in determining the work value of an E/M service.

Generally, the times indicated are not meant to be used to select the level of E/M service reported. An exception to this rule is in the case of visits that consist predominantly of counseling or coordination of care.

One of the least understood elements of E/M coding is using time as the key factor in selecting a code. When counseling and/or coordination of care constitute more than 50% of the physician-patient and/or family encounter, time may be considered the key or controlling factor to qualify for a particular level of E/M services. This includes time spent with those who have assumed responsibility for the care of the patient or decision making, whether or not they are family members (eg, child's parents, foster parents, person acting in locum parentis, legal guardian). The extent of counseling and/or coordination of care must be documented in the medical record.

Thus, it is the content of the E/M service that is used to select the appropriate level of service. This is true whether the E/M service involves a new or an established patient visit. The first question to be asked when coding E/M services is, "Did counseling or coordination of care dominate the visit?" If counseling and/or coordination of care did not constitute more than 50% of the encounter, then the level of service is selected on the basis of the key components that have been met. If counseling and/or coordination of care did dominate the visit, then the code should be selected on the basis of time.

> **CODING TIP**
>
> Professional services are characterized by face-to-face services performed by a physician and reported with specific CPT codes. Provided services such as telephone renewal of a prescription without a face-to-face encounter are not considered when patients are identified as new or established.

# Definitions of Commonly Used Terms

Words and phrases used throughout the E/M section are defined in the CPT code set to reduce the potential for differing interpretations and to increase consistency of reporting E/M services. It is very important to learn the definitions of these terms to appropriately report the codes within the E/M section.

## New Patient vs Established Patient

Solely for the purposes of distinguishing between new and established patients, professional services are characterized by face-to-face services rendered by a physician and reported by specific CPT code(s). A new patient is one who has received no professional services from the physician or another physician of the same specialty who belongs to the same group practice, within the past three years.

An established patient is one who has received professional services from the physician or another physician of the same specialty who belongs to the same group practice within the past three years.

If the patient has received a face-to-face professional medical service from the physician within the past three years and that encounter was coded by means of one or more CPT codes, the patient would not be considered a new patient but rather an established patient.

The definitions of new and established patient include professional services provided not only by a particular physician but also by other physicians of the same specialty belonging to the same group practice. This raises the question of subspecialty reporting within a given specialty (eg, electrophysiology specialists in a cardiology group, a hand surgeon in an orthopedic group). Although the CPT definitions do not explicitly address this question, it is possible for a patient receiving professional services from a subspecialist within the same group to be considered a new patient to another physician in the group.

For example, if the subspecialists within the group practice have a separate tax identification number for their subspecialty different from the general group tax identification number, the patient receiving professional services from the subspecialist may be considered a new patient.

What about the physician who leaves one group practice and joins a different group practice elsewhere in the state? Consider Dr A, who leaves his group practice in Frankfort, Illinois, and joins a new group practice in Rockford, Illinois. When he provides professional services to patients in the Rockford practice, will he report these patients as new or established?

If Dr A or another physician of the same specialty in the Rockford practice has provided no professional services to that patient within the past three years, Dr A would consider the patient new. However, if Dr A or another physician of the same specialty in the Rockford practice has provided any professional service to that patient within the past three years, the patient would be considered an established

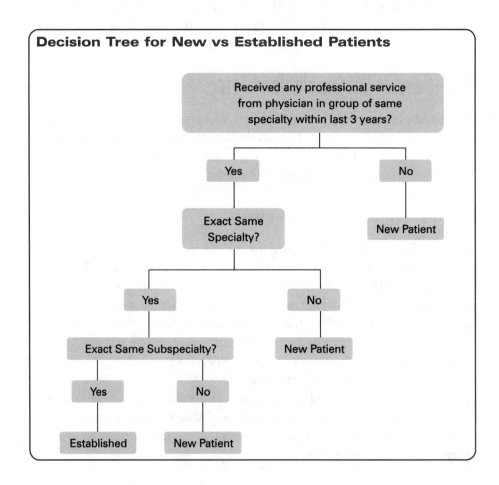

patient to Dr A. Remember, the definitions include professional services rendered by other physicians of the same specialty in the same group practice.

The decision tree on page 46 is provided to aid in determining whether to report the E/M service provided as a new or an established patient encounter.

## Concurrent Care

Concurrent care is the provision of similar services (eg, hospital visits) to the same patient by more than one physician on the same day. For CPT coding purposes, when concurrent care is provided, no special reporting is required. However, when concurrent care is provided, the *International Classification of Diseases, Ninth Revision, Clinical Modification* (ICD-9-CM) diagnosis code reported by each physician should reflect the need for the provision of similar services to the same patient by more than one physician on the same day. It is important to note that if the most specific ICD-9-CM diagnosis code should happen to be for the same condition, this does not preclude billing for concurrent care.

If Dr A, an endocrinologist, provides a hospital visit to manage the patient's type 2 uncontrolled diabetes mellitus while Dr B, an infectious disease specialist, provides a hospital visit to the same patient on the same day for management of the patient's pneumonia, each physician reports the appropriate level of E/M service based on the content of the service provided (eg, extent of the history obtained, extent of the examination performed, and the complexity of the medical decision making). The ICD-9-CM diagnosis code reported by each physician should reflect his or her role in the management of the patient.

## Counseling

CPT nomenclature defines counseling as it relates to E/M coding as a discussion with the patient and/or family or other caregiver concerning one or more of the following areas:
- Diagnostic results, impressions, and/or recommended diagnostic studies
- Prognosis
- Risks and benefits of management (treatment) options
- Instructions for management (treatment) and/or follow-up
- Importance of compliance with chosen management (treatment) options
- Risk factor reduction
- Patient and family education

Counseling, as defined previously, is not to be confused with psychotherapy, which is discussed in Chapter 9.

When it is evident that the reason for the patient's visit is to discuss laboratory test results, coders should prompt the practitioner for the length of time spent with the patient to allow accurate code selection.

## Nature of Presenting Problem

A presenting problem is a disease, condition, illness, injury, symptom, sign, finding, complaint, or other reason for encounter, with or without a diagnosis being established at the time of the encounter.

> **CODING TIP**
>
> Counseling includes discussion with the patient and/or family, guardian, or caretaker. Family members may receive counseling from the physician without the patient being present. Counseling of family members alone is reported with the various levels of E/M service.

| E/M Presenting Problems | |
|---|---|
| **Type** | **Definition** |
| Minimal | A problem that may not require the presence of the physician, but service is provided under the physician's supervision. |
| Self-limited or minor | A problem that runs a definite and prescribed course, is transient, and is not likely to permanently alter the health status or has a good prognosis with management/compliance. |
| Low severity | A problem where the risk of morbidity without treatment is low; there is little to no risk of mortality without treatment; full recovery without functional impairment is expected. |
| Moderate severity | A problem where the risk of morbidity without treatment is moderate; there is moderate risk of mortality without treatment; uncertain prognosis or increased probability of prolonged functional impairment. |
| High severity | A problem where the risk of morbidity without treatment is high to extreme; there is a moderate to high risk of mortality without treatment or high probability of severe, prolonged functional impairment. |

# Instructions for Selecting a Level of E/M Service

When selecting a level of E/M service, it is important to remember that it is ultimately the responsibility of the physician providing the E/M service to determine the level of service provided. Physician documentation in the patient's medical record is of utmost importance; it must support the level of service reported.

The following specific steps must be taken to select the appropriate level of E/M service:

1 Identify the category and subcategory of service.

2 Review the reporting instructions for the selected category or subcategory.

3 Review the E/M service code descriptors in the selected category or subcategory.

4 Determine the extent of history obtained.

5 Determine the extent of the examination performed.

6 Determine the complexity of medical decision making.

7 Select the appropriate level of E/M services.

Following is a comprehensive discussion of each of these steps.

## Step 1: Identify the Category and Subcategory of Service

The first step in selecting a level of E/M service is to identify the appropriate category and subcategory of service provided. Refer to the table of categories and subcategories of E/M services at the beginning of this chapter (eg, office or other outpatient services, new patient). A listing of the categories and subcategories of E/M service can also be found in the E/M guidelines of the CPT codebook.

## Step 2: Review the Reporting Instructions for the Selected Category or Subcategory

Once the appropriate category and subcategory of service have been identified, it is important to review the reporting instructions for the selected category and/or subcategory. Most of the categories and many of the subcategories of E/M service have special guidelines or instructions unique to that category or subcategory. It is important for users to read and be guided by these special instructions.

## Step 3: Review the E/M Service Code Descriptors in the Selected Category or Subcategory

Remember, the descriptors for the levels of E/M services recognize seven components (history, examination, medical decision making, counseling, coordination of care, nature of presenting problem, and time). The first six are used in defining the levels of E/M services. Take a minute to review the E/M code descriptors in the category or subcategory selected.

## Step 4: Determine the Extent of History Obtained

To select the appropriate level of E/M service, it is necessary to determine the extent of the key components performed (ie, extent of history obtained, extent of the examination performed, and the complexity of medical decision making). Start by determining the extent of history obtained.

The medical history provides essential information for diagnosis and management and varies based on the clinical judgment of the physician and each individual patient and problem(s).

The following are included in obtaining the history:
- Chief complaint (CC)
- History of present illness (HPI)
- Review of systems (ROS)
- Past, family, and/or social history (PFSH)

When some patient groups are considered (eg, newborn infants), not all components are available or appropriate to consider.

The CC is a concise statement describing the symptom, problem, condition, diagnosis, or other factor that is the reason for the encounter, usually stated in the patient's or parent's words.

The HPI is a chronological description of the development of the patient's present illness from the first sign and/or symptom to the present.

Patients usually express their problems as symptoms (eg, pain or discomfort) or signs (eg, a noticeable physical abnormality such as a lump, cut, bruise, or murmur), with the exception of a newborn, whose presenting complaint may be related to his or her mother's (eg, maternal fever during labor). The further elaboration of any symptom requires attention to some or all of the dimensions of the HPI. Signs are better described by physical findings. Problems can also be described as the status of one or more chronic conditions.

The CPT guidelines recognize seven dimensions of the HPI, including a description of the following:

- Location
- Quality
- Severity
- Timing
- Context
- Modifying factors
- Associated signs and symptoms

When an HPI is obtained, elaborating on the patient's CC(s) and other symptoms is most often accomplished by asking questions that focus on the seven dimensions. Following are examples of questions that the clinician may ask to elicit specific information regarding the dimensions of the HPI.

**Location**—What is the location of the pain or discomfort? Ask the patient to point to the specific symptomatic area. Is the pain diffuse or localized? Unilateral or bilateral? Does it radiate or is it referred to other location(s)?

**Quality**—Include a description of the quality of the symptom. For example, is the pain described as sharp, dull, throbbing, stabbing, constant or intermittent, acute or chronic, or stable, improving, or worsening?

**Severity**—The patient may be asked to describe the severity of the pain by using a crude self-assessment scale to measure subjective levels (ie, on a scale of 1 to 10, with 1 being no pain and 10 the worst pain experienced). Or the patient may be asked to compare the pain quantitatively with a previously experienced pain (eg, kidney stone or labor pains).

**Timing**—Timing involves establishing the onset of the pain and a rough chronology of the development of the pain. To accomplish this, the physician may ask if there is a repetitive pattern for the pain or if the pain primarily occurs in the evening or during daylight hours or if it is continuous.

**Context**—Where is the patient and what is he or she doing when the pain begins? Is the patient at rest or involved in an activity? Is the pain aggravated or relieved or does it recur with a specific activity? Has situational stress or some other factor preceded or accompanied the pain?

**Modifying factors**—What has the patient attempted to do to obtain relief or make himself or herself better? What makes the pain worse? For example, does the local application of heat or cold relieve or exacerbate the pain? Does eating relieve or exacerbate abdominal discomfort? Does coughing irritate the pain? Have over the counter or prescribed medications been attempted—with what results?

**Associated signs and symptoms**—A clinician's impressions formulated during the interview may lead to questioning about additional sensations or feelings. Examples might include diaphoresis (marked sweating) associated with indigestion or chest pain; tremulousness, weakness, and hunger pains in patients with diabetes; or blurring of vision accompanying a headache.

The following scenario is provided to further explain the elements of the HPI:

**EXAMPLE:** A 27-year-old man presents for evaluation of episodic cough and shortness of breath of two years' duration. He notes the latter to be exacerbated with exposure to smoke or dust. He has been employed at a feed mill for four years, which is dusty and exacerbates the symptoms. He has used no respiratory protection. He notes shortness of breath primarily with activity (eg, running up stairs) but otherwise feels he is able to keep pace with others his age and size without difficulty. He has noted some mild wheezing and has tried albuterol, which does not achieve prompt symptomatic relief. He is a lifelong nonsmoker with no history of asthma or other pulmonary disorder.

When the status of a chronic condition is being described, many of the same elements may apply as well as issues such as frequency of medication use, compliance, and associated measurements the patient reports (eg, home blood pressure, glucose). It is also common, especially in geriatric patients, to ascertain functional status related to activities of daily life (eg, ability to feed and clothe self, walk, shop, prepare food).

The ROS is an inventory of body systems obtained through a series of questions asked by the physician seeking to identify signs and/or symptoms that the patient may be experiencing or has experienced. This helps define the problem, clarify the differential diagnosis, identify testing needed, or serve as baseline data on other systems that might be affected by any possible management (treatment) options. An ROS may be highly dependent on the age of the patient and irrelevant for newborns and young infants.

The following elements of a system review have been identified in the CPT code set:

- Constitutional symptoms (fever, weight loss, etc)
- Eyes
- Ears, nose, mouth, throat
- Cardiovascular
- Respiratory
- Gastrointestinal
- Genitourinary

- Musculoskeletal
- Integumentary (skin and/or breast)
- Neurologic
- Psychiatric
- Endocrine
- Hematologic/lymphatic
- Allergic/immunologic

The past, family, and/or social history (PFSH) includes a review of past medical experiences of the patient and the patient's family.

*Past history* is a review of the patient's past experiences with illnesses, injuries, and treatments that may include significant information about the following:

- Prior major illnesses and injuries
- Prior operations
- Prior hospitalizations
- Current medications
- Allergies (eg, drug, food)
- Age-appropriate immunization status
- Age-appropriate feeding/dietary status
- Birth history (eg, birth weight, Apgar score)

*Family history* is a review of medical events in the patient's family, including significant information about the following:

- The health status or cause of death of parents, siblings, and children
- Specific diseases related to problems identified in the CC or HPI and/or ROS
- Diseases of family members that may be hereditary or place the patient at risk

*Social history* is an age-appropriate review of past and current activities that includes significant information about the following:

- Marital status and/or living arrangements
- Current/previous employment
- Use of drugs, alcohol, and tobacco
- Levels of education
- Sexual history
- Domestic violence
- Other relevant social factors

The levels of E/M services recognize four types of history. The types of history and their respective definitions are provided in the following table.

| E/M Patient Histories | |
| --- | --- |
| **Type of History** | **Definition** |
| Problem-focused | CC; brief HPI |
| Expanded problem-focused | CC; brief HPI; problem-pertinent ROS |
| Detailed | CC; extended HPI; problem-pertinent ROS including review of a limited number of additional systems; pertinent PFSH (directly related to the patient's problems) |
| Comprehensive | CC; extended HPI; ROS directly related to problem(s) identified in HPI plus review of all additional body systems; complete PFSH |

## Step 5: Determine the Extent of the Examination Performed

The next key component to consider is the extent of the examination performed. It depends on the clinical judgment of the physician and the nature of the patient's presenting problems.

The levels of E/M services recognize four types of examination. The types of examination and their respective definitions are provided in the following table.

| E/M Patient Examinations | |
| --- | --- |
| **Type of Examination** | **Definition** |
| Problem-focused | A limited examination of the affected body area or organ system |
| Expanded problem-focused | A limited examination of the affected body area or organ system and other symptomatic or related organ system(s) |
| Detailed | An extended examination of the affected body area(s) and other symptomatic or related organ system(s) |
| Comprehensive | A general multisystem examination or a complete examination of a single organ system |

For the purposes of the CPT definitions provided in the previous table, the following body areas are recognized:

- Head, including the face
- Neck

- Chest, including breasts and axillae
- Abdomen
- Genitalia, groin, buttocks
- Back
- Each extremity

For the purposes of the CPT definitions provided in the previous table, the following organ systems are recognized:

- Eyes
- Ears, nose, mouth, and throat
- Cardiovascular
- Respiratory
- Gastrointestinal
- Genitourinary
- Musculoskeletal
- Skin
- Neurologic
- Psychiatric
- Hematologic/lymphatic/immunologic

## Step 6: Determine the Complexity of Medical Decision Making

The final key component is the complexity of medical decision making. Medical decision making refers to the complexity of establishing a diagnosis and/or selecting a management option as measured by the three following elements:

- The number of possible diagnoses and/or the number of management options that must be considered
- The amount and/or complexity of medical records, diagnostic tests, and/or other information that must be obtained, reviewed, and analyzed
- The risk of significant complications, morbidity, and/or mortality as well as comorbidities associated with the patient's presenting problem(s), the diagnostic procedure(s), and/or the possible management options

Comorbidities or underlying diseases in and of themselves are not considered in selecting a level of E/M services unless their presence significantly increases the complexity of the medical decision making.

Four types of medical decision making are recognized in the CPT nomenclature. The following table lists them and the elements required to qualify for each type.

## Definitions of Types of Medical Decision Making

| Type of Medical Decision Making | Number of Diagnoses or Management Options | Amount and/or Complexity of Data to Be Reviewed | Risk of Complications and/or Morbidity or Mortality |
|---|---|---|---|
| Straightforward | Minimal | Minimal or none | Minimal |
| Low complexity | Limited | Limited | Low |
| Moderate complexity | Multiple | Moderate | Moderate |
| High complexity | Extensive | Extensive | High |

To qualify for a given type of medical decision making, two of the three elements in the above table must be met or exceeded.

A limited number of diagnoses or management options, moderate amount and/or complexity of data to be reviewed, and low risk of complications and/or morbidity or mortality constitute low-complexity medical decision making.

## Step 7: Select the Appropriate Level of E/M Services

Now that the appropriate category and subcategory of service have been identified, the guidelines for that specific category and/or subcategory have been reviewed, and the key components have been determined, it is time to select the appropriate level of E/M service. This selection is based on the key components performed by the physician and the number of key components required for the particular category/subcategory identified.

Some of the categories/subcategories of E/M service require all of the key components to meet or exceed requirements stated in the code descriptor to qualify for a level of E/M service. Other categories/subcategories of E/M service require only two of the three key components to meet or exceed the stated requirements to qualify for a particular level of service.

The following table indicates the categories and subcategories of service requiring all of the key components (ie, history, examination, and medical decision making) to meet or exceed the requirements stated in the code descriptor to qualify for a particular level of service.

## Categories and Subcategories of Service

| Category | Subcategory |
|---|---|
| Office or Other Outpatient Services | New Patient |
| Hospital Observation Services | |
| Hospital Inpatient Services | Initial Hospital Care |
| Observation or Inpatient Care Services (Including Admission and Discharge Services) | |
| Consultations | Office or Other Outpatient Consultations |
| | Initial Inpatient Consultations |
| Emergency Department Services | |
| Nursing Facility Services | Comprehensive Nursing Facility Assessments |
| Domiciliary, Rest Home (eg, Boarding Home), or Custodial Care Services | New Patient |
| Home Services | New Patient |

Finally, before selecting the level of E/M service, the content of the E/M service provided must be given careful consideration. This is true whether the E/M service involves a new or an established patient visit. If counseling and/or coordination of care do not constitute more than 50% of the encounter, the level of service is selected on the basis of the key components that have been met.

When counseling and/or coordination of care constitute more than 50% of the physician/patient and/or family encounter, time may be considered the controlling factor to qualify for a particular level of E/M services. This includes time spent providing counseling and/or coordination of care with those who have assumed responsibility for the care of the patient or decision making, whether or not they are family members (eg, foster parents, person acting in locum parentis, legal guardian).

When time is the controlling factor for selecting an E/M service, code selection for the encounter is based on the face-to-face physician-patient and/or family encounter time in the office or other outpatient setting, and unit/floor time in the hospital or nursing facility setting. The physician must document the extent of counseling/coordination of care services provided and distinguish between time spent on performing the key components of the encounter and the time spent providing counseling/coordination services by recording each time separately. The time spent performing the key components and the counseling/coordination services would be combined and this total time (face-to-face or unit/floor time in hospital or nursing facility) would be used to determine the appropriate code to select for the encounter, when counseling and/or coordination of care dominate the visit.

Consider the following scenario.

**EXAMPLE:** For several years, Dr Bravo has been treating Mrs George for type 2 diabetes, hypertension, and obesity. Three days before this appointment, blood work was performed to determine the status of her diabetes. She presents to the physician's office and the physician examines her for evidence of infection or circulatory problems. He then asks the patient about her compliance with the 1200-calorie diet she has been on for the past six months. After reviewing these findings, the physician indicates to the patient that she will have to begin using insulin, since her diabetes is not responding to the current treatment. Mrs George begins to sob uncontrollably. She tells Dr Bravo that this means she is going to die because her grandmother got gangrene from this kind of diabetes and died from it. After calming her, Dr Bravo explains that using insulin is not a death sentence. He discusses diet, insulin administration, and hypoglycemic reactions, as well as the symptoms of hyperglycemia. He refers Mrs George to an endocrinologist and provides instruction for proper foot and skin care and stresses the importance of seeing her ophthalmologist regularly. Mrs George is much calmer and feels that she will learn a lot from the booklets Dr Bravo has given her.

The total time Dr Bravo spent with Mrs George is 25 minutes, with 20 of those minutes spent providing counseling and/or coordination of care. Because more than 50% of the encounter was spent providing counseling and/or coordination of care, the total face-to-face time between Mrs George and Dr Bravo may be considered the key factor in selecting the level of E/M service. Therefore, since Mrs George is an established patient and 25 total minutes were spent with the patient, it would be appropriate to report code **99214**.

# A Review of the Categories and Subcategories of E/M Services

Within the E/M section of the CPT codebook there are several categories and subcategories of services. Generally, the categories of service vary depending on the site of service (eg, office or other outpatient, hospital inpatient services, emergency department services). Every category of E/M service has guidelines and instructional notes at the beginning of the category. Many of the subcategories have guidelines and instructional notes in addition to those that appear at the beginning of the category.

It is important for users to read and refer to this information for guidance in reporting the E/M codes. In the remainder of this chapter, an overview of the guidelines and instructional notes for the categories and subcategories of E/M services is provided. Please refer to the CPT codebook for the complete guidelines pertaining to each category and subcategory of service.

**CODING TIP**

A patient is considered an out-patient until inpatient admission to a health care facility occurs.

## Office or Other Outpatient Services (99201-99215)

The codes in the Office or Other Outpatient Services category (**99201-99215**) are used to report E/M services provided in the physician's office or other outpatient/ambulatory settings, including E/M services provided in an urgent care setting.

Within this category of E/M services there are subcategories of codes for new and established patient visits. When new patient visits within this category are reported, all three key components must meet or exceed the stated requirements to qualify for a particular level of E/M service. When established patient visits within this category are reported, two of the three key components must meet or exceed the stated requirements to qualify for a particular level of E/M service.

An important guideline to remember when reporting office visits is that if a patient is admitted to the hospital in the course of the office encounter, all E/M services provided by a physician in conjunction with the admission are considered part of the initial hospital care when performed on the same date as the admission. A separate code for the office visit is not reported. The initial hospital care level of service reported by the admitting physician should include the services related to the admission provided in the physician's office as well as the E/M services the physician provided on that same date in the inpatient setting.

**EXAMPLE:** A patient presents to Dr B's office with complaints of fever, chills, malaise, and a cough. The physician obtains the history from the patient, performs an examination, and orders a chest X ray. The patient is admitted to the hospital by Dr B on that same day for intravenous antibiotic therapy for treatment of pneumonia. After completion of his office hours that day, Dr B provides an E/M service to the patient in the hospital.

In the example, Dr B will not separately report the office visit and the initial hospital care. Rather, the initial hospital care level of service reported should include all the services related to the admission he provided in the office as well as in the inpatient setting.

The following two charts are provided to summarize the requirements for reporting office or other outpatient visits. In determining final code selection, be sure to refer to the E/M guidelines and the code descriptors in the CPT codebook.

## Office or Other Outpatient Services: New Patient

To qualify for a particular level of service, all three key components must be met or exceeded.

| Code | 99201 | 99202 | 99203 | 99204 | 99205 |
|---|---|---|---|---|---|
| **Key Components** | | | | | |
| **History** | Problem-focused | Expanded problem-focused | Detailed | Comprehensive | Comprehensive |
| **Examination** | Problem-focused | Expanded problem-focused | Detailed | Comprehensive | Comprehensive |
| **Medical Decision Making** | Straightforward | Straightforward | Low complexity | Moderate complexity | High complexity |
| **Contributory Factors** | | | | | |
| **Presenting Problem** | Self-limited or minor | Low to moderate severity | Moderate severity | Moderate to high severity | Moderate to high severity |
| **Counseling** | Counseling and/or coordination of care with other providers or agencies are provided consistent with the nature of the problem(s) and the patient's and/or family's needs | | | | |
| **Coordination of Care** | | | | | |
| **Time* Face-to-Face** | 10 minutes | 20 minutes | 30 minutes | 45 minutes | 60 minutes |

\* It should be recognized that the specific times expressed in the visit code descriptors are averages and therefore represent a range of times, which may be higher or lower depending on actual clinical circumstances.

If counseling and/or coordination of care dominate (more than 50%) the encounter, time may be used to select the code. This is the time physicians typically spend face-to-face with the patient and/or family.

## Hospital Observation Services (99217-99220)

The codes in the Hospital Observation Services category of service (**99217-99220**) are used to report E/M services provided to patients designated/admitted as "observation status" in a hospital. These patients are there to be observed to determine whether they should be admitted to the hospital, transferred to another facility, or sent home. Not all hospitals have a specific area designated for observation patients. The patient need not be located in an observation area designated by the hospital but rather designated/admitted as observation status.

Codes **99218-99220** are used to report the initial observation care. These codes may be reported for new or established patient visits. When these codes are reported, it is necessary for all three of the key components to meet or exceed the requirements stated in the code descriptor to qualify for a particular level of service.

## Office or Other Outpatient Services: Established Patient

To qualify for a particular level of service, two of the three key components must be met or exceeded.

| Code | 99211 | 99212 | 99213 | 99214 | 99215 |
|------|-------|-------|-------|-------|-------|
| **Key Components** | | | | | |
| **History** | NA | Problem-focused | Expanded problem-focused | Detailed | Comprehensive |
| **Examination** | NA | Problem-focused | Expanded problem-focused | Detailed | Comprehensive |
| **Medical Decision Making** | NA | Straightforward | Low complexity | Moderate complexity | High complexity |
| **Contributory Factors** | | | | | |
| **Presenting Problem** | Minimal | Self-limited or minor | Low to moderate severity | Moderate to high severity | Moderate to high severity |
| **Counseling** | Counseling and/or coordination of care with other providers or agencies are provided consistent with the nature of the problem(s) and the patient's and/or family's needs | | | | |
| **Coordination of Care** | | | | | |
| **Time* Face-to-Face** | 5 minutes | 10 minutes | 15 minutes | 25 minutes | 40 minutes |

NA = not applicable.

* It should be recognized that the specific times expressed in the visit code descriptors are averages and therefore represent a range of times, which may be higher or lower depending on actual clinical circumstances.

If counseling and/or coordination of care dominate (more than 50%) the encounter, time may be used to select the code. This is the time physicians typically spend face-to-face with the patient and/or family.

The codes in this category of service are not used to report hospital observation services involving admission and discharge services provided on the same date. Hospital observation services involving admission and discharge services provided on the same date are reported with codes **99234-99236**.

Only the physician admitting the patient to observation status may report the initial observation care code. For observation encounters provided by physicians other than the admitting physician, other E/M codes are reported, as appropriate.

For example, if a consultation is requested by the physician admitting the patient to observation status, the consulting physician would report the consultation by using the office or other outpatient consultation codes (**99241-99245**).

If the physician provides an E/M service on a given date in another site of service (eg, physician's office, hospital emergency department, nursing facility) and subsequently initiates observation status in a hospital for that patient on the same date, the physician reports only an initial observation care code for all E/M services provided on that date. The level of initial observation care reported by the supervising physician should include the services provided in the other site of service as well as those provided in the observation setting.

If a patient is designated as observation status on a given date and is subsequently admitted to the hospital on that date, only an initial hospital care code is reported for both of these E/M services provided on that date. The initial hospital care level of service reported should include all E/M services provided on that date.

Code **99217** is used to report observation care discharge day management. This code is used by the physician to report final examination of the patient, discussion of the observation stay, instructions for continuing care, and preparation of discharge records. Report this code only if the discharge from observation status is on a date other than the date of initial observation care.

No specific listing exists in the CPT codebook for reporting the middle day of an observation stay, since it was not envisioned that this would be a common occurrence. If the physician initiates observation status on Monday, continues to observe the patient on Tuesday, and discharges the patient from observation status on Wednesday, the E/M services provided on Tuesday are reported with unlisted code **99499**.

The hospital observation codes are not intended to be used to report physician services related to postoperative recovery of a patient. An E/M code is not reported for E/M services provided by the physician who performs a surgery and then routinely evaluates the patient in an observation area postoperatively. The global surgical package generally includes those evaluations immediately after surgery. (Refer to Chapter 4 for further discussion of the CPT surgical package definition.)

The following chart is provided to summarize the requirements for reporting hospital observation services. In determining final code selection, be sure to refer to the E/M guidelines and the code descriptors in the CPT codebook.

## Initial Observation Care: New or Established Patient

To qualify for a particular level of service, two of the three key components must be met or exceeded.

| Code | 99218 | 99219 | 99220 |
|---|---|---|---|
| **Key Components** | | | |
| **History** | Detailed or comprehensive | Comprehensive | Comprehensive |
| **Examination** | Detailed or comprehensive | Comprehensive | Comprehensive |
| **Medical Decision Making** | Straightforward or low complexity | Moderate complexity | High complexity |
| **Contributory Factors** | | | |
| **Presenting Problem** | Low severity | Moderate severity | High severity |
| **Counseling** | Counseling and/or coordination of care with other providers or agencies are provided consistent with the nature of the problem(s) and the patient's and/or family's needs | | |
| **Coordination of Care** | | | |
| **Time* Face-to-Face** | NA | NA | NA |

NA = not applicable.

* It should be recognized that the specific times expressed in the visit code descriptors are averages and therefore represent a range of times, which may be higher or lower depending on actual clinical circumstances.

If counseling and/or coordination of care dominate (more than 50%) the encounter, time may be used to select the code. This is the time physicians typically spend face-to-face with the patient and/or family.

## Hospital Inpatient Services (99221-99233)

The codes in the Hospital Inpatient Services category (**99221-99233**) are used to report E/M services provided to hospital inpatients. There are two subcategories of codes for hospital inpatient services: 1. Initial hospital care and 2. Subsequent hospital care.

Included in this range of codes are services provided to patients in a partial hospital setting. A partial hospital setting is used for crisis stabilization, intensive short-term daily treatment, or intermediate-term treatment of psychiatric disorders. The Centers for Medicare and Medicaid Services (CMS), for Medicare purposes, defines psychiatric facility partial hospitalization as follows:

**EXAMPLE:** A patient is admitted to a facility for the diagnosis and treatment of mental illness that provides a planned therapeutic program for patients who do not require full-time hospitalization, but who need broader programs than are possible from outpatient visits in a hospital-based or hospital-affiliated facility.

Initial Hospital Care

Let us first consider the guidelines for the Initial Hospital Care codes (**99221-99223**). These codes are used to report new or established patient E/M services. When initial hospital care is reported, all three of the key components must meet or exceed the requirements stated in the code descriptor to qualify for a particular level of service.

The guidelines for this series of codes indicate that they are intended to be reported for the first hospital inpatient encounter with the patient by the admitting physician. This date may not be the same as the date the patient was actually admitted to the hospital.

For example, the physician provides an E/M service to the patient in the office on Wednesday and subsequently admits the patient to the hospital on that same day. However, the physician does not have an inpatient encounter with that patient until Thursday morning. In this example, the appropriate office or other outpatient level of E/M service is reported for the E/M services provided on Wednesday. The date of service for the initial hospital care will be Thursday's date—the date the admitting physician had the first hospital inpatient encounter with the patient.

The initial hospital care level of service reported by the admitting physician should include all E/M services provided to that patient in conjunction with that admission on the same date. For example, if the physician provides an E/M service to the patient in the office (or other site of service) on Wednesday, admits the patient to the hospital, and subsequently has an inpatient encounter with that patient all on the same date, then the initial hospital care level of service reported should include all E/M services provided on that date. A separate code would not be reported for the E/M services provided in the office (or other site of service) on that date.

The following chart is provided to summarize the requirements for reporting initial hospital care. In determining final code selection, be sure to refer to the E/M guidelines and the code descriptors in the CPT codebook.

## Hospital Inpatient Services: Initial Hospital Care—New or Established Patient

To qualify for a particular level of service, two of the three key components must be met or exceeded.

| Code | 99221 | 99222 | 99223 |
|---|---|---|---|
| **Key Components** | | | |
| **History** | Detailed or comprehensive | Comprehensive | Comprehensive |
| **Examination** | Detailed or comprehensive | Comprehensive | Comprehensive |
| **Medical Decision Making** | Straightforward or low complexity | Moderate complexity | High complexity |
| **Contributory Factors** | | | |
| **Presenting Problem** | Low severity | Moderate severity | High severity |
| **Counseling** | Counseling and/or coordination of care with other providers or agencies are provided consistent with the nature of the problem(s) and the patient's and/or family's needs | | |
| **Coordination of Care** | | | |
| **Time\* Face-to-Face** | 30 minutes | 50 minutes | 70 minutes |

\* It should be recognized that the specific times expressed in the visit code descriptors are averages and therefore represent a range of times, which may be higher or lower depending on actual clinical circumstances.

If counseling and/or coordination of care dominate (more than 50%) the encounter, time may be used to select the code. This is the time physicians typically spend face-to-face with the patient and/or family.

### Subsequent Hospital Care

Subsequent Hospital Care codes (**99231-99233**) are used to report E/M services provided by the admitting physician on dates subsequent to the provision of initial hospital care. The codes in this series are also used to report subsequent as well as initial inpatient encounters by physicians other than the admitting physician. Whereas it is most common for other physicians to use inpatient consultation codes to report their services (refer to the discussion regarding consultations later in this chapter), the subsequent hospital care codes are also appropriate to use for the initial and subsequent inpatient encounters by physicians other than the admitting physicians.

When subsequent hospital care is reported, at least two of the three key components must meet or exceed the stated requirements to qualify for a particular level of E/M service.

The requirement for history in this subcategory of E/M service indicates "interval" history. Although this term is not specifically defined in CPT nomenclature, it refers to any new history information obtained since the last physician-patient encounter. The categories of service where the interval history concept applies are Subsequent Hospital Care (**99231-99233**); Subsequent Nursing

Facility Care (**99307-99310**); Other Nursing Facility Services (**99318**); Domiciliary, Rest Home (eg, Boarding Home), or Custodial Care Services, Established Patient (**99334-99337**); and Home Services, Established Patient (**99347-99350**).

An interval history focuses on the period of time since the physician last performed an assessment of the patient. For example, if the physician is providing subsequent hospital care to an inpatient and the physician reports CPT code **99232**, Subsequent hospital care, per day, for the evaluation and management of a patient, the key components listed in the code descriptor (of which the physician must perform two of the three) specify that an expanded, problem-focused interval history must be performed. An expanded, problem-focused interval history would address the CC, brief history of the present illness, and a problem-pertinent system review, focusing on the period of time since the physician last performed an assessment of the patient.

The following chart is provided to summarize the requirements for reporting subsequent hospital care. In determining final code selection, be sure to refer to the E/M guidelines and the code descriptors in the CPT codebook.

**Hospital Inpatient Services:** Subsequent Hospital Care—New or Established Patient

To qualify for a particular level of service, two of the three key components must be met or exceeded.

| Code | 99231 | 99232 | 99233 |
|---|---|---|---|
| **Key Components** | | | |
| **History** | Interval problem focused | Interval problem focused | Interval detailed |
| **Examination** | Problem-focused | Expanded problem-focused | Detailed |
| **Medical Decision Making** | Straightforward or low complexity | Moderate complexity | High complexity |
| **Contributory Factors** | | | |
| **Presenting Problem** | Stable, recovering, or improving | Responding inadequately or minor complication | Unstable or significant complication or new problem |
| **Counseling** | Counseling and/or coordination of care with other providers or agencies are provided consistent with the nature of the problem(s) and the patient's and/or family's needs | | |
| **Coordination of Care** | | | |
| **Time* Face-to-Face** | 15 minutes | 25 minutes | 35 minutes |

* It should be recognized that the specific times expressed in the visit code descriptors are averages and therefore represent a range of times, which may be higher or lower depending on actual clinical circumstances.

If counseling and/or coordination of care dominate (more than 50%) the encounter, time may be used to select the code. This is the time physicians typically spend face-to-face with the patient and/or family.

## Hospital Discharge Services (99238, 99239)

The codes in the Hospital Discharge Services series (**99238, 99239**) are used by the attending physician who provides care to patients being discharged, as long as the date of discharge is different from the date of admission. These codes do not recognize key components (ie, history, examination, and medical decision making), but rather are reported on the basis of the total time spent by the attending physician for final hospital discharge of the patient. The total time spent providing discharge services on that date is considered, even if that time is not continuous.

These codes may include, as appropriate, final examination of the patient, discussion of the hospital stay, instructions for continuing care to all relevant caregivers, and preparation of discharge records, prescriptions, and referral forms.

The hospital discharge services codes may be used to report discharge services provided to patients who die during the hospital stay. The attending physician will perform the final examination of the patient (pronouncing the patient dead), discuss the hospital stay with family members or others, and subsequently prepare discharge records (such as the discharge summary for the hospital record).

## Observation or Inpatient Care Services (99234-99236)

The E/M services provided to patients admitted and discharged on the same date of service are reported with the codes in the Observation of Inpatient Care Services series (**99234-99236**). These codes include admission and discharge services provided by the physician on the same date to patients receiving either observation or inpatient hospital care. Codes **99234-99236** can be used to report either observation for an outpatient (when such observation is performed in the hospital setting and the patient is admitted to observation status and discharged from observation status by the physician all on the same date, without becoming an inpatient) or inpatient services (when the patient receives inpatient admission and discharge services by the physician on the same date).

When the codes in this category of service are reported, all three of the key components must meet or exceed the requirements in the code descriptor to qualify for a particular level of service.

The following chart is provided to summarize the requirements for reporting observation or inpatient care services. In determining final code selection, be sure to refer to the E/M guidelines and the code descriptors in the CPT codebook.

## Observation or Inpatient Care Services (Including Admission and Discharge Services): New or Established Patient

To qualify for a particular level of service, all three key components must be met or exceeded.

| Code | 99234 | 99235 | 99236 |
|---|---|---|---|
| **Key Components** | | | |
| **History** | Detailed or comprehensive | Comprehensive | Comprehensive |
| **Examination** | Detailed or comprehensive | Comprehensive | Comprehensive |
| **Medical Decision Making** | Straightforward or low complexity | Moderate complexity | High complexity |
| **Contributory Factors** | | | |
| **Presenting Problem** | Low severity | Moderate severity | High severity |
| **Counseling** | Counseling and/or coordination of care with other providers or agencies are provided consistent with the nature of the problem(s) and the patient's and/or family's needs | | |
| **Coordination of Care** | | | |
| **Time\* Face-to-Face** | NA | NA | NA |

NA = not applicable.

\* Typical times have not been established for this category of services.

## Consultations

It is essential for the user to understand the following general guidelines that pertain to consultations before reporting this category of codes. The discussion that follows on the consultation guidelines is provided to show how these codes are reported when CPT coding guidelines are adhered to. Coders may wish to check with various payers in their area to be sure the payers' reporting and reimbursement policies for consultative services are consistent with CPT coding guidelines.

### General Guidelines

Let us first review the general guidelines pertaining to consultations. Developing a good understanding of these basic guidelines will help to ensure appropriate reporting of physician consultation services. The first general guideline pertains to how a consultation is defined in the CPT codebook:

> For purposes of CPT, a consultation is defined as a type of service provided by a physician whose opinion or advice regarding evaluation and/or management of a specific problem is requested by another physician or other appropriate source.

This definition raises the question of how "other appropriate source" is defined. CPT guidelines do not set restrictions regarding individuals who may be considered an other appropriate source. Some common examples include a physician assistant, a nurse practitioner, a doctor of chiropractic, a physical therapist, an occupational therapist, a speech-language therapist, a psychologist, a social worker, a lawyer, or an insurance company.

The written or verbal request for a consultation may be made by a physician or other appropriate source and documented in the patient's medical record. This documentation is necessary in the patient's record regardless of the site of service (eg, office, emergency department, hospital, nursing facility).

The consultant must document his or her opinion in the patient's medical record as well as any services ordered or performed. The consultant must also communicate his or her opinion and any services that were ordered or performed to the requesting physician or other appropriate source. On the basis of CPT guidelines, this information must be communicated by written report to the requesting physician or other appropriate source.

It is appropriate to report a consultation code when a consultative service between the same specialty in the same group practice is performed, provided the requirements for a consultative service are met as described previously. That is, a request for opinion and/or advice regarding evaluation and/or management of a specific problem is made by the attending physician, the written or verbal request for consultation is documented in the patient's medical record, and the consultant's opinion and/or advice is also documented in the patient's medical record and communicated by written report to the requesting physician.

The consulting physician may initiate diagnostic or therapeutic services at the same visit or a subsequent visit. These separately performed procedures usually stem from the decision-making components of the consultation and are based on the management option(s) chosen for that patient. Even though treatment is initiated, the initial service is still considered a consultative visit.

Another question readers may ask is, "What about the consultant who assumes responsibility for management of all or a portion of the patient's care?" When the consulting physician completes the consultation, he or she may indeed assume responsibility for management of a portion or all of the patient's care. The E/M services provided by the consulting physician after completion of the consultation should not be reported with the consultation codes. For example, in the hospital setting, the consultative service would be reported with the appropriate level of initial inpatient consultation code. The E/M services provided after completion of the consultation are reported with the appropriate level of subsequent hospital care code.

In the office setting, the appropriate level of office or other outpatient consultation code would be reported for the consultative service. The E/M services provided after completion of the consultation would be reported with the appropriate level of office or other outpatient services code. Consider the following scenario:

**EXAMPLE:** Dr A admits his patient, Mrs Miller, to the hospital for stabilization of her uncontrolled diabetes and aggressive treatment of her diabetic foot ulcer. Dr A requests Dr B's opinion and advice regarding evaluation and management of Mrs Miller's foot ulcer. The request and the need for the consultation are documented in Mrs Miller's medical record. Dr B performs the consultation, documents his opinion and advice in the medical record, and communicates this opinion and advice to Dr A. Dr B at the request of Dr A then assumes responsibility for management of Mrs Miller's foot ulcer.

In this scenario, Dr B reports his E/M services with the appropriate level of initial inpatient consultation (**99251-99255**) for the date of the consultative visit and reports the E/M services provided on subsequent dates with the appropriate level of subsequent hospital care code (**99231-99233**).

The following is a five-point summary of consultation requirements:
- A consultation is an E/M service provided by a physician whose opinion and/or advice regarding evaluation and/or management of a specific problem is requested by another physician or other appropriate source.
- The request and need for the consultation must be documented in the patient's medical record.
- The consultant's opinion and any services ordered or performed must be documented in the patient's medical record.
- A physician consultant may initiate diagnostic and/or therapeutic services at the same or a subsequent visit.
- The consulting physician must communicate his or her opinion and/or advice to the requesting physician or other appropriate source by written report.

### Documenting a Request for Consultation

Let us revisit the documentation of the request and need for consultation by the requesting physician or other source. This documentation should indicate the need for the opinion or advice, rather than "refer" to Physician X for evaluation.

## Consultation vs Referral

Much of the confusion in reporting consultative services begins with terms used to describe the service requested. The terms *consultation* and *referral* are mistakenly interchanged. However, CPT nomenclature recognizes these terms as different from each other. Careful documentation of the services requested and provided will alleviate much of this confusion.

When a physician refers a patient to another physician, it is not automatically a consultation. A consultation would be appropriate if the E/M service provided meets the above criteria for reporting a consultation. If a physician sends a patient to another physician for specialized care that is not in his or her domain and the physician to whom the patient is referred does not communicate his or her opinion or advice to the requesting physician, this is not a consultation.

To review the specific guidelines that pertain to each of the subcategories of consultation services:
- office or other outpatient consultations, new or established patient;
- initial inpatient consultations, new or established patient.

## Office or Other Outpatient Consultations (99241-99245)

Office or Other Outpatient Consultations codes (**99241-99245**) are used to report consultations provided in the office or other outpatient setting, including the following settings:

- The physician's office
- Hospital observation services
- Home services
- Domiciliary, rest home, or custodial care
- Emergency department
- Other ambulatory facility

Within this series of codes, there is no differentiation between new and established patient visits. When the codes in this subcategory of service are reported, all three key components must meet or exceed the stated requirements to qualify for a particular level of service.

Follow-up visits provided in the consultant's office or other outpatient facility including home, domiciliary, rest home, custodial care, or emergency department including hospital observation unit that are initiated by the consulting physician are reported by using codes in the office or other outpatient services category for established patient visits (**99211-99215**). A follow-up consultation usually consists of a visit to complete the initial consultation.

However, the office or other outpatient consultation codes may be reported again if this same physician receives a subsequent request from the attending physician to offer his or her opinion on the same patient again for the same problem in response to change in patient's status or availability of new information (eg, test results) or a completely different problem. If an additional request for an opinion or advice regarding the same or a new problem is received from the attending physician (or other appropriate source) and documented in the medical record, the office or other outpatient consultation codes may be reported again by the physician consultant. The need for this consultation must be documented in the patient's medical record along with the consultant's opinion or advice including written documentation to the requesting physician or source, which may consist of a new plan of care or patient management in response to changes in the patient's status.

The following chart is provided to summarize the requirements for reporting office or other outpatient consultations. In determining final code selection, be sure to refer to the E/M guidelines and the code descriptors in the CPT codebook.

## Office or Other Outpatient Consultations: New or Established Patient

To qualify for a particular level of service, all three key components must be met or exceeded.

| Code | 99241 | 99242 | 99243 | 99244 | 99245 |
|---|---|---|---|---|---|
| **Key Components** | | | | | |
| **History** | Problem-focused | Expanded problem-focused | Detailed | Comprehensive | Comprehensive |
| **Examination** | Problem-focused | Expanded problem-focused | Detailed | Comprehensive | Comprehensive |
| **Medical Decision Making** | Straightforward | Straightforward | Low complexity | Moderate complexity | High complexity |
| **Contributory Factors** | | | | | |
| **Presenting Problem** | Self-limited or minor | Low severity | Low to moderate severity | Moderate to high severity | Moderate to high severity |
| **Counseling** | Counseling and/or coordination of care with other providers or agencies are provided consistent with the nature of the problem(s) and the patient's and/or family's needs | | | | |
| **Coordination of Care** | | | | | |
| **Time* Face-to-Face** | 15 minutes | 30 minutes | 40 minutes | 60 minutes | 80 minutes |

\* It should be recognized that the specific times expressed in the visit code descriptors are averages and therefore represent a range of times, which may be higher or lower depending on actual clinical circumstances.

If counseling and/or coordination of care dominate (more than 50%) the encounter, time may be used to select the code. This is the time physicians typically spend face-to-face with the patient and/or family.

## Inpatient Consultations (99251-99255)

The Inpatient Consultation codes are used to report consultations provided to hospital inpatients, residents of nursing facilities, or patients in a partial hospital setting. Within this series of codes there is no differentiation between new and established patient visits. When the codes in this subcategory are reported, all three key components must meet or exceed the requirements of the code descriptor to qualify for a particular level of service.

Only one inpatient consultation per admission should be reported by a consultant per admission.

No separate category of codes is available for follow-up inpatient consultations provided in the inpatient or nursing facility. A follow-up consultation usually consists of a visit to complete the initial consultation. For example, if the consultant is unable to finish the initial consultation because certain test results are not available, the physician consultant may visit the patient again.

## Follow-up Inpatient Visits

Follow-up visits in the inpatient setting are reported with the subsequent hospital care codes (**99231-99233**). Similarly, follow-up consultative nursing facility visits should be reported with the subsequent nursing facility care codes (**99307-99310**).

If a subsequent inpatient or nursing facility consultation is requested by the attending physician for the same problem in response to change in patient's status or availability of new information (eg, test results) or a completely different problem in the same patient, this encounter should be coded using the subsequent hospital care codes (**99231-99233**) or subsequent nursing facility care codes (**99307-99310**) and not reported as an inpatient consultation. The consulting physician may report the inpatient consultation codes only once per patient admission or once per patient nursing facility visit.

The following chart is provided to summarize the requirements for reporting inpatient consultations. In determining final code selection, be sure to refer to the E/M guidelines and the code descriptors in the CPT codebook.

| **Consultations:** Inpatient Consultations—New or Established Patient | | | | | |
|---|---|---|---|---|---|
| To qualify for a particular level of service, all three key components must be met or exceeded. | | | | | |
| **Code** | 99251 | 99252 | 99253 | 99254 | 99255 |
| **Key Components** | | | | | |
| **History** | Problem-focused | Expanded problem-focused | Detailed | Comprehensive | Comprehensive |
| **Examination** | Problem-focused | Expanded problem-focused | Detailed | Comprehensive | Comprehensive |
| **Medical Decision Making** | Straightforward | Straightforward | Low complexity | Moderate complexity | High complexity |
| **Contributory Factors** | | | | | |
| **Presenting Problem** | Self-limited or minor | Low severity | Low to moderate severity | Moderate to high severity | Moderate to high severity |
| **Counseling** | Counseling and/or coordination of care with other providers or agencies are provided consistent with the nature of the problem(s) and the patient's and/or family's needs | | | | |
| **Coordination of Care** | | | | | |
| **Time* Face-to-Face** | 20 minutes | 40 minutes | 55 minutes | 80 minutes | 110 minutes |

* It should be recognized that the specific times expressed in the visit code descriptors are averages and therefore represent a range of times, which may be higher or lower depending on actual clinical circumstances.

If counseling and/or coordination of care dominate (more than 50%) the encounter, time may be used to select the code. This is the time physicians typically spend face-to-face with the patient and/or family.

## Emergency Department Services (99281-99285)

An *emergency department* is defined as an organized hospital-based facility for the provision of unscheduled episodic services to patients who present for immediate medical attention. E/M services provided in the emergency department are reported with the codes in this series. These codes are not limited to use by emergency department physicians.

No distinction is made between new and established patients. The reason for this is that many different physicians staff emergency departments and the service they provide is unscheduled and episodic. Also, previous information about a patient may not be readily available to physicians in the emergency department.

When the codes in this category of service are reported, all three key components must meet or exceed the requirements stated in the code descriptor to qualify for a particular level of service.

Note that code **99285** is unique in that it indicates that the three key components are required within the constraints imposed by the urgency of the patient's clinical condition and/or mental status. This means that code **99285** may be reported when the patient's condition requires this level of service but the physician is unable to complete a comprehensive level of history or examination because of the nature of the patient's clinical condition and/or mental status (eg, comatose patient). When this circumstance occurs, documentation should be used to specify the imposing constraints of the patient's clinical condition, and the diagnosis codes reported should be indicative.

Generally, when E/M services are provided by more than one physician to the same patient in the emergency department, only the emergency department physician should report his or her E/M services with the codes in this series. The other physician would report his or her services with the appropriate level of office or other outpatient services code, or with an office or other outpatient consultation code, as appropriate. Consider the following scenario:

**EXAMPLE:** A patient presents to the emergency department with a fracture of the arm. The emergency department physician provides E/M services, performing history, examination, and medical decision making. He then requests a consultation from an orthopedic specialist, documenting the need and request for the consultation in the patient's medical record. The orthopedic specialist performs the consultation in the emergency department. He documents his opinion and any services that were ordered or performed in the patient's medical record and communicates his findings to the emergency department physician.

In the previous example, the emergency department physician reports his E/M services with the appropriate level of service from the emergency department series of codes. The level of service is selected on the basis of the key component requirements (ie, extent of the history obtained, extent of the examination performed, and the complexity of the medical decision making).

The orthopedic specialist reports his E/M services with the appropriate level of office or other outpatient consultation. Again, the level of service selected is based on the key component requirements (ie, history, examination, medical decision making).

The following chart summarizes the requirements for reporting emergency department services. In determining final code selection, be sure to refer to the E/M guidelines and the code descriptors in the CPT codebook.

**Emergency Department Services: New or Established Patient**

To qualify for a particular level of service, all three key components must be met or exceeded.

| Code | 99281 | 99282 | 99283 | 99284 | 99285 |
|---|---|---|---|---|---|
| **Key Components** | | | | | |
| **History** | Problem focused- | Expanded problem-focused | Expanded problem-focused | Detailed | Comprehensive |
| **Examination** | Problem-focused | Expanded problem-focused | Expanded problem-focused | Detailed | Comprehensive |
| **Medical Decision Making** | Straightforward | Low complexity | Moderate complexity | Moderate complexity | High complexity |
| **Contributory Factors** | | | | | |
| **Presenting Problem** | Self-limited or minor | Low to moderate severity | Moderate severity | High severity | High severity |
| **Counseling** | Counseling and/or coordination of care with other providers or agencies are provided consistent with the nature of the problem(s) and the patient's and/or family's needs | | | | |
| **Coordination of Care** | | | | | |
| **Time\* Face-to-Face** | NA | NA | NA | NA | NA |

NA = not applicable.

\* It should be recognized that the specific times expressed in the visit code descriptors are averages and therefore represent a range of times, which may be higher or lower depending on actual clinical circumstances.

If counseling and/or coordination of care dominate (more than 50%) the encounter, time may be used to select the code. This is the time physicians typically spend face-to-face with the patient and/or family.

**CODING TIP**

When the neonate is transferred to another facility and the patient transport services code(s) **99289** and/or **99290** are reported, the initial neonatal intensive care code (**99295**) is reported only after the patient has been admitted to the critical care unit of the receiving facility.

## Pediatric Critical Care Patient Transport (99289, 99290)

The patient transport codes **99289** and **99290** apply only to pediatric patients who are critically ill or critically injured who receive face-to-face critical care services delivered by a physician during interfacility transport. A pediatric patient is defined in the CPT code set by the designation "24 months of age or less." Codes **99289** and **99290** are used to report the physical attendance and direct face-to-face care by a physician during the interfacility transport of a critically ill or critically injured pediatric patient. For the purpose of reporting codes **99289** and **99290**, face-to-face care begins when the physician assumes primary responsibility of the pediatric patient at the referring hospital/facility and ends when the receiving hospital/facility accepts responsibility for the pediatric patient's care. Only the time the physician spends in direct face-to-face contact with the patient during the transport should be reported. Pediatric patient transport services involving less than 30 minutes of face-to-face physician care should not be reported with codes **99289** and **99290**. Procedure(s) or service(s) performed by other members of the transporting team may not be reported by the supervising physician.

The following services are included when performed during the pediatric patient transport by the physician providing critical care and may not be reported separately:

- Routine monitoring evaluations (eg, heart rate, respiratory rate, blood pressure, and pulse oximetry), the interpretation of cardiac output measurements (**93561, 93562**), chest X rays (**71010, 71015, 71020**), pulse oximetry (**94760, 94761, 94762**), blood gases and information data stored in computers (eg, electrocardiograms, blood pressures, hematologic data) (**99090**)
- Gastric intubation (**43752, 91105**)
- Temporary transcutaneous pacing (**92953**)
- Ventilatory management (**94002-94004, 94660, 94662**)
- Vascular access procedures (**36000, 36400, 36405, 36406, 36410, 36415, 36540, 36600**).

Any services performed that are not listed above should be reported separately.

The direction of emergency care to transporting staff by a physician located in a hospital or other facility by two-way communication is not considered direct face-to-face care and should not be reported with codes **99289** and **99290**. Physician-directed emergency care through outside voice communication to transporting staff personnel is reported with code **99288**.

The emergency department services codes (**99281-99285**), initial hospital care codes (**99221-99223**), hourly critical care codes (**99291, 99292**), and initial date neonatal intensive care code (**99295**) are reported only after the patient has been admitted to the emergency department, the inpatient floor, or the critical care unit of the receiving facility.

Code **99289** is used to report the first 30 to 74 minutes of direct face-to-face time with the transport pediatric patient and should be reported only once on a given date. Code **99290** is used to report each additional 30 minutes provided on a given date. Face-to-face services less than 30 minutes should not be reported with these codes. Critical care of less than 30 minutes in total duration should be reported with the appropriate E/M code. The definition of critical care, as described in the Critical Care guidelines, also applies to the pediatric critical care patient transport codes.

## Critical Care Services (99291-99296)

Critical care is defined as the direct delivery by physician(s) of medical care for a critically ill or critically injured patient. A critical illness or injury acutely impairs one or more vital organ systems such that there is a high probability of

> **CODING TIP**
>
> Critical care and other E/M services may be provided to the same patient on the same date by the same physician. For example, a patient involved in a car accident is brought to the emergency department at 2 AM. The patient is immediately admitted to the critical care unit, where the attending critical care physician directs life-saving treatment. Later that same day at 8 PM when the patient is stabilized, the same critical care physician who attended the patient performs an E/M service to obtain a patient history and examination before transferring the patient out of the critical care unit to a medical floor. The critical care physician reports his critical care services provided earlier in the day as **99291** and **99292** and also reports a subsequent hospital care E/M service, code **99231**.

> **CODING TIP**
>
> Codes **99289** and **99290** may be reported separately from any other procedure/service (except for those services specifically described in the Pediatric Patient Transport guidelines) provided on the date of the transfer. The time spent by the physician performing separately reportable services or procedures should not be included in the face-to-face time reported by codes **99289** and **99290**.

imminent or life-threatening deterioration in the patient's condition. Critical care involves high-complexity decision making to assess, manipulate, and support vital system function(s) to treat single or multiple vital organ system failure and/or to prevent further life-threatening deterioration of the patient's condition. Examples of vital organ system failure include but are not limited to central nervous system failure, circulatory failure, shock, and renal, hepatic, metabolic, and/or respiratory failure. Although critical care typically requires interpretation of multiple physiologic parameters and/or application of advanced technologies, critical care may be provided in life-threatening situations when these elements are not present. Critical care may be provided on multiple days even if no changes are made in the treatment rendered to the patient, provided that the patient's condition continues to require the level of physician attention described above.

Providing medical care to a critically ill, injured, or postoperative patient qualifies as a critical care service only if both the illness or injury and the treatment being provided meet the above requirements. Critical care services include but are not limited to the treatment or prevention of further deterioration of central nervous system failure; circulatory failure; shock-like conditions; renal, hepatic, metabolic, or respiratory failure; postoperative complications; and overwhelming infection.

An important factor in reporting the critical care services codes **99291** and **99292** is that the codes describe the type of care provided, not the site in which the care is provided. Although critical care is usually given in a critical care area such as the coronary care unit, intensive care unit, respiratory care unit, or the emergency care facility, it is not required that the patient be physically located in such an area to receive critical care services. For example, critical care services provided in the outpatient setting (eg, emergency department or office) are reported using the critical care codes **99291** and **99292**. However, the pediatric and neonatal critical care service codes (**99293-99296**) and continuing intensive care for neonates/infants codes (**99298, 99299**) apply only to the inpatient setting.

In addition, simply because a patient happens to be in a critical care unit does not mean that the critical care codes should be reported. Services for a patient who is not critically ill but happens to be in a critical care unit are reported by means of other appropriate E/M codes (eg, initial or subsequent hospital care).

The following services are included in reporting critical care when performed during the critical period by the physician(s) providing critical care:

- The interpretation of cardiac output measurements (**93561, 93562**), chest X rays (**71010, 71075, 71020**), pulse oximetry (**94760, 94761, 94762**), blood gases, and information data stored in computers (eg, electrocardiograms, blood pressures, hematologic data) (**99090**)
- Gastric intubation (**43752, 91105**)
- Temporary transcutaneous pacing (**92953**)
- Ventilator management (**94002-94004, 94660, 94662**)
- Vascular access procedures (**36000, 36410, 36415, 36540, 36600**).

Any services performed that are not in this list should be reported separately.

Codes **99291** and **99292** are used to report physician attendance during the transport of a critically ill or critically injured patient and direct delivery of care by a physician for the critically ill or critically injured patient over 24 months of age. Code **99291** is used to report the first 30 to 74 minutes of critical care on a given date. It should be used only once per date, even if the time spent by the physician is not continuous on that date. Critical care of less than 30 minutes in total duration on a given date should be reported with the appropriate E/M code. Code **99292** is used to report additional blocks of time of up to 30 minutes each beyond the first 74 minutes. (See table that follows.)

## Critical Care Time Reporting

| Total Duration of Critical Care | Codes |
|---|---|
| Less than 30 minutes (less than 1/2 hour) | Appropriate E/M codes |
| 30–74 minutes (1/2 hour–1 hour 14 minutes) | 99291 × 1 |
| 75–104 minutes (1 hour 15 minutes–1 hour 44 minutes) | 99291 × 1 and 99292 × 1 |
| 105–134 minutes (1 hour 45 minutes–2 hours 14 minutes) | 99291 × 1 and 99292 × 2 |
| 135–164 minutes (2 hours 15 minutes–2 hours 44 minutes) | 99291 × 1 and 99292 × 3 |
| 165–194 minutes (2 hours 45 minutes–3 hours 14 minutes) | 99291 × 1 and 99292 × 4 |
| 195 minutes or longer. (3 hours 15 minutes or longer) | 99291 and 99292 as appropriate (see previous illustrated reporting examples above) |

### Reporting the Codes

The critical care services codes **99291** and **99292** are not based on the performance of the key components of history, examination, and medical decision making. Rather, they are time-based codes used to report the total duration of time on a given date spent by a physician providing critical care services to a critically ill or critically injured patient, even if the time spent by the physician on that date is not continuous. For any given period of time spent providing critical care services, the physician must devote his or her full attention to the patient and therefore cannot provide services to any other patient during the same period of time.

Time spent with the individual patient should be recorded in the patient's record. The time that can be reported as critical care is the time spent engaged in work directly related to the individual patient's care, whether that time was spent at the immediate bedside or elsewhere on the floor or unit. It is not necessary for the physician to be constantly at the bedside per se, but the physician should be engaged in work directly related to the individual patient's care.

For example, time spent on the unit or at the nursing station on the floor reviewing test results or imaging studies, discussing the critically ill patient's care with other medical staff or documenting critical care services in the medical record would be reported as critical care, even though it does not occur at the bedside. Also, when the patient is unable or clinically incompetent to participate in discussions, time spent on the floor or unit with family members or surrogate decision makers obtaining a medical history, reviewing the patient's condition or prognosis, or discussing treatment may be reported as critical care provided that the conversation bears directly on the management of the patient.

Time spent in activities that occur outside of the unit or off the floor (eg, telephone calls, whether taken at home, in the office, or elsewhere in the hospital) may not be reported as critical care since the physician is not immediately available to the patient. Time spent in activities that do not directly contribute to the treatment of the patient may not be reported as critical care, even if they are performed in the critical care unit (eg, participation in administrative meetings or telephone calls to discuss other patients).

Time spent performing additional services or procedures that are not included in the critical care codes is excluded from the determination of the time spent providing critical care. On the basis of CPT guidelines, if in the physician's clinical judgment the patient is no longer critically ill when the unbundled service or procedure is performed, it would not be appropriate to report critical care services for this time.

Code **99291** is used to report the first 30 to 74 minutes of critical care on a given date. It should be used only once per date, even if the time spent by the physician is not continuous on that date. Critical care of less than 30 minutes in total duration on a given date should be reported with the appropriate E/M code, not with code **99291**.

### Inpatient Pediatric Critical Care

Codes **99293** and **99294** are used to report inpatient services provided by a physician directing the care of a critically ill infant or young child from 29 days of postnatal age up through 24 months of age. Critical care services provided to neonates and pediatric patients in the outpatient setting (eg, emergency department or office) should be reported using the timed critical care codes **99291** and **99292**. However, pediatric critical care outpatient or emergency department services (**99291, 99292**) should not be reported separately when pediatric inpatient critical care services (**99293, 99294**) are provided later on the same day by the same physician. If a physician provides both outpatient (eg, office or emergency department) critical care services and inpatient critical care services to a pediatric patient on the same date of service, only the inpatient pediatric critical services should be reported (**99293**) on that day.

The services reported with codes **99293**, initial day of pediatric inpatient critical care, and **99294**, subsequent day(s) of inpatient pediatric critical care, include repetitive evaluation of the patient, therapy adjustment, and supervision of the health care team by the physician. These evaluations occur in both

**CODING TIP**

Code **99294** (subsequent pediatric critical care) may be reported on multiple days provided the patient's condition continues to require the level of physician attention necessary to care for critically ill patients, even if no changes are made in the treatment rendered to the patient.

brief and long encounters throughout the day (often representing a dozen or more encounters per day); for this reason, codes **99293** and **99294** are not time-based and are only to be used once per day, regardless of the number of encounters and services rendered.

Codes **99293** and **99294** should not be used for infants and young children who are no longer considered critically ill. Infants who are not critically ill but continue to require intensive observation, frequent interventions, and other intensive services should be reported according to the current or presenting body weight: less than 1500 g (**99298**), 1500–2500 g (**99299**), or 2501–5000 g (**99300**). Intensive care services provided to a noncritically ill infant/child over 5000 g (approximately 11.2 lbs) would be reported using the Subsequent Hospital Care codes (**99231-99233**). Critical care services to patients over 24 months of age would be reported with hourly (timed) critical care service codes (**99291, 99292**).

The following procedures are included (bundled) in codes **99293** and **99294** and should not be reported separately. Codes **99293** and **99294** also include any of the bundled procedures contained in the timed critical care codes (**99291, 99292**). Any services performed that are not bundled into these codes may be reported separately:

- Umbilical venous catheter (**36510**)
- Umbilical arterial catheters (**36660**)
- Central (**36555**) or peripheral (**36000**) vessel catheterization
- Vascular access procedures (**36400, 36405, 36406**)
- Other arterial catheters (**36140, 36620**)
- Oral or nasogastric tube placement (**43752**)
- Endotracheal intubation (**31500**)
- Lumbar puncture (**62270**)
- Suprapubic bladder aspiration (**51000**)
- Bladder catheterization (**51701, 51702**)
- Ventilatory management (**94002-94004**)
- Continuous positive airway pressure (CPAP) (**94660**)
- Surfactant administration (**94610**)
- Intravascular fluid administration (**90760-90761**)
- Transfusion of blood components (**36430, 36440**)
- Vascular punctures (**36420, 36600**)
- Invasive or noninvasive electronic monitoring of vital signs, bedside pulmonary function testing (**94375**)
- Monitoring or interpretation of blood gases or oxygen saturation (**94760-94762**)

Any services that are not listed here should be reported separately.

## Inpatient Neonatal Critical Care

Codes **99295** and **99296** are used to report inpatient services provided by a physician directing the care of a critically ill neonate, from birth through 28 days of postnatal age. Code **99295** is used only for the first date of inpatient critical

**CODING TIP**

Code **99295** may be used only once for the first day of neonatal critical care services, regardless of the number of visits/encounters the physician (single physician group) provides on that day. Code **99296** may be used multiple times, only once per day, up to the 30th day of postnatal age. If, after the 30th day of critical care services the patient still requires critical care, the pediatric critical care code **99293** should be reported for the first day (31st day of postnatal age) of care only, and then **99294** may be reported for subsequent days of care (beyond 31 days of age). If the patient status changes and intensive care rather than critical care is required, then the subsequent hospital care codes **99231-99233** should be reported unless the infant presents with a body weight of 5000 g or under. In this instance, the continuing intensive care services codes (**99298-99300**) would then apply.

care services. Critically ill neonates require cardiac and/or respiratory support (including ventilator or nasal CPAP when indicated), continuous or frequent vital sign monitoring, laboratory and blood gas interpretations, follow-up physician reevaluations, and constant observation by the health care team under direct physician supervision. Immediate preoperative evaluation and stabilization of neonates with life-threatening surgical or cardiac conditions are also included in code **99295**. Care for neonates with life-threatening surgical or cardiac conditions is included under this code. Code **99296** is used to report subsequent inpatient care of a critically ill neonate who continues to require cardiac and/or respiratory support (including ventilator or nasal CPAP when indicated), continuous or frequent vital sign monitoring, laboratory and blood gas interpretations, follow-up physician reevaluations throughout a 24-hour period, and constant observation by the health care team under direct physician supervision.

Codes **99295** and **99296** include repetitive evaluation of the patient, therapy adjustment, and supervision of the health care team by the physician. These evaluations occur in both brief and long encounters throughout the day (often representing a dozen or more encounters per day). For this reason, codes **99295** and **99296** are not time-based and are to be used only once per day, regardless of the number of encounters and services rendered.

The Neonatal Critical Care Services codes **99295** and **99296** should not be used for neonates who are no longer critically ill. Care for neonates/infants who no longer meet the definition of critically ill but require intensive observation, frequent interventions, and other intensive care services are reported with the Continuing Intensive Care Services codes (**99298**, **99299**, **99300**) according to present body weight (refer to list under explanation of codes **99298-99300**). When the present body weight of neonate or infant exceeds 5000 g and continued intensive care services are still required, the subsequent hospital care codes (**99231-99233**) should be used. Code **99497** should be reported for admission services for the first day of care for the neonate who requires intensive observation and monitoring.

The same procedures bundled into codes **99293** and **99294** (see list provided under codes **99293** and **99294**) are also bundled into codes **99295** and **99296** and should not be reported separately. Codes **99295** and **99296** also include any of the bundled procedures included in the timed critical care codes (**99291**, **99292**). Any services performed that are not bundled into these codes may be reported separately. Additionally, the initial day neonatal critical care code (**99295**) can be used in addition to standby services (**99360**) (see discussion of **99360**) or attendance at delivery upon request of delivering physician (**99440**) and/or when newborn resuscitation (**99440**) is required. Additionally, procedures performed as a necessary part of the resuscitation (eg, endotracheal intubation [**31500**]) may also be reported separately when performed as part of the preadmission delivery room care occurring prior to the initial inpatient neonatal critical care admission. To report these procedures separately, they must be performed as a necessary component of the resuscitation and not simply as a convenience before admission to the neonatal intensive care unit.

## Continuing Intensive Care Services (99298-99300)

Codes **99298-99300** are used to report intensive care (noncritical) services provided to neonates or infants with present body weight of 5000 g (approximately 11.2 lbs) or less (see the following list) who during any portion of a single calendar day are no longer considered critically ill but require intensive observation and frequent services and interventions only available in an intensive care setting.

| | |
|---|---|
| Body Weight Less Than 1500 g (approximately less than 3.3 lbs) | **99298** |
| Body Weight of 1500–2500 g (approximately 3.3–5.581 lbs) | **99299** |
| Body Weight of 2501–5000 g (approximately 5.582–11.2 lbs) | **99300** |

When the present body weight of neonate or infant exceeds 5000 g and continued intensive care services are still required, the subsequent hospital care codes (**99231-99233**) should be used.

Codes **99298**, **99299**, and **99300** represent subsequent day(s) of care and may be reported. Codes **99298-99300** are global codes with the same services included (bundled) under codes **99293-99296**.

The neonates/infants who receive continuing intensive care may or may not be (or have been) premature and are recovering from a variety of medical, cardiac, or surgical diagnoses (which occur in low-, normal-, and high-birth-weight infants). Code **99298** is used to report intensive care services to a neonate/infant presenting with a current body weight of less than 1500 g who is not critically ill but requires continuing intensive care services. Code **99299** is used to report intensive care services to a neonate/infant presenting with a current body weight of 1500–2500 g who is not critically ill but requires continuing intensive care services. Code **99300** is used to report intensive care services to a neonate/infant presenting with a current body weight of 2501–5000 g who is not critically ill but requires continuing intensive care services. The continuing intensive (noncritical) care of the neonate/infant who falls under this category of codes requires intensive cardiac and respiratory monitoring, continuous and/or frequent vital sign monitoring, heat maintenance, enteral and/or parenteral nutritional adjustments, laboratory and oxygen monitoring, and constant observation by the health care team under direct physician supervision.

### Reporting Conventional E/M Services and Nonpediatric Critical Care

Because the critical care patient is often incoherent or incapacitated, the critical care services codes do not include provision of conventional E/M services (eg, performing a history and physical examination).

Critical care and other E/M services may be provided to the same patient on the same date by the same physician. For example, an emergency department code or hospital E/M code can be reported early in the day when the patient

---

**CODING TIP**

Newborn resuscitation (**99440**) is not included in the listing of services included in reporting neonatal critical care codes (**99295**, **99296**). It is appropriate for a physician to report code **99440** (for the resuscitation immediately following the birth of the baby) and code **99295** for the initial neonatal critical care services. Both services should be clearly documented in the patient's medical record.

**CODING TIP**

Both codes **99436** (attendance at delivery) and **99295** (initial neonatal critical care) may be reported by the same physician on the same date. Both services should be clearly documented in the patient's medical record.

**CODING TIP**

A low-birth-weight baby weighs from 3.3 to 5.5 lbs (1500–2500 g). A very-low-birth-weight baby weighs less than 3.3 lbs (less than 1500 g). A low-birth-weight baby is typically 32 to 36 weeks of gestational age, and a very-low-birth-weight baby is typically 23 to 31 weeks of gestational age.

does not require critical care. If later that day the patient requires critical care services, a critical care code would be reported for these services in addition to the E/M code reported for the physician's services provided earlier in the day. Alternatively, the critical care services can occur before traditional E/M services are provided. Consider the following scenario:

**EXAMPLE:** A patient is brought to the emergency department with chest pains, and, before a traditional history and physical examination can be performed, he develops a full-blown myocardial infarction with cardiac arrest. During this medical emergency, the physician providing care to this patient would code the services provided during the medical emergency as critical care if they meet the duration criteria. The total time the physician spent in constant attendance would be reported with codes **99291** and **99292**, as appropriate. Also, any services not specifically listed in the critical care guidelines as being part of critical care services may be reported separately.

After a patient's medical crisis has resolved or stabilized and critical care services are no longer needed, the critical care service codes **99291-99296** should no longer be reported. If the patient is admitted to an intensive care area of the hospital or nonintensive medical floor of the hospital, the hospital inpatient services codes should be reported. However, the hospital inpatient service codes should not be used to report intensive care services provided to neonates or infants who require intensive management, observation, and frequent interventions (eg, infants born prematurely). Intensive (noncritical) care services provided to neonates/infants with present body weight of 5000 g or less should be reported with the Continuing Intensive Care Service codes **99298, 99299**, and **99300**.

Prolonged services cannot be used with the critical care codes. Prolonged services may be reported with other E/M services.

## Nursing Facility Services (99304-99318)

The codes in the Nursing Facility Services category of E/M services (**99304-99318**) are used to report services provided to patients in nursing facilities (eg, skilled nursing facilities, intermediate care facilities, or long-term care facilities). These codes are also used to report E/M services provided to patients in psychiatric residential treatment centers.

The Nursing Facility Services codes are divided into the following four subcategories:
- Initial nursing facility care (**99304-99306**)
- Subsequent nursing facility care (**99307-99310**)
- Nursing facility discharge services (**99315, 99316**)
- Annual nursing facility assessment (**99318**)

These subcategories of service are based largely on the responsibilities of nursing facilities to conduct thorough assessments of each resident's functional capacity by means of a resident assessment instrument. A resident assessment instrument is a form composed of a uniform minimum data set (MDS) and resident assessment protocols (RAPs).

As the term implies, the MDS is a set of assessment elements considered minimally necessary to evaluate skilled nursing facility and nursing facility residents. Assessments done by the facility must include at least the following:
- Medically defined conditions and prior medical history
- Medical status measurement
- Physical and mental functional status
- Sensory and physical impairments
- Nutritional status and requirements
- Special treatments or procedures
- Mental and psychosocial status
- Discharge potential
- Dental condition
- Activities potential
- Rehabilitation potential
- Cognitive status
- Drug therapy

RAPs supplement the MDS by providing the framework for seeking information beyond the MDS where MDS information shows it is needed.

The nursing facility must complete these assessments whenever one of the following events occurs:
- The patient is admitted to the facility
- Twelve months have passed since the previous assessment
- The patient has had a major permanent change in status

### Initial Nursing Facility Care (**99304-99306**)

Codes in the subcategory for initial nursing facility care are used to report the physician's involvement in providing admission or readmission services to nursing facility patients. There are three codes in this subcategory, one for each level of care that is provided dependent upon the patient's condition (eg, low, moderate, or high severity) and services provided (eg, detailed, comprehensive history or examination) by the physician.

Whether the patient is new or established is not pertinent in determining whether to select a code from the subcategory of initial nursing facility care or subsequent nursing facility care. It is important to note that the terms *new patient* and *established patient* in the heading relate to the physician-patient status, as they do for all E/M services. They do not relate to whether the patient is a new or established patient to the facility.

Nursing facility care may be performed at one or more sites in the assessment process. It is not mandatory that all of the assessments required for the admission of a patient to a nursing facility take place at the facility itself.

If the patient is admitted to the nursing facility in the course of an encounter in another site of service, the nursing facility level of service reported by the admitting physician should include the services related to the admission that were provided in the other sites of service as well as in the nursing facility setting, when performed on the same date as the admission or readmission.

An exception to this guideline is the reporting of hospital discharge or observation discharge services performed on the same date of nursing facility admission or readmission. It is appropriate to separately report hospital discharge or observation discharge services performed on the same date of nursing facility admission or readmission.

Let us review the three codes for reporting initial nursing facility care. Each of these three codes requires that all three of the key components meet or exceed the requirements in the code descriptor to qualify for a particular level of service.

Nursing facilities are required to conduct thorough assessments of all patients on admission and readmission to the nursing facility, including development of a new medical plan of care as determined by patient's status and required of facility. The initial nursing facility care codes include postservice coordination of care with nursing facility and other health care professionals involved in the patient's care (including telephone calls), discussions with family and/or surrogate decision makers (including preferred intensity of care/donot-resuscitate orders), review of laboratory data, and follow-up on medication effectiveness associated with the delivery of care to the patient until the next face-to-face physician encounter.

The first code in the series, **99304**, describes a physician's E/M service at the time of admission or readmission to the nursing facility. Reporting this code requires the performance and documentation of a detailed or comprehensive history or examination and medical decision making that is straightforward or of low complexity. Code **99305** requires the performance and documentation of a comprehensive history and examination that involves medical decision making of moderate complexity. Code **99306** also requires the performance and documentation of a comprehensive history and examination but involves medical decision making of high complexity. No typical unit times have been established for this series of codes.

The following chart is provided to summarize the requirements for reporting comprehensive nursing facility assessments. In determining final code selection, be sure to refer to the E/M guidelines and the code descriptors in the CPT codebook.

## Nursing Facility Services:
### Initial Nursing Facility Case Codes (99304-99306)

To qualify for a particular level of service, all three key components must be met or exceeded.

| Code | 99304 | 99305 | 99306 |
|---|---|---|---|
| **Key Components** | | | |
| **History** | Detailed or Comprehensive | Comprehensive | Comprehensive |
| **Examination** | Detailed or Comprehensive | Comprehensive | Comprehensive |
| **Medical Decision Making** | Straightforward or low complexity | Moderate complexity | High complexity |
| **Contributory Factors** | | | |
| **Presenting Problem** | Low severity | Moderate severity | High severity |
| **Counseling** | Counseling and/or coordination of care with other providers or agencies are provided consistent with the nature of the problem(s) and the patient's and/or family's needs | | |
| **Coordination of Care** | | | |
| **Time* Face-to-Face** | 25 minutes | 35 minutes | 45 minutes |

\* It should be recognized that the specific times expressed in the visit code descriptors are averages and therefore represent a range of times, which may be higher or lower depending on actual clinical circumstances.

If counseling and/or coordination of care dominate (more than 50%) the encounter, time may be used to select the code. This is the time physicians typically spend face-to-face with the patient and/or family.

### Subsequent Nursing Facility Care (99307-99310)

The codes in this series are used to report nursing facility care provided by a physician to a patient subsequent to the physician's initial and/or previous assessment of the patient. There are four levels of subsequent nursing facility care services involving straightforward to high-complexity medical decision making and requiring at least two of the three key components (history, examination, medical decision making) ranging in intensity from problem-focused to comprehensive. The history component required in each of these four levels of codes consists of an interval history.

It is important to note that certain facilities are licensed to provide inpatient hospital care, nursing facility care, and/or domiciliary, rest home, or custodial care services. If the coder is uncertain as to which code to use to report physician services, the facility should be asked how that patient was classified on the date the physician's service was provided.

The following chart is provided to summarize the requirements for reporting subsequent nursing facility care. In determining final code selection, be sure to refer to the E/M guidelines and the code descriptors in the CPT codebook.

**Nursing Facility Services:**
Subsequent Nursing Facility Care Codes (**99307-99310**)

To qualify for a particular level of service, two out of three key components must be met or exceeded.

| Code | 99307 | 99308 | 99309 | 99310 |
|---|---|---|---|---|
| **Key Components** | | | | |
| **History** | Problem-focused interval | Expanded problem-focused interval | Detailed interval | Comprehensive interval |
| **Examination** | Problem-focused | Expanded problem-focused | Detailed | Comprehensive |
| **Medical Decision Making** | Straightforward | Low complexity | Moderate complexity | High complexity |
| **Contributory Factors** | | | | |
| **Presenting Problem** | Stable, recovering, or improving | Responding inadequately to therapy or has developed a minor complication | Developed a significant complication or a significant new problem | Developed a significant new problem requiring immediate physician attention |
| **Counseling** | Counseling and/or coordination of care with other providers or agencies are provided consistent with the nature of the problem(s) and the patient's and/or family's needs | | | |
| **Coordination of Care** | | | | |
| **Time\* Face-to-Face** | 10 minutes | 15 minutes | 25 minutes | 35 minutes |

\* It should be recognized that the specific times expressed in the visit code descriptors are averages and therefore represent a range of times, which may be higher or lower depending on actual clinical circumstances.

If counseling and/or coordination of care dominate (more than 50%) the encounter, time may be used to select the code. This is the time physicians typically spend face-to-face with the patient and/or family.

### Nursing Facility Discharge Services (99315, 99316)

Codes **99315** and **99316** are time-based codes and are intended to be reported for the total duration of time spent (unit/floor time) by the physician for the final nursing facility discharge of the patient, even if the time spent providing the service is not continuous or provided during the course of one calendar day. Only one code is reported—code **99315** if the total time is 30 minutes or less, or code **99316** if the total duration of time is more than 30 minutes.

### Annual Nursing Facility Assessment (99318)

Code **99318** is used to report the annual assessment required by the nursing facility for its residents. This service requires a detailed interval history, a comprehensive examination, and medical decision making that is of low to moderate complexity. Code **99318** should not be used in conjunction with other nursing facility service codes and should occur as a separate service entailing only the annual nursing facility assessment dictated by the facility.

## Domiciliary, Rest Home (eg, Boarding Home), or Custodial Care Services (99324-99337)

The Domiciliary, Rest Home (eg, Boarding Home), or Custodial Care Services category of codes (**99324-99337**) is used to report E/M services provided in a facility that provides room, board, and other personal assistance services, generally on a long-term basis. These codes are also used to report E/M services in an assisted living facility. If the coder is uncertain whether this code series is applicable, the facility should be contacted to verify its classification.

There are separate codes for reporting new (**99324-99328**) and established (**99334-99337**) patient visits. When new patient visits are reported, all three key components must meet or exceed the requirements of the code descriptor to qualify for a particular level of service. When established patient visits are reported, two of the three key components must meet or exceed the requirements of the code descriptor to qualify for a particular level of service.

The following two charts summarize the requirements for reporting domiciliary, rest home (eg, boarding home), or custodial care services. In determining final code selection, be sure to refer to the E/M guidelines and the code descriptors in the CPT codebook.

## Domiciliary, Rest Home (eg, Boarding Home), or Custodial Care Services: New Patient

To qualify for a particular level of service, all three key components must be met or exceeded.

| Code | 99324 | 99325 | 99326 | 99327 | 99328 |
|---|---|---|---|---|---|
| **Key Components** | | | | | |
| **History** | Problem-focused | Expanded problem-focused | Detailed | Comprehensive | Comprehensive |
| **Examination** | Problem-focused | Expanded problem-focused | Detailed | Comprehensive | Comprehensive |
| **Medical Decision Making** | Straightforward | Low complexity | Moderate complexity | Moderate complexity | High complexity |
| **Contributory Factors** | | | | | |
| **Presenting Problem** | Low severity | Moderate severity | Moderate to high severity | High severity | Unstable or has developed a significant new problem requiring immediate physician attention |
| **Counseling** | Counseling and/or coordination of care with other providers or agencies are provided consistent with the nature of the problem(s) and the patient's and/or family's needs | | | | |
| **Coordination of Care** | | | | | |
| **Time* with Patient and/or Family or Caregiver** | 20 minutes | 30 minutes | 45 minutes | 60 minutes | 75 minutes |

NA = Non Applicable.

* Typical times have not been established for this subcategory of services.

## Domiciliary, Rest Home (eg, Boarding Home), or Custodial Care Services: Established Patient

To qualify for a particular level of service, two out of three key components must be met or exceeded.

| Code | 99334 | 99335 | 99336 | 99337 |
|---|---|---|---|---|
| **Key Components** | | | | |
| **History** | Problem-focused interval | Interval expanded problem-focused | Detailed interval | Comprehensive interval |
| **Examination** | Problem-focused | Expanded problem-focused | Detailed | Comprehensive |
| **Medical Decision Making** | Straightforward | Low complexity | Moderate complexity | Moderate to high complexity |
| **Contributory Factors** | | | | |
| **Presenting Problem** | Self-limited or minor | Low to moderate severity | Moderate to high severity | Moderate to high severity |
| **Counseling** | Counseling and/or coordination of care with other providers or agencies are provided consistent with the nature of the problem(s) and the patient's and/or family's needs | | | |
| **Coordination of Care** | | | | |
| **Time\* with Patient and/or Family or Caregiver** | 15 minutes | 25 minutes | 40 minutes | 60 minutes |

NA = Non Applicable.

\* Typical times have not been established for this subcategory of services.

## Domiciliary, Rest Home (eg, Assisted Living Facility), or Home Care Plan Oversight Services (99339-99340)

The Domiciliary, Rest Home (eg, Assisted Living Facility), or Home Care Plan Oversight Services codes **99339-99340** are intended to be reported for care plan oversight services of patients in the home, domiciliary, or rest home (eg, assisted living facility) under the individual supervision of a physician.

## Home Services (99341-99350)

The Home Services category of codes (**99341-99350**) is used to report provision of E/M services in the patient's private residence by the physician. There are separate subcategories of codes for new patient and established patient visits.

When new patient visits are reported, all three of the key components must meet or exceed the requirements stated in the code descriptor to qualify for a level of service. For established patient visits, two of the three key components must meet or exceed the stated requirements to qualify for a level of service.

The following two charts summarize the requirements for reporting home services. In determining final code selection, be sure to refer to the E/M guidelines and the code descriptors in the CPT codebook.

**Home Services:** New Patient

To qualify for a particular level of service, all three key components must be met or exceeded.

| Code | 99341 | 99342 | 99343 | 99344 | 99345 |
|---|---|---|---|---|---|
| **Key Components** | | | | | |
| **History** | Problem-focused | Expanded problem-focused | Detailed | Comprehensive | Comprehensive |
| **Examination** | Problem-focused | Expanded problem-focused | Detailed | Comprehensive | Comprehensive |
| **Medical Decision Making** | Straightforward | Low complexity | Moderate complexity | Moderate complexity | High complexity |
| **Contributory Factors** | | | | | |
| **Presenting Problem** | Low severity | Moderate severity | Moderate to high severity | High severity | Unstable or significant |
| **Counseling** | Counseling and/or coordination of care with other providers or agencies are provided consistent with the nature of the problem(s) and the patient's and/or family's needs | | | | |
| **Coordination of Care** | | | | | |
| **Time* Face-to-Face** | 20 minutes | 30 minutes | 45 minutes | 60 minutes | 75 minutes |

* It should be recognized that the specific times expressed in the visit code descriptors are averages and therefore represent a range of times, which may be higher or lower depending on actual clinical circumstances.

If counseling and/or coordination of care dominate (more than 50%) the encounter, time may be used to select the code. This is the time physicians typically spend face-to-face with the patient and/or family.

| **Home Services:** Established Patient | | | | |
|---|---|---|---|---|
| To qualify for a particular level of service, two out of three key components must be met or exceeded. | | | | |
| **Code** | **99347** | **99348** | **99349** | **99350** |
| **Key Components** | | | | |
| **History** | Problem-focused interval | Expanded problem-focused interval | Detailed interval | Comprehesive interval |
| **Examination** | Problem-focused | Expanded problem-focused | Detailed | Comprehensive |
| **Medical Decision Making** | Straightforward | Low complexity | Moderate complexity | Moderate to high complexity |
| **Contributory Factors** | | | | |
| **Presenting Problem** | Self-limited or minor | Low to moderate severity | Moderate to high severity | Moderate to high severity |
| **Counseling** | Counseling and/or coordination of care with other providers or agencies are provided consistent with the nature of the problem(s) and the patient's and/or family's needs | | | |
| **Coordination of Care** | | | | |
| **Time\* Face-to-Face** | 15 minutes | 25 minutes | 40 minutes | 60 minutes |

\* It should be recognized that the specific times expressed in the visit code descriptors are averages and therefore represent a range of times, which may be higher or lower depending on actual clinical circumstances.

If counseling and/or coordination of care dominate (more than 50%) the encounter, time may be used to select the code. This is the time physicians typically spend face-to-face with the patient and/or family.

## Prolonged Services

Within the Prolonged Services category of codes, there are separate subcategories of codes for reporting the following:

- Prolonged Physician Service With Direct (Face-to-Face) Patient Contact (**99354-99357**)
- Prolonged Physician Service Without Direct (Face-to-Face) Patient Contact (**99358, 99359**)
- Physician Standby Services (**99360**)

The following sections separately review the guidelines associated with reporting these codes.

### Prolonged Physician Service With Direct (Face-to-Face) Patient Contact (**99354-99357**)

The codes in the Prolonged Physician Service With Direct (Face-to-Face) Patient Contact series (**99354-99357**) are used when a physician provides prolonged service involving direct (face-to-face) patient contact that is beyond the usual service (ie, beyond the typical time) in either the inpatient or outpatient setting. The term *face-to-face* refers only to patient face-to-face contact.

These codes are time-based and reported for the total duration of face-to-face time spent by a physician providing prolonged services on a given date. It is not necessary for the time spent by the physician providing the prolonged service to be continuous.

These codes are all add-on codes in the CPT nomenclature. They are reported separately, in addition to the appropriate code for the E/M service provided. (Refer to Chapter 4 for further discussion of add-on codes.)

Codes **99354** and **99355** are used to report prolonged physician service with direct (face-to-face) patient contact in the office or other outpatient setting.

Code **99354** is used to report the first hour of prolonged service in the office or other outpatient setting. This code may also be used to report a total duration of prolonged service of 30 to 60 minutes on a given date. Prolonged service of less than 30 minutes in total duration on a given date is not reported separately. Less than 30 minutes of prolonged service is included in the E/M code reported for that date.

Code **99355** is used to report each additional 30 minutes beyond the first hour of prolonged services provided in the office or other outpatient setting. This code may also be used to report the final 15 to 30 minutes of prolonged service on a given date.

Prolonged service of less than 15 minutes beyond the first hour or less than 15 minutes beyond the final 30 minutes is not separately reported.

Codes **99356** and **99357** are used to report prolonged physician service with direct (face-to-face) patient contact in the inpatient setting.

Code **99356** is used to report the first hour of prolonged service in the inpatient setting. This code may also be used to report a total duration of prolonged service of 30 to 60 minutes on a given date. Prolonged service of less than 30 minutes in total duration on a given date is not reported separately. Less than 30 minutes of prolonged service is included in the E/M code reported for that date.

Code **99357** is used to report each additional 30 minutes beyond the first hour of prolonged services provided in the inpatient setting. This code may also be used to report the final 15 to 30 minutes of prolonged service on a given date. Prolonged service of less than 15 minutes beyond the first hour or less than 15 minutes beyond the final 30 minutes is not separately reported.

Following is an example of prolonged service with direct (face-to-face) patient contact:

**EXAMPLE:** Mrs Smith, an established patient of Dr Jones, periodically has an acute asthma attack. On the basis of her history, Dr Jones elects to treat her in his office. When Mrs Smith presents with an acute attack, Dr Jones performs an E/M service related to her presenting symptoms. Because Dr Jones knows Mrs Smith well, he does not need to perform the highest level of established patient office visit to treat her acute asthmatic attack. He performs the level of service based on her presenting problem that day. In order to treat the asthmatic attack, Dr Jones and his office staff initiate bronchodilators via an inhaler. Dr Jones evaluates her breath sounds at various intervals to determine the effectiveness of treatment. Once the acute attack is over and Mrs Smith's condition is stable, she is allowed to go home directly from Dr Jones' office rather than being seen in the emergency department. Dr Jones counsels Mrs Smith concerning her condition and the effects of the medication he has prescribed to treat this attack.

Dr Jones reports both the E/M service and the total time he spent face-to-face with the patient beyond the typical time associated with the basic E/M code, excluding the time he was not present during her visit to his office.

Dr Jones would not report the total time Mrs Smith spent in his office; only the time he spent in face-to-face contact with the patient would be included in the prolonged services time reported. These prolonged services include the time when he was not performing the history, physical examination, and medical decision making related to the level of E/M service he reported.

If time is considered the key or controlling factor in choosing the level of E/M service, the prolonged services codes (**99354-99357**) should be used in addition only if the service has exceeded 30 minutes beyond the highest level of E/M in the appropriate category. If the service does not exceed 30 minutes beyond the highest level of E/M, then modifier 21 (Prolonged Evaluation and Management Services) should be appended to the E/M code to indicate the extended service (rather than separately reporting the prolonged services codes). Consider the following example:

**EXAMPLE:** An E/M service for an established patient in the office setting in which counseling and/or coordination of care dominates lasts a total of 90 minutes. Code **99215** is reported for the first 40 minutes and code **99354** for the remaining 50 minutes. However, if the office visit lasts a total of 60 minutes, code **99215** would be reported for the first 40 minutes with modifier 21 appended to reflect the remaining 20 minutes. Modifier 21 is used when the extended service is less than 30 minutes beyond the time indicated in code **99215**. (Read more about the use of modifier 21 in Chapter 10.)

Some categories of E/M codes are not typically reported with codes **99354-99357**, either because no time is associated with the base E/M service and/or the services included in the E/M service already reflect an extensive duration of time and work. The following is an example:

- Hospital Observation Services (**99217-99220**)
- Emergency Department Services (**99281-99285**)
- Observation or Inpatient Care Services (Including Admission and Discharge Services) (**99234-99236**)
- Critical Care Services (**99291-99296**)
- Continuing Intensive Care Services for Infants (**99298-99300**)

## Prolonged Physician Service Without Direct (Face-to-Face) Patient Contact (**99358, 99359**)

Codes **99358** and **99359** are used to report prolonged services without direct (face-to-face) patient contact in either the inpatient or outpatient setting.

The total duration of time spent providing these services on a given date is reported, even if the time spent by the physician on that date is not continuous. Prolonged services of less than 30 minutes in total duration on a given date are not reported.

Both of these codes are considered add-on codes in the CPT code set and are reported separately in addition to the code(s) for other physician services and/or inpatient or outpatient E/M service. Code **99358** is intended to be reported separately in addition to code(s) for other physician service(s) and/or an inpatient or outpatient E/M service. Code **99358** must first be reported in order to report code **99359**.

Code **99358** is used to report the first hour of prolonged service on a given date, regardless of the place of service. This code may also be used to report a total duration of prolonged service of 30 to 60 minutes on a given date. It should be reported only once per patient, per date, even if the time spent by the physician is not continuous on that date.

Code **99359** is used to report each additional 30 minutes beyond the first hour of prolonged physician services, again regardless of the place of service. It may also be used to report the final 15 to 30 minutes of prolonged service on a given date. Prolonged service of less than 15 minutes beyond the first hour or less than 15 minutes beyond the final 30 minutes is not reported separately.

Following are a few additional points to consider:
- Telephone calls (**99371-99373**) should not be reported separately when codes **99358** and **99359** are reported.
- Communication with the family beyond the physician service rendered on a given date may be reported with codes **99358** and **99359**.
- If an additional service is rendered on the same date of service, it may be reported in addition to the prolonged services codes.

Following is an example of prolonged service without direct (face-to-face) patient contact:

**EXAMPLE:** A 16-year-old patient with a long history of clinical depression recently moved from New York to Virginia. The patient had previously been hospitalized at six institutions during a period of 10 years in New York. Before seeing the physician in Virginia, the patient and his family requested that his numerous records be sent from New York to the new physician in Virginia.

The physician in Virginia reviews the extensive records from the patient's prior hospitalizations, as well as the records from the physicians who treated this patient in New York. After reviewing the records, the physician in Virginia calls the last physician who treated the patient in New York to discuss the history and treatment of this patient. The physician in Virginia also calls the patient's father to discuss the current concerns the family expressed when setting up an appointment for their son.

The total time spent reviewing the records and tests as well as the time spent discussing the case is reported if the total time spent by the physician in Virginia exceeded 30 minutes on a given date. Code **99358** and code **99359** would be reported, as appropriate, on the basis of the total time the physician spent providing prolonged physician service without direct (face-to-face) patient contact. If later that day or week the physician provided E/M services (eg, an office or other outpatient visit), these services would be reported in addition to the prolonged services described.

### Physician Standby Services (**99360**)

Code **99360** is used to report physician standby services requiring prolonged physician attendance without direct (face-to-face) patient contact. Physician standby services are provided at the request of another physician.

The physician must be immediately available and/or physically present to provide care to the patient when reporting code **99360** but may not actually provide care. The physician providing the standby services cannot provide care or services to other patients during the period of standby.

This code is not reported by the standby physician if the period of standby ends with his or her performance of a procedure subject to a surgical package. It is also not appropriate to report this code for time spent proctoring another physician.

Code **99360** is used to report a total duration of 30 minutes of physician standby service on a given date. Standby service of less than 30 minutes on a given date is not reported separately. If an additional full 30 minutes of standby service is provided, it is appropriate to report code **99360** for each full 30 minutes of standby service.

The following is an example of standby services:

**EXAMPLE:** Dr Wise has provided all of Mrs White's prenatal care. The plan all along has been for Dr Wise, her family practitioner, to provide the prenatal care, deliver the baby, and provide all of the postpartum care. During her labor, Dr Wise notices decreased fetal heart tones. He requests Dr Kay, an obstetrician, to stand by during the delivery in the event of the need for an emergency cesarean section. Dr Kay provides physician standby services for a total duration of 40 minutes. During that time, Dr Kay provides no care or services to other patients. Mrs White has an otherwise uneventful delivery. Dr Wise delivers the baby without the need for Dr Kay's assistance.

In this example, Dr Kay reports his 40 minutes of standby services with code **99360** (this code will be reported only one time).

## Case Management Services (99363-99368)

As defined by the notes at the beginning of this category of service, physician case management is a process in which a physician is responsible for the following:
- Direct care of a patient
- Coordinating and managing access to health care services needed by the patient
- Initiating and/or supervising other health care services needed by the patient

There are three subcategories of case management services: anticoagulant management, medical team conference, direct (face-to-face) contact with patient and/or family and medical team conference without direct (face-to-face) contact with patient and/or family.

## Anticoagulant Management (99363-99364)

The Anticoagulant Management codes (**99363-99364**) are intended to describe the outpatient management of warfarin therapy, including ordering, review, and interpretation of International Normalized Ratio testing, communication with the patient, and dosage adjustments as appropriate. When reporting these services, the work of anticoagulant management may not be used as a basis for reporting an E/M service or Care Plan Oversight time during the reporting period.

Any period less than 60 continuous outpatient days is not reported. If less than the specified minimum number of services per period are performed, do not report the anticoagulant management services (**99363-99364**).

## Care Plan Oversight Services (99374-99380)

The Care Plan Oversight Services codes are used to report physician supervision of the following:
- A patient under the care of a home health agency (**99374**, **99375**)
- A hospice patient (**99377**, **99378**)
- A nursing facility patient (**99379**, **99380**)

All of the codes are time-based and used to report the complexity and approximate physician time of the care plan oversight services provided within a 30-day period of time. Only one physician may report care plan oversight services for a given period of time to reflect that physician's sole or predominant supervisory role involving regular physician development and/or revision of care plans; review of subsequent reports of patient status; review of related laboratory and other studies; communication (including telephone calls) for purposes of assessment or care decisions with health care professional(s), family member(s), surrogate decision maker(s) (eg, legal guardian), and/or key caregiver(s) involved in patient's care; integration of new information into the medical treatment plan; and/or adjustment of medical therapy, within a calendar month.

## Preventive Medicine Services (99381-99397)

Preventive Medicine Services (**99381-99397**) is a specific category of E/M codes for reporting preventive medicine services. This category of codes includes subcategories for reporting the following:
- Initial preventive medicine E/M service for new patient visits (**99381-99387**)
- Periodic preventive medicine reevaluation and management services for established patient visits (**99391-99397**)
- Preventive medicine counseling for individuals (**99401-99404**) and groups (**99411, 99412**)

The codes in this category of service include the ordering of appropriate immunization(s) and laboratory/diagnostic procedures. The performance of immunizations and ancillary studies involving laboratory, radiology, other procedures, or screening tests identified with a specific CPT code is reported separately.

The codes for initial and periodic preventive medicine E/M services are categorized by patient age. This is mainly because the types of services provided in a preventive visit vary by the age of the patient.

For example, E/M preventive services for a 28-year-old woman may include performing a pelvic examination, obtaining a Pap smear, breast examination, and blood pressure check. Counseling is provided regarding diet and exercise, substance use, and sexual activity.

On the other hand, an E/M preventive service for a 13-year-old girl who is an established patient may include a scoliosis screen; assessment of growth, development, and behavior; and review of immunizations. Anticipatory guidance may be given to the adolescent regarding good health habits and self-care, including problems with drugs, alcohol, and tobacco and other peer pressure issues. Alternatively, guidance may be given about sexual activity and the importance of educational activities and social interaction.

The preventive medicine E/M codes for new and established patients include a comprehensive history and a comprehensive examination. The comprehensive nature of the Preventive Medicine Services codes **99381-99397** reflects an age- and gender-appropriate history/examination and is not synonymous with the comprehensive examination required in E/M codes **99201-99350**.

The comprehensive history obtained as part of the preventive medicine E/M service is not problem-oriented and does not involve a CC or present illness. It does, however, include a comprehensive ROS and comprehensive or interval PFSH, as well as a comprehensive assessment/history of pertinent risk factors.

The comprehensive examination performed as part of the preventive medicine E/M service is multisystem, but the extent of the examination is based on the age of the patient and the risk factors identified.

Let us review the definitions of new and established patient as they apply to reporting preventive medicine services. Remember, a new patient is one who has received no professional services from the physician or another physician of the same specialty who belongs to the same group practice within the past three years.

The initial preventive medicine E/M codes are for reporting services provided to new patients. A common misconception is that the initial preventive medicine E/M service is reported for the first time the patient receives preventive medicine services, even if the patient has received problem-oriented services from that physician or another physician of the same specialty in the same group within the past three years.

Because codes **99381-99387** are used to report preventive medicine services provided to a new patient, these codes should not be reported if a patient received any professional services from this or another physician of the same specialty from the same group practice within the past three years.

**CODING TIP**

When reporting both a preventive medicine E/M service and a problem-oriented E/M service on the same day, pay close attention to the diagnosis codes submitted on the claim. The diagnoses reported should justify the reason for reporting both services on the same day.

**CODING TIP**

For nutrition services performed by a physician, see the E/M or preventive medicine service codes.

The guidelines specifically instruct users regarding how to report situations in which a problem or abnormal finding is encountered and addressed during a preventive services visit. If an abnormality is encountered or a preexisting problem is addressed in the process of performing the preventive medicine E/M service and the problem is significant enough to require additional work for the physician to perform the key components of a problem-oriented E/M service, the appropriate office/outpatient code (**99201-99215**) should be reported in addition to the appropriate code for the preventive E/M service.

The problem or abnormality encountered must require additional work and the performance of the key components of a problem-oriented service in order for the two E/M services to be reported on the same day. If a physician encounters an insignificant or trivial problem/abnormality in the process of performing the preventive medicine E/M service that requires no additional work and the performance of the key components of a problem-oriented service, it would not be appropriate to report the problem-oriented service in addition to the preventive services.

In the event that a problem or abnormality requires additional work and the performance of the key components of a problem-oriented E/M service, modifier 25 should be appended to the office/outpatient code reported. Appending modifier 25 indicates that a significant, separately identifiable E/M service (above and beyond the preventive medicine E/M service) was provided by the same physician on the same day as the preventive medicine service. (Read more about modifier 25 in Chapter 10.)

The codes for new and established patient preventive medicine E/M services (**99381-99397**) include counseling, anticipatory guidance, and risk factor reduction interventions that are provided at the time of the initial or periodic preventive medicine service. Counseling and/or risk factor reduction and behavior change interventions provided at a separate encounter for the purpose of promoting health and preventing illness or injury are reported with codes **99401-99412**.

Codes **99401-99412** are time-based codes. Code selection should be based on the approximate time spent providing counseling and/or risk factor reduction intervention services. Separate codes are available for reporting counseling and/or a risk factor reduction intervention(s) to an individual (**99401-99404**) or to individuals in a group setting (**99411, 99412**).

The preventive medicine counseling codes are not to be used to report counseling and risk factor reduction interventions provided to patients with symptoms or established illness. Counseling of individual patients with symptoms or established illness is reported with the appropriate hospital, office, consultation, or other E/M codes, as appropriate. The appropriate code for counseling groups of patients with symptoms or established illness is code **99078**. This code is located in the Medicine section of the CPT codebook.

The decision tree is provided to assist in determining appropriate reporting of preventive medicine and problem-oriented E/M services provided during the same encounter.

## Decision Tree

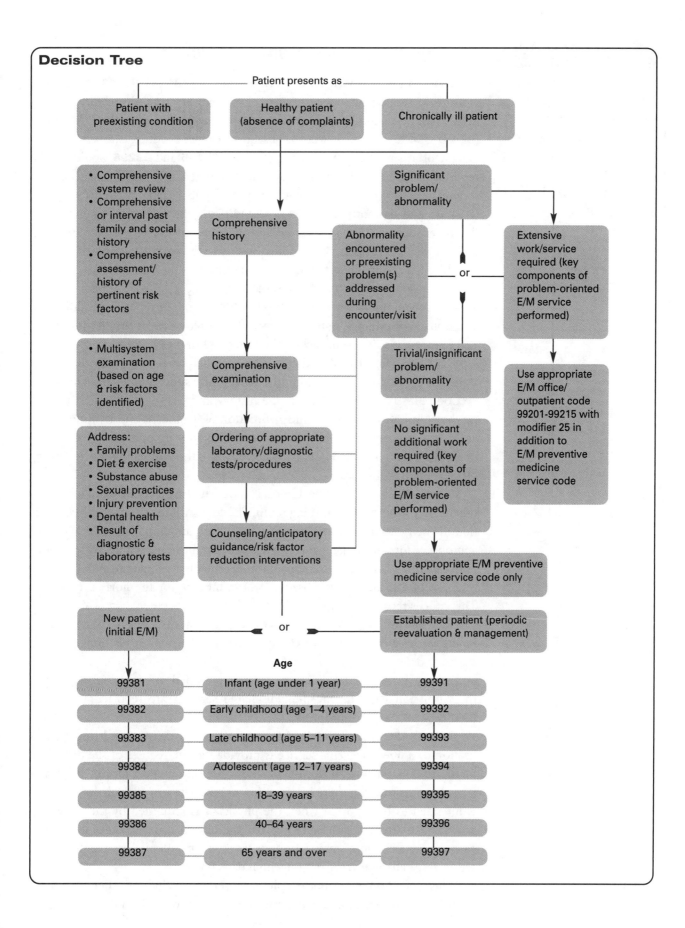

## Newborn Care (Normal) (99431-99440)

The codes in the Newborn Care (Normal) category (**99431-99440**) are used to report E/M services provided to normal (well) newborns in several different settings. If a critical condition is observed in the newborn during the E/M service (**99431-99435**) and the newborn subsequently receives critical care services in or outside of a neonatal critical care unit, codes **99295** and **99296** would also be reported as defined in the critical care subsection of this book. Physician standby services (**99360**), attendance at delivery and initial stabilization of newborn (**99436**), and newborn resuscitation (**99440**) may be used on the same day as the initial (neonatal intensive care unit admission) critical care service (**99295**). If the newborn is transferred to another facility to receive critical care services and the physician accompanies the newborn and manages the care of the patient during the transport, codes **99289** and **99290** should be reported. The pediatric critical care patient transport codes **99289** and **99290** may be reported in addition to the neonatal or pediatric initial (admission) critical care codes (**99293-99296**).

Following is a review of each of the codes within the Newborn Care category service. Note that critical and intensive care newborn and pediatric patient transport services are discussed in the critical care subsection of this chapter.

Code **99431** is used to report the history and examination of the normal newborn infant. This code includes initiation of diagnostic and treatment programs and preparation of hospital records. This code is appropriate for reporting E/M services provided to normal newborns in the hospital setting, including birthing room deliveries.

Code **99432** is used to report normal newborn care that is provided in settings other than the hospital or birthing room. The code includes the physical examination of the newborn and conference(s) with the parent(s). This code would be appropriate for reporting normal newborn care in the home setting. Normal newborn care provided in a freestanding birthing center is also reported with this code.

Code **99433** describes subsequent hospital care for the normal newborn. This code is reported only once per day.

Code **99435** is reported for history and examination of the normal newborn infant who is admitted and discharged from the hospital or birthing room on the same date.

For newborn hospital discharge services provided on a date subsequent to the admission date, the hospital discharge services are reported with code **99238** or **99239**, as appropriate.

Code **99436** is used for reporting attendance at delivery and initial stabilization of a newborn. This service is provided at the request of the delivering physician. The purpose of this physician service is to prepare for the delivery of a newborn who may require intervention or resuscitation after birth. This code is intended to be reported when the physician is requested by the delivering physician to attend the delivery because the newborn may require immediate care (eg, resuscitation, stabilization, or workup for potential problems such as sepsis, respiratory distress, or congenital defects).

When code **99436** is reported, physician services include changing into scrub clothes, hand scrub, obtaining maternal and fetal histories from the obstetrician, review of mother's chart and labor record, review of studies of newborn well-being, preparation of the radiant warmer, adjustment of wall suction, turning on wall oxygen and connecting to the self-inflating resuscitation bag, checking laryngoscope blade and light, and ensuring the availability of medications. Additionally, the physician reviews the medical and technical duties of the newborn resuscitation team that are present.

The physician is present during the birth of the child and provides any necessary assistance required to maintain the health of the child during the birthing process. Once the baby is born, additional physician services include receiving the newborn from the delivering physician, placing the child under the overhead warmer, drying, stimulating, bulb suctioning of the nose and mouth, a visual inspection of the child, obtaining a heart rate and respiratory rate, providing blow-by oxygen or brief application of CPAP as necessary, and assigning one- and five-minute Apgar scores.

The reporting of code **99436** also includes discussion of the care of the child with the obstetrician or delivering physician and parents as well as the completion of the delivery room attendance form and the Apgar scoring sheet.

Code **99436** does not include endotracheal intubation (**31500**) or direct laryngoscopy for aspiration (**31515**). If endotracheal intubation or direct laryngoscopy for aspiration is performed, then it would be appropriate to report these procedures additionally.

If the newborn requires resuscitation as described by code **99440**, then code **99436** would not be reported. In this case, it would be appropriate to report the newborn resuscitation (**99440**) instead of code **99436**.

As indicated in the parenthetical note following code **99436**, it is appropriate to report this code in addition to history and examination of the newborn (**99431** or other level of E/M services as appropriate). Code **99436** specifies that actual pediatric care and services are being provided during the period of attendance and that these services differ from those encompassed in CPT code **99431** for history and examination of a normal newborn or any other postdelivery procedural codes currently within the CPT nomenclature.

Code **99436** includes just the stabilization services rendered immediately after the delivery and a rapid visual assessment of the infant. The initial newborn history and examination in code **99431** (and other E/M categories) is a full history and examination with preparation of hospital records. Therefore, if E/M services are provided in addition to the attendance at delivery and initial stabilization of the newborn, then it would be appropriate to report the E/M services in addition to code **99436**.

Code **99440** describes the performance of newborn resuscitation. This code includes the provision of positive-pressure ventilation and/or chest compressions in a neonate who exhibits inadequate ventilation and/or cardiac output. The only procedures included are suctioning (without intubation to remove mucus, blood, or meconium), assisted ventilation (eg, bag and mask), and/or external cardiac massage (eg, chest compressions). Any other life support measures that are performed are reported separately.

If an intubation to suction meconium is performed at the time of delivery, code **31500** is the appropriate code to report to describe this service. Intubation alone is not considered a resuscitation. Intubation to evaluate for the presence of meconium at or below the vocal cords is not independently considered resuscitation. This should be coded as a distinct procedure.

### Non Face-to-Face Physician Services (99441-99443)

There are three codes within the Non Face-to-Face Physician Services subcategory (**99441-99443**) for reporting telephone calls by a physician. Each code includes examples of the type of service that may be provided when the code is reported.

### Special Evaluation and Management Services (99450-99456)

There are two subcategories of codes within the Special Evaluation and Management Services category of E/M services: (1) Basic Life and/or Disability Evaluation Services (**99450**) and (2) Work-Related or Medical Disability Evaluation Services (**99455, 99456**).

The codes in this category are used to report evaluations performed to establish baseline information before issuing life or disability insurance certificates.

Code **99450** for basic life and/or disability evaluation services includes a medical history as required by the life insurance company, an abbreviated examination consisting of height, weight, and blood pressure as well as collection of specimen samples required for laboratory tests, and the completion of necessary documentation and certificates.

Codes **99455** and **99456** for work-related or medical disability evaluation services include completion of medical history; performance of examination related to work or medical disability including formulation and assessment of diagnosis, stability, and impairment; development of future treatment plans; and completion of necessary documentation/certificates as required by work or medical disability insurance. These codes do not, however, include active management of the patient's condition. Codes **99455** and **99456** should not be used in conjunction with **99080** (special reports), as completion of forms is included (bundled) in codes **99455** and **99456**. These services are separate and distinct from other E/M services. If other E/M services and/or procedures are performed on the same date, the appropriate E/M or procedure code(s) can be reported in addition to the codes in this category. In this case, modifier 25 should be appended to the E/M service, if performed on the same date. (Refer to Chapter 10 for further discussion regarding modifier 25.)

## Procedures Included With E/M Codes

Are procedures included when E/M services are reported? Any procedure specifically identified with a CPT code performed on or subsequent to the date of initial or subsequent E/M services should be reported separately, with the exception of those procedures specifically identified as inclusive within the critical care services and neonatal and pediatric critical care sections of the CPT code set.

As indicated in the introduction of the CPT codebook, "Each procedure or service is identified with a five-digit code." This means that if a specific code number is assigned to a procedure or service, it is not the same as any other service. The reason it was given a separate code number is because the service or procedure represented by that code number is unique.

And what about the actual performance and/or interpretation of diagnostic tests or studies ordered during a patient encounter? Physician performance of H2 diagnostic tests or studies for which specific CPT codes are available may be reported separately, in addition to the appropriate E/M code. Physician interpretation of the results of diagnostic tests or studies may be reported separately with preparation of a separate distinctly identifiable signed written report. When the interpretation of diagnostic tests or studies is reported separately, modifier 26 is appended to the specific code for the diagnostic test or study reported. This will indicate that the professional component of the service is reported separately. (Refer to Chapter 10 for further discussion regarding use of modifier 26.)

Let us further explore the guideline pertaining to reporting the interpretation of diagnostic tests or studies. The key to this CPT guideline is that, for the physician to separately report the interpretation of the results of diagnostic tests or studies, he or she must prepare a separate, distinctly identifiable, signed written report. Physician review of diagnostic test or study results that have already been interpreted by another physician is considered an inherent part of the level of E/M service reported.

As discussed earlier in this chapter, one of the key components of the levels of E/M services is the complexity of medical decision making. *Medical decision making* refers to the complexity of establishing a diagnosis and/or selecting a management option. One of the elements by which the complexity of medical decision making is measured is the amount and/or complexity of medical records, diagnostic tests, and/or other information that must be obtained, reviewed, and analyzed. This review of test or study results would not be reported separately from the E/M service.

One final note: CPT guidelines for reporting procedures or services on the same date as an E/M service do not require different diagnoses to be reported for the E/M service and the procedure. Since the E/M service may be prompted by the symptom or condition for which the procedure or service is provided, different diagnoses are not required. When E/M services provided on the same date as another procedure or service are reported, use of CPT modifiers becomes necessary. Modifier 25 appended to an E/M code indicates that a significant, separately identifiable E/M service was provided by the same physician on the same day of the procedure or other services. Modifier 57 appended to an E/M code designates that the E/M service resulted in the initial decision to perform surgery. (Refer to Chapter 10 for further discussion of these modifiers.)

# Documentation Guidelines

Documentation guidelines are available from CMS that focus primarily on documentation of E/M services from a payer perspective and are a valuable tool for physicians. These guidelines can be found at www.cms.hhs.gov/. Although the

American Medical Association (AMA) was a key contributor in the development of these guidelines, the AMA does not provide clinical advice, nor does it dictate a payer's reimbursement policy.

## Who Can Report E/M Codes?

Again, the AMA does not dictate payers' reimbursement policies; therefore, some payers may allow nonphysicians (eg, psychologists, physical therapists) to report E/M codes. This is a payer policy issue that should be verified with individual payers.

# EXERCISES

**1** Name the three key components in selecting a level of E/M service.

**2** Define *new patient*.

**3** A physician makes a home visit to a 67-year-old established patient with hypertension and peripheral vascular disease. The patient is hemiplegic and has been homebound for two years after a stroke. The physician performs an expanded problem-focused interval history, a problem-focused examination, and straightforward medical decision making.

Identify the appropriate category/subcategory of E/M code(s) and assign the appropriate level of service for this encounter.

**4** A 55-year-old established male patient presents to the physician's office for periodic preventive medicine reevaluation and management. The patient has established diagnoses of hypertension (on beta blocker therapy), type 2 diabetes controlled with sulfonylurea, and chronic stable angina controlled with sublingual nitroglycerin as needed.

A comprehensive history and examination are performed as part of the preventive medicine service. The physician counsels the patient regarding diet, exercise, and injury prevention. Risk factors are identified and interventions discussed. Medically appropriate laboratory tests and diagnostic procedures are ordered. Anticipatory guidance counseling/risk factor reduction interventions are covered to the extent that they have not been covered in previous preventive medicine examinations.

Furthermore, specific history is taken and further examination is performed regarding the established diagnoses listed previously. The physician performs an expanded problem-focused history and examination addressing medication compliance, diet, and stress issues; performs an expanded problem-focused examination including vital signs, chest and heart examination, and checks for edema; and performs medical decision making of low to moderate complexity including counseling about medication and alternatives, a plan for appropriate laboratory work, a review of possible medication side effects, and a plan for ongoing management.

Identify the appropriate category/subcategory of E/M code(s) and assign the appropriate level of E/M code(s) and modifier(s) for this encounter.

**5** At the initial office visit for a new patient, a six-year-old boy with a two-day history of lower abdominal pain with occasional vomiting, a detailed history is obtained including gastrointestinal system, fever, appetite, and characteristics of pain and bowel movements. A detailed examination is performed, including examination of the chest and abdomen and rectal examination. Medical decision making is of low complexity. Ordering of appropriate laboratory studies and initiation of plans for surgical consultation are also performed.

Identify the appropriate category/subcategory of E/M services and assign the appropriate level of E/M code for this encounter.

**6** For several years, Dr Star has been treating Mrs Smith for type 2 diabetes, hypertension, and obesity. Before this appointment, blood work was performed to determine the status of her diabetes. Mrs Smith presents to the office and Dr Star examines her for evidence of infection or circulatory problems. He then asks her about her compliance with the 1200-calorie diet she has been on for the past six months. After reviewing these findings, Dr Star indicates to Mrs Smith that she will have to begin using insulin, since her diabetes is not responding to the current treatment. Mrs Smith begins to sob uncontrollably. She tells Dr Star that this means she is going to die because her grandmother got gangrene from this kind of diabetes and died from it. After calming the patient, Dr Star explains that using insulin is not a death sentence. He discusses diet, insulin administration, and hypoglycemic reactions, as well as the symptoms of hyperglycemia. He instructs Mrs Smith regarding proper foot and skin care and stresses the importance of seeing her ophthalmologist regularly. Mrs Smith is much calmer and feels that she will learn a lot from the booklets that Dr Star has given her to review.

The total time Dr Star spent with Mrs Smith is 25 minutes, with 20 of those minutes spent providing counseling and/or coordination of care. Assign the appropriate E/M code for this encounter.

**7** When reporting a level of E/M service from the Initial Hospital Care subcategory, how many key components must be met or exceeded to qualify for a particular level of service?

**8** True or False: A consultation is a type of service provided by a physician whose opinion or advice regarding evaluation and/or management of a specific problem is requested by another physician or other appropriate source.

**9** True or False: The emergency department services codes are restricted for use by the emergency department physicians.

**10** A five-year-old boy presents to the office with scaly lesions on his right forearm. They have been present for only a week. His father, whom he sometimes visits, has both a cat and a dog.

Within the scenario provided above, identify the following elements of the HPI:

Location:

Duration:

**11** A preterm infant is transported from the facility where he was born by a neonatologist and team from the receiving facility. The physician assumes responsibility for the neonate at the referring hospital, with the transport to the receiving facility neonatal intensive care unit (NICU) taking 1 hour 45 minutes. What code(s) should be reported?

**12**  In the previous scenario, may the neonatologist report the initial NICU code?

**13**  When the physician initiates diagnostic and/or therapeutic services at the time of the "consultative" service, is the encounter still considered a consultation?

**14**  If an anticoagulant management service is provided for a period less than 60 continuous outpatient days, is it appropriate to report codes 99363-99364?

**15**  True or False: If an immunization is administered at the same visit as a preventative medicine service, then it would be appropriate to report the immunization code, the associated administration code, and the preventive medicine service.

**16**  Which codes are used to report a consultation provided in the emergency department?

**17**  If a patient is admitted to the hospital on 10–23 and discharged on 10–26, what is the appropriate E/M code to report for the 10–26 discharge date?

# CHAPTER 4

# Surgery—General Guidelines

In Chapter 2, the placement of a code in the Current Procedural Terminology (CPT®) codebook was discussed. However, because CPT nomenclature is not a strict classification system, there may be some procedures that appear in sections other than those in which they may ordinarily be classified. The physician should select the name of the procedure or service that most accurately identifies the service performed.

When procedures for reporting, reimbursement, or other purposes are evaluated, it is essential that each procedure be considered on its own merits, and not simply based on the location or placement of the code in the CPT codebook. Also, the listing of a service or procedure and its code number in a particular subsection of the Surgery section does not restrict its use to a specific specialty group. Any procedure or service in any section of the CPT codebook or any subsection of service in the Surgery section may be used to report the services and procedures performed by any qualified physician or other qualified health care professional.

This chapter focuses on identifying the general layout of the Surgery section. In addition, the guidelines presented at the beginning of the Surgery section that define items that are necessary to appropriately interpret and report the procedures and services within that section will be reviewed.

## Subsections Within the Surgery Section

The following table provides a numeric listing of the subsections found in the Surgery section of the CPT codebook.

### Surgery Subsections and Code Ranges

| Subsection | Code Range |
|---|---|
| General | 10021-10022 |
| Integumentary System | 10040-19499 |
| Musculoskeletal System | 20000-29999 |
| Respiratory System | 30000-32999 |
| Cardiovascular System | 33010-37799 |
| Hemic and Lymphatic Systems | 38100-38999 |
| Mediastinum and Diaphragm | 39000-39599 |
| Digestive System | 40490-49999 |
| Urinary System | 50010-53899 |
| Male Genital System | 54000-55899 |
| Intersex Surgery | 55970-55980 |
| Female Genital System | 56405-58999 |
| Maternity Care and Delivery | 59000-59899 |
| Endocrine System | 60000-60699 |
| Nervous System | 61000-64999 |
| Eye and Ocular Adnexa | 65091-68899 |
| Auditory System | 69000-69979 |
| Operating Microscope | 69990 |

Coders should familiarize themselves with the subsections of Surgery and their number sequences, and take the time to obtain a general understanding of the layout of the Surgery section of the CPT codebook. As is seen in the Surgery section, there is a common layout within the subsections.

For example, in the Musculoskeletal System subsection, special notes are presented that are unique to this section. The next feature to notice is the anatomical arrangement of this subsection of the CPT codebook. The first heading in the Musculoskeletal System section is General, which precedes the following headings:

Head

Neck (Soft Tissues) and Thorax

Back and Flank

Spine (Vertebral Column)

Abdomen

Shoulder

Humerus (Upper Arm) and Elbow

Forearm and Wrist

Hand and Fingers

Pelvis and Hip Joint

Femur (Thigh Region) and Knee Joint

Leg (Tibia and Fibula) and Ankle Joint

Foot and Toes

Application of Casts and Strapping

Endoscopy/Arthroscopy

There is a "head-to-toe" arrangement of procedures and services in the musculoskeletal system subsection. Then, within each heading there is a consistent theme of the types of procedures or services described. Generally, there are codes to describe procedures involving the following:

Incision

Excision

Introduction or Removal

Repair, Revision, and/or Reconstruction

Fracture and/or Dislocation

Arthrodesis

Manipulation

Amputation

This format is repeated consistently throughout the Musculoskeletal System subsection. It is also apparent in the other Surgery subsections. It is important to take the time to develop an understanding of the general layout of the CPT codebook. This knowledge, used in conjunction with the CPT index, will assist coders in locating the appropriate code(s) for reporting the procedures and services provided.

Now that the general layout of the Surgery section has been described, next is an in-depth look at the Surgery Guidelines.

# CPT Nomenclature Surgical Package Definition

Let us begin by reviewing the definition of the "package" as defined in the CPT nomenclature. This definition can be found in the Surgery Guidelines, as follows:

*The services provided by the physician to any patient by their very nature are variable. The CPT codes that represent a readily identifiable surgical procedure thereby include, on a procedure-by-procedure basis, a variety of services. In defining the specific services "included" in a given CPT surgical code, the following services are always included in addition to the operation per se:*

- *Local infiltration, metacarpal/metatarsal/digital block or topical anesthesia*
- *Subsequent to the decision for surgery, one related E/M (evaluation and management) encounter on the date immediately prior to or on the date of procedure (including history and physical);*
- *Immediate postoperative care, including dictating operative notes; talking with the family and other physicians;*
- *Writing orders;*
- *Evaluating the patient in the postanesthesia recovery area;*
- *Typical postoperative follow-up care.*

This concept is referred to as a "package" for surgical procedures. This CPT definition indicates that when a surgical procedure is reported with a CPT code, the items listed in that guideline are included, if they were performed, and are not reported separately.

Examples of some of these variables include the following:
- The type of procedure performed
- The place where the surgery occurs
- The time (during hospitalization) the surgery is performed
- The insurance contract of each individual patient

Because it is not possible to address all of these variables in a code descriptor, only the preoperative E/M service related to the procedure performed on the date immediately before the date of the procedure (including the history and physical) is stated as inclusive of the CPT surgical package definition.

Also, a specific number of postoperative days are not indicated in the package definition. CPT guidelines provide specific instructions regarding follow-up care for diagnostic and therapeutic surgical procedures. However, these guidelines do not designate a set number of days in which this follow-up care may take place.

Unfortunately, there is no one standard definition of a global surgical package that is universally accepted. Services that are included in a global surgical package may differ for each third-party payer. It is important to become familiar with the reporting and reimbursement policies of the various insurance companies in the your area regarding the global surgical package.

# Follow-up Care

CPT guidelines separately address follow-up care for diagnostic procedures and follow-up care for therapeutic surgical procedures. Although a specific number of days is not described in the CPT guidelines pertaining to follow-up care, most insurance companies recognize a set number of days in which no separate payment will generally be made for services provided by the surgeon. Let us first consider the CPT guidelines for follow-up care for diagnostic procedures.

Follow-up care for diagnostic procedures includes only that care related to recovery from the diagnostic procedure itself. Care for the condition for which the diagnostic procedure was performed or care for other coexisting conditions is not included and may be reported separately. Some examples of diagnostic procedures include endoscopy, arthroscopy, and injection procedures for radiography.

Consider the following scenario:

**EXAMPLE:** A patient undergoes a diagnostic upper gastrointestinal endoscopy for suspected gastric ulcer disease. The findings of the endoscopy are positive for an acute gastric ulcer. At that time, the physician prescribes medication for treatment of the ulcer disease. The patient is instructed to return to the physician's office in one week for follow-up care related to the effectiveness of the medication prescribed.

In this scenario, the follow-up visit is separately reported with the appropriate level of E/M code based on key components that have been met during the encounter. Care for the condition for which the diagnostic procedure was performed or for other concomitant conditions is not included and may be reported separately. (Refer to Chapter 3 for further discussion of E/M coding.)

Now let us review the CPT guidelines for follow-up care for therapeutic surgical procedures.

Follow-up care for therapeutic surgical procedures includes only care that is usually a part of the surgical service. Complications, exacerbations, recurrence, or the presence of other diseases or injuries requiring additional services should be separately reported.

Code **99024**, located in the Medicine section of the CPT codebook, is available for reporting a postoperative follow-up visit for documentation purposes only. This code is useful to the reporting physician for tracking the number of postoperative visits provided that are included in the package for the procedure performed.

# Add-on Codes

Most of the procedures listed in the CPT nomenclature can be reported by themselves because they represent the total procedure that was performed. These codes "stand alone" to describe the total procedure or service. Under certain circumstances, it may be necessary to report two or more stand-alone codes to completely describe the procedures performed.

Some of the codes listed in the CPT code set describe procedures or services that must never be reported as a stand-alone code. These codes are referred to as add-on codes. Add-on codes describe procedures or services that are always performed in addition to the primary procedure or service. They describe additional intraservice work associated with the primary procedure or service.

Intraservice work varies on the basis of the type of service or procedure provided (eg, surgery, E/M services) and the location where the service or procedure is provided (eg, E/M services provided in the office vs hospital setting). For example, the intraservice period for an E/M service provided in the office setting includes the services provided while the practitioner is with the patient and/or family. This includes the time in which the practitioner obtains the history, performs an evaluation, and counsels the patient.

These additional or supplemental procedures are designated as "add-on" codes with a ✚ symbol and are listed in Appendix D of the CPT codebook. Add-on codes can also be readily identified by specific language in the code descriptor, which includes phrases such as "each additional" or "(List separately in addition to primary procedure)."

Modifier 51, Multiple Procedures, is not appended to add-on codes, since these codes are exempt from the multiple procedure concept.

The following criteria were used to identify add-on codes in CPT nomenclature:

- The service or procedure can never serve as a stand-alone code and must be reported in conjunction with another primary service or procedure.
- The service or procedure is commonly carried out in addition to the primary service or procedure performed. If not commonly performed in addition to the primary service or procedure, it is then defined as a stand-alone code; when performed in addition to another procedure, modifier 51 should be appended.
- The service or procedure must be performed by the same physician.
- The add-on code describes additional anatomical sites where the same procedure is performed (eg, reoperation, additional digit[s], lesion[s], neurorrhaphy/neurorrhaphies, vertebral segment[s], tendon[s], and joint[s]).
- The add-on code describes a special circumstance under which a specific service or procedure is performed in conjunction with the primary procedure.
- The add-on code describes an additional segment of time in a time-based code (eg, each additional 30 minutes).

- Add-on codes can be found in sections of the CPT codebook other than the Surgery section. Following are some examples in which add-on codes are used and specific codes describing the example.

## Additional Lesion(s)

**11100** Biopsy of skin, subcutaneous tissue and/or mucous membrane (including simple closure), unless otherwise listed (separate procedure); single lesion

**✚11101** each separate/additional lesion (List separately in addition to code for primary procedure)

(Use **11101** in conjunction with code **11100**)

Code **11100** is the primary procedure and code **11101** is the add-on code. Code **11101** would never be reported without first reporting code **11100**. As the code descriptor indicates, code **11101** is reported for each separate or additional lesion. The parenthetical note following code **11101** instructs the user regarding the code that is considered the primary procedure for that particular add-on code.

If biopsy is performed on three separate lesions of the skin, subcutaneous tissue, and/or mucous membrane, then code **11100** would be reported for the first lesion and code **11101** would be reported twice, once for the second lesion biopsied and again for the third lesion biopsied.

## Neurorrhaphy/Neurorrhaphies

**64831** Suture of digital nerve, hand or foot; one nerve

**✚64832** each additional digital nerve (List separately in addition to code for primary procedure)

(Use **64832** in conjunction with code **64831**)

Code **64831** is the primary procedure and code **64832** is the add-on code. Code **64832** would never be reported without first reporting code **64831**. As the code descriptor indicates, code **64832** is reported for each additional digital nerve that is sutured. The parenthetical note following code **64832** instructs the user regarding the code that is considered the primary procedure for that particular add-on code.

If two digital nerves of the hand and one digital nerve of the foot are sutured, then code **64831** would be reported for the first digital nerve sutured and code **64832** would be reported twice, once for the second digital nerve of the hand and again for the suture of the digital nerve of the foot.

## Joint(s)

**26860**    Arthrodesis, interphalangeal joint, with or without internal fixation;

**+26861**        each additional interphalangeal joint (List separately in addition to code for primary procedure)

        (Use **26861** in conjunction with code **26860**)

Code **26860** is the primary procedure and code **26861** is the add-on code. Code **26861** would never be reported without first reporting code **26860**. As the code descriptor indicates, code **26861** is reported for each additional interphalangeal joint that is fused (arthrodesis). The parenthetical note following code **26861** instructs the user regarding the code that is considered the primary procedure for that particular add-on code.

If arthrodesis of two interphalangeal joints is performed, then code **26860** would be reported for the first arthrodesis and code **26861** would be reported one time for the arthrodesis of the additional interphalangeal joint.

## Additional Time

**99291**    Critical care, evaluation and management of the critically ill or critically injured patient; first 30-74 minutes

**+99292**        each additional 30 minutes (List separately in addition to code for primary service)

        (Use **99292** in conjunction with **99291**)

Code **99291** is the primary service—used for reporting the first 30 to 74 minutes of critical care services. Code **99292** is the add-on code—used for reporting each additional 30 minutes of critical care service provided beyond the first 30 to 74 minutes. Code **99292** would never be reported to represent services provided to a particular patient without code **99291** being reported first. The parenthetical note following code **99292** instructs the user regarding the specific code that is considered the primary service when code **99292** is reported.

If the physician provides critical care services to a patient for a total duration of two hours on a given date, then code **99291** is reported for the first 30 to 74 minutes of service and code **99292** is reported twice, once for each additional 30 minutes of critical care services provided.

# Other CPT Codes Exempt from Modifier 51 (Appendix E)

The codes that appear in Appendix E are exempt from the use of modifier 51 but have not been designated as CPT add-on codes. These codes are identified throughout the text of the CPT codebook with a symbol ⊘ placed before the code.

The codes listed in Appendix E do not meet the criteria previously discussed to be designated as add-on codes. However, because of special circumstances, these codes are reported without appending modifier 51.

Before the implementation of the resource-based relative value scale (RBRVS), Medicare carriers automatically reduced the payment for secondary procedures. Since the implementation of the RBRVS, which uses work values, and the use of modifier 51 is specifically defined in the CPT nomenclature, the modifier 51-exempt codes (Appendixes D and E) do not require the use of the modifier to signal a payment reduction, as the work values for these services have already been reduced.

## Separate Procedure

Some of the codes listed in the CPT nomenclature have been identified by inclusion of the term *separate procedure* in the code descriptor. The separate procedure designation indicates that a certain procedure or service may be
- considered an integral component of another procedure or service,
- performed independently,
- unrelated,
- distinct from other procedure(s) or service(s) provided at that time.

Codes designated as separate procedures may not be additionally reported when the procedure or service is performed as an integral component of another procedure or service.

The following is an example of an integral component:

**58720**    Salpingo-oophorectomy, complete or partial, unilateral or bilateral (separate procedure)

**58150**    Total abdominal hysterectomy (corpus and cervix), with or without removal of tube(s), with or without removal of ovary(s)

When a total abdominal hysterectomy with removal of the tube(s) and ovary(s) is reported, it would not be appropriate to separately report code **58720** in conjunction with code **58150**. The procedure described by code **58720** is considered an integral component of the procedures described by code **58150**.

However, codes designated as separate procedures should be additionally reported when performed independently, unrelated, or distinct from other procedure(s) or service(s) provided.

The following is an example of a procedure performed independently:

**58720**    Salpingo-oophorectomy, complete or partial, unilateral or bilateral (separate procedure)

If removal of the fallopian tubes and ovaries is the only procedure performed, then it would be appropriate to report code **58720** to describe the procedure performed.

The following is an example of unrelated procedures:

**56605**   Biopsy of vulva or perineum (separate procedure); one lesion

**49505**   Repair initial inguinal hernia, age 5 years or older; reducible

Biopsy of the vulva or perineum is a procedure that is unrelated to repair of an inguinal hernia. In this example, if the same physician performed both of these procedures, then it would be appropriate to report both codes to fully describe the procedures performed. Modifier 59 would be appended to code **56605** to indicate that the biopsy was unrelated to the repair of the inguinal hernia. (Refer to Chapter 10 for further discussion of modifier 59.)

The following illustrates coding for a procedure that is distinct from another procedure or service:

**28110**   Ostectomy, partial excision, fifth metatarsal head (bunionette) (separate procedure)

**28292**   Correction, hallux valgus (bunion), with or without sesamoidectomy; Keller, McBride, or Mayo type procedure

Code **28292** describes correction of a bunion of the first metatarsophalangeal joint (big toe). Code **28110** describes partial excision of the bone of the fifth metatarsal head. In this example, code **28110** is considered a distinct and separate procedure from code **28292**. Therefore, it would be appropriate to report both codes to completely describe the procedures performed. Modifier 59 would be appended to code **28110** when these procedures are reported to indicate that a distinct procedure was performed.

When a procedure or service that is designated as a separate procedure is carried out independently or considered to be unrelated or distinct from other procedures or services provided at that time, the procedure or service designated as a separate procedure may be reported by itself or in addition to other procedures or services by appending modifier 59 to the specific separate procedure code reported. This indicates that the procedure is not considered a component of another procedure, but is a distinct, independent procedure. This may represent the following:
- Different session or patient encounter
- Different site or organ system
- Separate incision or excision
- Separate lesion
- Treatment of a separate injury (or area of injury in extensive injuries)

Modifier 59 is discussed in greater detail in Chapter 10.

# Endoscopic/Laparoscopic/Arthroscopic vs Open Procedures

The advent of endoscopes introduced a new method of exploration and treatment of conditions and diseases that had previously been viewed or treated through an open surgical incision. Many endoscopy procedure codes have been added to several systems in the CPT nomenclature over the years (eg, digestive system, female genital system, musculoskeletal system, respiratory system). There are also some codes for endoscopically assisted procedures.

In *CPT 2000*, the Laparoscopy/Hysteroscopy section of codes was deleted. All of these codes were renumbered and placed throughout the Surgery section of the CPT codebook within the appropriate anatomic subsection.

General guidelines for reporting endoscopic procedures are as follows:

1 Look up endoscopy/laparoscopy in the index and locate the organ/system being examined or treated by means of a scope.

2 Look at the codes in that system/organ section to find an endoscopy/laparoscopy heading.

3 If there is no endoscopy/laparoscopy heading in that section, look for a code with a descriptor that includes a suffix "-oscopy" and describes the procedure performed.

4 If there is no heading of endoscopy/laparoscopy or there is no specific code describing the use of an endoscope in its descriptor, the codes described in that section are open surgical procedures and should not be used to report a procedure using an endoscopic approach.

5 Clarify with the physician that the procedure was performed with an endoscope/laparoscope/arthroscope.

6 If it is determined that there is no specific code for the endoscopic/laparoscopic procedure, the unlisted procedure laparoscopy/endoscopy/arthroscopy code should be used to report the procedure. In this case, a copy of the operative report should be submitted to the insurance company when the claim is filed. (Refer to Chapter 2 for further discussion of unlisted codes.)

# Materials Supplied by the Physician

Supplies and materials provided by the physician (eg, sterile trays/drugs) over and above those usually included with procedures rendered are listed separately. The guideline indicates that the coder should list the drugs, trays, supplies, and materials provided by reporting code **99070** or the specific supply code.

CPT code **99070** is used to report supplies provided by the physician over and above those usually included with the services rendered. This code could be used to report, for example, a drug, special dressings used to pack a wound, wound irrigation equipment, or a pair of crutches.

CPT coding guidelines do not include listings of codes or procedures for which it is appropriate to separately report supply items (eg, surgical trays). Reimbursement of supplies and materials provided by the physician may vary from carrier to carrier.

# EXERCISES

1 True or False: The CPT nomenclature's definition of the global surgical package includes one related E/M encounter on the date immediately prior to or on the date of the procedure (including history and physical).

2 Which Category I CPT code is used to report a postoperative follow-up visit for documentation purposes only?

3 Define the CPT surgical package based on CPT guidelines.

4 What symbol is used to identify add-on codes in CPT nomenclature?

5 Supplies and materials provided by the physician over and above those usually included with the other service(s) rendered are reported separately by using which CPT code(s)?

6 True or False: The multiple procedure modifier (modifier 51) is not appended to an add-on code.

7 True or False: Category I, II, and III CPT add-on codes must never be reported as stand-alone codes.

8 List the appropriate Category I CPT code(s) for reporting suture of two digital nerves of the hand.

9 Assign the appropriate Category I CPT code(s) for the following procedure: diagnostic esophagoscopy with biopsy.

10 True or False: When using an add-on code, the service or procedure must be performed by the same physician.

11 True or False: Codes are placed in the CPT codebook based on use by specific specialty groups.

12 True or False: Codes designated as separate procedures may be additionally reported when the procedure or service is performed as an integral component of another procedure or service.

13 True or False: CPT includes listings of codes for supply items.

# CHAPTER 5

# Surgery

In Chapter 4, the general guidelines for reporting the codes in the Surgery section of the Current Procedural Terminology (CPT®) codebook are discussed. This chapter takes a closer look at some of the guidelines that are unique to the reporting of codes from specific subsections within the Surgery section.

The subsections within the Surgery section that are addressed in this chapter include the following:

- Integumentary System
- Musculoskeletal System
- Respiratory System
- Cardiovascular System
- Digestive System
- Urinary System
- Female Genital System
- Maternity Care and Delivery
- Eye and Ocular Adnexa
- Nervous System
- Auditory System

It is imperative that the coder responsible for reviewing the medical record and assigning CPT codes have a good understanding of the physician's practice and a solid understanding of how to use CPT codes and modifiers. In addition, it is essential that coders have a thorough understanding of medical terminology and anatomy to code accurately.

At the beginning of each section that follows, anatomy illustrations are provided. These illustrations serve as a quick anatomy reference to assist with understanding of the coding procedures under discussion. They are not intended as a replacement for an anatomy text and up-to-date medical dictionary, which are essential tools for accurate coding.

Before beginning this review of the specific subsections, let us first review some basic tips for coding surgical procedures described in an operative report.

# How to Code From an Operative Report

There is no quick way to code an operative report. One must read and reread the report to be sure the coding reflects all of the procedures and diagnoses contained in the report. To code only the preoperative diagnosis, postoperative diagnosis, and operation performed as listed at the beginning of the operative report would be incorrect. Additional procedures/diagnoses may be identified in the body of the operative report that are not indicated in the information provided at the top of the form. Coding directly from the text of the operative report will ensure that the coding reflects the procedures actually performed, as well as the diagnoses related to the procedures.

It is essential to communicate with the surgeon whenever there is a question about a procedure or the diagnosis related to it. It may also be necessary to refer to other portions of the patient's chart, such as the pathology report or history and physical examination, to correctly code the diagnosis for which a procedure was performed. For example, the pathology report will indicate whether a lesion that was removed was benign or malignant. Be sure to follow official *International Classification of Diseases, Ninth Revision, Clinical Modification (ICD-9-CM)* coding guidelines for coding and reporting when assigning diagnosis codes. Official guidelines for coding and reporting ICD-9-CM are available from the central office on ICD-9-CM at the American Hospital Association (telephone number 312 422-3000).

The following tips are offered to help with coding of the surgical procedures described in an operative report:

1 Look at the top of the operative report where it indicates the operation/procedures performed. When reading through the operative report, take note of the procedures that are described. Sometimes additional procedures may be coded; sometimes the procedures listed at the top of the operative report were not performed. Report only those services that are documented in the operative report. If there is a discrepancy, ask the physician to review the coding to ensure that it is accurate.

2 Make sure to be familiar with the terminology used throughout the operative report. Use a medical dictionary to learn the meaning of unfamiliar terms. For example, there is a big difference in meaning between *arthrectomy* and *atherectomy*. Major errors in coding can occur if one is unfamiliar with the terminology. Do not make an assumption about the meaning of terms.

3 Look in the index of the CPT codebook to locate the type of procedure that was performed.

4 If none of the CPT codes in a specific section identify the procedure performed, go back to the index to see if it refers to another series of codes. If, however, a code cannot be located that specifically identifies the procedure performed in the correct anatomy area related to the procedure that was performed, review the CPT modifiers to see if the procedure code needs to be modified. (Refer to Chapter 10 for further discussion of the use of CPT modifiers.)

5 Read the parenthetical notes in the section of codes being reviewed, as well as the guidelines for that section, to see what is included/excluded in that range of codes. If the parenthetical statements and guidelines are not helpful, ask the physician who performed the procedure to review the range of codes believed to be those most closely associated with the procedure. Two or more codes may need to be reported. If there is no procedure code or procedure code with a modifier that accurately describes the procedure performed, go to the end of that section of codes and report the unlisted procedure code. The service or procedure should be described when reported to third-party payers. (Refer to Chapter 2 for further discussion of unlisted procedure codes.)

6 Code only the procedures in the operative report verified in step 1. If, in discussion with the physician, he or she indicates that additional procedures were performed that are not reflected in the operative report, ask the physician to dictate an addendum to the operative report describing the performance of the additional procedures.

7 Once it has been determined which CPT code(s) to report for each surgical procedure performed, reread the operative note and isolate the diagnosis from the operative report. Look first at the preoperative diagnosis and then at the postoperative diagnosis at the top of the operative report. Reread the

entire report to see if there are additional findings to report that are not included in the preoperative and postoperative diagnosis listed. Be sure to follow official guidelines for coding and reporting ICD-9-CM.

Now that tips to help code from an operative report have been discussed, let us review and code an operative report by following the steps just outlined. Refer to the operative report on pages 129 and 130.

Looking at the top of the operative report where it indicates the operation performed, the following procedures are indicated by the physician:

- Exploratory laparotomy
- Sigmoid colon resection
- End-colostomy and creation of Hartmann pouch
- Appendectomy

The index of the CPT codebook is used to locate the type of procedure that was performed. In this case, an exploratory laparotomy, sigmoid colon resection, and appendectomy, are the major procedures. "Exploration, abdomen" directs you to **49000**, **49002**.

When referring to these codes, **49000** is shown to be a separate procedure. (Refer to the discussion of the *separate procedure* designation found in Chapter 4.) Since an open procedure such as the colon procedure may not be performed without a laparotomy, the exploratory laparotomy is considered an integral component of the colon surgery performed. The exploratory laparotomy is not reported in this case.

Code **49002** indicates that a previous recent laparotomy was performed. No prior laparotomy was performed, so this code is not selected. Even though the procedure "exploratory laparotomy" is listed in the "operation performed" section of the operative report, a separate code is not used to report this procedure, as it is part of another operative procedure.

The term *resection* in the index contains no entries for sigmoid or colon. In the medical dictionary, the term *resection* is defined as "excision." Excision of the colon is what was performed. The entry for "excision, colon" in the index lists three headings: partial; partial with anastomosis; and total. Codes **44140-44160** are the group of codes that should be referred to before codes are chosen to report the sigmoid colon resection.

The CPT codebook uses the term *colectomy*. This is defined as "excision of a portion of the colon (partial), or of the whole colon (complete or total)." Since this patient only had a part of the colon removed, the codes **44141-44147** are the ones that require further study. Each of these codes needs to be reviewed to see which one correctly matches the procedure described in the operative report.

Code **44140** indicates that a colectomy was done with anastomosis. *Anastomosis* is defined as "the joining together of two hollow organs or of two or more arteries or veins." In the operative report being discussed, the ends of the bowel that remained after the "mass" was removed were not joined together. The portion of the bowel connected to the rectum (the distal rectal stump) was tied off. A colostomy was created from the other portion of the bowel. Since there was no anastomosis, code **44140** is not the correct code to use to report the colectomy performed in this operative report.

Code **44141** indicates that a skin-level colostomy or cecostomy was performed after the colectomy. If an opening was made into the cecum, closing it around a tube that was brought out through the abdominal wall, it would be called a *tube cecostomy*. If the wall of the cecum was actually sutured to the skin, it would become a *cutaneous cecostomy*. In this operative report, a tube cecostomy or skin-level colostomy was not performed.

Code **44143** indicates that an end-colostomy and closure of distal segment (Hartmann-type procedure) was performed. This code represents what is described in this specific operative report. In the Hartmann procedure (operation), a portion of the sigmoid colon is resected, the distal end closed, and the proximal end brought out as an end-colostomy. In the procedure described in this operative report, the diseased sigmoid colon was removed without reanastomosis of the cut ends of the proximal colon and rectum.

In CPT code **44144**, creation of a mucofistula is described. An ostomy performed to prevent the passage of bowel contents to a more distal site is called a *diverting ostomy*. This is constructed by dividing the intestine so that bowel contents exit through the proximal end; nothing enters the distal end, which is now called a *mucous fistula*. For example, to allow a serious injury of the rectum to heal, a diverting sigmoid colostomy may be constructed to protect the healing rectum from the fecal contents. However, in this specific operative report, a mucofistula was not created.

Code **44145** indicates that a partial colectomy with coloproctostomy (low pelvic anastomosis) was performed. A coloproctostomy is an anastomosis between the colon and the rectum. As discussed previously, no anastomosis was performed. This code does not include creation of a colostomy; the operative report indicates that a colostomy was performed.

Code **44146** includes the components of **44145** and also includes a colostomy. Although a colostomy is included in this code, no anastomosis of bowel is recorded in the operative report, so this is not the correct code to report.

Code **44147** indicates that the approach used to perform the colectomy was abdominal and transrectal. (*Trans-* is a prefix denoting [1] through, across, or [2] to the other side.) In this operative report, the approach did not pass through or across the rectum. Also, code **44147** does not include a colostomy, which was performed in this operative report.

By examining all of the codes in the **44140-44147** series, code **44143** is selected as the code that describes the colectomy in this operative report. All of the other codes do not represent the type of colectomy with colostomy that was performed.

To code the appendectomy, the term *appendectomy* is checked in the index. Codes **44950-44960** are listed under this index entry. These three codes are reviewed, and code **44955** is selected, since the disease being treated involved the appendix and an appendectomy was required at the time of another major procedure. Note that code **44955** is an add-on code and cannot be reported alone. This code is to be reported separately, in addition to the code for the primary procedure. (Refer to Chapter 4 for further discussion of add-on codes.)

Thus, in this case, there are two codes that specify the procedures performed in this operative report (**44143** and **44955**).

**PT NAME:**

**ADM DATE:**

**DR NAME:**

**PREOPERATIVE DIAGNOSIS:**  Sigmoid colon obstruction

**POSTOPERATIVE DIAGNOSIS:**  Sigmoid colon obstruction with perisigmoid and pelvic abscess, and adherent appendix

**OPERATION PERFORMED:**  *Exploratory laparotomy*, sigmoid colon resection, end-colostomy and creation of *Hartmann pouch*, appendectomy

**DATE OF OPERATION:**

**SURGEON:**

**ANESTHESIOLOGIST:**

**ANESTHESIA:**  General endotracheal

**COMPLICATIONS:**  None

**OPERATIVE FINDINGS:** This patient had a long history of sigmoid colon stricture. She presented to the hospital several days prior to surgery with abdominal pain, and on studies had a nearly obstructing sigmoid stricture and pus in the colon. She was brought to the operating room to undergo a sigmoid resection and potential primary anastomosis, and was prepared for such a procedure with the usual bowel prep. On exploration, there was a large mass in the pelvis that appeared to be *diverticular*. On further exploration, there was free pus in an abscess cavity between the bladder and the sigmoid colon, adhesions were present, and the sigmoid was stuck down to the rectum. In addition, the mass involved the tip of the appendix, necessitating appendectomy. The *proximal* sigmoid and *distal* rectum were normal to palpation, as was the rest of the colon, and further exploration revealed the liver to be normal with no gallstones in the gallbladder and no lesions in the colon.

**OPERATIVE PROCEDURE:** After satisfactory induction of general endotracheal anesthesia, the patient was prepped and draped in the *lithotomy* position in the event that a stapling device would be needed for anastomosis. A long midline incision was made from the *pubic symphysis* to midway between the *xiphisternum* and the umbilicus. This was carried down to the anterior midline *fascia*, which was then divided, and the abdomen was entered. Exploration was carried out, which revealed the findings as noted previously. *Dissection* was begun to free the mass from the bladder with both *sharp* and *blunt* dissection. In the process of doing this, the abscess cavity was entered and cultures were taken and sent for analysis. With both blunt and sharp dissection, the mass was carefully encircled *anterolaterally*. The ureters were identified on both sides and followed completely down into the pelvis, and both of these were preserved carefully throughout the operation.

After the mass was freed completely on the anterolateral sides, a site was chosen on the *proximal sigmoid* for *transection*, and the *mesentery* was then taken down between clamps and ties of 3-0 Vicryl. After sufficient mesentery was divided, the GIA stapling device was used to divide the proximal sigmoid colon. In this fashion it was possible to retract the sigmoid in a *caudad* direction, allowing the posterior dissection of the mass from the sacrum. Some bleeding occurred, which was controlled with a combination of Bovie cautery and suture ligature when needed. With continued blunt and sharp dissection, the mass was finally freed from the attachments to the pelvic walls *posteriorly*, and the mass was isolated below where normal rectum was found. The rectum was then divided by means of a reticulator GIA stapling device, and the specimen was clamped on the proximal side and the colon divided at this level. The distal rectal stump was tied with 2-0 Prolene sutures and clips on the end of these for further identification. Bleeding was controlled in the pelvic area with Bovie cautery, and copious irrigation was performed. In the process of freeing the mass, it was necessary to separate the appendix from the mass, which was actually intimately adherent and could not be separated without injuring the appendiceal lumen. Therefore, appendectomy was performed by first dividing the mesoappendix between clamps and 3-0 Vicryl ties down at the base of the appendix. A purse-string of 3-0 silk suture was then placed in the cecum, and the appendix was crushed and tied with a 2-0 chromic tie. The stump was inverted and this purse-string tied. After this, the abdominal cavity was once again washed and checked for hemostasis, which was adequate. The *omentum* was then removed from the mid–transverse colon for a short distance and then divided to allow a segment of omentum to be placed in the pelvis near the site of the rectal stump. This was placed lateral to the side of the colostomy. At this point, the site for the *colostomy* was chosen, a button of skin was removed, the anterior and posterior fascia was divided in a vertical fashion, and the rectus muscle was spread. The sigmoid colon was then delivered through this opening, after further distance was attained by freeing the mesentery as required to allow it to reach the skin without tension. As mentioned before, this was passed *medial* to the omentum that was placed into the pelvis. After the end-colostomy was delivered through the opening, it was left in place and the wound closed with interrupted #1 Vicryl stitches in the midline fascia. Several interrupted vertical mattress sutures of 4-0 nylon were placed around the umbilicus, and the rest of the wound was left open and packed with Betadine-soaked gauze. The staple line on the colon was then removed and the colostomy matured with interrupted stitches of 4-0 chromic. A colostomy appliance was placed and the wound was cleaned, dried, and dressed sterilely. The patient tolerated the procedure well without any apparent complications. Sponge and needle counts were correct. She was taken to the recovery room in stable condition.

---

(Signature of Surgeon)

Date of Operation:

# I. Integumentary System

Since the Integumentary System section includes procedures for the whole body, it is important to pay attention to the code descriptor to ensure that the appropriate code is chosen for not only the procedure but also the correct anatomic area.

An understanding of CPT Basics outlined in Chapter 2 and Surgery Guidelines outlined in Chapter 4 is essential, as the Integumentary System section applies many of these basics (eg, indented codes and add-on codes). A thorough understanding of these procedures will help you use the codes in this section.

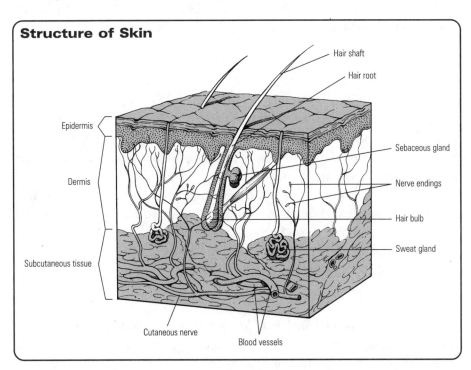

**Structure of Skin**

Hair shaft
Hair root
Epidermis
Sebaceous gland
Dermis
Nerve endings
Hair bulb
Sweat gland
Subcutaneous tissue
Cutaneous nerve
Blood vessels

The skin is the body's largest organ system, about 2500 to 3000 square inches in most adults. It is made up of two main layers: the epidermis, the thinner outer layer, and the dermis, the thicker inner layer. Below the dermis is subcutaneous tissue or superficial fascia. The integumentary system also contains the accessory organs of hair, nails, and several types of glands, including sebaceous, sweat (eccrine), and ceruminous (apocrine).

It is important to be familiar with the structure of the skin and medical terms associated with the skin. Use the CPT codebook in tandem with a medical dictionary to define unfamiliar words. An effort to understand these terms and their meanings early in the development of coding skills will serve the coder well.

## General

### Fine Needle Aspiration

Fine needle aspiration is reported with the codes from the **10021** series. A fine needle aspiration is performed when fluid or tissue is aspirated with a long, slender needle and the cells are examined cytologically. This is in contrast to a biopsy, in which a small piece of tissue is taken and examined for histologic architecture.

**CODING TIP**

An incision must be performed for an incision and drainage procedure to be reported so as to differentiate between an incision and drainage procedure and an aspiration procedure.

**CODING TIP**

Read operative reports carefully to accurately distinguish between a fine needle aspiration and a percutaneous needle biopsy.

The fine needle aspiration codes are not anatomy-specific. That is, any time a fine needle aspiration is performed anywhere in the body, regardless of the type of cells that are aspirated, one of these two codes is used. The distinguishing feature between the fine needle aspiration codes is imaging guidance. When a fine needle aspiration is performed without imaging guidance, code **10021** is reported. When imaging guidance is necessary for needle placement and the aspiration is performed, code **10022** is selected. If imaging guidance is performed, the codes for radiologic supervision and interpretation (S&I) are also reported. Codes **10021** and **10022** both include the preparation of smears, if smears are prepared. A cross-reference in the CPT codebook directs the coder to appropriate radiology codes (**76492**, **77002**, **77012**, **77021**). (Refer to Chapter 7 for further discussion of radiologic guidance.)

### Incision and Drainage

There are eight incision and drainage (I&D) codes in the Integumentary System section of the CPT codebook (**10060-10140**, **10180**). Many of these I&D procedures include one code for simple procedures and one code for complicated procedures; however, the terms *simple* and *complicated* are not defined in the CPT codebook. Rather, the choice of code is at the physician's discretion, based on the level of difficulty involved in the incision and drainage procedure. It is important to note that code **10060** should be reported for a simple or single I&D procedure and code **10061** should be reported for a complicated or multiple I&D procedure. Therefore, if a simple I&D procedure is performed on multiple lesions, the appropriate code is **10061**.

### Debridement

*Debridement* is defined by *Stedman's Medical Dictionary, 27th Edition*, as "excision of devitalized tissue and foreign matter from a wound." The debridement codes in the CPT code set are intended to be used for debridement procedures performed by surgical techniques chosen at the discretion of the physician. When a physician performs debridement, he or she intends to remove all foreign/dead material, reduce the number of bacteria in the wound, and leave intact the viable tissue. Debridement is performed to reduce the potential for complications that can jeopardize limb survival and become life threatening (eg, sepsis, embolism, gas gangrene, hemorrhage).

Debridement or repeated debridement procedures may be required depending on the extent of the skin injury, the degree of contusion and soft tissue crush, the fracture severity, the amount of dead and foreign material in the wound(s), and the amount of hemorrhage, swelling, and direct or indirect involvement of surrounding neurovascular ligamentous and tendinous structures. To describe the various types of debridement procedures, the CPT code set includes three sets of debridement codes.

The first set of debridement codes is specific to debridement of extensive eczematous or infected skin. Codes **11000** and **11001** may be reported for debridement of this type of skin on the basis of the percentage of the body surface debrided. Code **11000** is used for debridement of up to 10% of the body surface. Code **11001** is reported for each additional 10% of the body surface or fraction thereof. This means that debridement of a full 10% of the body area does not have to be additionally performed to report code **11001**. Rather, code **11001** can be reported for any fraction of 10% of body surface that is additionally debrided.

**EXAMPLE:** 11% of the body surface is debrided. This would be coded as:
> **11000** for the first 10%
> **11001** for the second 10% or fraction thereof

The second set of debridement codes is for reporting extensive tissue debridement for necrotizing soft tissue infection (eg, Fournier's gangrene). Codes **11004-11006** describe debridement procedures for specific areas that receive treatment. Add-on code **11008** describes removal of prosthetic material or mesh performed concurrently with the debridement procedures identified with codes **11004-11006**. Code **11008** should not be reported in conjunction with the other debridement procedure codes (**11000** and **11001, 11010-11044**).

The third set of debridement codes represents more extensive debridement procedures. Codes **11010-11012** describe services provided in preparation for treating an open or closed fracture (eg, to address the debridement of injuries sustained from blunt or penetrating trauma, motor vehicle accidents, or sports and recreational activity accidents). These three codes address fracture debridement procedures, not the type of fractures involved. They are intended to describe treatment of a number of injuries that require extensive preparation to adequately repair a wound site including both open and closed fractures and usually involve numerous layers of soft tissue and bone. Often, more than one injury (and more than one injury type) exists that requires multiple debridement procedures.

Codes **11010-11012** incorporate a number of procedures and can be staged and coded multiple times to indicate separate sites of fracture debridement or a separate service. Included as part of the services are prolonged cleansing of the contaminated site, removal of all foreign/dead material from the wound site, and irrigation of all tissue layers and exploration of the soft tissue injured (including neurovascular, ligamentous, and tendinous structures). The reason for performing these procedures is to leave viable tissue that may or may not be subsequently closed and to reduce the hemorrhaging and swelling usually associated with these types of wounds.

Although the descriptors of codes **11010-11012** state that the codes are for debridement associated with open fractures, codes **11010-11012** may be reported in cases in which debridement is necessary to treat a fracture site when no open fracture is present. For example, in a traumatic fracture injury, the skin is damaged extensively, causing massive involvement of the surrounding soft tissues, and requires significant debridement; however, the wound is not involved down to the fracture. An open fracture is typically defined as a fracture in which a wound, through the adjacent or overlying soft tissue, communicates with the site of the break; the fracture in this circumstance is not classified with the ICD-9-CM diagnosis code for open fracture. However, in this circumstance, it would be appropriate to report the relevant code from **11010-11012** to describe the debridement performed, as long as a fracture is present in the same area as the soft tissue injury.

For debridement procedures other than those described in codes **11000** and **11001** and **11010-11012**, the fourth set of debridement codes (**11040-11044**) would be reported. Examples of the use of these codes include stasis ulcers, superficial infected wounds, avascular necrotic tissue, and gangrene. As with codes **11010-11012**, codes **11040-11044** may be used more than one time for a single patient encounter when multiple sites are debrided. For each site, select the appropriate code on the basis of the intensity of the wound and append modifier 59 to the secondary code(s). These codes should not be reported in addition to codes **97597**, **97598**, and **97602** for active wound management. (See Chapter 9 for description of active wound management.) Note the following example:

**EXAMPLE:** Debridement is performed on wounds on the arm and leg. The debridement on the arm involves the skin and subcutaneous tissue, whereas the debridement on the leg involves not only skin and subcutaneous tissue but also muscle. For this example, code **11042 59** would be reported for the debridement of the arm and code **11043** would be reported for debridement of the leg.

## Paring or Cutting

Paring and cutting of benign hyperkeratotic lesions such as corns or calluses are reported with codes **11055-11057**. Notice that only one code from this series is reported for the total number of lesions that are pared or cut. Multiple codes should not be reported to equal the number of lesions, as these codes are not cumulative and are not designated as add-on codes. For example, if paring of three lesions is performed, only code **11056** (two to four lesions) is reported. It would not be appropriate to report both **11055** and **11056** for the paring of these three lesions, as code **11056** includes all lesions up to and including four.

## Biopsy

Codes **11100** and **11101** are general codes for biopsy of skin, subcutaneous tissue, and/or mucous membrane. It is important to note that these codes include simple closure when such closures are performed. Code **11100** is reported for biopsy of a single lesion. Code **11101** is an add-on code reported for each separate/additional lesion that is biopsied.

The guidelines clarify that obtaining the tissue for pathology during the course of certain surgical procedures in the integumentary system such as excision, destruction, or shave removals is a routine component of such procedures and is not considered a separate biopsy procedure and not separately reported. The biopsy procedure code (eg, **11100**, **11101**) should be reported for obtaining tissue for pathologic examination when performed independently or if unrelated or distinct from other procedures/services provided at that time. Such biopsies are not considered components of other procedures when performed on different lesions or different sites on the same date and should be reported separately.

As indicated in the CPT codebook, the user should select the code that most accurately identifies the service performed; codes **11100** and **11101** should be reported only if a more specific code of the anatomic area that is biopsied does not exist. However, if a code exists that describes both the biopsy and the anatomic area, that code should be selected. Be sure to check the index and other surgery sections corresponding to the biopsy area for additional biopsy codes. For example, biopsy of an eyelid involving lid margin, tarsus, and/or palpebral conjunctiva should be reported with code **67810** rather than **11100**.

## Removal of Skin Tags

Removal of skin tags by scissoring or any sharp method, ligature strangulation, electrosurgical destruction, or combination of treatment modalities including chemical or electrocauterization of wound is reported with codes **11200** and **11201**. These codes are reported for removal of skin tags from any area of the body.

Code **11200** is reported for the removal of skin tags up to and including 15 tags. Code **11201** is an add-on code to be reported for each additional 10 lesions removed.

### Shaving of Epidermal or Dermal Lesions

The CPT codebook defines *shaving* as the sharp removal by transverse incision or horizontal slicing to remove epidermal or dermal lesions without a full-thickness dermal excision. Epidermis is the thinner outer layer of the skin, and dermis is the thicker inner layer. Shaving is a procedure that involves slicing to remove the lesions, and it is reserved for those lesions at the upper layers of the skin—the epidermis and dermis.

Since the technique of shaving involves transverse incision or horizontal slicing, there is no need for suture closure. However, as stated in the guidelines, local anesthesia and any chemical cauterization or electrocauterization of the wound is included.

Codes **11300-11313** are reported on the basis of the anatomic area and the size of the lesion. When choosing a code, the first step is to pick the appropriate group of codes that includes the anatomic area where the lesion is located. For example, codes **11305-11308** are for lesions located on the scalp, neck, hands, feet, and genitalia. Next, the size of the lesion is chosen on the basis of the lesion diameter.

For example, a lesion on the leg measuring 1.0 cm in diameter is removed by shave technique. Because the lesion is located on the leg and has a diameter of 1.0 cm, code **11301** would be reported.

Each lesion shaved should be reported with a separate code, as the descriptors of codes **11300-11313** state *single lesion*. If more than one lesion is shaved, modifier 59 should be appended to the second and any subsequent codes to indicate a separate lesion(s).

> **CODING TIP**
>
> If a dermal or epidermal lesion is removed by shave technique, choose the appropriate code based on the anatomic site and size of the lesion from the **11300-11313** series.

## Nails

The nail is made up of structures such as the nail bed, nail plate, and matrix. The CPT codebook includes many procedures from excisions to avulsions of specific portions of the nail. It is essential to become familiar with these terms to assign the appropriate code for the procedure performed.

The most common nail procedures performed in many physician offices involve the trimming or debridement of nails. Code **11719** is used for trimming of nondystrophic nails. Code **11719** should be reported only once per visit, as the code descriptor states it is for any number of nails.

Codes **11720** and **11721** are for debridement of nails. Dystrophic changes are typically progressive and may result from defective nutrition of a tissue or organ. Code **11720** is reported for debridement of one to five nails, and code **11721** is for debridement of six or more nails. Only one code should be reported from **11720** and **11721** to describe the number of nails debrided, as code **11721** is not designated as an add-on code. For example, if eight nails are debrided, only code **11721** would be reported. It would not be appropriate to report codes **11720** and **11721**, as code **11721** includes nails up to six and any nails over six.

## Intralesional Injections

Lesions, such as keloids, psoriasis, acne (cystic or nodular), and others, may be treated by injecting drugs directly into the lesion itself. To report intralesional treatment, use codes **11900** and **11901**.

Code **11900** may be used when one to seven lesions are injected. Note that the code describes the number of lesions treated, not the number of injections. The code should be reported once when one to seven lesions are treated, even if a particular lesion is injected more than once.

When treating eight or more lesions, code **11901** should be reported only once to indicate the treatment of eight or more lesions. Do not use code **11901** in addition to code **11900**, as **11901** is not an add-on code. Again, the number of injections into a particular lesion is not a factor in code selection.

In addition, codes **11900** and **11901** should not be used for preoperative local anesthetic injection.

## Lesions

The CPT codebook includes several codes that describe the various techniques used to remove lesions. Codes for shaving of lesions, excision of lesions, and destruction of lesions can be found throughout the Integumentary System section. To correctly code the removal of lesions, start by choosing the group of codes that describes the technique used by the physician. (Refer to the flow chart on page 138 for Lesion Excision/Destruction.)

### Excision of Lesions

*Review of Benign and Malignant Lesion Guidelines*
The guidelines for excision of benign lesions state the following:

> Excision (including simple closure) of benign lesions of skin (eg, neoplasm, cicatricial, fibrous, inflammatory, congenital, cystic lesions) includes local anesthesia. See appropriate size and body area below. For shave removal, see **11300** et seq, and for electrosurgical and other methods, see **17000** et seq. Excision is defined as full-thickness (through the dermis) removal of a lesion, including margins, and

**CODING TIP**

For excision of benign lesions requiring more than simple closure, ie, requiring intermediate or complex closure, report **11400-11446** in addition to the appropriate intermediate (**12031-12057**) or complex (**13100-13153**) closure codes. For reconstructive closure, see **15002-15261** and **15570-15770**.

includes simple (non-layered) closure when performed. Report separately each benign lesion excised. Code selection is determined by measuring the greatest clinical diameter of the apparent lesion plus that
margin required for complete excision (lesion diameter plus the most
narrow margins required equals the excised diameter). The margins
refer to the narrowest margin required to adequately excise the lesion,
based on the physician's judgment. The measurement of lesion plus
margin is made prior to excision. The excised diameter is the same
whether the surgical defect is repaired in a linear fashion or reconstructed (eg, with a skin graft). The closure of defects created by
incision, excision, or trauma may require intermediate or complex
closure. Repair by intermediate or complex closure should be reported
separately. For excision of benign lesions requiring more than
simple closure, ie, requiring intermediate or complex closure, report
**11400-11446** in addition to appropriate intermediate (**12031-12057**)
or complex closure (**13100-13153**) codes. For reconstructive closure,
see **14000-14300, 15002-15261, 15570-15770**. See page 144 for
definition of intermediate or complex closure.

The guidelines for excision of malignant lesions state the following:

Excision (including simple closure) of malignant lesions of skin (eg,
basal cell carcinoma, squamous cell carcinoma, melanoma) includes
local anesthesia. See appropriate size and body area below. For destruction of malignant lesions of skin, see destruction codes **17260-17286**.
Excision is defined as full-thickness (through the dermis) removal of a
lesion including margins, and includes simple (non-layered) closure
when performed. Report separately each malignant lesion excised. Code
selection is determined by measuring the greatest clinical diameter of
the apparent lesion plus that margin required for complete excision
(lesion diameter plus the most narrow margins required equals the
excised diameter). The margins refer to the narrowest margin required
to adequately excise the lesion, based on the physician's judgment.

The measurement of lesion plus margin is made prior to excision. The
excised diameter is the same whether the surgical defect is repaired in a linear
fashion or reconstructed (eg, with a skin graft). The closure of defects created by
incision, excision, or trauma may require intermediate or complex closure.
Repair by intermediate or complex closure should be reported separately. For
excision of malignant lesions requiring more than simple closure, ie, requiring
intermediate or complex closure, report **11600-11646** in addition to appropriate intermediate (**12031-12057**) or complex closure (**13100-13153**) codes.
For reconstructive closure, see **14000-14300, 15002-15261, 15570-15770**.
See page 144 for definition of intermediate or complex closure. When frozen
section pathology shows that the margins of excision were not adequate, an
additional excision may be necessary for complete tumor removal. Use only one
code to report the additional excision and re-excision(s) based on the final

**CODING TIP**

For excision of malignant
lesions requiring more than
simple closure, ie, requiring
intermediate or complex closure, report **11600-11646**
in addition to appropriate intermediate (**13100-13153**)
closure codes. For reconstructive closure, see **14000-
14300, 15002-15261**,
and **15570-15770**.

widest excised diameter required for complete tumor removal at the same operative session. To report a re-excision procedure performed to widen margins at a subsequent operative session, see codes **11600-11646**, as appropriate. Append modifier 58 if the re-excision procedure is performed during the postoperative period of the primary excision procedure.

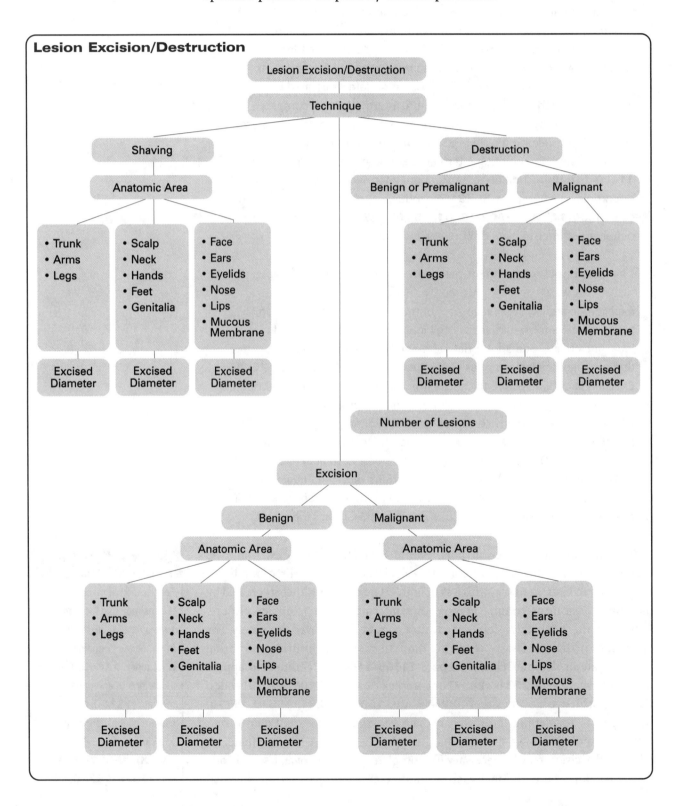

The codes for benign and malignant lesion excision are reported on the basis of the anatomic area and the size of the lesion. To properly code an excision of a lesion, the location of the lesion and size of the excised diameter must be documented.

When choosing a code, the first step is to pick the appropriate group of codes that includes the anatomic area where the lesion is located.

Next, the size of the lesion is determined by measuring the greatest clinical diameter of the apparent lesion plus that margin required for complete excision (lesion diameter plus the most narrow margins required equals the excised diameter). The *margins* refer to the narrowest margin required to adequately excise the lesion, based on the physician's judgment. The measurement of lesion plus margin is made prior to excision.

For example, if a benign lesion of the trunk measures 1.0 cm and the margin required to adequately excise the lesion includes 0.2 cm on both sides for a total margin of 0.4 cm, add 1.0 cm + 0.2 cm + 0.2 cm = 1.4 cm to determine the excised diameter. The appropriate group of codes would be **11400-11406**, because these are for benign lesions located on the trunk, arms, or legs. In this case, code **11402** should be reported to reflect the measurement of the benign lesion and necessary margins excised from the trunk. If the lesion is asymmetric or irregular, the maximum diameter is used to measure the lesion. The excised diameter is the same whether the surgical defect is repaired in a linear fashion or reconstructed (eg, with a skin graft). The physician should make an accurate measurement of the lesion at the time of the excision, and the size of the lesion should be documented in the operative report. A pathology report is less likely to contain an accurate measurement because of shrinkage or fragmentation of the specimen.

If more than one lesion is excised, report each lesion excised separately. For example, a malignant lesion with an excised diameter of 1.5 cm is excised from the left arm and another malignant lesion with an excised diameter of 2.0 cm is excised from the right arm. The appropriate method of reporting would be with code **11602** reported two times. Modifier 59 should be appended to the second code to indicate that a distinct procedure was performed on a different anatomic site.

The coding of the repair (closure) would follow the same guidelines as stated previously. Simple closure is included in excision of lesion(s); whereas intermediate or complex closure would be reported separately in addition to the excision code(s).

A common misconception is that multiple lesion excisions are added together and reported as one excision of lesion code, rather than reporting each lesion excision separately. The adding together of the lengths and reporting as a single item refers to the repair (closure) codes: if multiple wounds are repaired within the same classification, the lengths are added and the sum is reported as a single item.

## Measuring and Coding the Removal of a Lesion

Example: excision, malignant lesion of the back, 1.0 centimeters. Code 11606

margin
(2.0 cm)

1.0 cm
melanoma

Excised diameter
(lesion plus margins):
1.0 cm + 4.0 cm = 5.0 cm

margin
(2.0 cm)

Example: excision of benign lesion of the neck, 1.0 centimeter by 2.0 centimeters.
Code 11423.

margin (0.2 cm)

2.0 cm x 1.0 cm
benign lesion

Excised diameter
(lesion plus margins):
2.0 cm + 0.4 cm = 2.4 cm

margin (0.2 cm)

Example: excision, malignant lesion of the nose, 0.9 centimeters with skin margins of
0.6 centimeters. Code 11642.

Excised diameter
(lesion plus margins):
0.9 cm + 0.6 cm = 1.5 cm

margin (0.3 cm)

margin (0.3 cm)

0.9 cm malignant
lesion

*Lesions of Uncertain Morphology*

When excising a neoplasm of uncertain morphology (eg, melanoma or dysplastic nevus), the choice of the correct code is based on the final excised diameter as determined by the physician's judgment of the margins required for adequate excision. Generally, when excising lesions of uncertain behavior, larger margins may be required compared to clearly benign lesions that may require minimal margins. Excision of an ambiguous or moderately suspicious lesion with wider margins of surrounding grossly normal skin/soft tissue that subsequently pathology confirms was not malignant is appropriately reported using the excision of benign lesion codes **11400-11446**. Code selection is determined by measuring the greatest clinical diameter of the lesion plus the wider margins, which results in reporting the specific code that reflects the skill, time, and effort in treating such clinically uncertain lesions. If pathology confirms the presence of malignancy, codes **11600-11646** should be used to report the service. The operative report should document the clinical lesion size and margins, or the excised diameter.

Therefore, to ensure correct coding, a neoplasm that is yet to be definitely identified should be coded after the pathology report is received. When received, the CPT code for benign excision or malignant excision that best describes the procedure as performed and documented should be chosen.

### Coding Lesion Excision with Extended Margins

If a lesion is excised and during the same operative session the margins are extended after a positive pathologic diagnosis is made, then one excision of lesion code would be reported on the basis of the final widest excised diameter of the lesion that was removed.

### Coding Two Lesions Removed with One Excision

If two lesions are removed with one excision, only one excision of lesion code would be reported.

For example, if two benign skin lesions measuring 0.5 cm each are removed with one excision, then only one excision of lesion code would be reported. Since only one excision was performed, it would not be appropriate to report two separate excision of lesion codes. The excision of lesion code should accurately reflect the maximum excised diameter of the two lesions that were excised.

For example, two 0.5-cm facial lesions located 1 cm apart are excised through one excision. The maximum excised diameter is 0.5 cm + 1.0 cm + 0.5 cm = 2 cm. The code reported would be **11442**.

### Re-excision of Lesions

When a malignant lesion is excised and the patient returns for a re-excision for positive margins, the re-excision is reported as a malignant lesion, even though the pathology report may indicate that the re-excision reveals "no residual tumor."

As stated in the guidelines, when an additional excision is necessary for complete tumor removal and is performed during the same surgical session, only one code is used to report the additional excision and re-excision(s) based on the widest excised diameter required for complete tumor removal at the same operative session. Modifier 58 should be appended if the re-excision procedure is performed during the postoperative period of the primary excision procedure. Modifier 59 should be appended if the procedure is performed at a separate session on the same day of surgery.

For example, a patient had a 1.5 cm malignant lesion excised from his leg at a previous operative session. Subsequently, during the postoperative period, residual tumor was noted at the margin of the original excision and the margins were re-excised. The re-excision included a 1.0 cm excised diameter. In this example, code **11601 58** should be reported.

### Destruction of Lesions

*Destruction* is defined in the CPT codebook as the ablation of benign, premalignant, or malignant tissues by any method, with or without curettement, including local anesthesia, and not usually requiring closure.

"Any method" in these codes includes electrosurgery, cryosurgery, laser, and chemical treatment.

Types of lesions included in these codes are condylomata, papillomata, molluscum contagiosum, herpetic lesions, warts (ie, common, plantar, flat), milia, or other benign, premalignant (eg, actinic keratoses), or malignant lesions.

#### Premalignant Lesions

The first three codes in the destruction series are **17000**, **17003**, and **17004**. These three codes are used for destruction of premalignant lesions, for example, actinic keratoses by any of the described methods. Destruction of skin tags is reported with code[s] **11200** and **11201**; destruction of benign cutaneous vascular proliferative lesions is reported with codes **17106-17108**. Since plantar warts are not considered to be of premalignant nature, the parenthetical reference following code **17003** instructs users to report codes **17110** and **17111** for the destruction of these types of lesions. If codes exist in the CPT codebook for destruction of premalignant lesions in specific anatomic sites, then those specific codes should be used rather than **17000-17004**. If there is no code specific to the anatomic area where the premalignant lesion is located, then codes **17000**, **17003**, and **17004** should be used.

Code **17000** is reported for destruction of the first lesion. Code **17003** is an add-on code that is reported for destruction of each lesion from the second through the fourteenth. Code **17003** would be reported with code **17000** when up to 14 lesions are reported.

> **EXAMPLE:** Four actinic keratoses lesions on the face are destroyed by laser. Code **17000** would be reported for the first premalignant lesion and **17003** would be reported three times or with a 3 in the units column for the second through the fourth premalignant lesions. Remember that modifier 51 would not be appended to code **17003** as it is an add-on code.

Code **17004** is reported for destruction of 15 or more premalignant lesions. This code should not be reported in addition to codes **17000** and **17003**, as it encompasses all lesions up to and over 15. This code is a modifier 51 exempt code.

#### Benign Cutaneous Vascular Proliferative Lesions

Codes **17106-17108** are specific to destruction of benign cutaneous vascular proliferative lesions; for example, port wine stains. Unlike codes **17000-17004**, which are reported on the basis of the number of lesions, codes **17106-17108** are reported on the basis of square centimeters. When these codes are reported, only one code would be reported for the total square centimeters of the area treated. For example, if the treated area is 45 square centimeters, only code **17107** would be reported.

Very small vascular proliferative lesions may be treated by destruction techniques. Some coders have questioned whether modifier 52 for reduced services should be reported when lesions of a few millimeters in size are treated. Since the descriptor for code **17106** includes the phrase "less than 10 square centimeters," the use of modifier 52 is not necessary. The use of codes **17106-17108** is not appropriate for treatment of lesions such as telangiectasia, cherry angioma, verruca vulgaris, and telangiectasia associated with rosacea or psoriasis.

### Benign Lesions

Destruction of benign lesions other than skin tags or cutaneous vascular proliferative lesions is reported with codes **17110** and **17111**. These codes are reported for the destruction of common or plantar warts. Only one code from this series should be reported for the total number of lesions destroyed. For destruction of up to 14 lesions, only code **17110** should be reported. For 15 or more lesions, only code **17111** should be reported, as this code includes anything up to and more than 15 lesions.

### Malignant Lesions

The destruction of malignant lesions is reported with codes **17260-17286**. Similar to the excision of lesion codes, these codes are reported on the basis of the anatomic area of the lesion and the lesion diameter. Codes **17260-17286** are reported for each lesion destroyed and include any method of destruction as previously described.

## Repair

The repair of wounds may be classified as simple, intermediate, or complex. The complete definitions of simple, intermediate, and complex repairs can be found in the Repair guidelines.

The codes in the Repair section are used to designate wound closure utilizing sutures, staples, or tissue adhesives (eg, 2-cyanoacrylate), either singly or in combination with each other or in combination with adhesive strips. Wound closure utilizing adhesive strips as the sole repair material should be coded by means of the appropriate evaluation and management (E/M) code.

If during a single operative session more than one method of repair is used (eg, staples, sutures, and/or tissue adhesive), only one code is selected according to the classification of the repair performed, the size of the repair, and the location of the repair. The method of the repair plays a factor only if adhesive strips are used.

### Simple Repair

The simple repair codes are used for one-layer closure. Simple repair/closure is included when the excision of a benign or malignant lesion is reported and is not separately reported.

For example, a physician excises a 0.4-cm benign lesion on the skin of the arm with simple closure. To report this service, report only the code for the excised lesion, **11400**, as simple closure is included in the excision of the lesion.

### Intermediate Repair

Intermediate repair requires layered closure of one or more of the deeper layers of subcutaneous tissue and superficial (nonmuscle) fascia, in addition to the skin (epidermal or dermal) closure. Look at the diagram of the skin layers to see what structures are involved. The intermediate repair codes are also used for single-layer closure of heavily contaminated wounds that have required extensive cleaning or removal of particulate matter.

If a lesion is excised and intermediate closure is performed, report two codes, one code for the excision of lesion and the appropriate intermediate repair code (**12031-12057**).

For example, a physician excises a benign 2-cm lesion on the skin of the face and performs a 4-cm intermediate closure. Report the excision of lesion code (**11442**) in addition to the code for the intermediate closure of a wound as follows:

**12052**     for the intermediate repair, 2.6-5.0 cm

**11442 51**     for the excision of the facial lesion, 1.1-2.0 cm

Again, as the excision of lesion codes include only simple repair, the intermediate repair code would be reported in addition to the CPT code for the excision of lesion. In this instance, append modifier 51 to indicate that multiple procedures were performed. The primary procedure would be reported as listed, and the additional procedure is reported with modifier 51.

### Complex Repair

The complex repair codes include repair of wounds requiring more than one layered closure, scar revision, debridement (eg, traumatic lacerations or avulsions), extensive undermining, stents, or retention sutures. Necessary preparation includes creation of a defect for repairs. Complex repair does not include excision of benign (**11400-11446**) or malignant (**11600-11646**) lesions.

### Adding the Length of Repairs

Unlike the lesion excision codes, the repair codes are reported on the basis of the sum of lengths of repairs. When multiple wounds are repaired, the lengths of those wounds in the same classification (eg, simple, intermediate, and complex) and from all anatomic sites that are grouped together into the same code descriptor should be added together and reported as a single item.

For example, in the following scenario, the lengths of intermediate closures on the eyelid and face would be added together.

**EXAMPLE:** A patient has two benign lesions removed (one from the forehead and one from the cheek, each 1 cm in diameter) that require intermediate closure, with the length of one closure site being 4 cm and the other 6 cm. The lengths of these closures are added (4 cm + 6 cm = 10 cm), as the wound repair is within the same classification (intermediate) and the anatomic sites are grouped in the same code descriptor (codes **12051-12057**). In this instance, three codes are used—one for the total intermediate repair and two for the lesion excision:

**12054**

**11441 51**

**11441 59**

Do not add lengths of repairs from different groupings of anatomic sites (eg, face and extremities).

Do not add lengths of repairs from different classifications (eg, intermediate and complex repairs).

### More Guidelines on Reporting Repair (Closure) Codes
Determine whether the wound repair is simple, intermediate, or complex. The repair of the wound should be measured and recorded in centimeters, whether curved, angular, or stellate.

Debridement is reported separately only when gross contamination requires prolonged cleansing, when appreciable amounts of devitalized or contaminated tissue are removed, or when debridement is carried out separately without immediate primary closure.

The Repair (Closure) section in the CPT codebook should be referred to for the complete guidelines on reporting repairs (closures) of wounds.

## Adjacent Tissue Transfer or Rearrangement

Adjacent tissue transfer or rearrangement procedures (local flaps) are described by codes **14000-14350**. Note that these codes are for the "Excision (including lesion) and/or repair by adjacent tissue transfer or re-arrangement (eg, Z-plasty, W-plasty, V-Y plasty, rotation flap, advancement flap, double pedicle flap)." In other words, the excision of the lesion, whether it is benign or malignant, is included with codes **14000-14350** and should not be reported separately.

For example, a physician excises a 1.5-cm lesion on the cheek and performs an adjacent tissue transfer (4-sq cm defect). In this instance, only code **14040**, Adjacent tissue transfer or rearrangement, forehead, cheeks, chin, mouth, neck, axillae, genitalia, hands and/or feet; defect 10 sq cm or less, would be reported, as the excision of the lesion is included in the adjacent tissue transfer codes.

These guidelines give examples of adjacent tissue transfers and rearrangements such as Z-plasty and W-plasty. In these types of rearrangements, the repair of the defect is in the shape of the letters *Z* and *W*. To ensure that these codes are used appropriately, the guidelines point out that when lacerations are repaired, the procedures listed must be developed by the surgeon to accomplish the repair. For example, the surgeon plans on repairing the defect with a Z-plasty. If direct closure or rearrangement of traumatic wounds incidentally results in a configuration such as a *Z* or *W*, these codes should not be used.

As with many of the codes in the Integumentary System section, codes **14000-14350** are reported on the basis of the anatomic area and size. However, notice that the size refers to the defect, not the lesion size, as is seen in most other codes in this section of the CPT codebook. The term *defect* includes the primary and secondary defects. The primary defect, resulting from the excision, and the secondary defect, resulting from flap design to perform the reconstruction, are measured together to determine the code.

In addition, often the tissue transfer or rearrangement procedure creates an additional defect that must be coded. If a skin graft or another flap is necessary to close a secondary defect, this should be reported separately.

For example, a 5-cm benign lesion is excised from the neck and a transposition flap is used to close the 25-sq cm defect. The flap donor site is partially closed, but there is a remaining 10-sq cm defect, which requires a split-thickness skin graft:

**14041**     Adjacent tissue transfer

**15120 51**     Split-thickness autograft

The lesion excision is included in the adjacent tissue transfer code and is not coded separately. The skin graft necessary to close the flap donor site is coded in addition to the flap.

## Skin Replacement Surgery and Skin Substitutes

Procedures for harvesting of the graft, caring for the donor site, application of skin grafts, skin replacements, and skin substitutes by location and incremental units are reported with codes **15002-15431**.

The introductory language of the Skin Replacement Surgery and Skin Substitutes section specifies that the codes in this section are not intended to be reported for simple graft application alone or application stabilized with dressings (for example, by simple gauze wrap). The skin substitute or graft is anchored by the surgeon's choice of fixation to clarify the level of effort required to report these codes. Further language clarifies that supply of the skin substitute or graft should be reported separately, whereas routine dressing supplies should not be reported separately.

Definitions are as follows:
- **Skin replacement:** A tissue or graft that permanently replaces lost skin with healthy skin.
- **Skin substitute:** A biomaterial, engineered tissue, or combination of materials and cells or tissues that can be substituted for skin autograft or allograft in a clinical procedure.
- **Temporary wound closure:** Not the final resurfacing material but provides closure of the wound surface until the skin surface can be permanently replaced.

Skin grafts differ by their origin and, for autografts, by their anatomic source. Skin grafts, by origin, are as follows:
- **Autograft:** Tissue transplanted from one part of the body to another in the same patient.
- **Allograft (homograft):** Tissue transplanted from one individual to another of the same species.
- **Xenograft (heterograft):** Tissue transplanted from one species to an unlike species (eg, non-human, baboon to human).

An autograft is a skin portion removed from one site (donor site) of the patient's skin and placed on another site (recipient site) on the patient. Specifically, the skin removed and grafted originates from the patient and is therefore genetically identical. The purpose of the autograft is to replace the skin that was damaged or removed. The autograft can be of various thicknesses, shapes, and sizes. The configuration the graft takes depends on the nature of the defect. The range of codes used to report various autografts is **15100-15157, 15200-15261**. In some cases, the skin used for autografting may be a smaller skin portion that is cultured or grown in vitro to provide more graft material identical to the recipient site, which are tissue cultured autografts (reported with codes **15150-15157**). These codes are reported on the basis of the size and location of the recipient area. The size and location of the recipient site determines the correct code. Measurement in square centimeters is applicable to adults and children aged 10 and older whereas percentages of body area apply to infants and children younger than the age of 10.

Codes **15002-15005** describe burn and wound preparation or incisional or excisional release of scar contracture resulting in open wound requiring a skin graft. These codes are reported for the surgical preparation of the recipient sites of the trunk, arms and legs (**15002** and **15003**), face, scalp, eyelids, mouth, neck, ears, orbits, genitalia, hands, feet, and or/multiple digits (**15004** and **15005**). These codes are reported on the basis of surface area of 100 square centimeters applicable to adults and children aged 10 and older. The percentages of body surface apply to infants and children younger than the age of 10.

Codes **15002** and **15004** are stand-alone codes, reported for the first 100 square centimeters or 1% of body area of infants and children. Codes **15003** and **15005** are add-on codes reported for each additional 100 square centimeters or each additional 1% of body area of infants and children. Code **15003** would not be reported without first reporting code **15002**. The same principle applies to code **15005**, which would not be reported without code **15004**. Modifier 51 is not used with codes **15003** and **15005**. (Refer to Chapter 4 for further discussion of add-on codes.)

**EXAMPLE:** An excision of a burn wound on the trunk of an adult involving 130 sq cm would be reported with code **15002** for the first 100 sq cm. Code **15003** would be reported for the additional 30 sq cm, as this code includes excision of open wounds beyond the initial 100 sq cm up to and including the additional 100 sq cm.

Code **15040** is used for reporting the harvesting of skin for tissue-cultured skin autografts.

Code **15050** describes a pinch graft and is generally used to identify a relocated small portion of skin (a "pinch" of skin). The donor tissue is obtained by surgical excision from a different area. The tissue is then placed in the recipient site. As indicated in the code descriptor, this code would be used only once, regardless of the number of pinch grafts performed to cover a defect that measures 2 cm or less.

Codes **15100**, **15101**, **15120**, and **15121** are used for split thickness grafts. Split thickness grafts contain both the epidermal and dermal layers. Split thickness grafts are composed of epidermis and a portion of the underlying dermis.

Full-thickness skin grafts are described in codes **15200-15261**. Full-thickness grafts include epidermis, dermis, and, before trimming, usually some subcutaneous tissue.

Additional codes **15170-15176** are available for reporting acellular dermal replacements, which are also reported in the same way as the autografts, based on the size and location of the recipient area. The size and location of the recipient site determines the correct code. Measurement in square centimeters is applicable to adults and children aged 10 and older, whereas percentages of body area apply to infants and children younger than the age of 10.

Codes **15300-15366** are reported for the application of allografts and tissue-cultured allogeneic skin substitutes. Allografts are skin portions obtained from someone other than the patient receiving the graft (from a genetically different person). These grafts are not the final resurfacing material but provide a covering for the vulnerable surface until a more suitable graft material can be obtained. The purpose of the allograft is to protect the exposed recipient site from infection and to maintain overall viability of the underlying sensitive tissue for future transplant of an appropriate graft. Usually these types of free skin grafts are used when autograft material is not available because of extenuating circumstances, such as extensive burns. In these cases, the allograft may be placed until new skin can be cultured or obtained from an area capable of donating the needed skin at a later time. Allografts can be stored by means of refrigeration until they are needed. Codes **15330-15336** are specific for reporting acellular dermal allografts, and codes **15340-15366** are specific for reporting tissue cultured allogeneic skin/dermal substitutes.

Codes **15340** and **15341** are used to report tissue-cultured allogeneic skin substitutes used in smaller recipient sites for application in 25-sq cm increments. Modifier 58 may be used to delineate prospectively planned tissue-cultured allogeneic skin substitute procedures. It is important to note that the exclusionary parenthetical instruction following code **15341** precludes reporting **15340** and **15341** with the site preparation codes **15002-15005** and the debridement codes **11040-11042**.

Codes **15400-15421** are reported for the application of xenografts, which are similar to allografts in purpose. Xenografts (or heterografts) are free skin grafts obtained from a nonhuman source (eg, porcine tissue or pigskin) or a biologic wound dressing. The skin obtained serves as a temporary covering for the exposed surface and can be freeze-dried (eg, porcine graft) and used as needed. Acellular xenograft implants are reported with codes **15430** and **15431**. It is important to note that the exclusionary parenthetical instruction following code **15431** precludes reporting **15430** and **15431** with the site preparation codes **15002-15005**, Category III code **0170T**, and the debridement codes **11040-11042**. Category III code **0170T** is included in this exclusionary reference to indicate that repair of an anal fistula inherently includes placement of the porcine plug; therefore, the xenograft implantation should not be separately reported.

## Selecting the Appropriate Code

The following chart is provided to assist in the selection of the appropriate code.

| Code Range | Type of Graft | Definition and Product Examples |
|---|---|---|
| 15150-15157 | Tissue-cultured epidermal autograft | Cultured autologous skin with only an epidermal layer (eg, CEA, Epicel®, EpiDex®) |
| 15170-15176 | Acellular dermal replacement | A tissue-derived or manufactured device that provides immediate, temporary wound closure and that incorporates into the wound and promotes the generation of a neodermis that can support epidermal tissue (eg, Integra®) |
| 15300-15321 | Allograft skin | Cadaveric human skin allograft (eg, homograft—from skin banks) |
| 15330-15336 | Acellular dermal allograft | Decellularized allogeneic dermis may require immediate concurrent coverage with autologous tissue (eg, Alloderm®, Graft Jacket®) |
| 15340-15341 | Tissue-cultured allogeneic skin substitute | Cultured allogeneic skin with both a dermal and epidermal layer (eg, Apligraf®, Orcel™) |
| 15360-15366 | Tissue-cultured allogeneic dermal substitute | Cultured allogeneic neonatal dermal fibroblasts (eg, Transcyte®, Dermagraft®) |
| 15400-15421 | Xenogeneic dermis | Nonhuman dermis for temporary wound closure (eg, EZ Derm™, Mediskin®) |
| 15430-15431 | Acellular xenogeneic implant | Decellularized nonhuman connective tissue (eg, Oasis®, Surgisis®, PriMatrix®, etc) |

Note: This table represents examples only. Codes are based on the anatomic source and type of graft, not on the brand name of the material.

Other grafts included in this section have different compositions. These graft portions, similar to the previously mentioned autografts, serve a specific purpose according to their size, location, and physical makeup.

First, let us discuss composite grafts. Described by code **15760**, these grafts include more than one type of tissue, such as cartilaginous skin mixture found in the ear or nostrils. The "mixture" is assembled to fill in a defect to provide skin and structural support (cartilage) in the recipient site, therefore, minimizing scar contraction and distortion and mimicking as closely as possible the structure and function of the tissue of that area.

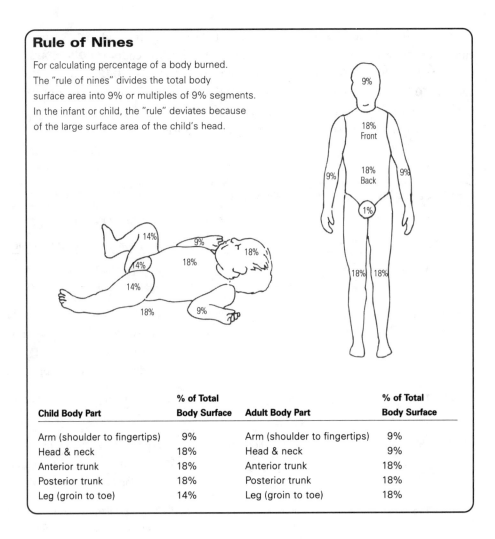

**Rule of Nines**

For calculating percentage of a body burned.
The "rule of nines" divides the total body
surface area into 9% or multiples of 9% segments.
In the infant or child, the "rule" deviates because
of the large surface area of the child's head.

| Child Body Part | % of Total Body Surface | Adult Body Part | % of Total Body Surface |
|---|---|---|---|
| Arm (shoulder to fingertips) | 9% | Arm (shoulder to fingertips) | 9% |
| Head & neck | 18% | Head & neck | 9% |
| Anterior trunk | 18% | Anterior trunk | 18% |
| Posterior trunk | 18% | Posterior trunk | 18% |
| Leg (groin to toe) | 14% | Leg (groin to toe) | 18% |

Code **15770** is used for a derma-fascia fat graft used in a similar manner to the composite grafts in that part of the purpose is to blend in blemishes or defects left behind by surgical excisions, atrophy, and other fleshy "standouts." The tissue used for the graft can be a continuous portion (containing all three of the layered components), individual parts (grafted layer-by-layer), or inserted in combination (such as fascia-fat layer, later covered by a dermal layer). The pockets and defects of the recipient area are therefore restored to their normal positioning as closely as possible. This code is reported once per graft site.

The last graft type included in the CPT code set is the punch graft as described in codes **15775** and **15776**. This is used typically for transplant of hairline to correct hair loss or for revision of scarring such as "ice-pick" acne scars. The graft is performed by removing small amounts of circularly excised donor tissue and transplanting the graft to an appropriately shaped recipient site. Only one code would be reported for the total number of punches performed. Code **15775** is used when a transplant of less than 15 punches is performed. If more than 15 punch grafts are performed, only code **15776** would be reported.

## Burns, Local Treatment

Codes **16000-16036** refer only to local treatment of burned surfaces. It is important that the physician document the percentage of body surface involved and the depth of the burn. To estimate the percentage of the body affected, the rule of nines is used. When using the rule of nines, one should be aware of the patient's age, since the surface area of an infant is estimated differently from that of an adult. The overall medical management of burn patients (other than the specific procedures in this section) is reported in the same way as other types of medical management, using the E/M codes.

Introductory language provides clarification that codes **16020-16030** include application of materials (eg, dressings) not described in the Skin Replacement Surgery and Skin Substitutes codes **15100-15431**.

The first code in the series, **16000**, is the only code that refers to the specific type of burn: first degree. First-degree burns are characterized by erythema and tenderness.

"Local treatment" refers to that which involves symptomatic relief for the patient. The code refers only to initial treatment of this type of injury, as follow-up treatments for first-degree burns are uncommon.

Codes **16020-16030** describe application and change of dressings for burn wounds and also include any associated debridement or curettement. Other debridement codes in the CPT codebook (eg, **11010-11044**) should not be reported to describe this type of debridement of burn wounds.

Codes in this section are categorized by assessing the size of the burn wound as small, medium, or large. These terms are further specified as follows:
- Small—less than 5% total body surface area
- Medium—5%–10% total body surface area
- Large—greater than 10% total body surface area

Because this series of codes refers to small, medium, and large wounds as well as body areas, the codes are to be used as a cumulative single code for each encounter to dress and/or debride burn wounds. That is, choose only one code in this series to represent the total service performed on that date.

For example, if dressings are changed on two extremities, report only code **16030** rather than **16025** two times. In this instance, modifier 59 for Distinct Procedural Services is not used when more than one area is treated during the same patient encounter. If for some reason the physician is required to perform dressings/debridement during different patient encounters on the same date, modifier 59 may be used to accurately identify this circumstance. Services in this category that are provided on different dates are, of course, reported separately.

The last codes in this series, **16035** and **16036**, describe escharotomy. Code **16035** describes the initial incision made into the eschar. Code **16036** is an add-on code to describe additional escharotomy incisions performed. Frequently, additional incisions are necessary in a circumferential burn, such as those involving an extremity or the chest. If more than one anatomic area requires escharotomy, use modifier 59 to identify each area treated.

## Mohs Micrographic Surgery

Mohs micrographic surgery is a specific technique used to treat malignant neoplasms of the skin. It is a technique for the removal of skin cancer in a critical location (periorbital, perioral, periauricular, perinasal, hands and feet, genitalia), recurrent tumors (tumors that have recurred after prior treatment), ill-defined skin cancer (tumor has ill-defined margins), large (greater than 2 cm) or aggressive tumors with histologic examination of 100% of the surgical margins (all of peripheral and deep margins are examined). This technique has the highest cure rate (97%–99% for primary tumors and 94% for recurrent tumors) and spares healthy tissue. When used, both the surgical and pathological services are combined into a specific group of CPT codes (**17311-17315**). In order to report these codes, the physician must act in two integrated but separate and distinct capacities: as surgeon and as pathologist. If either of these responsibilities is delegated to another physician who reports the services separately, it would not be appropriate to report these codes.

Mohs micrographic surgery is usually an outpatient procedure performed under local anesthesia (with or without sedation). Establishing effective sedation and anesthesia is critical to performance of the procedure. This procedure has the lowest recurrence rate. The overall procedure involves the following steps: tumor is identified and debulked; saucer-shaped piece of tissue is excised with 1–2 mm margin around and underneath curetted borders; the skin is marked for orientation; excised tissue is color-coded and mapped by sections for orientation; tissue sections are processed with frozen horizontal technique; Mohs surgeon evaluates slides for residual tumor; if residual tumor found, it is marked on map with proper orientation; second Mohs layer taken only in positive area; process is repeated until margins are clear; defect is repaired with appropriate technique.

The Mohs surgeon removes the tumor tissue and maps and divides the tumor specimen into pieces. Each piece is then embedded into an individual tissue block for histopathologic examination. After the specimen is taken during surgery, it is used to create tissue blocks. In the context of Mohs surgery, a tissue block is defined as an individual tissue piece embedded in a mounting medium for sectioning. This tissue block more accurately describes the unit of service in codes **17311-17315** rather than as specimens, as previously described.

Codes **17311-17314** are differentiated by the anatomic site and by the stage. Code **17311** is reported for first-stage Mohs surgery on the head, neck, hands, feet, genitalia, or any location with surgery directly involving muscle, cartilage, bone, tendon, major nerves, or vessels up to 5 tissue blocks. Add-on code **17312** is reported for each additional stage after the first for the same anatomic sites for up to 5 tissue blocks in conjunction with code **17311**. Code **17313** is reported for first-stage Mohs surgery of the trunk, arms, or legs up to 5 tissue blocks. Code **17314** is an add-on code used in conjunction with **17313** for reporting each additional stage beyond the first, up to 5 tissue blocks.

In Stage I (**17311**), under surgical lighting and magnification, the clinically evident tumor is outlined. A scalpel is used to incise along the planned borders of the excision. A beveled, slanted incision is made circumferentially (peripherally) around the resulting lesion to remove a uniformly thin (1–3 mm), saucer-like layer of tissue. This tissue is placed in a container such that orientation to the cutaneous defect can be maintained. A two-dimensional diagram, the Mohs micrographic surgery map (Mohs map), of the specimen is drawn, relating its orientation to the surgical defect. Following adequate hemostasis, the wound is dressed. Often the patient is guided to a waiting area/recovery room while the tissue is processed.

In the adjacent Mohs laboratory, the saucer-like specimen is subdivided, numbered, and color-coded. These steps are recorded on the Mohs map.

The subdividing of the single excisional specimen into smaller specimens (blocks) allows the beveled edges of the specimen to fall into the same horizontal plane as the deeper tissues upon sectioning the tissue. While maintaining the orientation of the specimens, the technician prepares horizontally oriented frozen sections and stains the glass-mounted sections with hematoxylin and eosin or toluidine blue. Each section is microscopically reviewed by the Mohs surgeon, who is trained in the interpretation of these horizontally oriented pathology specimens.

In cases where microscopic examination reveals tumor in one or more of the subdivided specimens, the Mohs surgeon makes a corresponding mark on the Mohs map. So marked, the Mohs map is used to precisely outline residual tumor within the surgical defect for subsequent resection in further stages of Mohs surgery. Subsequent stages are performed as outlined previously until all specimens processed are free of tumor.

The following case illustrates a typical example of a Mohs micrographic surgery case.

**EXAMPLE:** A facial basal cell carcinoma requiring three Mohs stages for eradication of tumor.

### Stage I (17311)

Mohs excision specimen (Mohs layer) was subdivided into four smaller specimens and each embedded in a block for pathologic processing. Upon microscopic review, tumor was identified in three of the four pathologic specimens, requiring another stage.

### Stage II (17312)

A second Mohs layer is excised, which includes the area containing residual tumor (identified from Mohs map of Stage I). This is subdivided into three smaller specimens and each embedded in a block for pathologic processing. Upon microscopic review, tumor was identified in one of the three pathologic specimens, requiring another stage.

### Stage III (17312)

A third Mohs layer is excised, which includes the area containing residual tumor (identified from Mohs map of Stage II). This is subdivided into two smaller specimens and each embedded in a block for pathologic processing. Upon microscopic review, no tumor was identified.

As previously described, in cases where additional Mohs micrographic surgical stages are required, codes **17312** and **17314** are used to report each additional stage.

Occasionally Mohs surgery is performed on larger tumors, which may require more than five tissue blocks to be examined per stage. For any stage in which there are more than the five tissue blocks for processing, code **17315** should be reported once for each additional tissue block beyond the first five tissue blocks (any stage, any lesion). For example, if a total of eight tissue blocks from the trunk were prepared and examined during the first Mohs stage, then it would be appropriate to report code **17313** one time and code **17315** three times. If in addition a total of six excised tissue blocks were prepared and examined during the second Mohs stage, then it would be appropriate to report codes **17314** one time and code **17315** one time.

It is desirable to confirm a pathologic diagnosis prior to Mohs surgery. If no pathology confirmation of a diagnosis had yet been performed and if a biopsy of a suspected lesion was performed prior to the more definitive Mohs procedure, it would be appropriate to separately report the codes for the diagnostic skin biopsy (**11100, 11101**) and the frozen section pathology (**88331**). Modifier 59 should be appended to distinguish the diagnostic biopsy from the more definitive Mohs procedure.

Furthermore, codes **88302-88309** on the same specimen should not be reported, as they are considered part of the Mohs surgery. In addition, code **88314** should not be reported in conjunction with codes **17311-17315** for routine frozen section stain (eg, hematoxylin and eosin or toluidine blue) performed during Mohs surgery. However, special stains (**88312-88314**), and immunohistochemistry (including tissue immunoperoxidase), each antibody (**88342**), may be reported in addition to the routine histopathologic preparation. Other procedures performed at the same session as Mohs surgery such as decalcification of bone (**88311**) may also be reported separately.

Finally, Mohs surgery may be performed on a tumor in one location and standard surgical or destructive techniques may be used to remove other tumor(s) in different locations on the same day. In this situation, surgical codes for the treatment of additional tumors with other modalities may be reported with modifier 59 in addition to the Mohs surgery codes.

## Reconstruction After Mohs Surgery

Some wounds after Mohs surgery are allowed to heal spontaneously by secondary intention without reconstruction of the wound; and, therefore, no Relative Value Units are included in the Mohs family of codes for surgical repair. Secondary intention is the spontaneous healing of a wound by granulation and new skin regrowth. If surgical repair is necessary, then the appropriate repair code would be separately reported.

Other procedures such as repair, flaps, and grafts may be performed concurrently with Mohs surgery by the same physician on the same day and are reported separately, as they are considered to be separate and distinct procedures. In addition, if reconstruction is performed after Mohs surgery, the corresponding reconstruction codes should be reported in addition to the Mohs surgery codes.

## Breast Procedures

Codes **19100-19499** describe surgical procedures performed on the breast. It is important to note that these procedures are considered unilateral procedures. When these procedures are performed bilaterally, modifier 50 Bilateral Procedure should be appended.

Breast biopsies are reported with codes **19100-19103**. There are two types of breast biopsies: percutaneous and open. Percutaneous needle core biopsy, which is aspiration or removal of tissue, is reported with codes **19100** and **19102** using imaging guidance. Open incisional biopsy, which is surgical removal of part of the lesion into the skin and exposure of the lesion, is reported with code **19101**.

Code **19105** describes cryosurgical ablation of a fibroadenoma using ultrasound guidance. Each fibroadenoma that is ablated is reported separately. Code **19105** includes ultrasound guidance; therefore, a separate code for ultrasound guidance should not be reported. A parenthetical note following code **19105** instructs users not to report codes **76940** or **76942** in conjunction with **19105**.

It is important to note that there are instances when two adjacent fibroadenomas are treated with one insertion of the cryoprobe. In such circumstances, code **19105** should only be reported one time.

Codes **19125** and **19126** describe excision of a breast lesion performed after being identified by preoperative placement of a radiological marker.

Codes **19300-19307** describe various mastectomy procedures. It is important to review the documentation in the medical record prior to selecting the appropriate mastectomy code. A partial mastectomy, also referred to as *lumpectomy, tylectomy, quadrantectomy,* and/or *segmentectomy,* is reported with codes **19301** and **19302**. Total mastectomy is described with various codes ranging from **19303-19307**, depending upon the structures being removed.

# II. Musculoskeletal System

Coding procedures and services from the Musculoskeletal System subsection of the CPT codebook can be challenging for even the advanced coder, largely because of the scope of the procedures in this section. Therefore, it is essential that one develop a clear understanding of the general guidelines in the Musculo-skeletal System subsection and of the additional guidelines that appear throughout the remainder of this section. One should become familiar with the arrangement of codes, since similar arrangements and sequences are common throughout this section.

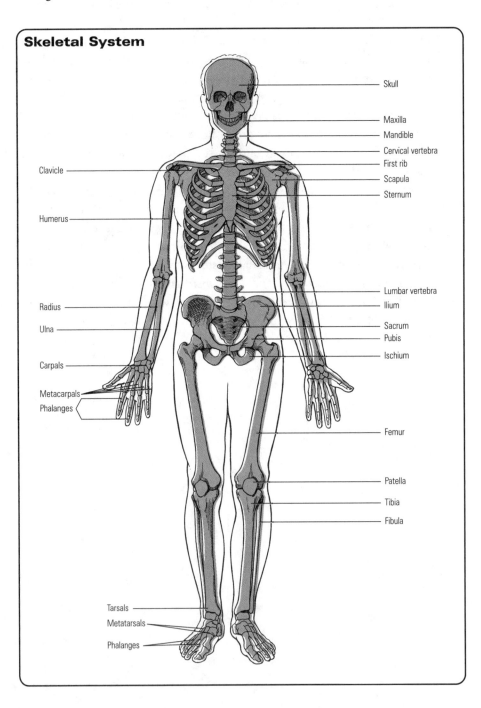

## Muscular System, Front

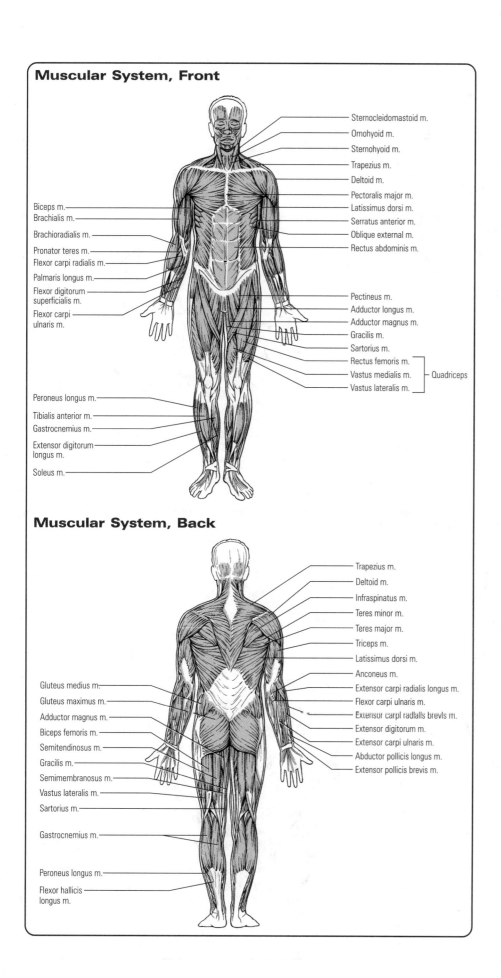

Sternocleidomastoid m.
Omohyoid m.
Sternohyoid m.
Trapezius m.
Deltoid m.
Pectoralis major m.
Latissimus dorsi m.
Serratus anterior m.
Oblique external m.
Rectus abdominis m.

Biceps m.
Brachialis m.
Brachioradialis m.
Pronator teres m.
Flexor carpi radialis m.
Palmaris longus m.
Flexor digitorum superficialis m.
Flexor carpi ulnaris m.

Pectineus m.
Adductor longus m.
Adductor magnus m.
Gracilis m.
Sartorius m.
Rectus femoris m.
Vastus medialis m.
Vastus lateralis m.

Quadriceps

Peroneus longus m.
Tibialis anterior m.
Gastrocnemius m.
Extensor digitorum longus m.
Soleus m.

## Muscular System, Back

Trapezius m.
Deltoid m.
Infraspinatus m.
Teres minor m.
Teres major m.
Triceps m.
Latissimus dorsi m.
Anconeus m.
Extensor carpi radialis longus m.
Flexor carpi ulnaris m.
Extensor carpi radialis brevis m.
Extensor digitorum m.
Extensor carpi ulnaris m.
Abductor pollicis longus m.
Extensor pollicis brevis m.

Gluteus medius m.
Gluteus maximus m.
Adductor magnus m.
Biceps femoris m.
Semitendinosus m.
Gracilis m.
Semimembranosus m.
Vastus lateralis m.
Sartorius m.
Gastrocnemius m.
Peroneus longus m.
Flexor hallicis longus m.

## Skull

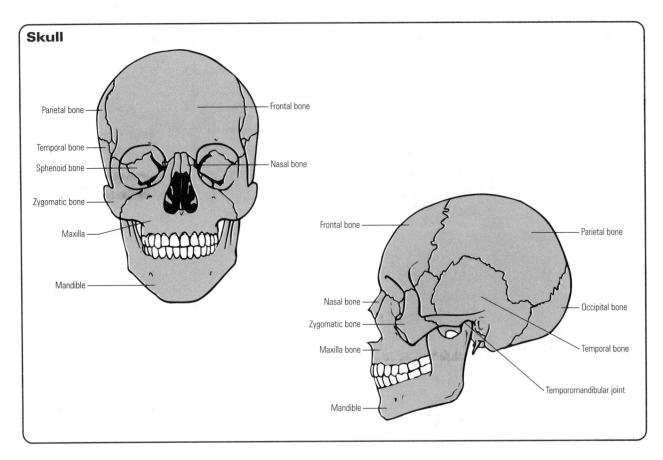

## Bones, Muscles, and Tendons of Hand

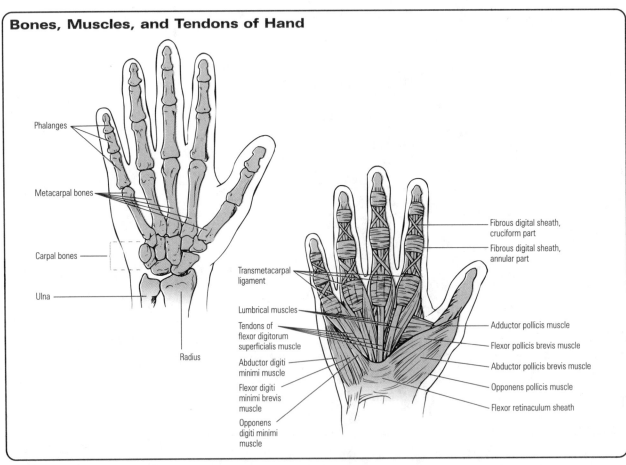

## Bones and Muscles of Foot

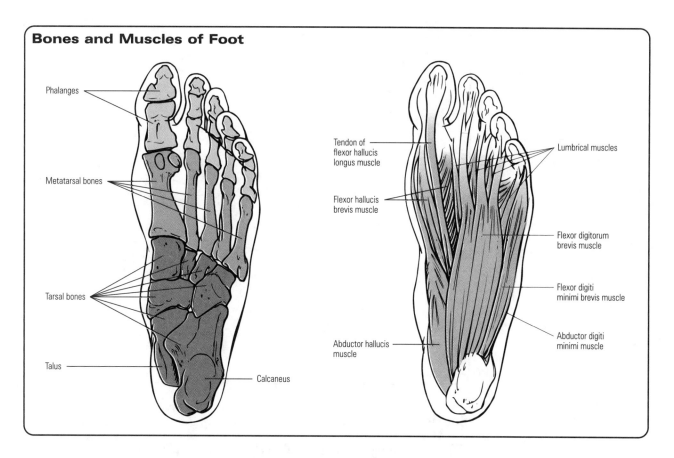

Phalanges

Metatarsal bones

Tarsal bones

Talus

Calcaneus

Tendon of
flexor hallucis
longus muscle

Flexor hallucis
brevis muscle

Abductor hallucis
muscle

Lumbrical muscles

Flexor digitorum
brevis muscle

Flexor digiti
minimi brevis muscle

Abductor digiti
minimi muscle

## Second Lumbar and 12th Thoracic Vertebrae

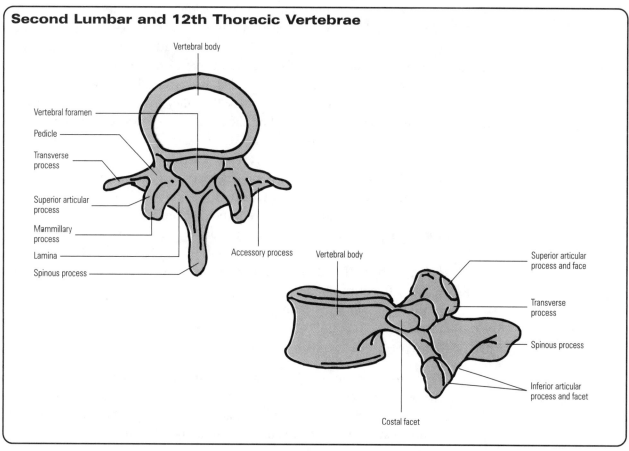

Vertebral body

Vertebral foramen

Pedicle

Transverse
process

Superior articular
process

Mammillary
process

Lamina

Spinous process

Accessory process

Vertebral body

Costal facet

Superior articular
process and face

Transverse
process

Spinous process

Inferior articular
process and facet

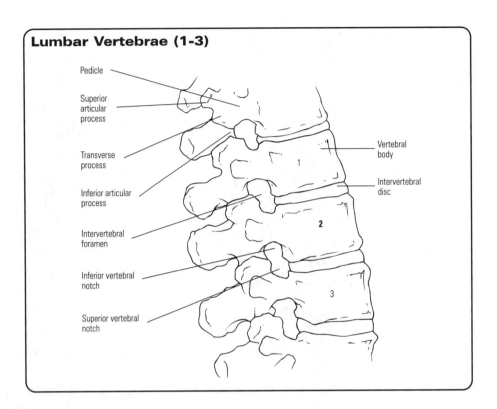

## Section Layout

The first heading in the Musculoskeletal System subsection is General. Some examples of the procedures found in this section include codes for wound exploration, codes describing replantation procedures, codes describing bone biopsy procedures, codes describing joint and tendon sheath injection, codes describing the application of external fixation, and codes to report obtaining autogenous bone, cartilage, tendon, fascia lata, or other tissue grafts. These codes typically may be applied to several anatomic locations; thus, they are not located in the specific anatomic subsections. This heading and its codes are followed by a "head-to-toe" arrangement of the remainder of the Musculoskeletal System subsection.

Within each anatomic heading, there is a consistent theme of the types of procedures/services described. Generally, there are codes to describe procedures involving incision; excision; introduction or removal; repair, revision, and/or reconstruction; fracture and/or dislocation; arthrodesis; and amputation. This format is repeated throughout the Musculoskeletal System subsection.

Now let us look at some of the highlights of the Musculoskeletal System subsection of the CPT codebook, reviewing some basic guidelines associated with reporting fractures and dislocations, spine surgery, bunion procedures, and the guidelines for reporting casting and strapping procedures.

## Fractures and Dislocations

When procedures for the treatment of fractures and dislocations are coded, the type of fracture (eg, closed, open) has no coding correlation with the type of treatment (eg, closed, open, or percutaneous) provided. For example, a closed fracture may require open treatment to accomplish the repair.

## Closed Treatment

Closed treatment of a fracture or dislocation specifically means that the fracture or dislocation site is not surgically opened (exposed to the external environment and directly visualized). Closed treatment is used to describe procedures that treat fractures by the following three methods:

- Without manipulation
- With manipulation
- With or without traction

## Open Treatment

Open treatment implies that the fracture is surgically opened (exposed to the external environment) and the fracture (denoted by bone ends) is visualized to allow internal fixation.

## Percutaneous Skeletal Fixation

Percutaneous skeletal fixation fracture treatment is neither open nor closed. In this procedure, the fracture fragments are not visualized directly, but fixation (eg, using pins) is placed across the fracture site, usually under X-ray imaging.

## Manipulation

The term *manipulation* is used throughout the musculoskeletal fracture and dislocation subsections to indicate the attempted reduction or restoration of a fracture or joint dislocation to its normal anatomic alignment by the application of manually applied forces. Orthopaedists typically refer to the manipulation of a fracture or dislocation as a *reduction*, which is the contracted form for the phrase *manipulative reduction*. Please note that although the term *manipulation* is used in other sections of the CPT codebook, this definition is used only for codes appearing in the Musculoskeletal System subsection.

## Injections

Codes **20550** and **20551** are used to report single or multiple injections per single anatomic tendon sheath or ligament. Thus, multiple injections to the same tendon would be reported only once, while injections to multiple tendon sheaths, ligaments, tendon origins, or tendon insertions would be reported one time for each injection.

Codes **20552** and **20553** are used to report trigger-point injections. These codes are intended to be reported once per session, regardless of the number of trigger points or muscles injected. The appropriate radiology codes (**77002**, **77021**, **76942**) should be reported in addition to the injection codes for imaging guidance.

# Spine Surgery

When coding for spine surgery, there are many sets of guidelines for the coder to consider. At the beginning of the Spine subsection, there are general guidelines that apply to the entire section. Additional guidelines throughout the remainder of the Spine subsection can be found under various subheadings. Read and apply these guidelines carefully when coding for spine surgery procedures. Careful review of each code descriptor is also imperative to ensure that the correct codes are selected.

The vertebral column (spine) consists of a series of bones known as *vertebrae*. An adult human possesses 33 vertebrae divided into the following five types:

**1** Seven cervical vertebrae (C1-C7)—neck area

**2** Twelve thoracic vertebrae (T1-T12)—upper back area

**3** Five lumbar vertebrae (L1-L5)—lower back area

**4** Five sacral vertebrae (S1-S5)—the sacrum

**5** Four coccygeal vertebrae—the coccyx or tailbone

The sacral vertebrae are typically fused into a single bone known as the *sacrum*. The coccygeal vertebrae are sometimes fused into a single bone known as the *coccyx*. Therefore, the actual number of bones in the vertebral column may be 26 to 29, depending on whether the coccygeal vertebrae are fused. Between each pair of vertebrae is a disc (intervertebral disc) that cushions the spinal column.

Vertebrae are commonly named by a letter that corresponds to the region of the vertebral column to which the vertebra belongs, followed by a number that indicates where in the region the vertebra is located. For example, the most superior cervical vertebra is called C1, with the next cervical vertebra down designated as C2. The most superior thoracic vertebra is T1, with the next one down designated as T2.

A vertebral interspace is the nonbony compartment between two adjacent vertebral bodies that contains the intervertebral disc and includes the nucleus pulposus, annulus fibrosus, and two cartilaginous endplates.

A vertebral segment describes the basic constituent part into which the spine may be divided. It represents a single complete vertebral bone with its associated articular processes and laminae.

A good understanding of medical terminology pertaining to spine anatomy is important for accurate coding of spine procedures. Review the illustrations provided in this chapter as well as any standard anatomy text. Become familiar with the anatomy of the vertebral column. Learn the various components of the vertebrae, including the vertebral bodies, spinous processes, laminae, facets, and intervertebral discs. Learn the difference between a vertebral segment and an interspace. Developing this basic knowledge will assist in understanding the code descriptors and appropriately reporting the codes for spine surgery.

Take a few minutes to review this section of the CPT codebook. Notice the various subheadings and the code descriptors within each. Codes can be found to describe procedures that involve excision, osteotomy, fracture and/or dislocation, manipulation, arthrodesis, exploration, and spinal instrumentation.

Additional codes for reporting procedures of the spine and spinal cord can be found in the Nervous System subsection of the Surgery section. Codes in the **62263-64999** series are available for reporting various procedures of the spine and spinal cord.

In some instances, to completely code for spinal procedures performed, it will be necessary to report codes from the Nervous System subsection in addition to codes from the Musculoskeletal System subsection. Read and follow the guidelines, instructional notes, and parenthetical notes found throughout both of these sections of the CPT codebook. Some of the specific guidelines for reporting procedures of the spine (vertebral column) follow. However, always refer to the current CPT codebook for complete code descriptors and guidelines.

### Co-surgeon Reporting—Using Modifier 62

Co-surgery may be required because of the complexity of the procedure(s), the patient's condition, or both. The additional surgeon does not act as an assistant at surgery in these circumstances but performs a distinct portion of the procedure as stated in the language for modifier 62. The definition of this modifier indicates the following:

*Two surgeons*: When two surgeons work together as primary surgeons performing distinct parts of a procedure, each surgeon should report his or her distinct operative work by adding modifier 62 to the procedure code and any associated add-on codes for that procedure, as long as both surgeons continue to work together as primary surgeons. Each surgeon should report the co-surgery once using the same procedure code. If additional procedures (including add-on procedure[s]) are performed during the same surgical session, separate code(s) may also be reported with modifier 62 added. Note: If a co-surgeon acts as an assistant in the performance of an additional procedure(s) during the same surgical session, those services may be reported using separate procedure code(s) with modifier 80 or modifier 82 added, as appropriate.

Modifier 62 is not to be used with instrumentation or bone graft codes. Documentation to establish medical necessity for both surgeons is required for some services.

It is suggested that before a scheduled surgery, the approach and spine surgeon discuss what portion of the operation each is expected to perform on the basis of case complexity. If because of complexity it is agreed that the approach surgeon is needed as a co-surgeon (both the spine and approach surgeon serve as primary surgeons) to perform additional procedures, modifier 62 can be appended to these agreed-on procedures.

When an approach surgeon only opens and closes the patient, then modifier 62 should be appended to the distinct principal procedure along with any additional level(s) that require approach work by only the approach surgeon.

Modifier 62 can be added to additional procedural codes only if both surgeons agree to continue to work together as primary surgeons on the basis of the complexity of the case. Modifier 80 can be appended to additional procedural code(s) by the approach surgeon if both surgeons agree that the approach surgeon is needed to continue to work as an assistant to the spine surgeon.

**EXAMPLE:** Procedure: Anterior Thoracic Two-Level Arthrodesis, Anterior Single-Level Discectomy, Anterior Plate Instrumentation, Structural, Autograft Iliac Crest Bone Graft

> **CODING TIP**
>
> Modifier 62 can be added to additional procedural codes only if both surgeons agree to continue to work together as primary surgeons on the basis of the complexity of the case.

**Example 1**
Approach Surgeon Performs Approach and Closure Only

*Surgeon Performing Approach Only*
**22556 62**

**22585 62**

*Surgeon Performing the Spine Procedure*
**22556 62**

**22585 62**

**63077 51**

**22845**

**20938**

**Example 2**
Approach Surgeon Performs as Co-surgeon with Spine Surgeon for Entire Case

*Surgeon Performing Approach and Serving as Co-surgeon for Entire Case*
**22556 62**

**22585 62**

**63077 62 51**

*Surgeon Performing the Spine Procedure*
**22556 62**

**22585 62**

**63077 62 51**

**22845**

**20938**

**Example 3**
Approach Surgeon Performs Approach and Closure and Performs Rest of Case as Assistant to Spine Surgeon

*Surgeon Performing Approach and Serving as Assistant for Entire Case*
**22556 62**

**22585 62**

**63077 80 51**

*Surgeon Performing the Spine Procedure*

**22556 62**

**22585 62**

**63077 51**

**22845**

**20938**

## General Guidelines for Spine Surgery

*Osteotomy*

When two surgeons work together as primary surgeons performing distinct parts of an anterior spine osteotomy, each surgeon should report his or her distinct operative work by adding modifier 62 to the procedure code. In this situation, modifier 62 may be appended to the procedure code(s) (**22210-22214, 22220-22224**), as appropriate, and to the associated additional segment add-on code(s) (**22216, 22226**), as long as both surgeons continue to work together as primary surgeons.

*Fracture and/or Dislocation*

When two surgeons work together as primary surgeons performing distinct part(s) of open fracture and/or dislocation procedure(s), each surgeon should report his or her distinct operative work by adding modifier 62 to the procedure code. In this situation, modifier 62 may be appended to the procedure code(s) (**22318-22327**), as appropriate, and to the associated additional fracture vertebrae or dislocated segment add-on code (**22328**), as long as both surgeons continue to work together as primary surgeons.

*Vertebral Body, Embolization or Injection*

Percutaneous vertebroplasty is a minimally invasive, radiologically guided vertebral augmentation procedure that uses radiologic imaging to identify a fractured vertebral body and monitor the injection of polymethylmethacrylate (PMMA), an acrylic polymer cement. In addition to injection of the PMMA, vertebroplasty also involves fluoroscopic or computed tomography (CT) guidance, which is separately reportable, to aid in proper needle placement before injection of the polymer cement. In addition to stabilizing the fractured vertebral body, vertebroplasty often immediately alleviates the pain caused by the fracture. Osteoporotic compression fractures comprise about 90% of the vertebroplasty candidate cases. The other 10% of cases are either metastatic lesions of myeloma or painful hemangiomas.

**CODING TIP**

Codes **22520** and **22521** are reported for a single vertebral body only. If percutaneous vertebroplasty is performed on additional thoracic or lumbar vertebral bodies during the same session, then add-on code **22522** should be additionally reported for vertebroplasty of each additional vertebral body.

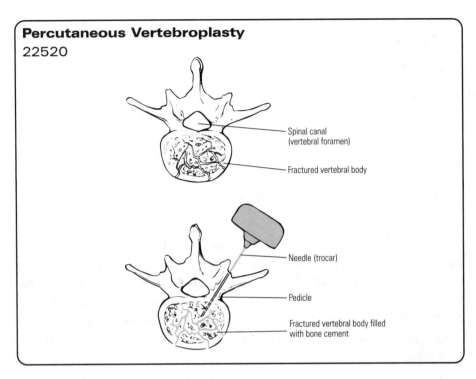

**Percutaneous Vertebroplasty**
22520

- Spinal canal (vertebral foramen)
- Fractured vertebral body
- Needle (trocar)
- Pedicle
- Fractured vertebral body filled with bone cement

Percutaneous vertebroplasty is a significantly different procedure from "open" surgical augmentation using PMMA, which is reported with code **22851**. (Refer to Spinal Instrumentation, discussed on page 170.) Since percutaneous vertebroplasty does not require creation of an open surgical wound, it is not appropriate to report this procedure using code **22851**.

| | |
|---|---|
| **22520** | Percutaneous vertebroplasty, one vertebral body, unilateral or bilateral injection; thoracic |
| **22521** | lumbar |
| **22522** | each additional thoracic or lumbar vertebral body (List separately in addition to code for primary procedure) |

Selecting the appropriate code depends on the anatomic area of the spine undergoing the vertebroplasty. Code **22520** is reported for percutaneous vertebroplasty performed on the thoracic spine, whereas code **22521** is reported for vertebroplasty of the lumbar spine.

**EXAMPLE:** Vertebroplasty is performed on T6, T7, and T8. The physician would report code **22520** one time for the first level. Code **22522** would be reported twice, one time for each additional level. Since code **22522** is an add-on code, modifier 51 would not be appended to report the additional levels. (Refer to Chapter 4 for further discussion of add-on codes.)

Radiologic S&I is separately reported by means of codes **72291** and **72292**. The S&I code selected should accurately reflect the type of guidance used and be reported for each vertebral body for which vertebroplasty is performed.

Open vertebral procedures are sometimes followed by arthrodesis and may include bone grafts and instrumentation. Bone grafting procedures are reported separately and in addition to the vertebral procedure, arthrodesis, and instrumentation, when performed.

Add-on codes **20930-20938** are used to report the various types of bone grafts used for spine surgery. These codes are located under the heading of General Musculoskeletal Procedures in the Surgery section of the CPT codebook. As indicated in the code descriptors, these codes apply only to bone grafts used for spine surgery. For other bone grafts, see the General category.

Understanding the terms used in the bone graft code descriptors is essential to choosing the correct code. As mentioned, the term *allograft* refers to donor bone usually obtained from a bone bank. *Autograft* is cancellous bone or cortical bone surgically removed from another area of the patient's own body. A morselized bone graft consists of small pieces of bone, often cancellous, removed from the patient's own body or obtained from a bone bank. A structural bone graft consists of a whole piece of cancellous and/or bone cortex, obtained either from the patient's own body or from a bone bank, used to reconstruct and support vertebral segments or spinal arthrodesis.

The bone graft codes **20900-20938** are reported without appending modifier 51. Modifier 62 should also not be appended to bone graft codes **20900-20938**.

If bone marrow is aspirated for grafting in an arthrodesis, CPT code **38220** is used to report the separate aspiration procedure. The placement of the bone marrow aspirate is included as part of the arthrodesis procedure reported.

Percutaneous intradiscal electrothermal annuloplasty (**22526, 22527**) is performed by insertion of a needle or catheter (subsequently heated) into a disc to effect a thermal change in the annular tissue, modulating nerve fibers in a disrupted disc's annulus, and stabilizing the collagen of the annulus as a treatment for back pain. When performed bilaterally, code **22526** is reported once. Code **22527** is also reported only one time regardless of the number of additional levels treated in a single session. Since fluoroscopic guidance is an inclusive component of codes **22526** and **22527**, it would not be appropriate to use codes **77002** or **77003**. Category III codes **0062T** and **0063T** should be reported for percutaneous intradiscal annuloplasty by a method other than electrothermal. Again, since fluoroscopic guidance is included in codes **0062T** and **0063T**, codes **77002** and **77003** are not reportable. However, CT (**77012**) and magnetic resonance imaging (MRI) (**77021**) guidance and localization for needle placement and annuloplasty are additionally reportable, when performed.

## Spinal Arthrodesis

Arthrodesis is defined as the surgical fusion/fixation of a joint by a procedure designed to firmly join joint surfaces by promoting the proliferation of bone cells and new bone. Spinal arthrodesis is performed on vertebral segments of the spine.

Arthrodesis performed for spinal deformities such as scoliosis or kyphosis is reported with codes **22800-22812**. When two surgeons work together as primary surgeons performing distinct part(s) of an arthrodesis for spinal deformity, each surgeon should report his or her distinct operative work by adding modifier 62 to the procedure code. In this situation, modifier 62 may be appended to the procedure code(s) (**22800-22819**), as long as both surgeons continue to work together as primary surgeons.

If the arthrodesis is performed for a reason other than to correct a spinal deformity, the codes used to report arthrodesis are categorized by the anatomic approach, as follows, used by the physician:

- Anterior or anterolateral approach (**22548-22585**)
- Posterior, posterolateral, or lateral transverse process technique (**22590-22632**)
- Lateral extracavitary approach technique (**22532-22534**)

Spinal arthrodesis may be performed in the absence of other spinal procedures. When arthrodesis is combined with another definitive procedure (eg, osteotomy, fracture care, vertebral corpectomy, or laminectomy), then modifier 51 should be appended to the arthrodesis code reported. When the code for arthrodesis is listed as the primary procedure, modifier 51 is not appended.

The arthrodesis codes **22585**, **22614**, **22632**, and **22534** are add-on codes, indicating that modifier 51 should not be used with these codes. (Refer to Chapter 4 for further discussion of add-on codes.)

When two surgeons work together as primary surgeons and perform distinct part(s) of anterior interbody arthrodesis, each surgeon should report his or her distinct operative work by adding modifier 62 to the procedure code. In these situations, modifier 62 may be appended to the procedure code(s) (**22554-22558**), as appropriate, and to the associated additional interspace add-on code (**22585**), as long as both surgeons continue to work together as primary surgeons.

Excision of an intervertebral disc may be performed at the same operative session as an arthrodesis. Separate CPT codes are used to report the disc excision. To report an intervertebral disc excision by laminotomy or laminectomy, one would report codes in the **63020-63035** series. However, intervertebral disc excision performed to prepare the vertebral surface for the bone graft is considered part of the arthrodesis procedure and not reported separately.

For both codes **22554** and **22630**, if the surgeon removes a disc and/or a bony endplate only to prepare the vertebrae for fusion, then no additional code(s) in the **63000** series should be reported. The appropriate code(s) **63045-63048**, **63075-63078** should be reported when, in addition to removing the disc and preparing the vertebral endplate, the surgeon removes posterior osteophytes and decompresses the spinal cord or nerve root(s), which requires work in excess of that normally performed when a posterior lumbar interbody fusion (PLIF) is performed.

To report code **22554** in addition to code **63075**, the surgeon must perform the additional procedure(s) and work that leads to the decompression of neural elements. In most cases, the dura and/or neural elements are exposed to ensure decompression, which, for reporting purposes, is considered over and above the work described by code **22554**. Therefore, the decompression procedure **63075** (with modifier 51 appended) would be reported in addition to code **22554**. Examples of types of additional procedures include drilling off the posterior

**CODING TIP**

When performing the discectomy, code **63075**, the operating microscope code **69990** should not be reported since use of the operating microscope is considered to be inclusive.

osteophytes with the use of the operating microscope, opening the posterior longitudinal ligament to look for free disc fragments (decompressing the spinal cord), or removing far lateral disc fragments to decompress the nerve roots.

To report code **22630** in addition to code **63047 51**, again, additional procedure(s) must be performed. For example, in spinal procedures performed on patients with lateral lumbar stenosis, the surgeon may perform additional work above and beyond that described by the PLIF, such as facetectomy and/or foraminotomy, to adequately decompress the nerve roots. In this case, one would report **63047 51** in addition to code **22630**.

A common question relates to the issue of laterality (unilateral vs bilateral procedures), and the response is that codes **22554** and **63075** relate to operations that involve a midline anterior approach. It would not be appropriate to use modifier 50 or report these codes twice, once for each side. These codes should be reported only one time per interspace. Code **22554** describes when a surgeon removes as much disc as necessary to prepare the disc space, whereas with code **22630**, the physician performs a technique that involves a bilateral posterior approach. Surgical practice has evolved to the point where the procedure is now performed from a unilateral approach. Unilaterality and bilaterality have never been part of the descriptor of code **22630**. Code **22630** should be reported without modifier 50 appended, since there is no separation in the descriptor to differentiate whether the procedure was performed with a unilateral or a bilateral approach.

To further clarify, code **22630** may also require that the physician perform a posterior fusion, which involves bone grafting and placement of posterior spinal instrumentation. These additional procedures should be reported. If the surgeon uses a threaded bone dowel or prosthetic device in the disc space, he or she should report code **22851**. If any other type of bone graft is performed, the appropriate bone graft code should be reported.

The anterior fusion procedure described by code **22554** may require bone grafting and placement of anterior spinal instrumentation. Again, in this circumstance, the appropriate bone grafting code and anterior spinal instrumentation code should be reported in addition to code **22554**.

Codes **63040-63044** are the only codes that can be reported for procedures performed on a recurrent herniated nucleus pulposus at each previously explored cervical or lumbar interspace. The term *reexploration* describes the repeat surgical exposure of a surgical tract and target at the same site on the same patient at a time after an initial surgical procedure(s) was performed. As with other CPT code descriptors, the time frame associated with the reexploration procedure is not specifically stated. Should reexploration be required within the operative period of an initial procedure, then the appropriate reexploration code(s) should be reported with modifier 78 appended.

### Reexploration Procedures

To allay misinterpretation of the reporting of spinal reexploration procedures, the **63040-63044** code series delineates the following conditions:

- That reexploration laminotomy or hemilaminectomy is considered a unilateral procedure. Anatomically, either the right and/or left lamina or disc

> **CODING TIP**
>
> If the operating microscope is required, report code **69990**.

material may be excised. Therefore, if right and left hemilaminectomies are performed at a cervical or lumbar interspace, codes **63040-63044**, as appropriate, should be reported with modifier 50 appended.

- That the reexploration procedure involves a single interspace, as opposed to an entire region of the spine (eg, cervical, lumbar). In certain instances, other spinal procedures may be performed at the time of the reexploration procedure that involve vertebral segment(s) or interspace(s) not previously explored. Therefore, the appropriate bone graft, arthrodesis, and/or spinal instrumentation codes should be additionally reported. In this circumstance, modifier 51 should be appended to code **63040** or **63042**. It is not appropriate to append modifier 51 to add-on codes **63043** or **63044**.

For example, if a laminectomy, facetectomy, and foraminotomy are performed concurrently (unilaterally or bilaterally) with decompression of the spinal cord, cauda equina, and/or nerve roots on a single vertebral segment at the lumbar level and this segment has not been previously explored, then it would be appropriate to report CPT code **63047**. CPT code **63048** is an add-on code that may be reported only when **63047** has been reported for the first lumbar vertebral segment procedure and it is necessary to report procedures for one or more additional segments. For coding purposes, a segment is defined as a single complete vertebral bone with associated articular processes and laminae.

When two surgeons work together as primary surgeons performing distinct part(s) of a spinal cord exploration/decompression operation, each surgeon should report his or her distinct operative work by adding modifier 62 to the procedure code (and any associated add-on codes for that procedure code, as long as both surgeons continue to work together as primary surgeons). In this situation, modifier 62 may be appended to the definitive procedure code(s) (**63075**, **63077**, **63081**, **63085**, **63087**, **63090**) and, as appropriate, to associated additional interspace add-on code(s) (**63076**, **63078**) or additional segment add-on code(s) (**63082**, **63086**, **63088**, **63091**), as long as both surgeons continue to work together as primary surgeons.

When two surgeons work together as primary surgeons and perform distinct parts of an anterior or anterolateral approach for an intraspinal excision, each surgeon should report his or her distinct operative work by adding modifier 62 to the single definitive procedure code. In this situation, modifier 62 may be appended to the definitive procedure code(s) (**63300-63307**), as appropriate, and to the associated additional segment add-on code (**63308**), as long as both surgeons continue to work together as primary surgeons.

(Refer to the Nervous System subsection in Chapter 5 for further discussion of other spinal cord, vertebrectomy, or intraspinal excision codes.)

### Spinal Instrumentation

Instrumentation procedure add-on codes **22840-22848** and **22851** are reported without appending modifier 51. Insertion of spinal instrumentation is reported separately and in addition to arthrodesis and any definitive procedure(s) performed. In addition, modifier 62 may not be appended to the definitive or add-on spinal instrumentation procedure code(s) (**22840-22848**, **22850-22852**).

**CODING TIP**

Codes **22840-22855** should be separately reported when performed in conjunction with code(s) for fracture, dislocation, arthrodesis, or exploration of fusion of the spine **22325-22328**, **22532-22534**, **22548-22812**, and **22830**. Add-on codes **22840-22848, 22851** are reported in conjunction with code(s) for the definitive procedure(s) without modifier 51.

Code **22849**, for reinsertion of spinal fixation, and code **22855**, for removal of anterior spinal instrumentation, should not be reported with modifier 62 appended. The Spine subsection guidelines reflect the use of modifier 62 with the spinal instrumentation codes. The notes preclude the use of modifier 62 with the spinal instrumentation codes **22840-22848** and **22850-22852**.

Codes **22840-22855** should be separately reported when performed in conjunction with code(s) for fracture, dislocation, arthrodesis, or exploration of fusion of the spine **22325-22328**, **22532-22534**, **22548-22812**, and **22830**. Add-on codes **22840-22848**, **22851** are reported in conjunction with code(s) for the definitive procedure(s) without modifier 51.

The guidelines further clarify that codes **22849**, **22850**, **22852**, and **22855** for reporting revisions of previous instrumentation procedures do not have modifier 51-exempt status. Hence, modifier 51 should be appended when reported in addition to another definitive procedure (eg, arthrodesis, decompression, and exploration of fusion). In addition, the guidelines state that code **22849**, Reinsertion of spinal fixation device, should not be reported in conjunction with the instrumentation removal codes **22850**, **22852**, and **22855** when performed at the same spinal level. It is also specified that when code **22830**, Exploration of spinal fusion, is performed in conjunction with a definitive procedure, including arthrodesis and decompression, code **22830** should be reported separately with modifier 51.

*Segmental instrumentation* is defined as fixation at each end of the construct and at least one additional interposed bony attachment.

*Nonsegmental instrumentation* is defined as fixation at each end of the construct and may span several vertebral segments without attachment to the intervening segments. Notice that fusion of two adjacent vertebrae is considered nonsegmental, even when using pedicle screws.

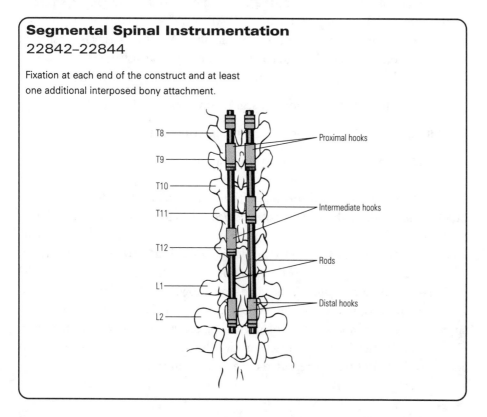

**Segmental Spinal Instrumentation**
22842–22844

Fixation at each end of the construct and at least one additional interposed bony attachment.

T8 — Proximal hooks
T9
T10
T11 — Intermediate hooks
T12
L1 — Rods
L2 — Distal hooks

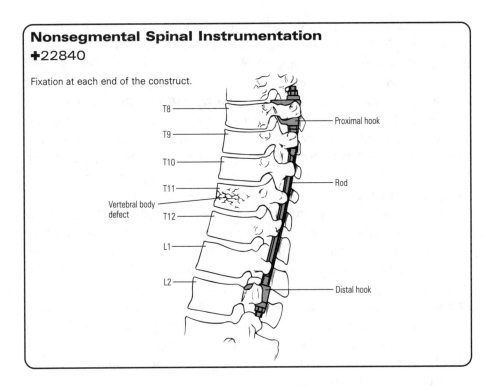

**Nonsegmental Spinal Instrumentation**
**+22840**

Fixation at each end of the construct.

T8 — Proximal hook
T9
T10 — Rod
T11
Vertebral body defect
T12
L1
L2 — Distal hook

Codes are available for reporting the following:

- Posterior nonsegmental instrumentation (**+22840**)
- Posterior segmental instrumentation (**+22842-22844**)
- Anterior instrumentation (**+22845-22847**)
- Pelvic fixation (**+22848**)

A special note about add-on code **22841** (internal spinal fixation by wiring of spinous processes): Do not report this code when wiring is performed with other types of segmental or nonsegmental instrumentation. Minimal wiring is considered an inclusive component of the segmental and nonsegmental instrumentation codes.

Three codes are available for reporting removal of instrumentation:

**22850**, Removal of posterior nonsegmental instrumentation

**22852**, Removal of posterior segmental instrumentation

**22855**, Removal of anterior instrumentation

Code **22849** is used to report reinsertion of a spinal fixation device. The type of instrumentation in this code is not specified. Therefore, it would be used for all types of devices. It is appropriate to separately report removal of spinal instrumentation (**22850, 22852, 22855**) in addition to code **22849** for the reinsertion.

Code **22851** is used to report application of an intervertebral biomechanical device(s) (eg, synthetic cage[s], threaded bone dowel[s], methylmethacrylate) to a vertebral defect or interspace. This code is to be reported only one time per interspace, regardless of the number of devices placed at that interspace. However, if, for example, metal cages are placed at two different vertebral interspaces, then add-on code **22851** may be reported once for each interspace.

Consider the following two examples:

**EXAMPLE 1:** Two metal cages are placed at the L3-L4 interspace. Add-on code **22851** would be reported one time.

**EXAMPLE 2:** A metal cage is placed at the L3-L4 interspace and another metal cage is placed at the L5-S1 interspace. Add-on code **22851** would be reported two times.

It is important to note that a single cage or methylmethacrylate used to cover a defect spanning two or more interspaces is reported with add-on code **22851** one time. For example, a single metal cage spanning the L3-L5 interspaces would be reported with add-on code **22851**, times one.

Codes **22857**, **22862**, and **22865** describe variations of anterior approach lumbar disc replacement surgery involving placement of an artificial disc anchored to the vertebral end plates on the vertebrae above and below a single lumbar intradiscal space. The anterior approach (through the abdomen to access the anterior portion of the spine, without disruption of the spinal cord area) and the fluoroscopic imaging are not reported separately. However, any procedures for spinal cord or nerve root decompression are not included, and therefore are appropriately reported with codes **63001-63048**.

Initial placement of a lumbar artificial disc in a single interspace is reported with code **22857**. Do not additionally report the lumbar arthrodesis (**22558**), anterior instrumentation (**22845**), applications of intervertebral biomechanical devices (**22851**), nor exploration of the retroperitoneal area (**49010**) when performed at the same level. Should a lumbar artificial disc procedure be performed at an additional lumbar interspace, Category III code **0163T** is reported for each additional interspace.

The revision and replacement of an existing lumbar artificial disc at a single level is reported by code **22862**. Codes **22558**, **22845**, **49010**, and **22851** are not reported in addition to **22862** when performed at the same level. Also not additionally reported is code **22865** for the removal of the previously placed artificial disc, as removal is inherent in code **22862**. Category III code **0165T** is reported for revision of other previously placed discs at other interspaces.

Removal of an existing lumbar artificial disc at a single level is reported using code **22865**. Code **49010** for exploration of the retroperitoneal area is included in **22865**; however, removal of the disc requires other surgical interventions (ie, fusion) to stabilize the former site of the artificial disc. Therefore, codes **22558**, **22845**, and **22851** are not excluded from reporting with code **22865**. Category III code **0164T** is reported for removal of lumbar artificial disc performed at additional levels.

Codes **0163T-0165T** are not reported with codes **22851** or **49010** when performed at the same level.

### Approach for Spine Surgery

Under certain circumstances, one surgeon performs the approach procedure for spine surgery, including making the incision and exposing the area requiring surgery. Another surgeon then performs the definitive procedure on the spine.

**CODING TIP**

Codes **22857-22865** represent single lumbar interspace procedures. For additional interspace procedures, use Category III codes **0163T-0165T**. Anterior approach is an inclusive component of codes **22857-22865** and **0163T-0165T**, as is fluoroscopic guidance, if performed.

After the completion of the definitive procedure, the first physician returns to perform the closure of the operative site.

The approach and the closure are considered inclusive components of the definitive procedure performed. Only one total procedure listed in the CPT codebook is performed by two surgeons. This circumstance is reported by means of modifier 62.

Each surgeon reports his or her services by reporting the primary procedure code and appending modifier 62. If one surgeon does not use modifier 62, the third-party payer may assume that the physician reporting the procedure without a modifier performed the entire procedure, despite the second surgeon's reporting the procedure with modifier 62.

Alternatively, if a co-surgeon acts as an assistant in the performance of additional procedures during the same surgical session, those services may be reported by means of separate procedure code(s) with modifier 80 or modifier 82 added, as appropriate.

Therefore, the two-surgeon modifier 62 may indicate the following circumstances:

- That two surgeons continued to work together as primary surgeons performing distinct part(s) of a procedure and any associated add-on code(s) for that procedure; and
- That, in addition to either of the above instances where modifier 62 is used, the co-surgeon acts as an assistant (see modifiers 80 and 82) in the performance of additional procedure(s) during the same surgical session.

Both physicians should document their individual level of involvement with the surgery in separate operative reports and include copies of their reports when the procedure is reported to the third-party payer. This will allow the third-party payer to determine reimbursement for each surgeon based on the level of involvement of each surgeon in performing the procedure.

**EXAMPLE 1:** Co-surgeon involvement for exposure/closure of procedure and associated add-on codes.

A patient's surgery includes arthrodesis of two interspaces of the thoracic spine by anterior interbody technique, with anterior instrumentation of three vertebral segments. Morselized autograft is used, which is obtained through a separate incision. Physician A performs a thoracotomy at the start of the surgical session, carefully preserving major vasculature to expose the vertebral segments. Physician B performs the arthrodesis and spinal instrumentation. On completion of the arthrodesis and spinal instrumentation, Physician A closes the operative site.

The physicians in this example would code the services as follows:

| | |
|---|---|
| Physician A | **22556 62** |
| Physician B | **22556 62** |
| | **+22585** |
| | **+22845** |
| | **+20937** |

**EXAMPLE 2:** Co-surgeon involvement for exposure/closure of procedure and associated add-on codes, and continued involvement as an assistant.

A patient's surgery includes arthrodesis of two interspaces of the thoracic spine by anterior interbody technique, with anterior instrumentation of three vertebral segments. Morselized autograft is used, which is obtained through a separate incision. Physician A performs a thoracotomy at the start of the procedure, carefully preserving major vasculature to expose the vertebral segments. Physician B performs the arthrodesis and spinal instrumentation. Physician A continues to work with Physician B as a co-surgeon for the multiple arthrodesis procedures and elects to act as an assistant for the bone graft and spinal instrumentation procedures. On completion of the arthrodesis and spinal instrumentation, Physician A closes the operative site.

The physicians in this example would code their services as follows:

| Physician A | **22556 62, 22585 62, 22845 80, 20937 80** |
|---|---|
| Physician B | **22556 62** |
| | **22585 62** |
| | **+22845** |
| | **+20937** |

Note: Modifier 62 is not appended to either the spinal instrumentation (**22845**) or the bone graft (**20937**) code.

## Distal Radius and Ulnar Styloid Fracture Treatment

Distal radial fractures occur with various degrees of complexity. Open treatment is differentiated by the type of repair required: intraarticular (**25608, 25609**); extraarticular (**25607**); and the number of fragments requiring internal fixation—**25608** describes fractures that require the fixation of two fragments, while **25609** describes fractures that require the fixation of three or more fragments.

When closed treatment of a distal radial fracture is performed, the closed repair of the ulnar styloid is included when performed on the same extremity. Therefore, it is not appropriate to report code **25600** or **25605** in conjunction with **25650**.

To differentiate, even though fractures of the distal radius are often associated with ulnar styloid fractures, ulnar styloid fracture treatment is usually not performed at the time of treatment of the radial fracture. Therefore, neither percutaneous nor open treatment of an ulnar styloid fracture is included in the work of percutaneous skeletal fixation of a distal radial fracture or epiphyseal separation (**25606**). Percutaneous (**25651**) and open (**25652**) ulnar styloid repairs should be reported in addition to codes **25606, 25607,** and **25609**. External fixation (**20690**) should be reported separately if performed in addition to the internal fixation described by code **25606**.

**CODING TIP**

Closed treatment of an ulnar styloid fracture (**25650**) should not be reported in addition to the distal radial fracture codes 25600, 25605, 25607-25609.

**CODING TIP**

For application of external fixation in addition to internal fixation, use **20690** and the appropriate internal fixation code.

## Bunion Procedures

Hallux valgus (bunion) is a common deformity of the first metatarsophalangeal (MTP) joint. Coding for the correction of a bunion and its associated deformities can be challenging. Not all bunion deformities are the same, and different techniques are needed to repair different levels of deformity. CPT codes **28290-28299** are available to describe the various techniques used to correct bunion deformities.

To code appropriately for the treatment of bunion deformities, one must understand the specific procedures included when reporting the codes for bunion (hallux valgus) correction. All of the codes in the **28290-28299** series include the following procedures when performed at the first MTP joint. These are integral components of the operation and are not to be reported separately:

- Capsulotomy
- Arthrotomy
- Synovial biopsy
- Neuroplasty
- Synovectomy
- Tendon release
- Tenotomy
- Tenolysis
- Excision of medial eminence
- Excision of associated osteophytes
- Placement of internal fixation
- Scar revision
- Articular shaving
- Removal of bursal tissue

In addition to learning the inclusive components of bunion correction procedures, the following illustrations of various techniques of bunion correction will assist in coding for these procedures.

**28290** Correction, hallux valgus (bunion), with or without sesamoidectomy; simple exostectomy (eg, Silver-type procedure)

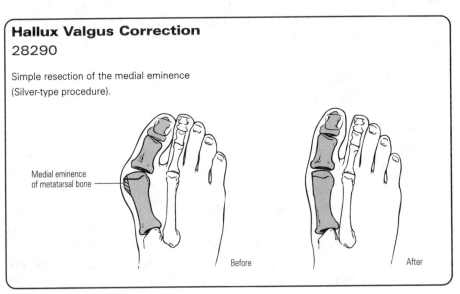

**Hallux Valgus Correction**
28290

Simple resection of the medial eminence (Silver-type procedure).

Medial eminence of metatarsal bone

Before    After

**CODING TIP**

As per the parenthetical instruction following code **28760**, "(For hammertoe operation or interphalangeal fusion, use **28285**)," code **28285** may be reported for interphalangeal fusion involving partial or total phalangectomy for other than hammertoe (ie, mallet toe repair).

**28292**    Correction, hallux valgus (bunion), with or without
sesamoidectomy; Keller-, McBride-, or Mayo-type procedure

### Keller-Type Procedure
28292

Simple resection of the base of the proximal
phalanx with removal of the medial eminence.

A hemi-implant is optional.

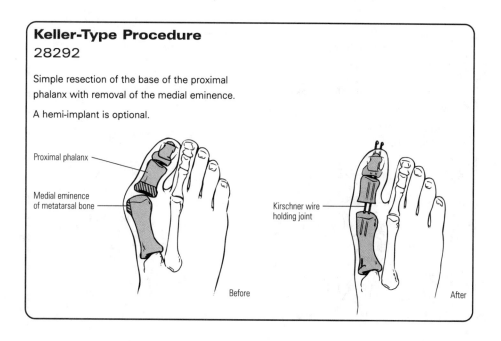

Proximal phalanx

Medial eminence
of metatarsal bone

Kirschner wire
holding joint

Before

After

**28294**    Correction, hallux valgus (bunion), with or without
sesamoidectomy; with tendon transplants (eg, Joplin-type
procedure)

### Joplin Procedure
28294

Tendon transplant is an important part of procedure.

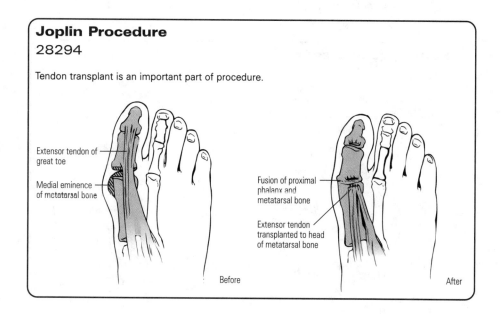

Extensor tendon of
great toe

Medial eminence
of metatarsal bone

Fusion of proximal
phalanx and
metatarsal bone

Extensor tendon
transplanted to head
of metatarsal bone

Before

After

**28296**    Correction, hallux valgus (bunion), with or without sesamoidectomy; with metatarsal osteotomy (eg, Mitchell-, Chevron-, or concentric-type procedures)

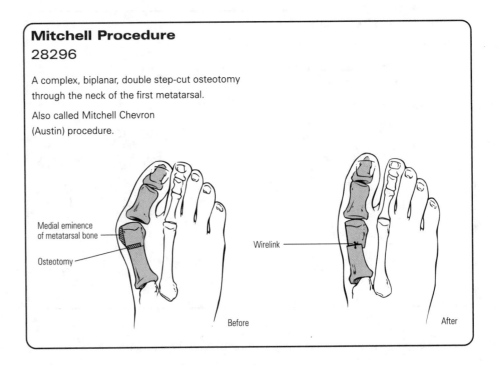

**Mitchell Procedure**
28296

A complex, biplanar, double step-cut osteotomy through the neck of the first metatarsal.

Also called Mitchell Chevron (Austin) procedure.

Medial eminence of metatarsal bone

Osteotomy

Wirelink

Before

After

**28297**    Correction, hallux valgus (bunion), with or without sesamoidectomy; Lapidus-type procedure

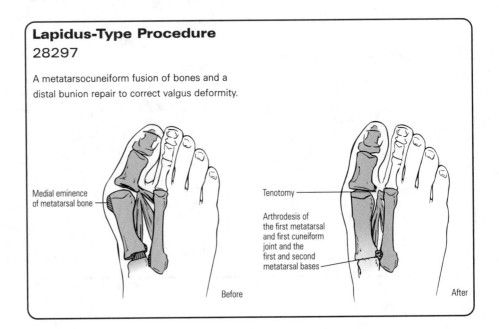

**Lapidus-Type Procedure**
28297

A metatarsocuneiform fusion of bones and a distal bunion repair to correct valgus deformity.

Medial eminence of metatarsal bone

Tenotomy

Arthrodesis of the first metatarsal and first cuneiform joint and the first and second metatarsal bases

Before

After

**28298**    Correction, hallux valgus (bunion), with or without
sesamoidectomy; by phalanx osteotomy

## Phalanx Osteotomy
## 28298

The Akin procedure involves removal of a
bony wedge from the base of the proximal
phalanx to reorient the axis.

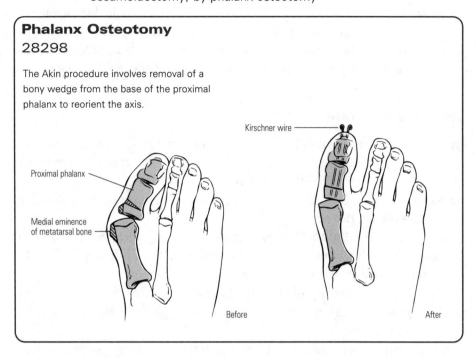

Kirschner wire

Proximal phalanx

Medial eminence
of metatarsal bone

Before                                   After

**28299**    Correction, hallux valgus (bunion), with or without
sesamoidectomy; by other methods (eg, double osteotomy)

## Double Osteotomy
## 28299

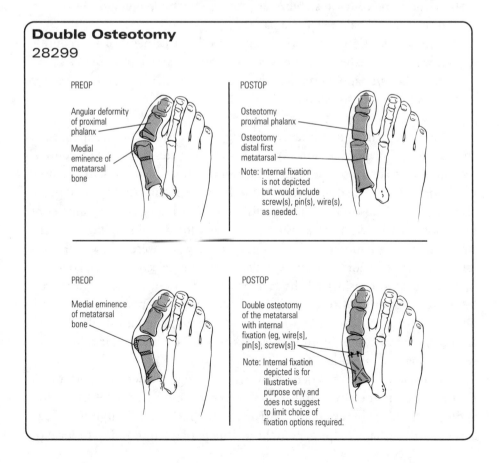

PREOP

Angular deformity
of proximal
phalanx

Medial
eminence of
metatarsal
bone

POSTOP

Osteotomy
proximal phalanx

Osteotomy
distal first
metatarsal

Note: Internal fixation
is not depicted
but would include
screw(s), pin(s), wire(s),
as needed.

PREOP

Medial eminence
of metatarsal
bone

POSTOP

Double osteotomy
of the metatarsal
with internal
fixation (eg, wire[s],
pin[s], screw[s])

Note: Internal fixation
depicted is for
illustrative
purpose only and
does not suggest
to limit choice of
fixation options required.

Code **28299** represents a combination of codes **28296** and **28310-28315**. Bunion surgery has evolved, and it is now common practice to perform a double osteotomy. For the correction of hallux valgus deformities with double osteotomy, two operative procedures must be performed. The first is a chevron osteotomy of the distal first metatarsal with correction of the hallux valgus, followed by an osteotomy of the proximal phalanx to correct additional angular deformity.

## Casting and Strapping

The guidelines at the beginning of the Musculoskeletal System subsection indicate that the services listed in this section of the CPT codebook include the application and removal of the first cast or traction device only. Subsequent replacement of a cast and/or traction device may require an additional listing with the **29000-29799** series of codes.

The codes in the **29000-29799** series have specific guidelines pertaining to their use. It is important to develop a good understanding of these guidelines to appropriately code for the application of casts and strapping.

Following is a summary of the guidelines for reporting the application of casts and strapping. The application of casts and strapping codes may be used to report the following:

- A replacement cast/strapping procedure, during or after the period of normal follow-up care
- An initial service performed without restorative treatment or musculoskeletal section procedure to stabilize or protect a fracture, injury, or dislocation and/or to afford pain relief to a patient
- An initial cast/strapping service when no other treatment or procedure is performed or is expected to be performed by the same physician
- An initial cast/strapping service when another physician provides a restorative treatment or procedure(s)

Before reporting an initial cast/strapping with a casting and strapping code, consider the following questions: Will any restorative treatment or procedure(s) (eg, surgical repair, closed or open reduction of a fracture or joint dislocation) be performed, or is treatment expected to be performed? Will the same physician assume all subsequent fracture, dislocation, or injury care? By answering these questions, you will establish a good basis for deciding if the casts and strapping codes should be reported. Once you have answered these questions, refer to the general guidelines for specific rules when selecting a final code.

Remember to consider all the facts when making the decision to use the **29000-29799** series of codes for initial cast/strapping application. When it is not clear if the same physician who places the cast/strapping will also provide all subsequent care, it is appropriate to ask the physician to confirm his or her role in managing the patient's care.

Another important consideration when deciding whether to report a code for the application of casts and strapping vs a code for treatment of fracture and/or dislocation is the surgical "package" concept. The CPT surgical package, as discussed in Chapter 4, applies to the treatment of fracture and/or dislocation

---

**CODING TIP**

The **29000-29799** series of codes is also used to report the application of replacement casts used during or after the period of follow-up care.

codes found throughout the Musculoskeletal System subsection of the CPT codebook. By reporting a treatment of fracture code, the physician is reporting the service of a surgical package.

If the cast is placed after some type of restorative surgical treatment of a fracture, dislocation, or other injury (open treatment or closed manipulation), do not report the cast separately with the **29000-29799** series of codes. The first cast/splint or strapping application is included in the treatment of fracture and/or dislocation code.

Generally, codes for treatment of fracture and/or dislocation are reported only if the same physician is responsible for the initial cast, follow-up evaluation(s), and the management of the fracture/dislocation until healed.

The casting and strapping guidelines also address the application of temporary casts/strapping placed preoperatively. A temporary cast/splint/strap is not considered part of preoperative care. Therefore, the use of modifier 56 for preoperative management is not appropriate. A physician who applies the initial cast, strap, or splint and assumes all subsequent restorative fracture, dislocation, or injury care cannot use the application of casts and strapping codes as an initial service, since this is included in the restorative treatment of fracture and/or dislocation codes.

The codes for application of casts and strapping include the removal procedure. Therefore, codes for removal of casts are to be reported only when the physician is removing a cast that was applied by another physician.

If the cast/strapping is applied in the office, supplies/materials can be billed separately by means of CPT code **99070** or Healthcare Common Procedure Coding System (HCPCS) Level II codes, as appropriate. In addition, if the key components of an E/M service are met at the time of a cast/strapping application, the appropriate level of E/M service is also reported with modifier 25 appended.

## Endoscopy/Arthroscopy

The last category of codes in the Musculoskeletal System subsection includes codes for reporting endoscopic/arthroscopic procedures. The guidelines at the beginning of this category of codes indicate that surgical arthroscopy always includes a diagnostic arthroscopy. This is also indicated by the *separate procedure* designation of the diagnostic scope codes. As discussed in Chapter 4, this designation may indicate that a procedure or service is considered an integral component of another procedure/service—that is, diagnostic arthroscopy is considered an integral component of surgical arthroscopy.

Review the codes in this section and become familiar with the various endoscopy/arthroscopy codes available in the Musculoskeletal System subsection.

General guidelines for coding endoscopic procedures are as follows:

**1** Look up endoscopy/laparoscopy in the index and locate the organ/system being examined or treated with a scope.

**2** Look at the codes in that system/organ section to find an endoscopy/laparoscopy heading.

**3** If there is no endoscopy/laparoscopy heading in that section, look for a code with a descriptor that includes a suffix "-oscopy," and describes the procedure performed.

**4** If there is no heading of endoscopy/laparoscopy or there is no specific code describing the use of an endoscope in its descriptor, one may be certain the codes described in that section are open surgical procedures and should not be used to report a procedure using an endoscopic approach.

**5** Clarify with the physician that the procedure was performed with an endoscope/laparoscope.

**6** If it is determined there is no specific code for the endoscopic/laparoscopic procedure one is attempting to code, use the unlisted procedure laparoscopy/endoscopy/arthroscopy code to report the procedure. In this case, a copy of the operative report should be submitted to the insurance company when the claim is filed. (Refer to Chapter 2 for further discussion of unlisted codes.)

# III. Respiratory System

The Respiratory System subsection of the CPT codebook contains codes for reporting procedures of the following:
- Nose
- Accessory sinuses
- Larynx
- Trachea and bronchi
- Lungs and pleura

Following the illustrations are some highlights of procedures and guidelines in the Respiratory System subsection. This section includes a review of some of the basic guidelines associated with reporting the nasal endoscopy, laryngoscopy, and bronchoscopy codes.

# Respiratory System

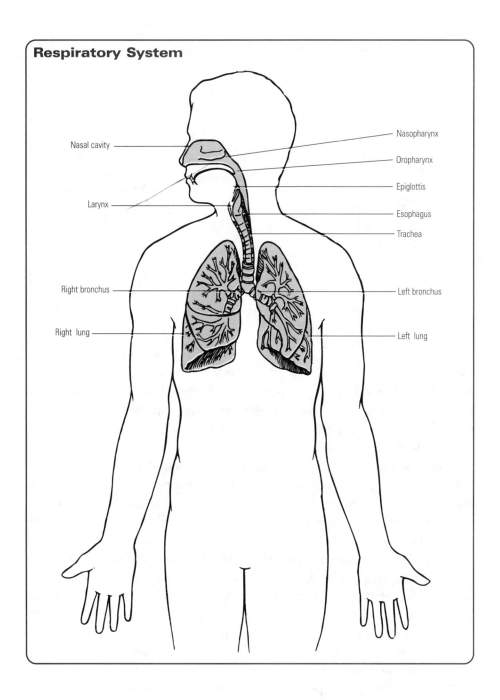

Nasal cavity

Larynx

Right bronchus

Right lung

Nasopharynx

Oropharynx

Epiglottis

Esophagus

Trachea

Left bronchus

Left lung

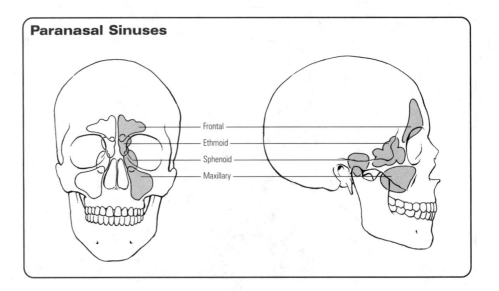

**Paranasal Sinuses**

Frontal
Ethmoid
Sphenoid
Maxillary

## Nasal Endoscopy

Four separate sinus cavities exist on each side of the face. (Please refer to the illustrations provided.) The maxillary sinus (also called the maxillary antrum) is below the eye, the ethmoid sinus is between the eye and the nose or nasal cavity, the sphenoid sinus is behind the nasal cavity, and the frontal sinus is above the eye in the forehead region.

Since these sinuses are in separate anatomic locations, there is a separate and significant amount of work involved with each sinus on which surgery is performed. Surgery on the sinuses can be performed through an incision on the face or forehead. This type of sinus surgery is reported with the codes in the **31000-31230** series.

Surgery on the sinuses can also be performed through the nose by means of a fiberoptic telescope or endoscope. Codes for endoscopic sinus surgery are located in the **31231-31294** range. Separate codes are available for reporting diagnostic nasal/sinus endoscopy and surgical nasal/sinus endoscopy.

Codes **31231-31294** are used to report unilateral procedures unless otherwise specified in the code descriptor. If one of the procedures listed in this range of codes is performed bilaterally and the code does not specify bilateral procedure, modifier 50, Bilateral procedure, should be appended to the appropriate code.

Codes **31231-31235** for diagnostic nasal/sinus endoscopy refer to the use of a nasal/sinus endoscope to inspect the following:

- The interior of the nasal cavity
- The middle and superior meatus
- The turbinates
- The sphenoethmoid recess

Whenever a diagnostic evaluation is performed, typically all of these areas would be inspected. A separate code is not reported for each area inspected.

Codes **31237-31294** are used to report surgical nasal/sinus endoscopy. A surgical sinus endoscopy includes a sinusotomy, when appropriate, and diagnostic endoscopy. When surgical and diagnostic endoscopies are performed at

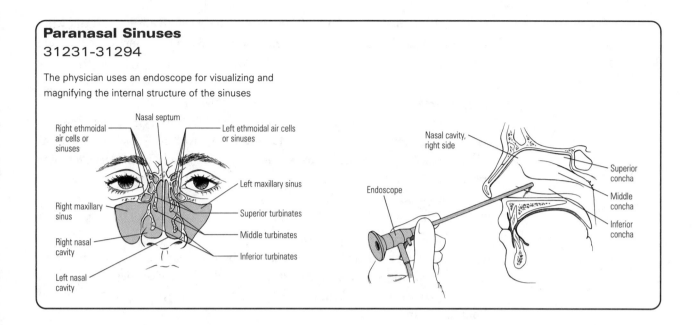

**Paranasal Sinuses**
31231-31294

The physician uses an endoscope for visualizing and magnifying the internal structure of the sinuses

the same session, only the surgical endoscopy would be reported, since the diagnostic procedure is considered an integral part of any therapeutic procedure.

## Laryngoscopy

Codes **31505-31579** are used to report various laryngoscopic procedures. This range of codes includes both diagnostic and therapeutic procedures. When a diagnostic procedure is performed with a therapeutic laryngoscopic procedure, only the therapeutic procedure is reported. The diagnostic procedure is considered an inclusive component of the therapeutic procedure.

### Operating Microscope (69990)

Many of the codes in this section include the use of an operating microscope (**31526**, **31531**, **31536**, **31541**, **31561**, and **31571**) to perform microsurgical techniques, which are inclusive when these codes are reported. The parenthetical notes that appear after each of these codes indicate that code **69990** is not to be reported separately. Code **69990** is an add-on code, which means that it is reported for the use of an operating microscope in addition to the primary procedure code. This separate code is reported only when the use of the operating microscope is not considered an inclusive component of the procedure performed.

### Diagnostic Direct Laryngoscopy of Newborn
### (Use of Modifier 63)

Code **31520** describes diagnostic direct laryngoscopy of a newborn, with or without tracheoscopy. Performing this procedure on a newborn requires additional skill and time. Unless otherwise designated, modifier 63, Procedure Performed on Infants, may be appended to procedures/services listed in the **20000-69999** series to indicate that the procedures performed on neonates and infants up to a present body weight of 4 kg have resulted in significantly increased complexity and physician work. The parenthetical note following code **31520** advises users not to append modifier 63 to this code, since the code already reflects the increased complexity associated with this type of patient.

### Approach Techniques—Indirect and Direct

There are separate codes to report indirect and direct laryngoscopy. Indirect laryngoscopy, reported with codes **31505-31513**, involves the use of a mirror to visualize the larynx (ie, the larynx is not directly visualized). Direct laryngoscopy, reported with codes **31515-31571**, is performed with a lighted scope to allow direct visualization of the larynx.

### Flexible Fiberoptic Laryngoscopy

Laryngoscopy performed with a flexible fiberoptic laryngoscope is reported with the codes in the **31575-31578** series. Specific services described in this series of codes include diagnostic laryngoscopy, biopsy, removal of a foreign body, and removal of a lesion.

If laryngoscopy is performed with the patient under general anesthesia, then it would be appropriate to append modifier 23, Unusual Anesthesia, which indicates the use of unusual anesthesia. Occasionally, because of unusual circumstances, a procedure that usually requires either no anesthesia or local anesthesia may be performed under general anesthesia. This circumstance is reported by appending modifier 23 to the procedure code of the basic service.

For example, if a diagnostic direct laryngoscopy with tracheoscopy were performed on a 3-year-old child under general anesthesia, this would be reported as **31525-23**.

### Flexible Fiberoptic Swallowing Evaluation and Laryngeal Sensory Testing

Evaluation of swallowing and laryngeal sensory testing with a flexible fiberoptic endoscope is not described by this series, as indicated by the multiple parenthetical notes following code **31578** that direct users to codes **92612-92617** to report those services.

## Bronchoscopy

Bronchoscopy is reported with the codes in the **31622-31656** series. A number of different codes are available describing various procedures performed via bronchoscopy. If more than one bronchoscopic procedure is performed, it would be appropriate to report these procedures separately.

It is important to note that all of the codes in the **31622-31640** series include fluoroscopic guidance. Therefore, it would not be appropriate to separately report fluoroscopic guidance when performed in conjunction with the **31622-31640** bronchoscopy codes.

CPT code **31622** describes diagnostic bronchoscopy. This code is used to describe a procedure that involves the use of a bronchoscope with visualization of all major lobar and segmental bronchi. It may also include the obtaining of diagnostic specimens as part of the examination.

**CODING TIP**

Bronchoscopy is considered an inherently bilateral procedure.

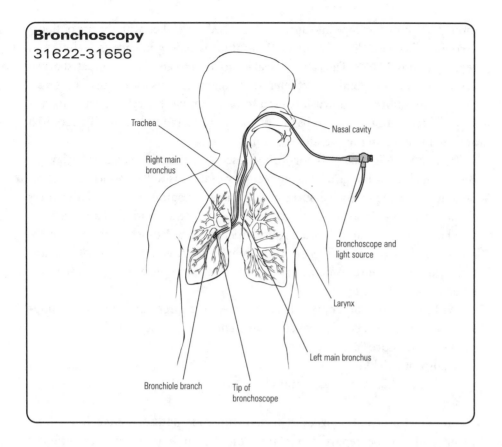

**Bronchoscopy**
31622-31656

Trachea

Nasal cavity

Right main bronchus

Bronchoscope and light source

Larynx

Left main bronchus

Bronchiole branch

Tip of bronchoscope

Code **31622** is designated as a separate procedure. Diagnostic bronchoscopy is not separately reported when performed as an integral component of another procedure/service. Surgical bronchoscopy always includes diagnostic bronchoscopy when performed by the same physician. (Refer to Chapter 4 for further discussion of the *separate procedure* designation.)

The following clinical vignette is provided as an example of the appropriate use of code **31622**:

**31622**   Bronchoscopy, rigid or flexible, with or without fluoroscopic guidance; diagnostic, with or without cell washing (separate procedure)

**EXAMPLE:** A 72-year-old man undergoes a diagnostic fiberoptic bronchoscopy for evaluation of hemoptysis. His chest X ray is normal. The physician inserts the bronchoscope through the upper airway, noting any abnormalities. The vocal cords are visualized, and the structure and function are noted. The bronchoscope is advanced into the tracheobronchial tree. The patient has mild erythema throughout the tracheobronchial tree. In the right lower lobe, blood is seen coming from the right posterior basilar segment. Sterile saline washings of this bronchus are obtained and sent for culture and cytologic examination.

Code **31623** describes bronchoscopy with brushings or protected brushings. Brushings or protected brushings take significantly more time to perform than bronchoscopy with cell washing. Protected brushings involve passing a catheter through the bronchoscope into an area of diseased lung, often with the use of fluoroscopic guidance. When performed, the fluoroscopic guidance is included in reporting code **31623**. The catheter seal is broken and an uncontaminated brush is then advanced beyond the catheter to obtain specimens for culture and sensitivity, or an unprotected brush is used to take samples for cytology and microscopic examinations. Several passes of the unprotected brush may be required and are included in the overall procedure.

Code **31624** is used to report bronchoscopy with bronchial alveolar lavage. Bronchial alveolar lavage allows the recovery of cells as well as noncellular components from the epithelial surface of the lower respiratory tract. This differs significantly from "washings," which refer only to the aspiration of secretions or small amounts of instilled saline from larger airways. Bronchial alveolar lavage involves repeated instillations of sterile saline occurring in aliquots with aspiration into one or more containers. Sequential and separate aspirations are numbered for laboratory testing.

Within the bronchoscopy code family, there are three distinct types of biopsies that are performed via bronchoscopy. They are as follows:
- Bronchial mucosal
- Transbronchial lung
- Transbronchial needle aspiration

Bronchial mucosal biopsies, reported with code **31625**, are taken by direct vision and can be reported one time only, even if performed at different anatomic sites.

Transbronchial lung biopsies, reported with code **31628**, are taken peripherally with fluoroscopic guidance of the biopsy forceps. It is important to note that when the transbronchial lung biopsies are taken from different lobes, they represent new procedures with independent risk factors such as biopsy forceps location of the lesion, bleeding, pneumothorax, or air embolism. Add-on code **31632** is reported in conjunction with code **31628** for the performance of a transbronchial lung biopsy performed in each additional lobe. A critical element to the appropriate application of these codes is that while add-on code **31632** may be reported for each biopsy performed in a separate lobe, it would not be appropriate to report multiple biopsies within the same lobe.

The third type of biopsy performed via bronchoscopy is transbronchial needle aspiration. Reported with code **31629**, transbronchial needle aspiration biopsies are taken centrally by penetration of a large airway with a specially designed biopsy needle and aspiration of a lymph node or central mass lesion. This represents a less invasive approach that otherwise would require an invasive surgical approach with additional potential risks of an open approach procedure. Add-on code **31633** is reported in conjunction with code **31629** for the performance of a needle aspiration biopsy performed in each additional lobe after the initial lobar needle aspiration procedure. As stated previously, a critical element to the appropriate application of these codes is that while add-on code **31633** may be reported for each aspiration biopsy performed in a separate lobe, it would not be appropriate to report multiple biopsies within the same lobe.

The possible sites for a bronchoscopic biopsy include the upper airway, which extends from the vocal cords to the lobar bronchi, and each of the five lobes of the lungs and their bronchi: the right upper, middle, and lower lobes and the left upper and lower lobes.

Code **31643** describes bronchoscopy with placement of catheter(s) for intracavitary radioelement application for clinical brachytherapy. This code includes only the bronchoscopy and placement of catheter(s). It does not include the clinical brachytherapy portion of the procedure. When performed, intracavitary radioelement application is reported separately with the appropriate code from the **77761-77763** series. Remote afterloading high-intensity brachytherapy is also reported separately with the appropriate code from the **77781-77784** series. (Refer to Chapter 7 for further discussion of brachytherapy.)

Code **31656** describes bronchoscopy with injection of contrast material for segmental bronchography. This code does not include the radiological portion of the procedure. When performed, the radiological S&I of the bronchography are reported separately with either code **71040** (unilateral procedure) or code **71060** (bilateral procedure).

## Thoracoscopy

Thoracoscopy is reported with the codes in the **32601-32665** series. A separate series of codes report diagnostic thoracoscopy (**32601-32606**) and surgical thoracoscopy (**32650-32665**).

Thoracoscopy is the direct examination of the pleural cavity using an endoscope. To insert the thoracoscope into the pleural cavity, pneumothorax must first be completed. This pneumothorax is included in the thoracoscopy code reported.

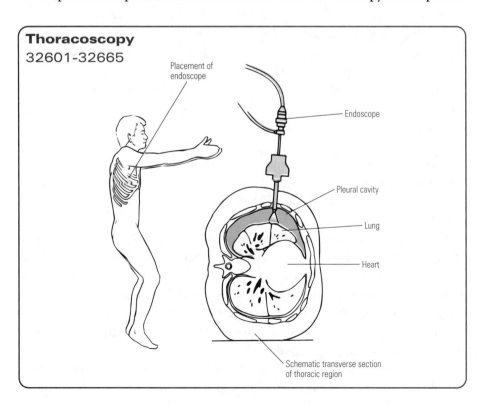

**Thoracoscopy**
32601-32665

Placement of endoscope

Endoscope

Pleural cavity

Lung

Heart

Schematic transverse section of thoracic region

Examination of the pleural cavity is possible only if the pleural space between the lung and chest wall is sufficiently large enough to manipulate the instruments easily and to visualize all important areas of the thoracic cavity. Depending on the location of the pleural lesion, the point of entry of the scope may vary for the affected area to be viewed, biopsied, or treated.

When thoracoscopy is enhanced with video-assisted techniques, the procedure is called video-assisted thoracic surgery (VATS). VATS requires additional incisions for the introduction of retractors and instruments used for exposure and dissection of lesions. VATS expands the intrathoracic image of conventional thoracoscopy (which is limited to the surgeon and restricted by the keyhole view from the thoracoscope) to multiple viewers. VATS allows the image obtained via the thoracoscope to be seen by multiple viewers by continuous video image display on a monitor in the surgical suite.

Diagnostic thoracoscopy involves examination and biopsy only. Surgical thoracoscopy, in addition to examination and possible biopsy, always includes a therapeutic operative procedure. Surgical thoracoscopy always includes diagnostic thoracoscopy. For example, thoracoscopic examination, biopsy, and decortication are all included when code **32651** is reported.

If more than one thoracoscopic procedure is performed during the surgical thoracoscopy, report all procedures separately. The primary procedure is reported without a modifier. Modifier 51 is appended to the secondary procedure(s) performed. Modifier 51 is used to report multiple procedures (other than E/M services) performed at the same session by the same provider. (Refer to Chapters 2 and 10 for further discussion of modifiers.)

If the thoracoscopic procedure that was performed is not specifically listed in the **32601-32665** series of codes, use the unlisted procedure code (**32999**). When reporting an unlisted code to describe a procedure or service, it will be necessary to submit supporting documentation (eg, procedure report) along with the claim to provide an adequate description of the nature, extent, need for the procedure, and the time, effort, and equipment necessary to provide the service. (Refer to Chapter 2 for an expanded discussion regarding unlisted codes.)

## Pneumonectomy

Codes for excision of a lung (pneumonectomy) are in the **32420-32525** series. Total pneumonectomy is reported with the codes in the **32420-32445** series. Removal of the lung involving other than total pneumonectomy is reported with codes in the **32480-32500** series.

A total pneumonectomy, as described by code **32440**, is removal of the entire lung. Code **32442** describes a sleeve pneumonectomy. A sleeve pneumonectomy involves a total pneumonectomy and also includes resection of the tracheal carina with end-to-end anastomosis of the trachea and contralateral (opposite side) mainstem bronchus. Extrapleural pneumonectomy, described by code **32445**, includes resection of the parietal pleura, which is the thoracic lining of the ribs, diaphragm, and mediastinum.

A lobectomy is the removal of a single lobe of the lung. Code **32480** reports a single lobectomy. This code describes either the removal of one of the three lobes in the right lung (right upper lobe, right middle lobe, or right lower lobe) or removal of one of two lobes in the left lung (left upper lobe, left lower lobe).

A bilobectomy, as described by code **32482**, is removal of two lobes of the right lung (eg, right upper and right middle or right middle and right lower). A bilobectomy is not removal of one lobe from the right lung and one lobe from the left lung. Bilobectomy is not a bilateral procedure. Bilobectomy is not performed on the left lung, since there are only two lobes on the left side. When both lobes of the left lung are removed, this operation is a pneumonectomy.

Each lobe of the lung has multiple segments. A segmentectomy, as described by code **32484**, is removal of one of the divisions of a lobe. Code **32486** is used to report a sleeve lobectomy. A sleeve lobectomy is similar to a lobectomy but also includes removal of a portion of the bronchus going to the remaining lung. Most commonly, sleeve lobectomies are upper lobectomies that include removal of the upper lobe plus a portion of the bronchus going to the lower lobe(s).

Completion pneumonectomy is reported with code **32488**. A completion pneumonectomy is a secondary operation in which the lung tissue remaining after previous lung excision surgery is entirely removed. For example, a portion of a right lung (eg, a lobe) has been removed previously for a cancerous tumor. The cancer recurs, and it is necessary to remove all of the remaining right lung tissue. This subsequent removal of the remaining lung tissue on the right lung is a completion pneumonectomy.

Code **32491** describes the excision of bullous or nonbullous emphysematous lung(s) for lung volume reduction. This code is specifically for procedures performed on patients with severe emphysema who are undergoing the procedure to reduce lung volume. Although this is generally a bilateral procedure, the word *lung* contains a parenthetic "(s)" because this procedure can be performed unilaterally. Therefore, code **32491** reflects both unilateral and bilateral procedures.

Code **32500** is used to report a wedge resection of the lung. A wedge resection is the removal of a portion of lung less than an anatomic segment. A wedge resection may also be referred to as a *limited resection* in that the lesion is excised as well as a margin of the surrounding normal lung. A wedge resection may be made in any portion of a diseased lung.

Code **32501** is an add-on code used to describe resection and repair of a portion of the bronchus when performed at the time of a lobectomy or segmentectomy. This code is used when a portion of the bronchus to the preserved lung is removed. A plastic closure is required to allow functional preservation and is not to be used for closure for the proximal end of a resected bronchus. Code **32501** is never to be reported as a stand-alone code. This code is intended to be reported in conjunction with codes **32480**, **32482**, and **32484**. (Refer to Chapter 4 for further discussion of add-on codes.)

## Lung Allotransplantation

Solid organ transplantation has rapidly evolved since the first living donor kidney transplantation was performed in the United States in 1954. Multiple factors have contributed to this evolution, including increased interest from living donors. Yet despite this interest, a discrepancy still exists between the number of potential recipients and the number of donors, which has resulted in increasing the utility of organs from deceased donors, thereby widening the pool of transplant organs available today. Technological advancements and better surgical skills allow today's transplant surgeons to salvage organs that would have previously been discarded.

To understand the complexity of lung allotransplantation, it may be helpful to review the three distinct components of physician work involved with this procedure. They are as follows:

- Cadaver donor pneumonectomy(s) (**32850**)
- Backbench work (**32855-32856**)
- Recipient lung allotransplantation (**32851-32854**)

The first component of the lung allotransplantation process is the cadaver donor pneumonectomy. This step involves preparation of the organ, including harvesting the allograft and cold preservation of the allograft (perfusing with cold preservation solution and cold maintenance), and is reported with procedure code **32850**. It is important to note that the harvest of the lung allograft may be from either a cadaver or living donor. However, when performing a heart and heart-lung transplant combination, grafts may be harvested from cadaver donors only.

The second component of physician work of the lung allotransplantation process is backbench work. This step involves standard preparation of a cadaver or living donor allograft prior to transplantation. Backbench work may include tailoring or reconstruction, ie, alteration of arteries and/or veins in order to render the allograft transplantable. Procedure codes **32855-32856** describe standard backbench work (eg, the dissection and removal of surrounding soft tissues) and reconstruction work (eg, alteration of organs) and reflect the expertise involved in the effort to render the organs usable.

The third and final component of physician work is allotransplantation, reported with codes **32851-32854**, as appropriate. This step includes the appropriate organ removal (if required) prior to transplantation, transplantation of the allograft, and care of the recipient.

In addition to the lung, the following organs may also be harvested from living or cadaver donors: kidney, intestine, liver, and pancreas, all of which have established transplantation reporting mechanisms in their respective anatomic code sections of the CPT codebook. See section V of Chapter 5 for an expanded transplantation discussion regarding the intestines, liver, and pancreas and section VI for an expanded discussion of renal transplantation.

# IV. Cardiovascular System

The Cardiovascular System section of the CPT codebook contains codes for reporting procedures of the heart and pericardium and arteries and veins.

This portion of Chapter 5 reviews the CPT guidelines associated with reporting pacemaker and defibrillator procedures and coding for coronary artery bypass procedures.

**Cardiac Anatomy**

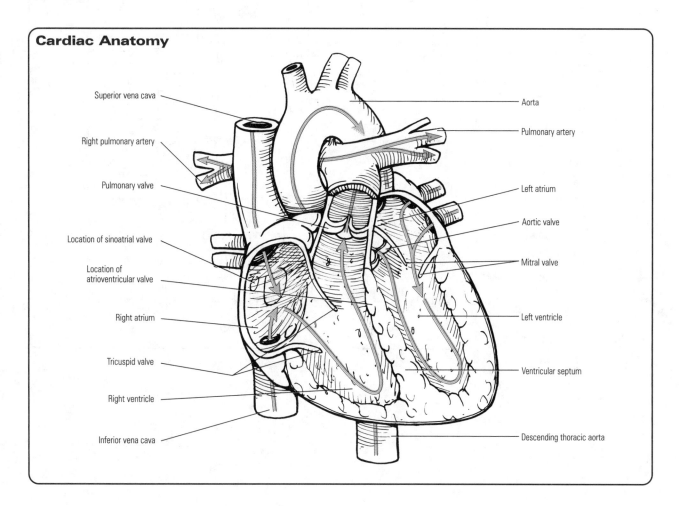

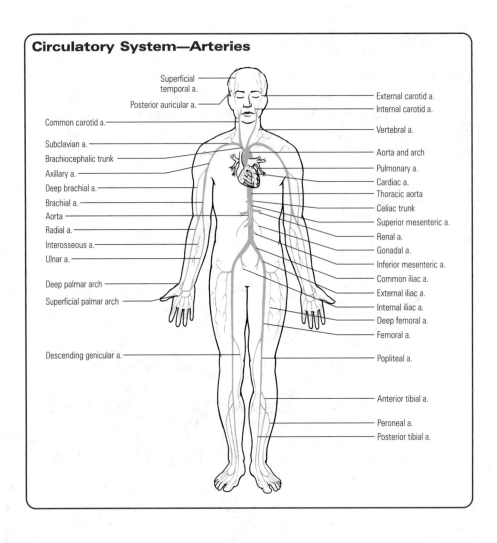

**Circulatory System—Arteries**

Superficial temporal a.
Posterior auricular a.
Common carotid a.
Subclavian a.
Brachiocephalic trunk
Axillary a.
Deep brachial a.
Brachial a.
Aorta
Radial a.
Interosseous a.
Ulnar a.
Deep palmar arch
Superficial palmar arch
Descending genicular a.

External carotid a.
Internal carotid a.
Vertebral a.
Aorta and arch
Pulmonary a.
Cardiac a.
Thoracic aorta
Celiac trunk
Superior mesenteric a.
Renal a.
Gonadal a.
Inferior mesenteric a.
Common iliac a.
External iliac a.
Internal iliac a.
Deep femoral a.
Femoral a.
Popliteal a.
Anterior tibial a.
Peroneal a.
Posterior tibial a.

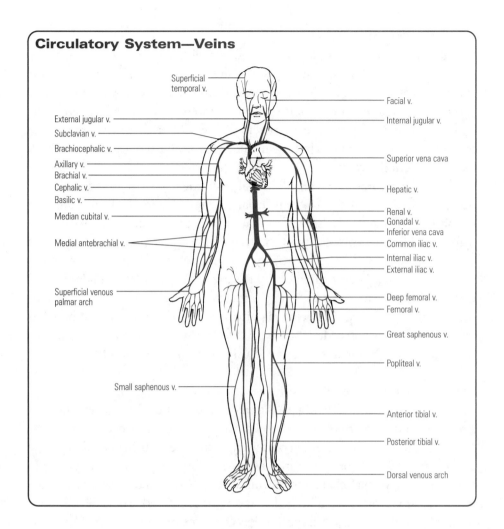

**Circulatory System—Veins**

Superficial temporal v.

Facial v.

External jugular v.

Internal jugular v.

Subclavian v.

Brachiocephalic v.

Superior vena cava

Axillary v.

Brachial v.

Cephalic v.

Hepatic v.

Basilic v.

Renal v.

Median cubital v.

Gonadal v.

Inferior vena cava

Medial antebrachial v.

Common iliac v.

Internal iliac v.

External iliac v.

Superficial venous palmar arch

Deep femoral v.

Femoral v.

Great saphenous v.

Popliteal v.

Small saphenous v.

Anterior tibial v.

Posterior tibial v.

Dorsal venous arch

## Transmyocardial Revascularization

Code **33140** describes a procedure performed on a beating heart that includes thoracotomy with opening of the pleural space or a sternotomy and opening of the pericardium to provide laser channels into the epicardium to vaporize tissue and create channels through the ventricular wall to the ventricular cavity to relieve angina. When performed as an adjunct to other cardiac procedures (eg, coronary artery bypass grafts), add-on code **33141** is reported.

## Pacemaker or Pacing Cardioverter-Defibrillator Guidelines

A pacemaker system includes a pulse generator (containing electronics and a battery) and one or more electrodes (leads). The pulse generator is placed in a subcutaneous pocket created either in a subclavicular site or underneath the abdominal muscles just below the rib cage. Electrodes (leads) may be inserted through a vein (transvenous) or placed on the surface of the heart (epicardial). Epicardial placement of electrodes requires a thoracotomy for electrode insertion.

## Types of Pacing Systems

In addition to the various placement methods, different types of systems may also be inserted. A single-chamber pacemaker system includes a pulse generator and one electrode inserted in either the atrium or ventricle. A dual-chamber pacemaker system includes a pulse generator and one electrode inserted in the right atrium and one electrode inserted in the right ventricle. Each of these electrodes is then connected to a pulse generator capable of pacing and sensing both the atrium and the ventricle.

In certain circumstances, an additional electrode may be required to achieve pacing of the left ventricle (bi-ventricular pacing). The implant procedure for the biventricular system is similar to that of a single- or dual-chamber system, with the additional complexity of the transvenous placement of the lead in a cardiac vein to reach the left ventricle. Implantation of a biventricular system requires a coronary guide catheter and the use of venography to guide the lead through the coronary sinus and into a cardiac vein for placement in the left ventricle. Transvenous (cardiac vein) placement of the electrode should be separately reported using code **33224** or **33225**. Epicardial placement of the electrode should be separately reported using code **33202** or **33203**.

## Pacing Cardioverter-Defibrillator Systems

Similar to a pacemaker system, a pacing cardioverter-defibrillator system includes a pulse generator and electrodes, although pacing cardioverter-defibrillators may require multiple leads, even when only a single chamber is being paced. A pacing cardioverter-defibrillator system may be inserted in a single chamber (pacing in the ventricle), in dual chambers (pacing in the atrium and ventricle), or as a biventricular system (pacing in the left and right ventricles). These devices use a combination of antitachycardia pacing, low energy cardioversion, or defibrillating shocks to treat ventricular tachycardia or ventricular fibrillation.

Pacing cardioverter-defibrillator pulse generators may be implanted in a subcutaneous infraclavicular pocket or in an abdominal pocket. Removal of a pacing cardioverter-defibrillator pulse generator requires opening of the existing subcutaneous pocket and disconnecting the pulse generator from its electrode(s). A thoracotomy (or laparotomy in the case of abdominally placed pulsed generators) is not required to remove the pulse generator.

The electrodes (leads) of a pacing cardioverter-defibrillator system are positioned in the heart via the venous system (transvenously), in most circumstances. However, in certain circumstances, an additional electrode may be required to achieve pacing of the left ventricle (biventricular pacing). In this event, transvenous (cardiac vein) placement of the electrode should be separately reported using code **33224** or **33225**. Epicardial placement of the electrode should be separately reported using code **33202** or **33203**.

## Epicardial Lead Placement

Electrode positioning on the epicardial surface of the heart requires thoracotomy, or thoracoscopic placement of the leads. Removal of electrode(s) may first be attempted by transvenous extraction (**33244**). However, if transvenous extraction is unsuccessful, a thoracotomy may be required to remove the electrodes (**33243**). Use codes **33212**, **33213**, **33240**, as appropriate, in addition to the thoracotomy or endoscopic epicardial lead placement codes to report the insertion of the generator if done by the same physician during the same session.

The generator is placed at a session other than that of the electrode placement. Codes **33202** and **33203** separate the services of lead placement from generator placement and allow reporting for lead placement in scenarios in which the cardiologist places the generator and one or more of the electrodes by a transvenous route. For cases of biventricular generator placement, left ventricular lead placement is performed by another physician at a different session. In these cases, the surgeon is asked to place the additional leads via thoracotomy, median sternotomy, thoracoscopic approach, or subxiphoid approach. In addition, there are times when new leads are required via transthoracic placement but no new pacemaker is required. Codes **33202** and **33203** allow these services to be reported separately and represent the variations that occur in the approach techniques used for epicardial lead placement.

**CODING TIP**

Codes **33202** and **33203** also represent left ventricular epicardial lead placement.

### Change of Pulse Generator (Battery)

When the "battery" of a pacemaker or pacing cardioverter-defibrillator is changed, it is actually the pulse generator that is replaced. Please note that a code for the removal of the pulse generator (eg, **33233**, **33241**) and a separate code for the insertion of the new pulse generator (eg, **33212**, **33213**, **33240**) are reported for the replacement.

### Device Replacement

If removal and replacement procedures are performed, then both procedures are reported separately. In most circumstances, the electrodes of a pacing cardioverter-defibrillator system are positioned in the heart via the venous system (transvenously). Removal of the electrode(s) may first be attempted by transvenous extraction, described by code **33244**. If transvenous extraction is unsuccessful, a thoracotomy may be required to remove the electrodes (as described by code **33243**). Replacement of a pacemaker electrode, pacing cardioverter-defibrillator electrode(s), or a left ventricular pacing electrode is reported using codes **33206-33208**, **33210-33213**, or code **33224**.

### Repositioning

Repositioning of a pacemaker electrode, pacing cardioverter-defibrillator electrode(s), or a left ventricular pacing electrode is reported with code **33215** or **33226**.

### Electrophysiologic Services

The codes in this section do not include the electrophysiologic evaluation of defibrillator systems or electronic analysis and monitoring of pacemakers or defibrillators. Electrophysiologic services are reported separately with codes in the Medicine section of the CPT codebook. (Refer to Chapter 9 for further discussion of reporting electrophysiologic services.)

### Radiological Supervision and Interpretation

Radiological supervision and interpretation (S&I) (eg, fluoroscopy) used for insertion of a pacemaker is a separately reportable service. The physician responsible for this portion of the procedure reports his or her services separately with CPT code **71090**. If the same physician is responsible for the radiological S&I and the insertion of the pacemaker/pacing cardioverter-defibrillator, that physician will report a code for the pacemaker insertion from the **33200** series of codes and code **71090** for the radiological S&I.

### Surgical Creation of a Pocket for Pulse Generator (Use of Modifier 62)

Surgical creation of a pocket for the pulse generator is included when the codes for pacemaker and pacing cardioverter-defibrillator procedures are reported. Use of modifier 62 becomes necessary when two physicians participate as primary surgeons during the single procedure. If one physician creates the pocket and a second physician inserts the device, each physician should report his or her distinct operative work by appending modifier 62, Two Surgeons, to the single definitive procedure code.

> **CODING TIP**
>
> Surgically creating a pocket for the pulse generator is included when the codes for pacemaker and defibrillator procedures are reported.

**EXAMPLE:** Physician A performs the surgical creation of the pocket for the pulse generator. Physician B inserts a permanent pacemaker with transvenous atrial and ventricular electrodes. The following codes would be reported:

Physician A:    **33208-62**

Physician B:    **33208-62**

Each physician should separately document his or her involvement in the performance of the single definitive procedure performed. This documentation should be submitted when the claim is filed with the insurance company. (Refer to Chapter 10 for further discussion regarding the use of modifier 62.)

Now that the various guidelines for reporting the pacemaker or pacing cardioverter-defibrillator codes have been reviewed, let us review the codes in this section of the CPT codebook.

### Pacemaker or Pacing Cardiodefibrillator Codes

Pacemakers are most commonly inserted using a transvenous approach, described by codes **33206-33208**. These codes include the subcutaneous insertion of the pulse generator and transvenous placement of electrode(s) and are specific to the chamber of the heart in which the transvenous leads are positioned (atrial; ventricular; atrial and ventricular). All three approaches require surgical creation of a pocket for placement of the pulse generator.

The use of the word *replacement* in the **33206-33208** code series is not meant to imply that the removal of an existing device is included in the replacement procedure. If an existing permanent pacemaker is replaced, then codes **33206-33208** are used to describe the insertion of the replacement pacemaker and transvenous electrode(s), while removal of the existing pacemaker is reported separately with a code from the **33233-33237** series.

## Insertion/Replacement of Temporary Transvenous Pacemaker/Electrode

Code **33210** describes the insertion or replacement of a single temporary transvenous pacing catheter, atrial or ventricular. Code **33211** describes the insertion or replacement of two temporary transvenous pacing catheters, atrial and right ventricular. These pacing catheters are then attached to an external pulse generator. Note that both of these codes have the *separate procedure* designation. (Refer to Chapter 4 for further discussion of this designation.)

## Insertion/Replacement of Pulse Generator

Codes **33212** and **33213** describe the insertion or replacement of only the pacemaker pulse generator. The code selection depends on whether one or two leads are reconnected to the pulse generator and tested for pacing and sensing parameters. In both instances, the pacemaker pocket is surgically reentered, the pulse generator is disconnected from the leads, the leads are tested to verify proper functioning, and a new pulse generator is attached and placed in the pacemaker pocket.

## Upgrade of Implanted Pacemaker System

Code **33214** is used to report the conversion of an implanted pacemaker system from a single-chamber to a dual-chamber system. This code includes removal of the previously placed pulse generator, testing of the existing lead, insertion of a new lead, and insertion of a new dual-chamber system pulse generator.

## Repositioning of Previously Implanted Pacemaker/Pacing Cardioverter-Defibrillator

Code **33215** describes repositioning of a previously implanted right atrial or right ventricular transvenous pacemaker or pacing cardioverter-defibrillator electrode. This code may be used to report repositioning of electrodes implanted for either single- or dual-chamber systems and may be reported at any time after the initial placement of the electrode. Remember to append the appropriate modifier (eg, modifier 59 for the same date of service or modifier 76, 77, 78, as appropriate) when repositioning is performed within the postoperative period.

> **CODING TIP**
>
> The appropriate method for reporting the repair of only one transvenous electrode for a dual-chamber device is to append modifier 52, Reduced Services, to code **33220**.

## Insertion of Transvenous Electrode(s)

Codes **33216** and **33217** describe the insertion of transvenous electrodes for either a single- or dual-chamber system. The single-chamber system requires insertion of one electrode (**33216**) and the dual-chamber system requires insertion of two electrodes (**33217**), one in the atrium and one in the right ventricle.

## Transvenous Electrode Repair

Codes **33218** and **33220** describe repair of pacemaker electrode(s). Correct code selection is based on whether a single electrode for a single-chamber device is repaired (**33218**) or two electrodes for a dual-chamber device are repaired (**33220**). If pulse generator replacement is required at the same session, either code **33212** or **33213** should be reported separately in addition to the code for the electrode repair.

### Revision/Relocation

Codes **33222** and **33223** are used to report revision and/or relocation of the skin pocket for a pacemaker or implantable cardioverter-defibrillator. Code **33222** describes revision or relocation of the skin pocket for a pacemaker, while code **33223** describes the revision of the skin pocket for a single- or dual-chamber pacing cardioverter-defibrillator.

### Insertion/Repositioning of Cardiac Venous System (Left Ventricular) Pacing Electrode

Codes **33224-33226** are used to report lead placement procedures in the cardiac venous system of the left ventricle to achieve biventricular pacing. This technique differs greatly from the simple, direct-lead positioning used for pacing of the right atrium or ventricle. Insertion of a left ventricular pacing electrode uses a transcatheter technique that provides access through the coronary sinus into a cardiac vein. Accurate placement of the electrode requires the use of venography to identify and map the cardiac venous system prior to placement of the lead.

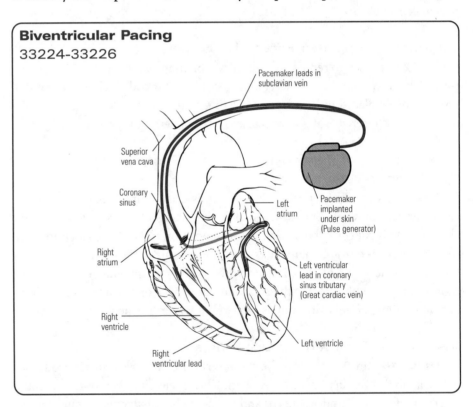

**Biventricular Pacing**
33224-33226

Pacemaker leads in subclavian vein

Superior vena cava

Coronary sinus

Left atrium

Pacemaker implanted under skin (Pulse generator)

Right atrium

Left ventricular lead in coronary sinus tributary (Great cardiac vein)

Right ventricle

Left ventricle

Right ventricular lead

**CODING TIP**

Code **33225** should never be reported as a stand-alone code, because of its designation as an add-on code.

Code **33224** describes the insertion of a pacing electrode into the cardiac venous system for left ventricular pacing and includes attachment to a previously placed pacemaker or pacing cardioverter-defibrillator pulse generator. Revision of the pacemaker pocket, removal, insertion, and/or re-insertion of the existing pulse generator are included in the procedure, if performed. When epicardial electrode(s) are inserted at the same session, code **33224** should be reported in addition to code **33202** or **33203**.

Code **33225** is an add-on code that is reported when insertion of a left ventricular pacing electrode is performed at the time of insertion of a pacing cardioverter-defibrillator or pacemaker pulse generator in the right atrium and/or ventricle. The parenthetical note following code **33225** lists the codes with which it may be reported.

Code **33226** is used to report repositioning of a previously implanted cardiac venous system left ventricular pacing electrode. This code also includes revision of the pacemaker pocket, removal, insertion, and/or re-insertion of the existing pulse generator and may be reported at any time after the initial placement of the electrode. The appropriate modifier (eg, modifier 59 for the same date of service, or modifier 76, 77, 78, as appropriate) should be appended when repositioning is performed within the postoperative period.

## Removal Procedures

Code **33233** describes removal of a permanent pacemaker pulse generator. Codes **33234** and **33235** describe removal of transvenous pacemaker electrode(s) from either a single-lead system with atrial or right ventricular lead placement (**33234**), or removal of a transvenous electrode(s) from a dual-lead system (**33235**).

Codes **33236**, **33237**, and **33238** describe thoracotomy as the surgical approach for the removal of a pacemaker pulse generator and pacing electrodes of an epicardial single-chamber system (**33236**) or epicardial dual-chamber system (**33237**), and the removal of permanent transvenous electrodes (**33238**). Removal of a single epicardial lead system (**33236**) requires exposure of a small area of the heart. Removal of a dual epicardial lead system (**33237**) usually requires more extensive exposure. The procedure described by code **33238** is used in cases where an infected transvenous lead has to be removed but attempts to remove it via the usual mechanisms (ie, **33234**) are unsuccessful. For a failed attempt at transvenous extraction, it would be appropriate to use (with the modifier 52, Reduced Services, appended) in addition to code **33238**.

## Pacing Cardioverter-Defibrillator Pulse Generator/Electrode(s)

The codes in the **33240-33249** series describe the techniques used for insertion, removal, and repair of implantable cardioverter-defibrillator generator and/or lead systems. Implantable cardioverter-defibrillators can be inserted by using an open surgical approach (eg, sternotomy or thoracotomy) or a transvenous approach for insertion of electrodes.

Code **33240** describes the insertion of a single- or dual-chamber pacing cardioverter-defibrillator pulse generator. This code may be reported for the initial insertion of the pulse generator or replacement of a previously placed device. If the pulse generator is replaced (ie, removal of an existing pulse generator and insertion of a new generator), then the removal of the existing implantable cardioverter-defibrillator pulse generator is reported separately.

Code **33241** describes the subcutaneous removal of a single- or dual-chamber pacing cardioverter-defibrillator pulse generator. Because the pulse generator is located outside the thoracic cavity (eg, in a pocket under the abdominal muscles), the removal does not require a thoracotomy. The removal of the electrode(s) is a separately reportable service with codes **33243** and **33244**, as appropriate.

Code **33243** is reported for the removal of single- or dual-chamber pacing cardioverter-defibrillator electrode(s) by thoracotomy or sternotomy. Code **33244** is reported for the removal of a single- or dual-chamber pacing cardioverter-defibrillator electrode(s) by transvenous extraction. Rather than creating a thoracotomy incision, the lead is removed through the blood vessel. Since trans-venous extraction is not always successful, a failed attempt at transvenous extrac-tion followed by removal by thoracotomy would be reported with code **33244** appended by modifer 52, *Reduced Services,* and code **33243**.

Code **33249** describes the insertion or repositioning of electrode lead(s) for single- or dual-chamber pacing cardioverter-defibrillator and insertion of the pulse generator by other than a thoracotomy approach.

## Electrophysiologic Operative Procedures

Supraventricular arrhythmias originate above the bundle of His. Surgical treat-ment of atrial fibrillation or flutter may be performed by either open incisional (**33254-33256**) or endoscopic approach (**33265-33266**). These families of codes describe combinations of surgical and electrophysiologic (radiofrequency, cryo-therapy, microwave, ultrasound, laser) techniques to place lesions that interrupt the intra-atrial reentrant pathways that support dysrhythmia (no rhythm) to create a mazelike pathway for sinus activation of the atria and the atrioventric-ular (AV) node. Any of the surgical methods described are utilized to create the new impulse pathways, in which excision or isolation of the left atrial appendage is accomplished. Stapling, oversewing, ligation, or plication are included and not separately reported.

If excision or isolation of the left atrial appendage by any method, including stapling, oversewing, ligation, or plication, is performed in conjunction with any of the atrial tissue ablation and reconstruction (maze) procedures (**33254-33259**, **33265**, and **33266**), it is considered part of the procedure and not sep-arately reported. The appropriate atrial tissue ablation add-on code (**33257**, **33258**, **33259**) should be reported in addition to a open cardiac procedure requiring sternotomy or cardiopulmonary bypass if performed concurrently.

*Limited* operative ablation and reconstruction (**33254** and **33265**) involves surgical isolation of supraventricular dysrhythmia triggers in the left or right atrium. Code **33254** describes a closed-heart operation for paroxysmal or short duration atrial fibrillation/flutter, using atrial incision(s) and adjunctive ablation techniques that are limited to the left atrium or do not extend to the AV annulus. Code **33265** describes a closed-heart, endoscopic operation for paroxysmal or short duration atrial fibrillation/flutter, using atrial incision(s) and adjunctive ablation techniques that are limited to the left atrium or do not extend to the AV annulus.

*Extensive* operative ablation and reconstruction (**33255**, **33256**, and **33266**) includes both those services included in the "limited" service description and any additional ablation of atrial tissue to eliminate sustained supraventricular dysrhythmias. To be considered *extensive*, the procedure must include operative ablation that involves either the right atrium, the atrial septum, or left atrium in continuity with the AV annulus.

Code **33255** describes a closed-heart operation for chronic atrial fibrillation or flutter, Cox Maze III or variation, atrial incision(s) and adjunctive ablation techniques that include extensive lesion sets and annular lesions. Only **33256** is reported if cardiopulmonary bypass is performed in addition to the maze procedure. Code **33253** was extensively revised and renumbered to code **33256**. Code **33266** describes a closed-heart endoscopic operation for chronic atrial fibrillation or flutter, Cox Maze III or variation, atrial incision(s) and adjunctive ablation techniques that include extensive lesion sets and annular lesions.

### Patient-Activated Event Recorder

Codes **33282** and **33284** describe the implantation and removal of an insertable loop recorder device that extends the cardiac monitoring period sufficiently to evaluate infrequent, recurrent symptoms. The implantation (**33282**) includes the initial programming of the device. Code **93727** is reported for subsequent or periodic electronic analysis, as well as any necessary reprogramming.

### Cardiac Valve Procedures

Code **33410** is used to report the performance of cardiac valve replacement involving suturing at both the inlet and outlet portions of the valve. The stentless tissue valve lacks the rigid stent and sewing ring of valves described by code **33405**.

## Coronary Artery Bypass Procedures

### Venous Grafting or Arterial Grafting

Coronary artery bypass graft (CABG) procedures may be reported in three ways, depending upon the type of operation performed. The first two reporting methods require only a single code as follows:

- A bypass operation performed with only venous grafts. This is reported with a single code from the **33510-33516** series, reflecting the number of distal anastomoses performed.
- A bypass operation performed with only internal mammary arteries or other arteries. This is reported with a single code from the **33533-33536** series, with code selection again reflecting the number of distal anastomoses performed. The codes in this series are also used to report coronary artery bypass procedures with a combination of arterial and venous grafts.

### Combined Arterial-Venous Grafting

- Bypass operations performed with a combination of venous and arterial grafts for distal anastomoses.

The third reporting method requires the use of two codes:

- A code from the **33517-33523** series to indicate that both arteries and veins were used. The appropriate code should describe the number of distal venous anastomoses used for the bypass; and
- An arterial graft code from the **33533-33536** series to indicate the number of distal arterial anastomoses required for the bypass procedure.

Codes in the combined arterial-venous grafting for coronary bypass series (**33517-33523**) are not to be reported alone. The appropriate vein graft code from this series is used in conjunction with a code from the arterial grafting

> **CODING TIP**
>
> Codes **33533-33536** are used for reporting arterial grafting for coronary artery bypass. These codes include the use of the internal mammary artery, gastroepiploic artery, epigastric artery, radial artery, and arterial conduits procured from other sites. However, for harvesting the radial artery, use code **35600**.

series (**33533-33536**) to completely describe combined arterial-venous grafting for coronary bypass. As indicated by the symbol placed before each code, codes **33517-33523** are add-on codes and exempt from the use of modifier 51, Multiple Procedures.

### Open Procurement of Graft Material

Open procurement of the saphenous vein graft is included in the description of work for codes **33510-33516** and **33517-33523** and should not be reported as a separate service or co-surgery. Arterial graft procurement is included in the description of work for codes **33533-33536** and should not be reported as a separate service or co-surgery. When a surgical assistant performs arterial and/or venous graft procurement, the assistant reports his or her services by appending modifier 80, Assistant Surgeon, to the appropriate code from the **33510-33516**, **33517-33523**, or **33533-33536** series.

Open procurement of these three types of graft material is reported separately as follows:

- Upper extremity vein (**+35500**)
- Femoropopliteal vein (**+35572**)
- Upper extremity artery (**+35600**)

The procurement of these vessels for graft material requires additional decision making and more technically difficult surgical work. These procedures may be indicated for patients who, for example, have had previous bypass surgery or severe vascular disease, resulting in a lack of suitable superficial autogenous vessels for graft material.

Codes **35500** and **35572** are designated as add-on codes and, as such, would not be reported alone. Code **35500** may be reported with CABG codes **33510-33536** and bypass graft codes **35556, 35566, 35571, 35583-35587**; code **35572** may be reported in conjunction with codes **33510-33516, 33517-33523, 33533-33536, 34502, 34520, 35001, 35002, 35011-35022, 35102, 35103, 35121-35152, 35231-35256, 35501-35587, 35879-35907**. Code **35600** is an add-on code. Modifier 51 should not be appended to codes **35500, 35572,** or **35600**.

## Endoscopic (Minimally Invasive) Venous Conduit Harvest

Harvesting of venous conduit using a minimally invasive endoscopic approach is not considered part of the CABG procedures (**33510-33523**) and is reported separately using the add-on code **33508**. Endoscopic harvesting of venous conduit includes the use of a trocar to establish the approach and video assistance for intraoperative visualization of the venous and tissue structures. These integral procedural components are not separately reportable.

## CABG Coding Examples

Let us review two examples of coding for CABG procedures.

**EXAMPLE 1:** A patient undergoes two CABGs including aortocoronary saphenous vein grafts to the right coronary artery (RCA) and the left anterior descending (LAD) artery.

---

**CODING TIP**

Procurement of the saphenous vein graft is included in the description of work for codes **33510-33516** and **33517-33523** and is not reported separately. However, procurement of an upper extremity vein for coronary artery bypass procedure is a separately reportable service. Procurement/harvest of an upper extremity vein for coronary artery bypass is reported with code **35500**, Harvest of upper extremity vein, one segment, for lower extremity or coronary artery bypass procedure (List separately in addition to code for primary procedure). For harvesting of an upper extremity artery (eg, radial artery), use code **35600**.

The following code is used to report this procedure:

**33511**   Coronary artery bypass, vein only; two coronary venous grafts

**EXAMPLE 2:** A patient undergoes three CABGs including aortocoronary saphenous vein grafts to the right coronary artery and the left circumflex artery. A left internal mammary artery bypass graft to the LAD artery is also performed. A total of three bypass grafts are performed, including two venous grafts and one arterial graft.

The following codes are used to report the bypass grafting described:

**33533**   Coronary artery bypass, using arterial graft(s); single arterial graft

**33518**   Coronary artery bypass, using venous graft(s) and arterial graft(s); two venous grafts (List separately in addition to code for arterial graft)

## Redo Operations

Code **33530** is an add-on code used to report coronary artery bypass or valve reoperation procedures performed more than one month after the original operation. Code **33530** is not reported alone; it is reported in addition to the appropriate code(s) to describe the bypass or valve procedure performed. Specifically, it is reported in conjunction with codes **33400-33496, 33510-33536, 33863**.

Code **33530** is reported to reflect the increased difficulty associated with the redo procedure.

Repeat sternotomy requires removal of previously placed wire sutures, which sometimes become embedded in the bony portion of the sternum. Because the anterior cardiac chambers, great vessels, and other mediastinal structures may be densely adherent to the posterior table of the sternum, the sternal incision must be made with extreme care to avoid potential hemorrhage. Once the mediastinum has been entered, the scarring and adhesions from previous surgery usually obscure the anatomic landmarks and make dissection both difficult and hazardous.

When a redo coronary artery bypass procedure is reported, only the number and type of bypass grafts used in the redo procedure are reported. Nothing from the first operation gets reported for redos. The removal of embedded sternal wires is considered inclusive in the redo operation and should not be reported separately. Supportive procedures (eg, Swan-Ganz catheter insertion and removal, arterial line insertion and removal, placement and removal of pacemaker wires, placement and removal of chest tubes) are also included in the coronary artery bypass operation codes and should not be reported separately. However, reoperation for bleeding, intra-aortic balloon insertion, and removal, as well as other services related to complications of the surgery would be reported if they occurred.

Consider the following example:

**EXAMPLE:** A redo triple coronary bypass operation is performed two years after the original procedure, with a combination of two saphenous veins and an internal mammary artery used for the redo. The original operation involved the use of only saphenous veins.

The redo procedure involved the use of two venous grafts and one arterial graft. Therefore, the appropriate codes for reporting the redo procedure are as follows:

**33533**   Coronary artery bypass, using arterial graft(s); single arterial graft

**+33518**   Coronary artery bypass, using venous graft(s) and arterial graft(s); two venous grafts (List separately in addition to code for arterial graft)

**+33530**   Reoperation, coronary artery bypass procedure or valve procedure, more than one month after original operation (List separately in addition to code for primary procedure)

## Cardiac Assist

Codes **33967** and **33968** are reported for percutaneous insertion (**33967**) and removal (**33968**) of an intra-aortic balloon assist device (IABAD) percutaneously through a femoral puncture in the groin. IABAD insertion, performed as an adjunct pumping assist measure, may be performed in addition to other cardiac procedures (eg, coronary artery bypass graft) for maintenance of hemodynamic stability and should be reported with modifier 51 appended.

## Endovascular Repair of Abdominal Aortic, Descending Thoracic Aortic, or Iliac Aneurysm

### Component Codes

Codes **33880-33881**, **34800-34826**, **34833-34834**, and **34900** represent a family of component procedure codes used to report placement of an endovascular graft for repair of an abdominal aortic aneurysm or for treatment of aneurysm, pseudoaneurysm, arteriovenous malformation (AVM), or trauma of the infrarenal abdominal aorta, descending thoracic aorta, or the iliac artery.

Component coding systems require the use of multiple codes to fully describe the total procedure performed. There are specific codes to describe open femoral or iliac artery exposure, catheterization of the vessel, device manipulation and deployment, associated radiological S&I services, and closure of the arteriotomy sites.

### Inclusive Procedures

Because a collapsed endoprosthesis is placed within the targeted treatment zone, balloon angioplasty and/or stent deployment within the target treatment zone, either before or after endograft deployment, are not separately reportable procedures. Introduction of guide wires and catheters should be reported separately (eg, **36140**, **36200**, **36245-36248**), but catheter manipulations during the procedure are necessary for device placement and deployment and are not reported separately. Extensive repair or replacement of an artery should be separately reported (eg, **35226** or **35286**).

### Radiological Supervision and Interpretation

Fluoroscopic guidance for placement of the graft, as well as radiological supervision for angioplasty/stent deployment in the target zone, are included in the radiological supervision and interpretation (S&I) codes (**75952**, **75953**, **75954**). Therefore, fluoroscopic guidance is not separately reported.

---

**CODING TIP**

The aortorenal bypass code 35560 is a unilateral code. Modifier 50 should be appended in the event that a bilateral procedure is performed.

---

**CODING TIP**

When applying the concepts of component coding to endovascular repair of abdominal and thoracic aortic and iliac artery aneurysms, be careful not to confuse the use of the term *component* when reporting these procedures. *Component coding* refers to the use of multiple codes to describe various procedures performed. Unrelated to component coding, the prosthetic device placed to accomplish aneurysm treatment may have one or more component(s), or modules.

### Separate Interventional Procedures

Other interventional procedures performed at the time of endovascular abdominal aortic aneurysm repair should be additionally reported. Examples include renal transluminal angioplasty, arterial embolization, intravascular ultrasound, balloon angioplasty, and stenting of native arteries outside the endoprosthesis target zone, when performed before or after deployment of the graft.

### Open (Direct) vs Endovascular Repair

While the graft material used in the repair may be similar to that used in an open repair, the method of attachment differs. In open (direct) repair of an abdominal aortic aneurysm (**35081, 35102**), the prosthesis is sutured proximally and distally to the artery undergoing repair.

During endovascular repair, the device is anchored above and below the aneurysm, thus sealing off the aneurysmal sac. Balloon dilatation and/or stent placement may be necessary within the device to ensure proper seating and expansion of the device. The endovascular approach uses minimally invasive techniques as opposed to the large incisions required to perform the open (direct) repair.

### Endoprosthesis Devices

Codes **34800-34805** are used to report the placement of the primary prosthesis for endovascular repair of an infrarenal aortic aneurysm. The main difference between these codes is the device shape and number of components.

Code **34800** describes placement of an endovascular tube graft, which can be placed through a single groin incision but frequently requires bilateral incisions for accurate placement. A closely related procedure to code **34800** is **34805**. Both are reported for endovascular aortic aneurysm repair. The primary differences are the length and shape of prosthesis required for effective aneurysm treatment. Code **34800** describes a tubular-shaped prosthesis that lies only within the abdominal aorta. Alternatively, code **34805** describes a procedure that requires the use of a longer prosthesis that extends into one iliac artery, therefore requiring a tapered cylindrical shape that is smaller in diameter at the distal end. All angioplasty performed within the target zone of the prosthesis deployment is included in **34805**, and therefore is not separately reported, as are any stent placements within the body of the graft, completion arteriograms, and pressure measurements.

---

**CODING TIP**

If the endovascular aortic or iliac repair procedure requires extensive repair or replacement of an artery, this should also be reported separately (eg, **35226, 35286**).

**Endovascular Repair of Abdominal Aortic Aneurysm**
34802

Using fluoroscopic guidance, a "compressed" prothesis is introduced through arteries in the groin and advanced into position with the aneurysm. Once in the aorta, the prothesis is expanded.

Renal arteries

Modular bifurcated prosthesis

Abdominal aortic aneurysm

Common iliac arteries

Code **34802** is reported for placement of a modular (two-piece) bifurcated aortic endograft. Code **34802** differs from code **34805** in description of the configuration, length, and shape of the prosthesis required to treat the aneurysm effectively. The prosthesis described by code 34802 is constructed of two separate pieces that are joined inside the patient's body during placement to make the ultimate configuration of an inverted "Y."

Code **34803** is reported for an endovascular abdominal aortic aneurysm repair using a modular bifurcated two-docking limb device. This code describes an inverted-*Y*-shaped three-piece modular prosthesis, which spans the infrarenal abdominal aorta with the limbs extending into each iliac artery. The proximal ends of the limbs are joined to the main prosthesis component in a modular fashion after the main body component of the prosthesis is deployed within the aneurysm during the procedure. The distal ends of each limb are extended into the iliac arteries.

Code **34804** is used to report use of a one-piece bifurcated (not modular) endoprosthesis. This code is most similar to **34802** with the *Y* configuration, but differs in that it is a one-piece construction.

Code **34900** describes introduction, positioning, and deployment of an endovascular graft for treatment of aneurysm, pseudoaneurysm, or arteriovenous malformation (AVM), or trauma of the iliac artery.

Code **34808** describes the placement of an iliac artery occlusion device for prevention of retrograde blood flow into the aneurysm sac. Often this requires restoration of blood flow beyond the occlusion device by performance of a femoral-femoral bypass crossover graft, reported with CPT code **34813**. Since open exposure of both femoral arteries is required to perform the femoral-femoral crossover, code **34812** should also be reported, appended by modifier 50, Bilateral Procedure.

Radiological S&I for aortic endograft repair is **75952**, including all types of endograft devices described by codes **34800** through **34808**. For endovascular repair of an isolated iliac aneurysm treated with an iliac endograft, **75954** is used for the radiological S&I provided for the procedure.

## Open Surgical Exposure of Arteries

Open surgical exposure of the access arteries is often required to accommodate the large delivery sheaths used for placement of the endovascular prostheses and may be necessary when the arteries are diseased or of an inadequate diameter to allow passage of the large endovascular sheaths. Therefore, artery exposure and catheterization (**36140**, **36200**, **36245-36248**) for delivery of aortic endovascular prosthesis are separately reportable.

Open femoral artery exposure by groin incision is reported with code **34812**. Since this is a unilateral code, modifier 50, Bilateral Procedure, should be appended if surgical exposure is performed bilaterally. Surgical exposure of the iliac artery through a retroperitoneal or abdominal incision is reported with code **34820**.

Code **34833** describes open surgical exposure of the iliac artery but also includes suturing of a temporary, large-diameter synthetic conduit onto the iliac artery. The endovascular repair is performed through this conduit, which is removed following completion of the procedure.

Brachial artery exposure, reported using code **34834**, may be performed when an alternate access is indicated (eg, during repair of a dissected aorta or for a patient with very tortuous iliac arteries).

## Proximal or Distal Extension Prosthesis

When an infrarenal aortic or iliac endograft is not long enough or the intraprocedural angiogram indicates the presence of an endoleak at the time of the original endovascular repair, codes **34825** and **34826** are reported to describe the placement of an extension graft or cuff to complete the repair. Code **34825** represents placement of a proximal or distal extension prosthesis in the initial vessel; code **34826** is reported for each additional vessel. Reporting is based on the number of vessels requiring extension prosthesis placement, not the number of extensions/cuffs placed in a single vessel.

The radiological S&I for cuff placement is coded as **75953**, used once for each vessel treated with cuffs/extensions. Endovascular extension placement performed during the postoperative period of the original procedure is reported with modifier 78, Unplanned Return to the Operating/Procedure Room by the Same Physician Following Initial Procedure for a Related Procedure, appended.

## Conversion to Open Surgical Procedure

In the event that complications arise during the endovascular repair procedure (eg, endoleak, dissection, occlusion of major arterial branches such as the renal arteries, acute occlusion of the aortic or iliac flow, device failure), codes **34830-34832** are reported to describe the conversion to an open surgical procedure for repair of complications involving a previously placed endoprosthesis.

These procedures differ from direct (open) aneurysm repair procedures, as the direct aneurysm repair codes are intended to report the initial open repair of a

> **CODING TIP**
>
> When thrombectomies are performed on anatomically different vessels through the same incision, each thrombectomy is separately reported, and modifier 59 is appended to the second procedure to indicate performance of the procedure on a different vessel.

ruptured or nonruptured aortic aneurysm and do not include removal of the failed endograft or repair of damage associated with failed placement of an endograft.

### Bypass Graft and Composite Graft

Procurement of the upper extremity vein is not included when a coronary artery bypass graft (CABG) or lower extremity bypass procedure is reported. Code **35500** is separately reported in addition to the grafting procedure (codes **33510-33536, 35556, 35566, 35571, 35583-35587**) for the harvest of a single vein segment for use in a lower extremity bypass or CABG procedure.

Code **35600** is intended to report the harvest of an upper extremity artery for use in coronary artery bypass grafting (CABG). This includes the procurement, implantation, and management of the free radial artery graft. Use of other arteries listed in the Coronary Artery Bypass Guidelines are included within the CABG procedure.

Codes **35682-35683** are intended to report the harvest of two or more vein segments from a limb other than that undergoing bypass for use as bypass graft conduit, reported with codes **35556, 35566, 35571**, and **35583-35587**, as appropriate.

### Excision, Exploration, Repair, Revision

Codes **35879, 35881** describe work performed on established lower extremity arterial bypass grafts in order to prevent thrombosis of the graft and possible subsequent limb loss. Codes **35879** and **35881** describe open revision of graft-threatening stenoses of lower extremity arterial bypass graft(s) (previously construction with autogenous vein conduit) using vein patch angioplasty or segmental vein interposition techniques. To differentiate, code **35876** should be used for thrombectomy with revision of any noncoronary arterial or venous graft, including those of the lower extremity (other than hemodialysis graft or fistula).

Codes **35883** and **35884** represent the revision of the femoral anastomosis of a synthetic arterial bypass graft typically performed to treat an arterial narrowing (stenosis) at the site where a synthetic bypass graft has been sewn (anastomosed) to the native femoral artery (groin). This type of stenosis may occur within a few months or many years after the original placement of the bypass graft.

The open femoral artery synthetic bypass revision codes **35883** and **35884** are unilateral procedures differentiated by use of an autogenous or nonautogenous graft to repair the stenotic graft site. Modifier 50, Bilateral Procedure, should be appended to report bilateral procedures. Codes **35883** and **35884** should not be reported for the same session.

The procedures described by **35700, 35875**, and **35876** are inclusive of codes **35883** and **35884** and would not be separately reportable.

Code **35700** would not be separately reported, as codes **35883** and **35884** would always be performed in a reoperative field.

Code **35500** would not be reportable if directly associated with code **35884**, because the harvest of a short segment of vein from a distant site is included in the work of the open synthetic bypass revision using an autogenous graft.

# Vascular Injection Procedures

Code **36002** is intended to report the treatment of iatrogenic pseudoaneurysms of the upper and lower extremities. Thrombin solution is introduced by needle injection into the pseudoaneurysm cavity until arterial bleeding has been demonstrably thrombosed.

## Insertion of Central Venous Access Device Procedures

To qualify as a central venous access catheter or device, the tip of the catheter/device must terminate in the subclavian, brachiocephalic (innominate), or iliac veins, the superior or inferior vena cava, or in the right atrium. The venous access device may be either centrally inserted (jugular, subclavian, femoral vein, or inferior vena cava catheter entry site) or peripherally inserted (eg, basilic or cephalic vein). The device may be accessed using either an exposed catheter (external to the skin) or using a subcutaneous port or subcutaneous pump.

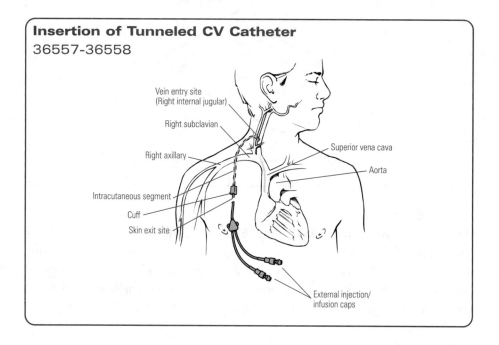

**Insertion of Tunneled CV Catheter**
36557-36558

Vein entry site
(Right internal jugular)

Right subclavian

Right axillary

Intracutaneous segment

Cuff

Skin exit site

Superior vena cava

Aorta

External injection/
infusion caps

The procedures involving these types of devices fall into the following five categories:

- Insertion
- Repair
- Partial replacement of only the catheter component associated with a port/pump device, but not entire device
- Complete replacement of entire device via same venous access site (complete exchange)
- Removal of entire device.

There is no coding distinction based on catheter size or between venous access achieved percutaneously (through the skin) or by cutdown technique (open exposure of venous access site).

### Device Insertion

Insertion (**36555-36571**) requires placement of the device through a newly established venous access site. Insertion procedures are further distinguished according to patient age. With the exception of the tunneled, centrally inserted central venous access device with subcutaneous pump (**36563**), separate codes are provided for patients under 5 years of age and those who are age 5 years or older.

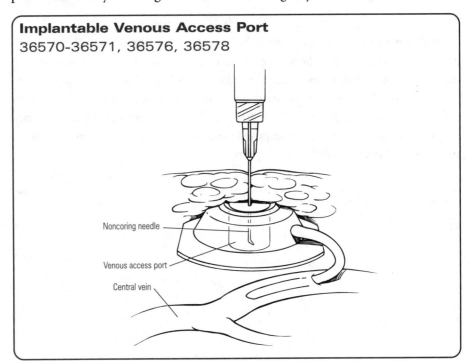

**Implantable Venous Access Port**
36570-36571, 36576, 36578

Noncoring needle
Venous access port
Central vein

### Repair of Device

When repair procedures (**36575**, **36576**) are performed, the existing catheter and/or pump/port device(s) are restored to proper function and reinserted using the same access site. Repair of a device does not include either pharmacologic or mechanical correction of intracatheter or pericatheter occlusion. When performed, these procedures should be reported using codes **36595** or **36596**, as appropriate.

### Replacement

Complete (**36580-36585**) and partial (**36578**) replacement of a device are performed using the existing venous access site. Complete device replacement involves the removal of the entire catheter and associated components and complete exchange using the same venous access site. Partial replacement involves exchange of only the catheter component of a port or pump device but not the port or pump device itself. This is performed using the existing venous access site. The same code is used whether or not a new tunnel is created and whether or not a new subcutaneous pocket is created. The determination of replacement depends upon use of the existing venous access.

### Removal

If an existing central venous access device is removed and a new one is placed using a separate venous access site, both the removal of the old device (**36589-36590**) and insertion of the new device should be separately reported. The removal codes apply to catheters that are tunneled or have a subcutaneous port and involve typically sharp and/or blunt dissection to remove the catheter.

## Multicatheter Devices

The codes used for reporting repair and replacement (partial and complete) reflect procedures performed on single-catheter devices. If these procedures are performed for multicatheter devices, use the appropriate code describing the service reported with a frequency of two. Replacement of the catheter portions only of a dual catheter subcutaneous pump involving two separate access sites should be reported by using code **36578** once for each separate catheter replaced. Insertion of a multicatheter device, requiring two catheters placed using two separate venous access sites, is reported using codes **36565-36566**.

## Radiological Guidance

When imaging is used for these procedures, either for gaining access to the venous entry site or for manipulating the catheter into final central position, use **76937** or **77001**, as appropriate, in addition to the code for the procedure(s) performed. The previous fluoroscopic guidance code (**75998**) has been replaced with **77001**. The new code includes contrast injection and venography if done from the same puncture as catheter placement. Venography may be coded separately only if the procedure requires venography for diagnostic purposes to allow placement of the central venous catheter and only if it must be done from a separate venipuncture site.

### Arterial

Code **36640** describes physician access for arterial catheterization that acts as a portal and remains in place until the completion of continuous prolonged chemotherapy infusion. Cutdown does not involve venoarterial cannulization, use of a membrane oxygenator/perfusion pump, or the chemotherapy infusion. Infusion is additionally reported by codes **96420-96425**, as appropriate.

### Extracorporeal Circulation Membrane Oxygenation (ECMO) Access

Code **36822** describes the bedside adaptation of cardiopulmonary bypass similar to that used during open heart surgery, wherein blood pumped by the heart is diverted from the lungs so that the lungs have a chance to rest and heal. Code **36822** also describes the use of portable percutaneous cardiopulmonary support systems for the provision of rapid, temporary, complete support of cardiac and pulmonary function in critically ill patients who are unresponsive to conventional therapy. The machine removes the blood from the body to eliminate carbon dioxide, oxygenate the blood, and return it to the body for systemic circulation.

### Regional Chemotherapy Access

Code **36823** describes placement of venoarterial cannulation for chemotherapy perfusion (supported by a membrane oxygenator/profusion device) to an isolated region of an extremity to treat a neoplastic process and includes calculation and administration of the chemotherapy agent injected directly into the perfusate, thus not requiring additional reporting of the chemotherapy administration code(s) **96408-96425**.

### Thrombectomy

The CPT Nomenclature has several codes that describe various procedures for thrombectomy procedures in the management of arterial or venous grafts. Code **35875** describes an open procedure for thrombectomy of nonhemodialysis grafts or fistulae. This procedure is typically performed in arterial or venous bypass grafts that have been placed for relief of limb ischemia or repair of extremity aneurysm or arterial trauma.

In contrast, codes **36831** and **36833** are reported for the performance of open thrombectomy of autogenous or nonautogenous dialysis grafts, in which a balloon catheter or other device is passed in both the proximal and distal directions to remove the thrombus. Code **36833** is further distinguished by the concurrent performance of an arteriovenous (A-V) access revision in addition to the thrombectomy procedure. Code **36832** is reported when an A-V access revision only is performed without thrombectomy at the operative session.

Code **36870** is reported for the procedure in which the approach for the autogenous or nonautogenous graft thrombectomy is performed percutaneously. The removal of the thrombus, as reported by this code, can be performed by any technology, including mechanical and/or pharmacologic thrombolysis in any combination of techniques or devices. Administration of a pharmacological thrombolytic agent, when performed by any technique, is an inherent component of this procedure. Procedures performed in addition to the thrombectomy (eg, access into graft or fistula, angioplasty, imaging, stenting, infusion outside the graft) are reported separately.

Codes **36860** and **36861** describe thrombectomy procedures performed on external types of dialysis devices. External dialysis devices are devices that contain dual-lumen central lines that have external ports. These types of catheters do not require open incisional techniques to remove the clots. This revision differentiates these procedures from thrombectomy procedures that require open procedures to perform (ie, procedures that require opening the vessel to remove the thrombus, coded as **36831**).

### Hemodialysis Access Creation

Code **36818** is reported for the performance of an open upper arm cephalic vein transposition to include tunneling for brachiocephalic anastomosis. This procedure requires two upper-arm incisions, one medial over the brachial artery, the other lateral to expose the vein. A tunnel is created between the incisions, and complete dissection of a substantial portion of the cephalic vein is required to allow it to be moved to a more superficial location and pulled through the tunnel for anastomosis with the brachial artery on the medial aspect of the upper arm. This approach is often performed in patients with large or obese arms.

Code **36819** is reported for direct A-V anastomosis by basilic vein transposition. The result of this procedure is the creation of permanent hemodialysis access. This extensive procedure includes the dissection of the basilic vein from the antecubital crease to the axilla. It also includes the associated nerve preservation, tunnel creation, vein relocation, and anastomosis.

Code **36818** differs from code **36819** in that the procedure described by code **36819** consists of the basilic vein transposition for brachiobasilic anastomosis.

Additionally, code **36820** consists of forearm vein transposition performed in the lower arm between the elbow and the wrist.

Code **36821** describes a less extensive procedure that includes direct anastomosis of a vein to an artery. This procedure is typically performed at the wrist and involves only a moderate amount of arterial and venous dissection.

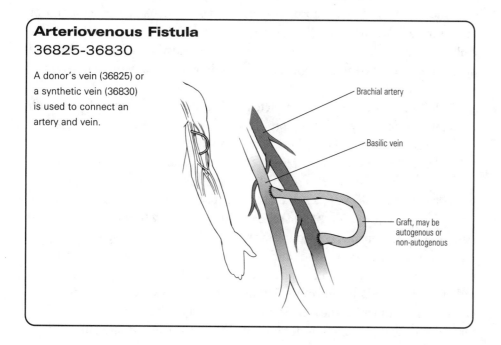

**Arteriovenous Fistula**
36825-36830

A donor's vein (36825) or a synthetic vein (36830) is used to connect an artery and vein.

Brachial artery

Basilic vein

Graft, may be autogenous or non-autogenous

Code **36830** is the most commonly performed hemodialysis access operation and is used to report placement of a synthetic subcutaneous tube graft in which one end is anastomosed to the brachial artery and the other to a large vein. This is most often performed when patients do not have large, visible wrist veins for the performance of a native (eg, Cimino) fistula reported with code **36821**.

## Transcatheter Procedures

Code **37204** describes performance of therapeutic occlusion of nonhead/nonneck and non-CNS arteries or veins (for head/neck and CNS embolization, see **61624** and **61626**). The embolization material is delivered through small catheters to temporarily or permanently stop flow to the area supplied by a blood vessel.

Common indications for embolization include the presence of abnormal arteries or veins or a combination of both (AVMs); life-threatening bleeding in the lungs, gastrointestinal tract, or pelvis; and tumors that are supplied by a large number of blood vessels. Some transcatheter embolization agents used when reporting **37204** include gelatin sponge, polyvinyl alcohol, coils, and ethanol and glue.

Embolization procedures are reported with component coding. The selective catheterization code for the desired vessel(s), angiography (injecting contrast), if not previously performed, S&I embolization code (**75894**), and surgical embolization code **37204** are reported for a transcatheter embolization procedure. Both of the embolization codes (**37204** and **75894**) are reported one time each for embolotherapy performed in a single operative field, regardless of the number of vessels or numbers of embolization agents required to complete the embolization.

However, the embolization codes **37204** (surgical component) and **75894** (S&I component) are reported for each operative field treated (eg, right and left kidney, right and left lung). In this case, modifier 59, Distinct Procedural Service, should be appended to designate the separate sites treated.

In addition to the embolization codes, codes for diagnostic angiogram or venogram are reported if the diagnostic study is done at the time of the embolization. Code **75898**, angiogram through an existing catheter, is also used once for each field treated for the angiogram done to document completion of the embolization.

Code **37210** describes the complete procedure to treat uterine fibroids with bilateral uterine artery embolization. This procedure is an exception to the previously listed rules for coding therapeutic embolizations.

Codes **37215** and **37216** are reported for percutaneous stent placement in the cervical portion of the extracranial carotid artery. The codes are further distinguished by the use of or lack of employment of an embolic protection system.

Unlike procedure code **37204**, codes **37215** and **37216** are inclusive of all aspects of the therapeutic procedure, including catheterization, diagnostic angiography of the ipsilateral carotid, and all radiologic supervision and interpretation. It is important to note that the appropriate codes for reporting carotid catheterization and imaging of the ipsilateral carotid only are reported for those circumstances in which the carotid catheterization and imaging have been performed and stent placement is not indicated for treatment. Additionally, all arteriographic imaging of the ipsilateral cervical and cerebral carotid arteries is included and not separately reported. Therefore, codes **37215** and **37216** include the following:

- Selective ipsilateral carotid access
- All diagnostic imaging for ipsilateral common carotid bifurcation and cerebral vessels
- All related radiological S&I interpretation required to complete the therapeutic stent placement.

When the initial ipsilateral carotid arteriogram (including imaging and access) confirms the need for carotid stenting, codes **37215** and **37216** are inclusive of these services. If carotid stenting is not indicated, then the appropriate codes for carotid catheterization and imaging would be reported in lieu of codes **37215** and **37216**.

# V. Digestive System

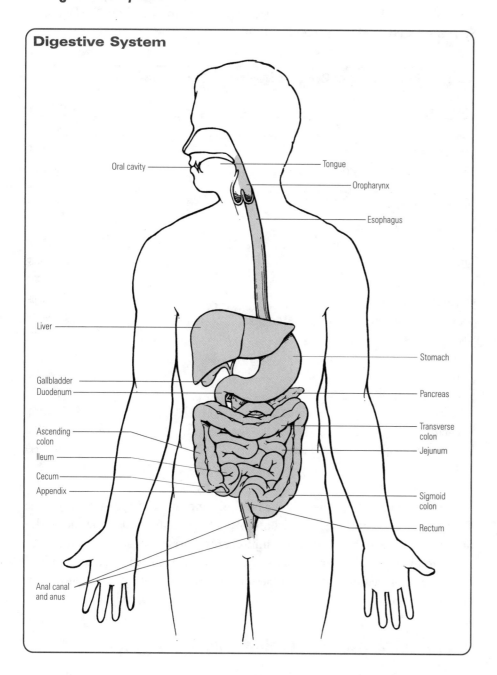

**Digestive System**

Oral cavity

Tongue

Oropharynx

Esophagus

Liver

Stomach

Gallbladder

Duodenum

Pancreas

Ascending colon

Transverse colon

Ileum

Jejunum

Cecum

Appendix

Sigmoid colon

Rectum

Anal canal and anus

## Section Layout

The following table indicates the categories of codes found within the Digestive System subsection of the Surgery section.

| Digestive System Categories and Code Ranges | |
|---|---|
| **Category** | **Range of Codes** |
| Lips | 40490-40799 |
| Vestibule of Mouth | 40800-40899 |
| Tongue and Floor of Mouth | 41000-41599 |
| Dentoalveolar Structures | 41800-41899 |
| Palate and Uvula | 42000-42299 |
| Salivary Gland and Ducts | 42300-42699 |
| Pharynx, Adenoids, and Tonsils | 42700-42999 |
| Esophagus | 43020-43499 |
| Stomach | 43500-43999 |
| Intestines (Except Rectum) | 44005-44799 |
| Meckel's Diverticulum and the Mesentery | 44800-44899 |
| Appendix | 44900-44979 |
| Rectum | 45000-45999 |
| Anus | 46020-46999 |
| Liver | 47000-47399 |
| Biliary Tract | 47400-47999 |
| Pancreas | 48000-48999 |
| Abdomen, Peritoneum, and Omentum | 49000-49999 |

Take a few moments to review the headings and subheadings in the Digestive System subsection of the CPT codebook. Attention will be focused on the guidelines associated with reporting the common procedures of tonsillectomy and adenoidectomy, enterectomy, appendectomy, various gastrointestinal endoscopy and laparoscopy procedures, lysis of adhesions, intraperitoneal catheter placement, and hernia repair.

## Allotransplantation/Transplantation

Similar to the endoscopy general guidelines, there is a common template of guidelines and codes for reporting allotransplantation or transplantation procedures performed on the intestines (except rectum), liver, and pancreas.

The guidelines for transplantation procedures performed on these organs are structured according to three physician work components and follow the template described later. The guidelines should be reviewed carefully before attempting to code the following procedures:

- Removal of donor organ (eg, donor enterectomy, donor hepatectomy, etc)
- Backbench work
- Recipient transplantation/allotransplantation

Backbench work is the preparation of the donor organ graft for transplantation to the recipient site. The specific work involved in backbench work is defined in the guidelines. This preparation of the graft is performed on a backbench in the operating room, hence the term *backbench work*.

To code these three components of physician work, one must first go to the appropriate anatomic site within the Digestive System subsection of the CPT codebook. Once there, notice that each of these components is separately reported with specific codes. This is a common theme among the three anatomic sites—intestines, liver, and pancreas. However, it is important to note that there are subtle variations to the reporting of these procedures for each anatomic site.

In the Intestines (Except Rectum) subsection, guidelines for all three components of physician work are listed under the Excision heading. Notice that the donor enterectomy codes (**44132** and **44133**) and allotransplantation codes (**44135** and **44136**) are listed under the Excision heading, and the backbench work codes (**44715**, **44720**, and **44721**) are listed under the Other Procedures heading.

In the Liver subsection, the same template of guidelines is listed under the Transplantation heading. The donor hepatectomy codes (**47133**, **47140-47142**), backbench work codes (**47143-47147**), and the allotransplantation codes (**47135** and **47136**) are all listed under the Transplantation heading.

Similarly, the guidelines for the same physician work components involving the pancreas are listed in the Pancreas subsection under the Transplantation heading. Codes for donor pancreatectomy (**48550**), backbench work (**48551**, **48552**, and **48554**), and allotransplantation (**48554**) are listed here as well.

The operative report for backbench preparation of an intestine allograft should document the mobilization and fashioning of the mesenteric artery and vein.

When coding backbench work for liver graft, review the operative report carefully for the type of backbench preparation performed, as there are three codes to choose from for backbench preparation (**47143**, **47144**, or **47145**).

Standard backbench work to prepare a pancreas allograft (following donor pancreatectomy and prior to allotransplantation to recipient site) includes a splenectomy, duodenotomy, ligation of bile duct, ligation of mesenteric vessels, and Y-graft arterial anastomoses from the iliac artery to the superior mesenteric artery and to the splenic artery. This work should be documented in the operative report and is an integral part of code **48551**.

Backbench preparation may include additional reconstruction of the graft such as venous and/or arterial anastomosis(es) prior to transplantation. This additional work is reported separately and is identified by codes **44720** and **44721** (intestine allograft), **47146** and **47147** (liver graft), and **48552** (pancreas allograft). The operative report should be reviewed for this additional work and the appropriate code reported based on the additional work performed.

## Lips

### Repair (Cheiloplasty)
Code **40650** describes a full thickness repair of the vermilion ("pink lip") only. This repair involves all layers of tissue (ie, mucosa, submucosa, and subcutaneous tissue).

## Tonsillectomy and Adenoidectomy

Codes for reporting tonsillectomy and adenoidectomy procedures are found in the **42820-42836** series. Separate codes are listed to describe the following:

- Tonsillectomy and adenoidectomy (**42820-42821**)
- Tonsillectomy alone, whether primary or secondary (**42825-42826**)
- Adenoidectomy alone, primary (**42830-42831**)
- Adenoidectomy alone, secondary (**42835-42836**)

Once the range of codes for the type of procedure performed has been identified, the appropriate code is then selected on the basis of the age of the patient. Separate codes are reported for procedures performed on patients under age 12 and age 12 or older. This criterion of age is fairly uncommon in the CPT code set and is meant to serve as an indication of the level of difficulty of the procedure.

A primary procedure is one in which no prior tonsillectomy or adenoidectomy has been performed. A secondary procedure is one that is performed to remove residual or regrowth of tonsil or adenoid tissue. The medical record should be carefully reviewed for information on prior tonsillectomy or adenoidectomy, in the event that the surgeon does not indicate the operation as primary or secondary.

All of the codes in this section are intended to represent bilateral procedures. Do not append modifier 50, Bilateral Procedure, to these codes. If the procedure is performed as a unilateral procedure, modifier 52, Reduced Services, should be appended to the code.

Separate codes are available within the Pharynx, Adenoids, and Tonsils category for reporting control of hemorrhage after tonsillectomy and adenoidectomy procedures. Codes **42960-42962** are used to report control of oropharyngeal hemorrhage after tonsillectomy. Codes **42970-42972** are used to report control of nasopharyngeal hemorrhage after adenoidectomy. The appropriate code should be chosen on the basis of the specific procedure performed to control the hemorrhage. These circumstances are reported by appending modifier 78, Unplanned Return to the Operating/Procedure Room by the Same Physician Following Initial Procedure for a Related Procedure During the Postoperative Period, to the code reported for the control of hemorrhage.

## Intestines (Except Rectum)

### Lysis of Adhesions

The guiding principle in reporting lysis of adhesions (**44005**, **44180**) separately is the complexity involved in performing this procedure. Many patients have some adhesions, and while it may be necessary to lyse them when doing another surgical procedure, it is not always appropriate to report the lysis procedure separately.

When the adhesions are few, are reasonably easy to lyse, and add very little additional time and effort to the primary surgery, the lysis is generally not reported as an additional procedure. If, however, the adhesions are multiple or dense, cover the primary operative site, or add considerable time to the operative procedure and increase the risk to the patient, the procedure may be reported.

This can be done either by appending modifier 22, Increased Procedural Services, to the primary surgical code or by reporting the appropriate lysis code appended by modifier 51, Multiple Procedures.

If lysis of adhesions is performed independent of any other procedure, then code **44005** or **44180** should be reported.

### Excision

Codes **44126** and **44127** and add-on code **44128** describe the surgical techniques for correcting small intestinal atresias, a congenital anomaly unique to newborns and preterm infants. Code **44126** describes resection of a segment of small intestine in which an atresia is present and does not involve tapering of the intestine. Code **44127** also describes resection of a segment of a small intestine where an atresia is present but that also involves tapering of the intestine. Add-on code **44128** describes resection of each additional intestinal segment in which an atresia is present.

### Laparoscopy

Codes **44202-44213** reflect the complexity of performing different types of laparoscopic intestinal resections (ie, small bowel vs colon vs rectum), such as in the treatment of Crohn's colitis, colonic polyps, diverticulosis with or without hemorrhage, diverticulitis, colon obstruction, rectal prolapse, sigmoid/cecal volvulus, angiodysplasia of the colon, and colon cancer.

If the open procedure counterpart of a laparoscopic procedure is performed, then the code that describes the open procedure should be reported.

If a laparoscopic procedure is performed but there is not a CPT code that accurately describes the laparoscopic procedure, the open procedure code should not be reported. Instead, the unlisted laparoscopic code (**44238** for the intestine except rectum or **45499** for the rectum) should be reported. An open procedure code should never be reported to describe a procedure that was performed laparoscopically.

### Appendectomy

There are four codes listed in the CPT code set for reporting appendectomy procedures. Codes **44950-44960** describe open surgical appendectomy procedures. Code **44970** is used to report laparoscopic appendectomy. Careful review of each code descriptor and the parenthetical notes following the codes is necessary to make the appropriate code selection.

Code **44950** is used to report an appendectomy. The parenthetical note that follows this code indicates that an incidental appendectomy during intra-abdominal surgery usually does not warrant a separate identification. Thus, when an incidental appendectomy is performed, a separate code is usually not reported for the appendectomy. However, if it is necessary to report the incidental appendectomy, modifier 52, Reduced Services, should be appended to procedure code **44950**.

Code **44955** describes an appendectomy performed for an indicated purpose at the time of another major procedure. This code describes an appendectomy

> **CODING TIP**
>
> Do not report diagnostic laparoscopy or laparoscopic lysis of adhesions in addition to the laparoscopically assisted small bowel resection, as these services are included.

not performed as an independent procedure. The add-on code designation associated with this code indicates that it is to be listed separately in addition to the code for the primary procedure performed. This code would never be reported alone.

Code **44960** is specifically used to report an appendectomy performed for a ruptured appendix with abscess or generalized peritonitis.

Finally, if the appendectomy is performed laparoscopically, then code **44970** is reported to describe this procedure.

## Endoscopy—General Guidelines

Within the Digestive System subsection of the CPT codebook, a number of codes are available for reporting endoscopy procedures. When reporting the endoscopy procedures, remember that surgical endoscopy always includes diagnostic endoscopy.

In reviewing the codes and definitions for reporting the various endoscopy procedures, one will recognize a common template used for each of the endoscopy code families discussed. This template has been used to list a consistent set of procedures within each procedural family of codes.

The template is based on the specific technique used during the procedure. Codes are available to describe the following:

• Biopsy
• Removal of foreign body
• Dilation
• Hot biopsy or bipolar cautery treatment
• Snare treatment
• Ablation of lesion not amenable to treatment by hot biopsy, bipolar treatment, or snare
• Control of bleeding

Several endoscopic procedures listed in the CPT codebook deal with the endoscopic control of bleeding. The codes are intended to be used when treatment is required to control bleeding that occurs spontaneously or as a result of traumatic injury (noniatrogenic), and not as a result of another type of operative intervention.

For example, if a sigmoidoscopy with endoscopic biopsy is performed and the excision of the tissue specimen causes bleeding that is controlled endoscopically, this would be reported only with code **45331** (for the sigmoidoscopy with biopsy). In this case, it is incorrect to report code **45334** (sigmoidoscopy with control of bleeding) to describe the situation, because any control of iatrogenically caused bleeding is included within the biopsy procedure.

Notice that when two distinct procedures are performed on the same day or at the same session, it is appropriate to report these procedures separately. This guideline also applies in the instance when multiple procedures identified by different indented codes within the same family of codes are performed. Consider the following two examples:

**EXAMPLE 1:** Two or more procedures from the same family of codes are performed on the same patient by the same physician at the same session.

An esophagogastroduodenoscopy (EGD) with biopsy (code **43239**) and an EGD with dilation of gastric outlet for obstruction (code **43245**) are performed. The physician reports the codes as follows:

**43245**

**43239 59**

In this case, both codes are reported to completely describe the procedures performed. The primary procedure is reported without the use of a modifier. Modifier 59, Distinct Procedural Service, is appended to indicate that the procedures were performed during different sessions. (Refer to Chapters 2 and 10 for further discussion of the use of modifiers.)

**EXAMPLE 2:** An upper gastrointestinal endoscopy and lower gastrointestinal endoscopy are performed on the same patient by the same physician on the same day.

A diagnostic colonoscopy (code **45378**) and a diagnostic EGD (code **43235**) are performed on the same patient by the same physician on the same day (not during the same session). The physician would report the codes as follows:

**45378**

**43235 59**

In this case, both codes are reported to completely describe the procedures performed. The primary procedure is reported without the use of a modifier. Modifier 59, Distinct Procedural Service, is appended to indicate that the procedures were performed during different sessions. (Refer to Chapters 2 and 10 for further discussion of the use of modifiers.)

## Biopsy and Excision of Same Lesion

When endoscopic procedures are performed, if the same lesion is biopsied and subsequently removed during the same operative session, only the code for the removal of the lesion would be reported. However, if one lesion is biopsied and a separate lesion is removed during the same operative session, report a code for the biopsy of one lesion and an additional code for the removal of the separate lesion. Consider the following examples:

**EXAMPLE 1:** A colonoscopy with biopsy of a lesion in the transverse colon is performed. That same lesion is removed later in the same operative session by snare technique. In this example, only code **45385** is reported.

**EXAMPLE 2:** An EGD is performed with biopsy of two separate lesions, one in the stomach and one in the esophagus. During the procedure, the lesion in the stomach is subsequently removed by bipolar cautery.

In this example, it would be appropriate to report two codes; code **43239** is reported for the biopsy of the lesion in the esophagus and code **43250** for the removal of the lesion in the stomach. The biopsy of the lesion in the stomach is not separately reported. In this case, the use of modifier 59, Distinct procedural service, is necessary to indicate that two separate areas were involved. (Refer to Chapter 10 for further discussion regarding the use of modifier 59.)

**EXAMPLE 3:** A colonoscopy is performed with biopsy of a lesion in the transverse colon and removal of a lesion by hot biopsy forceps in the ascending colon. In this example, it is appropriate to report two codes: code **45384** for the removal of the lesion in the ascending colon and code **45380**, with modifier 59 appended, for the biopsy of the lesion in the transverse colon.

> **CODING TIP**
>
> Code **44361**, should be reported to describe a "push enteroscopy of the distal duodenum and jejunum with gastric biopsy" using a pediatric colonoscope.

When the biopsy of one lesion and the removal of another lesion using a different technique from a different site during the same operative session is performed, the use of modifier 59, Distinct Procedural Service, is essential to report the different procedures. Modifier 59 is used to indicate that there was a separate incision/excision, separate lesion. If one lesion is biopsied and a separate lesion is removed, it would be appropriate to append modifier 59 to the code reported for the biopsy procedure. (Refer to Chapters 4 and 10 for further discussion regarding the use of modifier 59.)

Now that some of the guidelines that are common to all of the endoscopy families of codes have been reviewed, let us take a closer look at some of the specific endoscopic code families. The following table indicates the various endoscopy series of codes that will be discussed in this chapter.

## Endoscopy Types and Code Ranges

| Type of Endoscopy | Code Range |
| --- | --- |
| Esophagoscopy | 43200-43232 |
| Esophagogastroduodenoscopy (EGD) | 43234-43259 |
| Proctosigmoidoscopy | 45300-45327 |
| Sigmoidoscopy | 45330-45345 |
| Colonoscopy | 45378-45392 |
| Anoscopy | 46600-46615 |

### Esophagoscopy

Codes **43200-43232** describe various esophagoscopy procedures. Esophagoscopy is limited to study of the esophagus. When the endoscope passes the diaphragm into the stomach, the procedure is esophagogastroscopy. When the pyloric channel is traversed, it is described as esophagogastroduodenoscopy. Codes **43200-43272** include moderate (conscious) sedation when performed.

In reviewing this series of codes, keep in mind the template used for endoscopy procedures. The information provided regarding single or multiple biopsies; removal or ablation of tumors, polyps, or other lesions; and control of bleeding can be applied to the codes in other endoscopy families with similar code descriptors.

The parent code in this series (code **43200**) describes a diagnostic esophagoscopy, where an endoscope is passed through the mouth into the esophagus. When performed, the collection of specimens by brushing or washing is included in reporting this code. Code **43200** has been designated as a "separate procedure." If a surgical endoscopy is performed during the same session, the diagnostic endoscopy is not separately reported. (Refer to Chapter 4 for further discussion of the separate procedure designation.)

Code **43201** describes esophagoscopy with directed submucosal injection(s), any substance. The code descriptor includes an "(s)" at the end of the word injection. Therefore, this code should be reported only one time, regardless of the number of injections performed. Examples of substances that may be injected are India ink, botulinum toxin, saline, and corticosteroid solutions. This code is not used to report injection sclerosis of esophageal varices (varicose veins in the esophagus), which is reported using code **43204**. Code **43227** is used to report injection of substances to control bleeding.

Code **43202** describes esophagoscopy with biopsy. The code descriptor indicates "single or multiple." Therefore, this code should be reported only one time regardless of the number of biopsies performed.

Codes **43204** and **43205** describe esophagoscopy procedures with treatment of esophageal varices. Code **43204** describes esophagoscopy with injection sclerosis of esophageal varices. Code **43205** is used to report esophagoscopy with band ligation of esophageal varices.

Code **43215** is used to report esophagoscopy with removal of foreign body. If the procedure is performed with radiological guidance, a separate code from the **70000** series is reported for the radiological guidance or radiological S&I. The parenthetical note following code **43215** directs the user to code **74235** for radiological S&I. (Refer to Chapter 7 for further discussion of radiological S&I.)

**CODING TIP**

The "⊙" symbol that is found next to many of the endoscopy codes indicates that these codes include moderate (conscious) sedation when performed, and moderate (conscious) sedation should not be reported separately.

**CODING TIP**

Trans-nasal endoscopy, a procedure where a thin flexible endoscope is passed through the nares into the esophagus, is coded as **43499**, unlisted procedure esophagus.

Codes **43216**, **43217**, and **43228** are used to report esophagoscopy with removal of tumor(s), polyp(s), or other lesion(s). The appropriate code is selected based on the technique of removal. The wording of these codes indicates that they are to be reported only once per operative session, regardless of the number of lesions treated using that treatment method. Check the operative report carefully to verify the technique used to remove the lesion(s). In some instances, multiple lesions may be removed by different techniques. If this is the case, choose the codes that describe each technique used. The second and/or third techniques are reported with modifier 59 to identify separately reportable procedures.

Code **43216** describes removal of lesion(s) by hot biopsy forceps or bipolar cautery. Hot biopsy forceps use monopolar current, requiring the use of a grounding pad placed somewhere on the patient's body. Bipolar current does not require a grounding pad, as current runs simply from one portion of the tip of the device to another portion.

Code **43217** is used to report removal of lesion(s) by snare technique. A snare is a wire loop that is used to encircle tissue rather than simply grabbing it.

Code **43228** is used when other techniques, such as laser treatment or other thermal therapies, are used for the ablation of a lesion. This code describes esophagoscopy with ablation of tumor(s), polyp(s), or other lesion(s) not amenable to removal by hot biopsy forceps, bipolar cautery, or snare technique.

Code **43220** is used to report esophagoscopy with balloon dilation (less than 30 mm in diameter). The measurement in this code refers to the maximum diameter of the balloon itself, not the diameter of the esophagus. This code describes those cases where a through-the-scope-type balloon dilator is used. The endoscope remains in place as a balloon-tipped catheter is passed through its instrument channel and dilation is performed while the balloon is inflated under direct endoscopic observation.

Code **43226** describes esophagoscopy with insertion of a guidewire and subsequent dilation of the esophagus over the guidewire. This code includes both the insertion of the guidewire and the dilation of the esophagus. This procedure involves the passage of the endoscope, after which a flexible-tipped guidewire is passed through the endoscope into the stomach. The endoscope is then withdrawn, leaving the guidewire in place. A series of dilators is passed over the guidewire, each with a small central lumen created to accommodate the guidewire into the esophagus. After the largest desired dilator has been used, the guidewire and the dilators are then removed. The endoscope has been removed by the time the actual dilation is performed.

The parenthetical notes that appear after code **43220** direct the user to code **43458** for endoscopic dilation with a balloon 30 mm in diameter or larger. Codes **43450** and **43453** are reported for dilation without visualization. Although these codes are not included in the endoscopy series of codes, following is a review of their intended use.

Code **43458** is used in those cases where larger esophageal dilation balloons are used, specifically to treat achalasia. Typically this would involve fluoroscopic observation, which is reported separately using code **74360** in addition to the code for the dilation. Code **43458** does not include endoscopy, which is reported separately when performed.

Code **43450** is reported whenever esophageal dilation is performed by unguided sound or bougie. Code **43453** is used in the case where a guidewire is passed, generally under fluoroscopic observation, without the use of an endoscope. A separate code (**74360**) is used to report the fluoroscopic observation of esophageal dilation.

Code **43227** is used to report esophagoscopy with control of bleeding. Bleeding can be treated by several endoscopic techniques including, but not limited to, application of cautery with heater probe or bipolar or monopolar probe, injection of vasoconstrictive or irritant liquids, or laser cautery. All methods used to control bleeding are reported with this one code.

Code **43231** is used to report esophagoscopy, with endoscopic ultrasound examination limited to the esophagus, to allow assessment of the lesion(s).

Code **43232** is used to report esophagoscopy with endoscopic ultrasound examination limited to the esophagus whenever transendoscopic ultrasound-guided fine needle biopsy(s) through or across the esophagus is performed in search of any abnormalities. The actual pathology test performed on the specimen(s) obtained would be separately reported by using the appropriate laboratory code (codes **88172-88173**). As indicated in the parenthetical note that follows code **43232**, the radiological S&I for gastrointestinal endoscopic ultrasound is included when reporting codes **43231** and **43232**. Therefore, code **76975** is not to be reported with codes **43231** and **43232**.

Code **43234** is used to report an upper gastrointestinal endoscopy, simple primary screening examination using a small-diameter flexible endoscope that is swallowed by the patient. Unlike code **43235**, this procedure is often performed without moderate sedation.

### Esophagogastroduodenoscopy (EGD)

The EGD family of codes begins with code **43235**. Remember, EGD describes a procedure in which the endoscope is swallowed through the mouth and the pyloric channel is traversed with the endoscope.

Take a few minutes to review the code descriptors in the EGD series. Become familiar with the various codes available for reporting these procedures. Because of the common template used for the endoscopy codes, the code descriptors should already look familiar. Also, the guidelines provided previously for esophagoscopy regarding single or multiple biopsy; removal or ablation of tumors, polyps, or other lesions; submucosal injections; and control of bleeding can be applied to the codes in the EGD series.

A common question related to the reporting of codes in the EGD series is how to code for an EGD that involves testing for *Helicobacter pylori*. A number of commercial kits are available that are designed to detect the presence of urease produced by *H pylori*. These tests typically involve obtaining a tissue biopsy via the endoscope. The appropriate way to report the EGD portion of the procedure is with code **43239**.

The actual laboratory test for detection of *H pylori* would be reported separately. Generally, code **87076** or **87077** would be reported. Notice that other endoscopic and/or laboratory procedures may be performed as well. The appropriate code(s) should be selected and reported on the basis of the specific service(s) provided and procedure(s) performed.

Code **43236** describes EGD with directed submucosal injection(s), any substance. The code descriptor includes an "(s)" at the end of the word injection. Therefore, this code should be reported only one time, regardless of the number of injections performed. Code **43236** describes the submucosal injection of any substance. Examples of substances that may be injected are india ink, botulinum toxin, saline, and corticosteroid solutions.

Codes **43237** and **43238** differ from the other codes in this series in that they describe EGD procedures that include an endoscopic ultrasound examination, which is limited to the esophagus. It is important to note this distinction particularly between codes **43238** and **43242**. Both codes **43238** and **43242** describe EGD with transendoscopic ultrasound-guided procedures. However, code **43242** includes an endoscopic ultrasound examination of the esophagus, stomach, and either the duodenum and/or jejunum, while the endoscopic ultrasound examination in code **43238** is limited to the esophagus.

Code **43240** describes an endoscopically guided drainage of a pancreatic pseudocyst performed through the gastric wall. This code includes insertion of the drainage tube into the pseudocyst, when performed.

Code **43242** describes an EGD with endoscope ultrasound and transendoscopic ultrasound-guided intramural or transmural fine needle aspiration/biopsy of the upper gastrointestinal tract wall, including the esophagus, stomach, and either the jejunum and/or duodenum, as appropriate. As stated in the parenthetical note that follows this code, the radiological S&I for gastrointestinal endoscopic ultrasound is included when reporting code **43242**. Therefore, codes **76942** and **76975** should not be reported. The actual pathology test performed on the specimen(s) obtained would be separately reported by using the appropriate laboratory code (**88172**, **88173**).

Next, let us review the codes available for reporting percutaneous gastrostomy tube placement. Nonendoscopic percutaneous placement of a gastrostomy tube is reported using **49440**. Code **43246** is used to report percutaneous endoscopic gastrostomy (PEG) tube placement. When a PEG tube is placed by two physicians, each physician reports code **43246** with modifier 62, Two Surgeons, appended. Modifier 62 indicates two surgeons. In separate procedure notes, each physician should indicate his or her involvement in the procedure. (Refer to Chapter 10 for further discussion of the use of modifier 62.)

Percutaneous endoscopic gastrostomy tube placement (code **43246**) may be performed by one of several methods. An example of one such method follows:

**EXAMPLE:** With the patient placed in the supine position and the room lights dimmed, the endoscope is passed into the patient's stomach. Once the light of the endoscope enters the stomach, it transilluminates the abdominal wall.

A second physician presses a finger to create an indentation on the portion of the abdominal wall selected for gastrostomy tube insertion while the endoscopist views the indentation through the scope. A polypectomy snare is passed through the endoscope and maneuvered over the bulge created by the assistant's finger. Through a small incision at the insertion site, a cannula is inserted into the stomach, the inner stylet of the cannula is removed, and a suture is threaded through the cannula. The endoscopist grasps the suture tightly with the wire snare and then removes the endoscope, pulling the suture along with it and out of the patient's mouth. Next, the suture is tied to the tapered end of the gastrostomy tube. The opposite end of the gastrostomy tube is mushroom-shaped, which allows the gastrostomy tube to remain in the stomach after the procedure is completed. The second physician pulls the suture at the abdominal incision site and the gastrostomy tube follows, traversing the esophagus and entering the stomach. The proximal end of the gastrostomy tube then exits the stomach at the abdominal incision site. When five or six inches of the tube have been pulled out onto the abdomen, the endoscope is reinserted to assess the position of the mushroom-shaped end of the gastrostomy tube within the stomach. When the gastrostomy tube lightly contacts the stomach wall, a crossbar is slipped over the external portion of the tube and advanced to contact the skin of the abdomen, securely positioning the tube. Depending on the type of gastrostomy tube, it may be sutured in place. The endoscope is then removed.

Code **43256** describes transendoscopic gastroenteral stent placement, including predilation for patients with duodenal obstruction or gastric outlet strictures caused by conditions such as malignant neoplasms. Gastroenteral stenting represents an important nonsurgical treatment alternative for palliation of these patients.

## Bariatric Surgery

Bariatrics is the branch of medicine concerned with the management (prevention or control) of obesity and allied diseases. When conservative means of weight reduction such as dieting, exercise, behavioral modification, and pharmacological therapy have been unsuccessful for individuals suffering from clinically severe obesity, surgical treatment based on established principles for weight control are considered. These procedures involve the stomach, duodenum, jejunum, and/or ileum.

Laparoscopic techniques to perform gastric restrictive procedures for morbid obesity are reported by code **43644**, which describes the Roux-en-Y gastric bypass; code **43645** describes small bowel reconstruction to limit absorption; code **43770** describes gastric restrictive procedures that identify laparoscopic placement of the adjustable restrictive device (eg, gastric band and subcutaneous port components). Typical postoperative follow-up care after gastric restriction using the adjustable gastric band technique includes subsequent band adjustment(s) through the postoperative period for the typical patient. Band adjustment refers to changing the gastric band component diameter by injection or aspiration of fluid through the subcutaneous port component. Code **43771** describes laparoscopic revision of the restrictive device, code **43772** describes laparoscopic removal of the restrictive device, code **43773** describes laparoscopic removal and replacement of the restrictive device component, and code **43774** describes laparoscopic removal of the restrictive device and subcutaneous port components.

Open procedures are reported by code **43845**, which describes the gastric restrictive procedure with partial gastrectomy, pylorus-preserving duodenoileostomy, and ileoileostomy; code **43846** describes the gastric restrictive procedure, with gastric bypass; short limb Roux-en-Y; gastroenterostomy; code **43848** describes the revision, open, of gastric restrictive procedure for morbid obesity, other than an adjustable gastric resrictive device; code **43886** describes the revision of the subcutaneous port component; code **43887** describes the open removal of the subcutaneous port component; and code **43888** describes the open removal and replacement of the subcutaneous port.

> **EXAMPLE:** In a gastric bypass for morbid obesity (code **43846**), the stomach is partitioned with a staple line on the lesser curvature (no band, no gastric transection). A short limb of small bowel (less than 100 cm) is divided and anastomosed to the small upper stomach pouch.

### Gastric Stimulation for Gastroparesis and Morbid Obesity

The treatment of gastroparesis via electrical stimulation to the stomach is performed by implantation or replacement of gastric neurostimulator electrodes in the antrum of the stomach. Because implantation of these electrode devices may require any of a number of procedures to complete the treatment, separate codes have been included in the CPT codebook to identify the placement of the pulse generator device (**64590**), the implantation of electrodes, or the revision or removal of the implanted devices. Placement of electrodes is performed by either laparoscopic (**43647**) or open exposure (**43881**) of the anatomic site near the gastric antrum. The revision or removal of the gastric neurostimulator electrodes is also performed via laparoscopic (**43648**) or open (**43882**) techniques. For insertion of gastric neurostimulator pulse generator, use code **64590**. Code **64595** is reported for the revision or removal of a gastric neurostimulator pulse generator. Electronic analysis and programming of gastric neurostimulator pulse generator for gastroparesis is reported using **95980-95982**, as appropriate.

The treatment of morbid obesity via electrical stimulation to the stomach is performed by implantation or replacement of gastric neurostimulator electrodes in the lesser curvature of the stomach. Because implantation of these electrode devices may require any of a number of procedures to complete the treatment, separate codes have been included in the CPT codebook to identify the placement of the pulse generator device (**64590**), the implantation of electrodes, or the revision or removal of the implanted devices. Category III code **0155T** describes laparoscopic implantation of gastric stimulator electrodes in the lesser curvature for morbid obesity. Code **0156T** describes laparoscopic revision or removal of gastric stimulator electrodes for morbid obesity. Code **0157T** describes open laparotomy with implantation or replacement of gastric neurostimulator electrodes in the lesser curvature for morbid obesity. Code **0158T** describes open laparotomy with revision or removal of gastric neurostimulator electrodes for morbid obesity. For insertion of gastric neurostimulator pulse generator, use **64590**. Electronic analysis, programming, and reprogramming of a gastric neurostimulator pulse generator, lesser curvature for morbid obesity is reported using Category III code **0162T**.

## Proctosigmoidoscopy

Proctosigmoidoscopy is the examination of the rectum and sigmoid colon.

The proctosigmoidoscopy family of codes begins with code **45300**. Codes for rigid proctosigmoidoscopy should be used only when a stiff hollow tube, or proctoscope, is used for the examination. If a flexible instrument is used, the codes for flexible sigmoidoscopy should be used, as described in the **45330-45345** code series. A rigid instrument may be used to perform some simple surgical procedures or to examine only the rectum and most distal sigmoid colon. The flexible sigmoidoscope reaches substantially farther into more proximal regions of the sigmoid colon than the rigid proctoscope.

Become familiar with the codes in this series. Notice that code **45300** describes diagnostic rigid proctosigmoidoscopy. When performed, collection of specimen(s) by brushing or washing is included in reporting code **45300**. This code is designated as a separate procedure. (Refer to Chapter 4 for further discussion of the *separate procedure* designation.) Code **45303** is used to report rigid proctosigmoidoscopy with dilation.

Code **45305** describes proctosigmoidoscopy with biopsy. The number of biopsy specimens taken is not considered when code **45305** is reported. This code is reported only once regardless of whether single or multiple biopsies are performed.

The proctosigmoidoscopy family of codes has a unique convention for reporting removal of tumors, polyps, or other lesions that is not seen in the flexible endoscopy families of codes. Code **45308** describes proctosigmoidoscopy with removal of a single tumor, polyp, or other lesion by hot biopsy forceps or bipolar cautery. Code **45309** describes proctosigmoidoscopy with removal of a single tumor, polyp, or other lesion by snare technique.

Removal of multiple tumors, polyps, or other lesions by hot biopsy forceps, bipolar cautery, or snare technique through the proctoscope is reported with code **45315**. Code **45315** is reported only one time regardless of the number of lesions removed by these techniques. In all other endoscopy code families, with the exception of the anoscopy family, only one code is used to describe single or multiple lesions.

Code **45320** describes the ablation of lesions not amenable to removal by hot biopsy forceps, bipolar cautery, or snare technique. This code is reported once to include any number of tumors, polyps, or other lesions that are ablated.

## Sigmoidoscopy

Sigmoidoscopy is the examination of the entire rectum and sigmoid colon and may include examination of a portion of the descending colon.

Sigmoidoscopy procedures are reported with the **45330-45345** series of codes. This family of codes also includes the template of procedures. Remember, the guidelines previously discussed for single or multiple biopsies; removal or ablation of tumors, polyps, or other lesions; submucosal injections; and control of bleeding are also applied to the codes in the sigmoidoscopy series.

Code **45335** describes use of a flexible sigmoidoscope with directed submucosal injection(s), any substance. The code descriptor includes an "(s)" at the end of the word injection to indicate that this code should be reported only one time regardless of the number of injections performed. Examples of substances that may be injected are India ink, botulinum toxin, saline, and corticosteroid solutions.

### Colonoscopy

Colonoscopy is the examination of the entire colon, from the rectum to the cecum, and may include examination of the terminal ileum. As indicated in the Endoscopy guidelines, an incomplete colonoscopy, with full preparation for a colonoscopy, should be reported with a colonoscopy code with modifier 52, Reduced Services, appended. Documentation should be provided to indicate the reason for the incomplete procedure. (Refer to Chapter 10 for further discussion of modifier 52.) Note that the reporting guidelines differ for Medicare patients. Modifier 53, Discontinued Procedure, should be appended to the CPT code for an incomplete colonoscopy. Colonoscopy procedures are reported with the **45378-45387** series of codes. These codes describe an endoscopy in which a colonoscope is inserted in the anus and moved through the colon "proximally" past the splenic flexure (meaning the examiner is able to advance the colonoscope beyond the splenic flexure) to visualize the lumen of the transverse and ascending (right side) to the cecum and/or terminal ileum. Like the other endoscopy families of codes, this code family also includes the template procedures.

Code **45381** describes a flexible colonoscopy proximal to the splenic flexure, with directed submucosal injection(s), any substance. The code descriptor includes an "(s)" at the end of the word injection to indicate that this code should be reported only one time, regardless of the number of injections performed. Code **45381** describes the submucosal injection of any substance. Examples of substances that may be injected are India ink, botulinum toxin, saline, and corticosteroid solutions.

Colonoscopy with removal of tumor(s), polyp(s), or other lesion(s) is described by codes **45383**, **45384**, and **45385**. Each of these codes describes different removal techniques. Code **45380** describes colonoscopy with single or multiple biopsies. When coding forceps removal of a polyp as a cold biopsy, code **45380** should be reported. It is important to note that the terms *forceps*, *cold biopsy*, *cold biopsy forceps*, and *biopsy* do not describe the same technique that the term *snare* does. As such, code **45385** should not be reported for removal of polyps using cold or hot biopsy forceps; this code describes only removal of a polyp using a snare technique.

When reviewing an operative report for a colonoscopy with removal of tumor(s), polyp(s), or other lesion(s), one may see phrases such as "removed in its entirety" and "piecemeal removal." These phrases are not relevant to code selection, as coding the procedures is based upon the technique used to remove the tissue. Depending upon the circumstances, the surgeon may choose to remove the tissue in pieces, or he or she may remove the entire lesion with one application of the technique used. Codes **45380**, **45383**, **45384**, and **45385** are reported one time per colonoscopy procedure, regardless of whether the technique used is applied to multiple polyps or multiple times on a single polyp.

When the biopsy of one lesion and the removal of another lesion using a different technique from a different site during the same operative session is performed, the use of modifier 59, Distinct Procedural Service, is essential to report the different procedures. Modifier 59 is used to indicate that there was a separate incision/excision, separate lesion. If one lesion is biopsied and a separate lesion is removed using a snare technique, it would be appropriate to append modifier 59 to the code reported for the biopsy procedure. (Refer to Chapters 4 and 10 for further discussion regarding the use of modifiers 51 and 59.)

### Anus/Incision

Code **46020** describes anal seton placement, which is commonly performed to treat fistula in ano, Crohn's fistula in ano, and anoperineal or anovaginal fistulas. Codes **46060** and **46280** describe placement of the seton in addition to other surgical procedures. Code **46020** should be reported when placement of the seton is the only procedure performed. Code **46020** should not be reported in addition to codes **46060** and **46280**, as these codes include placement of a seton, when performed. When a diagnostic anoscopy is performed as described by code **46600** in addition to placement of a seton, only code **46020** should be reported. Code **46600** should not be reported, as it is designated as a separate procedure.

### Anoscopy

Codes for reporting anoscopy are found within the **46600-46615** series. This family of codes uses the same template format as the other endoscopy families. Like the proctosigmoidoscopy family of codes, the anoscopy code family has separate codes to describe the removal of a single lesion by hot biopsy forceps or bipolar cautery, removal of a single lesion by snare technique, and removal of multiple lesions by any of these techniques. In addition, one code describes single and multiple lesions, as in the other code families.

## Biliary Tract

### Excision

There are occasions when the provider will perform a cholecystectomy and exploration of the common bile duct as well as a cholangiogram. Code **47605** describes a cholecystectomy with cholangiography. Code **47610** describes a cholecystectomy with exploration of the common bile duct. Cholangiogram is considered an inclusive component of code **47610**. Therefore, when these three procedures are performed at the same session, only code **47610** should be reported. The same principle applies to the laparoscopic equivalent, **47564**.

## Abdomen, Peritoneum, and Omentum

Introduction, Revision, and/or Removal

Code **49419** describes the insertion of an intraperitoneal cannula or catheter and includes placement of a permanent subcutaneous reservoir. Intraperitoneal chemotherapy is commonly administered through this device. Code **49420** describes the temporary insertion of an intraperitoneal cannula or catheter without the placement of a subcutaneous reservoir. It is important to carefully review the documentation to determine whether a subcutaneous reservoir was placed, as code selection depends upon this information.

Code **49421** describes the permanent insertion of an intraperitoneal cannula or catheter for drainage or dialysis. For laparoscopic insertion of a permanent intraperitoneal cannula or catheter, code **49324** is reported.

Code **49325** is used to report the revision of an intraperitoneal cannula/catheter and includes the removal of obstructive material around the catheter when performed. This procedure is often considered as the next step in the management sequence for catheter inflow pain. Some causes of pain include the jet effect of the dialysate due to the malposition of the end hole of the tubing and the catheter tip against the abdominal wall; entrapment of the catheter by omentum, epiploic appendices, uterine tubes, compartmentalizing adhesions; and bowel distention, peristalsis, or tubing resiliency forces (shape memory effects) from mechanical stresses created at the time of catheter implantation. To relieve omental entrapment of the catheter tip, an omental tacking procedure is performed. Add-on code **49326** describes the laparoscopic omental tacking procedure performed to avert omental entrapment. Procedurally, code **49326** describes an intervention wherein the omentum is displaced from the pelvis into the upper abdomen and attached to the abdominal wall or falciform ligament of the liver. Add-on code **49326** may be reported in addition to codes **49324** and **49325**.

Add-on code **49435** is reported in conjunction with codes **49324** and **49421** and describes the attachment of a subcutaneously implanted extension tubing component to the external end of an intraperitoneal catheter. This procedure is performed to allow the catheter exit site to be located in the upper chest (presternal, parasternal) area, away from the usual lower abdominal region. This code can be used with either an open (**49421**) or laparoscopic (**49324**) insertion of the intraperitoneal cannula or catheter. A presternal catheter dialysis catheter system (**49435**) allows the remote location of the dialysis catheter exit site in the chest region while maintaining the proper deep pelvic positioning of the intraperitoneal component for normal hydraulic function of the device and reduced risk of infectious complications.

Code **49436** is reported for the delayed creation of an exit site from a previously embedded (buried) subcutaneous segment of an intraperitoneal catheter. Peritoneal dialysis catheter infection-related complications include subcutaneous tunnel tract infections and peritonitis resulting from the progression of a tunnel tract infection. Totally embedding the catheter in the abdominal wall (reported in a previous session with code **49421**) at the time of the implantation procedure allows the site of implantation a sterile environment and time to heal without the potential contamination of the transmural segment from the catheter skin exit-site wound. After at least a 3-week interval, the external limb of the catheter superficial to the subcutaneous polyester cuff is retrieved through a small skin incision (**49436**) and the patient is started on full-volume peritoneal dialysis without requiring a break-in period.

## Hernia Repair

The codes for reporting open surgical hernia repair are found in the **49491-49611** series. The codes in this series identify surgical intervention for the hernia repair. The intent of the surgical repair is to permanently close off the orifice through which the organs protrude.

In addition to the codes in the **49491-49611** series for reporting open surgical hernia repair procedures, codes **49650-49659** are available for reporting various laparoscopic hernia repairs. Codes **49650** and **49651** describe laparoscopic repair of an initial and a recurrent inguinal hernia, respectively.

Code **49659** is used to report unlisted laparoscopy procedures for hernioplasty, herniorrhaphy, or herniotomy.

The initial treatment of a hernia can be medical, whereby the hernia can be reduced (the organ[s] put back into normal body cavity) without surgical intervention. The medical reduction is a temporary measure and does nothing to cure the underlying pathology; it is used to alleviate the problems associated with the hernia. No separate code exists to describe the medical reduction of a hernia, nor does it constitute surgical treatment.

Generally, this reduction is performed as part of an E/M service and is not reported separately. Note: When a manual reduction is the only service performed, unlisted code **49999** may be reported with a report to indicate the service provided.

Code **49495** describes repair of an initial reducible inguinal hernia, and code **49496** describes repair of an initial incarcerated or strangulated inguinal hernia in a full-term infant under age 6 months, or preterm infants over 50 weeks of postconception age and under age 6 months at the time of surgery, with or without hydrocelectomy.

The hernia repair codes are categorized primarily by the type of hernia.

> **CODING TIP**
>
> Postconception age equals gestational age at birth plus age of the infant in weeks at the time of the hernia repair. Initial inguinal hernia repairs performed on preterm infants who are over 50 weeks of postconception age and under age 6 months at the time of surgery should be reported with codes **49495** and **49496**.

## Types of Hernias and Code Ranges

| Type of Hernia | Code Ranges |
| --- | --- |
| Inguinal | 49491-49525; 49650, 49651 |
| Lumbar | 49540 |
| Femoral | 49550-49557 |
| Incisional or ventral | 49560-49566 |
| Epigastric | 49570-49572 |
| Umbilical | 49580-49587 |
| Spigelian | 49590 |
| Omphalocele | 49600-49611 |

Repair of diaphragmatic or hiatal hernia is not reported with the codes in this series. Rather, codes **39502-39541** from the Mediastinum and Diaphragm subsection of Surgery are used to report this type of hernia repair.

When a code indicates "repair recurrent inguinal hernia, any age, reducible," this means that the hernia has been previously surgically reduced (put back into its normal body cavity) and the hernial orifice has been surgically repaired. If a hernia is manually reduced and not surgically repaired, the reprotrusion of the hernial contents does not constitute a recurrence.

Some of the types of hernias are further categorized as initial or recurrent on the basis of whether the hernia has required previous repair(s).

Some of the codes reflect the patient's age and whether the hernia is reducible, incarcerated, or strangulated. The age of the patient is indicated when the type of procedure (technique) used to repair the hernia varies based on the patient's age.

A reducible hernia is one that can be corrected by manual manipulation; there is free mobility of the hernia contents through the hernial orifice.

*Incarcerated* refers to the abnormal entrapment of a part (ie, a hernia that is nonreducible). A nonreducible hernia is one that cannot be reduced by manipulation. In these types of hernias, the hernial contents are fixed in the hernial sac.

Strangulation is the most serious complication related to a hernia. Congestion or strangulation at the hernial ring impairs the blood supply to the herniated part. Once the vessels are obstructed, a simple incarceration becomes a strangulation.

The hernia repair codes represent the repair of the hernia only. The excision or repair of strangulated organs or structures is reported with a separate code(s) in addition to the code for the hernia repair. Generally, the greater service is listed first on the claim form. An additional procedure(s) is identified by appending modifier 51, Multiple Procedures, to the secondary procedure(s) reported. (Refer to Chapters 2 and 10 for further discussion of the use of modifiers.)

Code **49568** is used to report implantation of mesh or other prosthesis. The implantation of mesh or other prosthesis is reported separately only with the incisional or ventral hernia repair codes (codes **49560-49566**). Mesh or other prostheses are commonly used to repair other types of hernias. However, the use of mesh or other prostheses with other types of hernia repair is not reported separately.

Take the time to review the descriptors for the hernia repair codes. Notice that in codes **49491-49501** the code descriptor indicates "with or without hydrocelectomy." This means that this hernia repair can occur with or without a hydrocelectomy being performed at the same operative session. However, these codes include the hydrocelectomy when performed. Hydrocelectomy is not reported with an additional, separate code when performed with the hernia repair described by codes **49491-49501**.

However, a hydrocelectomy performed with hernia repair described by codes **49505-49507** requires the reporting of code **55040** for the excision of the hydrocele in addition to the appropriate hernia repair code (code **49505** or **49507**).

# VI. Urinary System

The Urinary System subsection of the CPT codebook contains codes for reporting procedures of the following:
- Kidney
- Ureter
- Bladder
- Urethra

Generally, under each anatomic heading, codes can be found for reporting procedures involving incision, excision, introduction, repair, and endoscopy procedures.

This section contains discussion of some of the procedures and guidelines associated with reporting renal transplantation, lithotripsy, renal tumor ablation, laparoscopy procedures, bladder catheter insertion, urodynamics, endoscopy procedures, and prostate procedures.

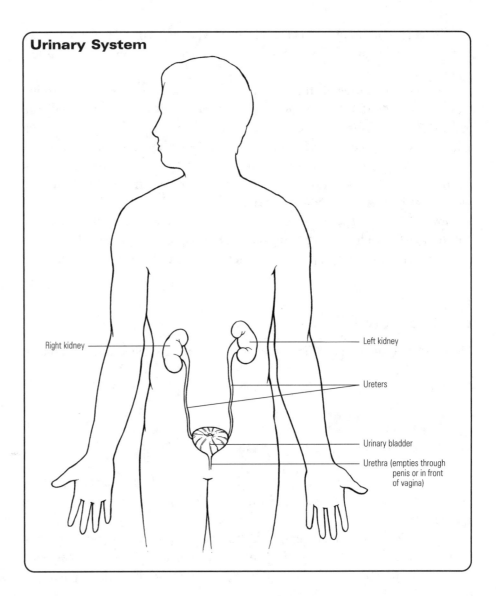

**Urinary System**

Right kidney

Left kidney

Ureters

Urinary bladder

Urethra (empties through penis or in front of vagina)

## Renal Transplantation

Codes and guidelines for reporting renal allotransplantation are structured to identify the following three separate components of physician work:
- Cadaver donor nephrectomy, unilateral or bilateral
- Backbench work
- Recipient renal allotransplantation

Backbench work is the preparation of the donor organ graft for transplantation to the recipient site. The specific work involved in backbench work is defined in the guidelines. This preparation of the graft is performed on a back bench in the operating room, hence the term *backbench work*. Standard backbench work varies based upon whether the donor kidney is from a cadaver (**50323**) or a living donor (**50325**). The operative report should be carefully reviewed to determine whether the donor organ is from a living or a cadaver donor. Additional backbench work to prepare the donor kidney prior to transplantation may include venous, arterial, and/or ureteral anastomosis(es). This additional work is separately reported with a code from **50327** through **50329** as appropriate.

## Renal Pelvis Catheter Stent Procedures

Renal pelvic catheter stent procedures are most often performed for the treatment of ureteral strictures and obstructions. They are differentiated by approach (percutaneous and transurethral) and type (internally dwelling and externally dwelling). Codes **50382-50389** are reported for the removal of ureteral stents.

Code **50382** describes the removal as well as replacement of an internally dwelling ureteral stent when performed through a percutaneous transnephric approach. This procedure involves removal of an indwelling, entirely internal double-J ureteral stent. Code **50384** is reported for procedures involving only the removal of an internally dwelling ureteral stent via a new percutaneous transnephric approach (the stent is not replaced). Code **50387** is reported for removal and replacement of an externally accessible (the stent catheter has a portion that lies external to the patient) ureteral stent via the transnephric approach.

Code **50389** is reported for those instances in which a previously placed nephrostomy tube catheter must be removed using fluoroscopic guidance. This procedure may be needed for an encrusted nephrostomy tube catheter that is resistant to removal or a damaged nephrostomy tube catheter that may completely fracture during removal (so a safety wire is used to maintain access as the catheter is removed while observing under fluoroscopy).

## Lithotripsy

Code **50590** describes extracorporeal shockwave lithotripsy of the kidney. As code **50590** is an inherently unilateral code, modifier 50 should be appended when the procedure is performed bilaterally. (Refer to Chapter 10 for further discussion of modifier 50.)

## Renal Tumor Ablation

There are specific codes for renal tumor ablation, depending on the surgical approach: laparoscopic, open, or percutaneous. Code **50542** describes laparoscopic ablation of renal mass lesion(s) by any method (eg, cryoablation or radiofrequency ablation). This code is reported one time regardless of the number of lesions treated. The code for open ablation of renal mass lesion(s), **50250**, is specific to cryoablation. Tumors treated by nephrectomy are coded using the appropriate nephrectomy code (**50220-50240**). Renal mass lesion(s) ablated by any open method other than cryoablation or treated by nephrectomy, such as open radiofrequency ablation of renal tumor(s), would be reported using the unlisted code **53899**. Both the laparoscopic, any method and open, cryoablation renal mass lesion(s) codes **50542** and **50250**, respectively, include intraoperative ultrasound guidance if provided.

For renal tumor(s) ablation procedures from a percutaneous approach, there are specific codes based on the method of tumor ablation. Code **50592** is used to report percutaneous radiofrequency ablation of renal tumor(s). Code **50593** is used to report percutaneous cryoablation of renal tumor(s). As different modes of imaging may be used depending on the patient's specific clinical circumstances, imaging for the guidance and monitoring of the percutaneous renal tumor ablation procedure is separately reported. The modality-specific imaging codes for the guidance and for monitoring of ablation are **76940**, **77013**, and **77022** (ultrasound, computed tomography, magnetic resonance, respectively). Percutaneous renal tumor ablation is an inherently unilateral code. Therefore, modifier 50 should be appended when the procedure is performed bilaterally.

## Insertion of Bladder Catheter

Codes **51701-51703** describe insertion of bladder catheters. Code **51701** differs from codes **51702** and **51703** in that it describes the insertion of a nonindwelling bladder catheter used for intermittent catheterization or catheterization to obtain postvoid residual urine or to obtain a clean-catch urine specimen, after which the catheter is removed. Codes **51702** and **51703** describe the insertion of a temporary indwelling bladder catheter, which remains in place for a period of time.

## Endoscopic Procedures

Some of the most frequently used procedures listed in the Urinary System subsection of the CPT codebook are endoscopic, including the use of cystoscopy, urethroscopy, cystourethroscopy, ureteroscopy, pyeloscopy, and renal endoscopy. An endoscopy can be used as a diagnostic tool performed before proceeding with a more intensive surgical procedure or to check on the progress, completion, or a complication during the surgical procedure.

CPT descriptors will indicate whether an endoscopic procedure is included in the surgical procedure. Examples of the use of cystourethroscopy before, after, or during a urological procedure are a sling operation for stress incontinence as described in code **57288**, to check status of sutures in the bladder or transperineal placement of needles or catheters into the prostate as described in code **55875**, or to check for radioactive seeds that may have become dislodged during the procedure. The use of cystourethroscopy in these examples would not be reported separately.

There are times, however, when one endoscopic procedure must be performed before a more extensive endoscopic procedure due to anatomical locations. In this case, one would append modifier 51 to indicate that multiple procedures were performed at the same session by the same provider. (Refer to Chapter 10 for further discussion of modifier 51.)

Consider the following example:

**EXAMPLE:** A patient presents for a cystourethroscopy and removal of a calculus that is located in the ureter. However, in order to be able to remove the calculus, the urethral stricture must be dilated for access to the calculus.

To accurately reflect these services, the following codes should be reported:

**52352**   Cystourethroscopy, with ureteroscopy and/or pyeloscopy; with removal or manipulation of calculus (ureteral catheterization is included)

**52281 51**   Cystourethroscopy, with calibration and/or dilation of urethral stricture or stenosis, with or without meatotomy, with or without injection procedure for cystography, male or female

The CPT codes in this section are also listed with a primary or base code with more extensive codes listed in sequential order or in anatomical order. For example, codes **52351-52355** describe cystourethroscopy, with ureteroscopy and/or pyeloscopy, beginning with a diagnostic procedure and ending with a resection of a renal pelvic tumor.

In some instances, the main surgical procedure is identified in the CPT descriptor along with minor related procedures that therefore cannot be reported separately. For example, code **52601** describes transurethral electrosurgical resection of the prostate, including control of postoperative bleeding, complete (vasectomy, meatotomy, cystourethroscopy, urethral calibration and/or dilation, and internal urethrotomy are included). The minor procedures indicated in the descriptor would need to be performed before, during, or after the surgery and cannot be reported separately.

## Laterality of Cystourethroscopy Codes

Cystourethroscopy codes that are inherently unilateral are as follows:

**52005**, **52007**, and **52320-52355**.

When unilateral procedures are performed bilaterally, modifier 50 should be appended to the appropriate code(s). (Refer to Chapter 10 for further discussion of modifier 50.)

Cystourethroscopy codes that should never be reported with modifier 50 are as follows:

**52000**, **52010**, **52204-52285**, **52305-52318**, **52402**.

A careful review of each code descriptor is necessary when selecting the appropriate endoscopy code(s). Be sure to distinguish codes for ureteral versus urethral procedures. Also note that when multiple endoscopic procedures are performed at the same session by the same provider, it is appropriate to separately report them. In this case, one would append modifier 51 to indicate that multiple procedures were performed at the same session by the same provider. (Refer to Chapter 10 for further discussion of modifier 51.)

Consider the following example:

**EXAMPLE:** Dr New performs cystourethroscopy with fulguration and resection of a medium bladder tumor (code **52235**). During the same endoscopic session he also performs a steroid injection into a urethral stricture (code **52283**).

To accurately report his services during that session, Dr New will report the following codes:

**52235**   Cystourethroscopy, with fulguration (including cryosurgery or laser surgery) and/or resection of; MEDIUM bladder tumor(s) (2.0 to 5.0 cm)

**52283 51**   Cystourethroscopy, with steroid injection into stricture

### Stent Insertion

Codes in the **52320-52355** series include the insertion and removal of a temporary stent during diagnostic or therapeutic cystourethroscopic intervention(s). The insertion of a temporary stent refers to those types of stents that are used during the cystoscopy procedure and removed at the completion of that intervention. A temporary stent may be used during a procedure and then removed and replaced with a self-retaining or indwelling stent during the same intervention.

Codes in the **52320-52355** series, with the exception of code **52332**, do not include the placement of a self-retaining or indwelling stent.

Placement of a self-retaining or indwelling stent is not required in all cases, but when performed via cystourethroscopy, it should be reported separately with code **52332**. In these cases, code **52332** is reported in addition to the primary procedure(s) performed with modifier 51 appended. (Code **50605** is used to report ureterotomy with stent insertion.)

The insertion and removal of a temporary ureteral catheter (**52005**) during diagnostic or therapeutic cystourethroscopic with ureteroscopy and/or pyeloscopy is included in **52320-52355** and should not be reported separately.

To report insertion of a self-retaining, indwelling stent performed during diagnostic or therapeutic cystourethroscopy with ureteroscopy and/or pyeloscopy, report **52332**, in addition to primary procedure(s) performed (**52320-52355**), and append modifier 51. Code **52332** is used to report a unilateral procedure unless otherwise specified.

It is possible to place indwelling or self-retaining stents in both ureters through the same cystoscope during the same cystourethroscopic diagnostic and/or therapeutic intervention. When bilateral ureteral stents are placed, modifier 50 is appended to code **52332**.

In addition, stents may be placed percutaneously without the use of a cystoscope. Code **50393** is used to report the initial percutaneous placement of a ureteral stent through the renal pelvis. Imaging services provided in conjunction with ureteral stent placement may vary according to the patient's specific clinical circumstances and may be reported using code **74480**, **74475**, or **76942**, **77002**, or **77012**. Unlike the initial placement code, imaging is specifically an included service for the percutaneous exchange of an internally dwelling ureteral stent (code **50382**) and for the exchange of an externally accessible transnephric ureteral stent (code **50387**), and therefore imaging guidance would not be reported separately.

The exchange of a ureterostomy tube or externally accessible ureteral stent via the ileal conduit is reported with code **50688**. If imaging guidance is performed, code **75984** is additionally reported.

When bilateral percutaneous ureteral stent services are performed, modifier 50 should be appended.

Indwelling stent(s) are removed at the discretion of the physician. The removal procedure may or may not require the use of an endoscope. If the indwelling stent is inserted via ureterotomy or other procedure that is subject to the surgical package concept, no additional reporting is warranted when the stent is removed during the normal postoperative follow-up period.

Cystourethroscopy with removal of a self-retaining/indwelling ureteral stent, planned or staged during the associated normal postoperative follow-up period of the original procedure, is reported by means of code **52310** or **52315** with modifier 58 appended, as appropriate. (Refer to Chapter 10 for further discussion of modifier 58.) If the indwelling stent is inserted via ureterotomy or other procedure that is subject to the surgical package concept, no additional reporting is warranted when the stent is removed during the normal postoperative follow-up period.

For the removal of an internally dwelling ureteral stent from a percutaneous approach, code **50384** is reported. For the percutaneous removal of a nephrostomy tube with concurrent indwelling ureteral stent removal, code **50389** is reported. Both **50384** and **50389** include radiological S&I services.

For the removal (without replacement) of a nephrostomy tube or an externally accessible ureteral stent that does not require fluoroscopic guidance and is not subject to a surgical package, report the appropriate level of E/M service provided.

The use of endoscopy and other instrumentation to treat noncalculous ureteral strictures that may be associated with hydronephrosis is reported by code **52341** or **52344**, as appropriate; in the ureteropelvic junction by code **52342** or **52345**; and in the intrarenal area by code **52343** or **52346**. Codes **52320** and **52352** differ in that these codes describe procedures to treat calculous diseases and should be used to describe removal or manipulation of ureteral calculus.

Codes **52341-52343** describe the use of a cystoscope that is passed through the urethra and into the bladder to allow the physician to visualize the ureteral orifice to allow the passage of guide wires to direct balloons or enable other interventions (eg, laser, electrocautery, or incisional devices) in the strictured area.

Codes **52344-52346** describe the use of a ureteroscope passed through the urethra to the bladder and directly into the ureter. The ureteroscope is used to directly visualize the stricture and to pass guide wires to direct the use of laser, balloons, or incisional or electrocautery devices.

Code **52351** describes a diagnostic cystourethroscopy with ureteroscopy and/or pyeloscopy. This code is not routinely reported with codes **52341-52346** and **52352-52355**, as it describes a diagnostic cystourethroscopy when performed on the same side. However, there are instances when a diagnostic cystourethroscopy and a procedure described by a code from the **52341-52346** or **52352-52355** series are performed on contralateral (opposite) sides of the body. In this case, it would be appropriate to report code **52351** separately with modifier 59 appended. (Refer to Chapter 10 for further discussion of modifier 59.)

## Prostate Procedures

Codes in the **52450-52700** series are used to report transurethral procedures of the vesical neck and prostate. Codes **53850-53853** are also used to report transurethral destruction of prostatic tissue.

Let us take a few moments to review the differences between these codes, which are used for reporting prostate procedures.

Code **52601** is used to report procedures commonly referred to as TURP (transurethral resection of the prostate). This procedure uses electrical current to heat a wire loop on a resectoscope that slices through urethral/prostatic tissue like a knife. Two settings exist to regulate the current. The high voltage current is used to cut the tissue and the low voltage current to coagulate the bleeding. As indicated in the code descriptor, when code **52601** is reported, vasectomy, meatotomy, cystourethroscopy, urethral calibration and/or dilation, and internal urethrotomy are included, when performed, and not reported separately. This code is intended to describe an initial resection of the prostate. Also, this code describes a complete TURP.

Codes **52612** and **52614** are used to report prostate resection performed in two stages. Code **52612** is used to report the first stage of a two-stage resection. Code **52614** describes the second stage of a two-stage resection procedure and is reported when the resection is completed.

Code **52630** describes the removal or resection of obstructive tissue that has regrown longer than 1 year postoperatively after the initial resection of the prostate.

Code **53852** describes transurethral destruction by radiofrequency thermotherapy where low power radiofrequency energy is used to cause tissue ablation and coagulation of prostate tissue. Insulated needles are pierced through the prostatic urethra to deliver radiofrequency energy directly into the prostate while the insulation on the needles protects the urethra. This procedure creates areas of necrosis within the prostate while preserving the urethral tissue.

The related code defines the procedure by the energy source used to avoid the inclusion of proprietary procedures (eg, "the TUNA System") in the CPT Nomenclature.

Code **53853** describes transurethral destruction of prostate tissue by water-induced thermotherapy, where water is heated outside the body and circulated through the prostate in heat-shielded catheters; only the balloon emits heat. At 60° C, coagulative necrosis of the prostatic tissue occurs to an average depth of 1.0 cm from the urethra. As water is heated and pumped from outside the body, there is no need to use internal temperature probes as is necessary with benign prostatic hypertrophy (BPH) treatments such as microwave (code **53850**) and radiofrequency-based (code **53852**) procedures.

Code **52647** describes noncontact laser coagulation of the prostate. This code is intended to describe laser procedures that primarily heat the prostate and require sloughing for the treatment to be complete. This code should be used even if an incision or small amount of vaporization is done in combination with the coagulation. In this case, it is not appropriate to separately report code **52648** for the small amount of vaporization performed.

Code **52648** describes contact laser vaporization with or without transurethral resection of the prostate (TURP). This code is used to report laser procedures that use a contact tip or high-power density laser. Contact vaporization is usually accomplished by moving a laser tip across the surface of the prostate, causing immediate vaporization of tissue and an end result that looks like a cavity (similar to the effect of a TURP).

Another technique for laser treatment of BPH involves placing the laser fiber within the prostatic substance with tissue destruction and delayed cavitation (eg, Indigo system for interstitial laser ablation). Although this technique might appear to be most appropriately reported with code **52648**, in fact, it should be reported with code **52647**, as the tissue undergoes coagulative necrosis and not immediate vaporization and cavitation.

Code **53850** describes transurethral microwave thermotherapy, which is the selective destruction of prostate cells by therapeutic levels of heating. Transurethral microwave thermotherapy is a process of delivering sufficient microwave heating to destroy prostatic tissue without causing unnecessary damage to surrounding structures. The technique combines the principles of microwave radiation heating and conductive cooling to destroy tissue deep within the prostate while preserving surrounding structures such as the bladder neck, urethral mucosa, and distal sphincter.

Cryosurgical ablation of the prostate is a procedure that is an alternative to radical prostatectomy or radiation therapy in the treatment of prostate cancer. Code **55873** describes this procedure, which uses a cryosurgical probe to destroy diseased tissue by freezing. The cryosurgical probes are placed through the perineum into the prostate with the use of ultrasonic guidance imaging. The ultrasound probe is placed in the rectum. Real-time images from the ultrasound are used to place the cryoprobes and to monitor the treatment.

> **CODING TIP**
>
> Ultrasonic guidance is included when code **55873** is reported.

Transurethral resection of residual obstructive tissue after 90 days postoperatively is reported with code **52620**. This code describes a procedure in which the physician removes the remaining obstructive tissue after the initial resection of the prostate.

## Radiation Treatment

Code **55875** describes transperineal placement of needles or catheters into the prostate for interstitial radioelement application, with or without cytoscopy. Code **55876** describes placement, by needle or any approach, of interstitial device(s) in the prostate for radiation therapy guidance. This may be done with the aid of fiducial markers to improve the accuracy for seed migration and a reduction in organ deformation, or with dosimeter for safe dose escalation with external beam radiation therapy. This therapeutic procedure is for men with malignant neoplasms of the prostate.

# VII. Female Genital System

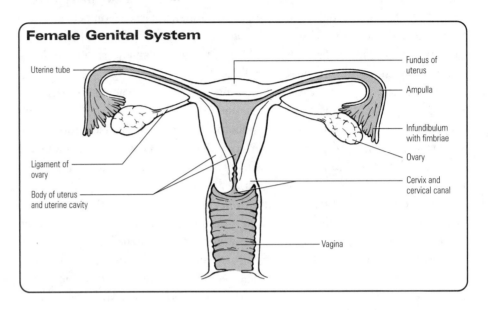

**Female Genital System**

Uterine tube

Fundus of uterus

Ampulla

Infundibulum with fimbriae

Ovary

Ligament of ovary

Cervix and cervical canal

Body of uterus and uterine cavity

Vagina

## Gynecologic Surgery

Codes for reporting procedures of the female genital system are found in the **56405-58999** series.

Specific codes are available for reporting procedures of the following anatomy:

- Vulva, Perineum, and Introitus (**56405,56821**)
- Vagina (**57000-57425**)
- Cervix Uteri (**57452-57820, 57800**)
- Corpus Uteri (**58100-58579**)
- Oviduct/Ovary (**58600-58770**)
- Ovary (**58800-58960**)

In addition, there is a separate series of codes (**58970-58976**) for reporting procedures related to in vitro fertilization.

A series of codes also exists for reporting procedures related to laparoscopic/hysteroscopic surgery of the uterus (**58541-58579**) and laparoscopic surgery related to procedures on the oviduct or ovaries (**58660-58679**). (Refer to Chapter 4 for further discussion of laparoscopic procedures.)

Code **58999** is available for reporting unlisted (nonobstetrical) procedures of the female genital system. (Refer to Chapter 2 for further discussion of unlisted codes.)

The *separate procedure* designation is used throughout the female genital system codes. Become familiar with the guidelines associated with reporting codes that have the separate procedure designation. (These guidelines are discussed extensively in Chapter 4.)

Browse through this subsection of the CPT codebook. Become familiar with its layout and the various codes available for reporting the procedures of the female genital system. Now a few minutes will be taken to review some of the specific guidelines throughout this subsection.

Within each anatomic subsection, Vulva, Perineum and Introitus; Vagina; Cervix Uteri; Corpus Uteri; Oviduct/Ovary; and Ovary, there are specific listings for procedures that involve incision, destruction, excision, repair, etc. At the beginning of the first anatomic heading, the following definitions that are applicable to the vulvectomy codes (**56620-56640**) appear:

A *simple* vulvectomy procedure is the removal of skin and superficial subcutaneous tissues.

A *radical* vulvectomy procedure is the removal of skin and deep subcutaneous tissue.

Removal of less than 80% of the vulvar area is defined as a *partial vulvectomy*.

Removal of greater than 80% of the vulvar area is defined as a *complete vulvectomy*.

When coding for vulvectomy procedures, one must determine the extent of the procedure performed from the operative report. If this information is not clearly documented, consult with the physician for clarification before code assignment.

Codes **56605** and **56606** describe biopsy of the vulva or perineum. Code **56605** is reported for biopsy of one lesion. Biopsy of each separate additional lesion is reported with code **56606**. Code **56606** is designated as an add-on code. This code would never be reported without first reporting code **56605**. (Refer to Chapter 4 for further discussion of add-on codes.)

Code **56820** describes endoscopic examination and magnification of the vulva to evaluate for viral lesions, neoplasia, or malignancy. Code **56821** describes the same service with biopsy(s). If multiple biopsies are performed on the vulva during the same session, then code **56821** should only be reported one time, as indicated by the optional plural form of biopsy(s). Additional endoscopic examinations of other sites should be reported separately with modifier 51 appended. It would not be appropriate to append modifier 50 for multiple vulvar biopsies.

Within the series of codes for reporting procedures of the vagina (**57000-57425**), specific listings are given for procedures that involve incision, destruction, excision, introduction, repair, manipulation, and endoscopy.

Codes **57022** and **57023** describe incision and drainage of a vaginal hematoma differentiated as a hematoma occurring in an obstetrical patient as a result of delivery (**57022**) or a nonobstetrical condition resulting from trauma or injury (**57023**). An injury resulting in a vaginal hematoma that occurs in a pregnant woman who sustains an injury before and unrelated to delivery (eg, bicycle mishap) should be reported with code **57023**.

Codes **57061** and **57065** are used to report destruction of vaginal lesion(s) by any method. Code **57061** describes a simple destruction procedure. Code **57065** is used to report an "extensive" destruction procedure. The determination of whether a procedure is simple or extensive is based on the clinical judgment of the physician. The method/technique of destruction listed in codes **57061** and **57065** includes but is not limited to laser surgery, electrosurgery, cryosurgery, and chemosurgery.

The introduction codes in this anatomic site include diaphragm or cervical cap fitting (**57170**), fitting and insertion of a pessary or an intravaginal support device (**57160**), and introduction/irrigation of medication or hemostatic agents into the vagina for injuries or infection (**57150** and **57180**). Also, code **57155** is available for insertion of a tandem (hollow cylinder) and/or a vaginal ovoid (empty capsule into which a radioactive element can be placed) in preparation for radiation therapy (brachytherapy) for cervical cancer. The actual insertion of the radioactive element and radiation therapy is performed by the radiologist, and a series of codes is included in the Radiology section under the Clinical Brachytherapy subsection (**77761-77763**, **77781-77784**) to report these procedures.

The repair codes pertaining to the vagina include vaginal/perineal injuries not occurring during delivery (**57200-57210**), vaginal repairs involving urinary and rectal structures (**57220-57260**), repair of vaginal hernias (**57265-57270**), correction of vaginal prolapse and stress urinary incontinence (**57282-57288**), closure of rectovaginal/urethrovaginal fistulas (**57300-57330**), and construction of artificial vagina (**57291-57292**). Laparoscopic colpopexy is reported using code **57425**. Open colpopexy procedure codes should never be used when the laparoscopic approach is performed. If mesh or other prosthesis is used when a vaginal repair is performed, then it would be appropriate to report add-on code **57267**.

Also, notice that some of the code descriptors for listings in the repair series of codes include the parenthetical statement "nonobstetrical." If these procedures are performed as an obstetric procedure, then the appropriate code from the Maternity Care and Delivery subsection should be used to report the procedure.

The codes under the Manipulation heading include codes to report pelvic examinations (**57410**), dilation of vagina (**57400**), and removal of vaginal foreign body (**57415**) performed under general anesthesia. A pelvic examination performed with a local anesthetic or without anesthesia is not reported separately; it is included in the level of E/M service reported for the visit. (Refer to Chapter 3 for further discussion of E/M coding.) Similarly, removal of impacted foreign body performed without anesthesia is included in the level of E/M service for the visit.

Under the Endoscopy heading, codes **57420** and **57421** are intended to report endoscopic examination and magnification of the surface of the vagina, performed for those patients with conditions that include abnormal Pap smear or prior hysterectomy with cervix removal and abnormal Pap smear. Examination of contiguous portions of the cervix performed as a part of the endoscopic vaginal examination are included and not separately reported.

Codes **57452-57461** are used to report various cervical colposcopic procedures. Code **57452** describes a diagnostic colposcopic examination. Code **57454** describes colposcopy with biopsy(s) of the cervix and endocervical curettage. Note that the language of the code indicates *biopsy(s)*. Therefore, this code is reported only one time, whether one or multiple cervical biopsies are performed. If only a biopsy of the cervix is performed, it would be appropriate to report code **57455**. If only endocervical curettage is performed, it would be appropriate to report code **57456**. Codes **57454-57461** are further differentiated according to the biopsy method (ie, excisional, loop electrode).

Code **57460** is used to report a loop electrode biopsy procedure of the cervix performed at the same operative episode as a colposcopy. In this procedure, the physician views the vagina and cervix through a colposcope. A hot cautery wire is used to excise a cone or section of cervical tissue and cauterize the area at the same time. The loop electrode conization procedure, described by code **57461**, consists of a procedure performed to obtain a large tissue specimen from patients with abnormal Pap smears in which a portion of the endocervix (most typically in the transformation zone) is excised where a discrete lesion has been visualized on the exocervix. It typically involves use of a loop electrode to excise a lesion on the ectocervix with adequate margins and subsequent use of a second loop to remove the involved portion of the endocervix. Code **57461** is not reported in addition to code **57456**, as the endocervical curettage reported by code **57456** is an inclusive component of the loop electrode conization.

Within the cervix uteri series of codes (**57452-57800**), one will find subcategories of codes for procedures that describe endoscopy, excision, repair, and manipulation. Code **57520** is used to report excision of a cone shape of endocervical tissue (conization) of the cervix by means of a cold knife or laser without a colposcopy. When this code is reported, any fulguration, dilation and curettage (D&C), or repair performed is also included and not reported separately.

Code **57522** also describes conization of the cervix; however, the technique is by loop electrode excision. This code is used to report the excision of a cone shape of endocervical tissue by means of a loop electrode. Since a conization of the cervix by the loop electrode procedure is a different, less complex procedure than conization with cold knife or laser, separate codes are listed to differentiate between these techniques. If a loop electrode biopsy is performed with a colposcopy, code **57460** would be reported. Colposcopic loop electrode conization would be reported with code **57461**.

Codes in the corpus uteri series (**58100-58579**) describe procedures involving excision, introduction, repair, and laparoscopy/hysteroscopy.

Codes **58140-58146** describe open vaginal and abdominal approach procedures for excision of intramural myomas (uterine fibroids). The myomectomy codes are further differentiated by the total weight of the excised lesions. A myomectomy performed laparoscopically is reported with codes **58545-58546**.

Note that various hysterectomy procedures are described here. Code **58150** describes a total abdominal hysterectomy, with or without removal of tube(s), with or without removal of ovary(s). Codes in the **58260-58294** series describe various vaginal hysterectomy procedures.

Removal of the fallopian tube(s) and/or ovary(s), when performed with an abdominal hysterectomy procedure, is not reported separately. The code descriptors for abdominal hysterectomy procedures include the language "with or without removal of tube(s), with or without removal of ovary(s)." If a salpingectomy (**58700**), salpingo-oophorectomy (**58720**), or oophorectomy (**58940**) is performed as a separate procedure without an abdominal or vaginal hysterectomy, then codes **58700**, **58720**, and **58940** are reported, as appropriate, to describe these procedures. (Refer to Chapter 4 for further discussion of the separate procedure designation.) In addition, if an enterocele or urethrocystopexy repair is performed at the same session as a vaginal hysterectomy procedure, it should be determined whether the appropriate codes in the **58260-58294** series are available before referring to procedures from the **57200-57330** series of codes.

The introduction codes within the corpus uteri series include insertion and removal of intrauterine devices (IUDs) (**58300-58301**) and introduction of catheters for diagnostic purposes (eg, hysterosalpingography, hysterosonography) or to establish patency of fallopian tubes (**58340** and **58345**). The radiological component of these two procedures is listed in the Radiology section of the CPT codebook and includes codes **76831**, **74740**, and **74742**. Several codes also exist within this anatomical heading related to fertility medicine, including artificial insemination (**58321**, **58322**) and sperm washing for artificial insemination (**58323**). The remainder of the codes under Introduction include chromotubation of oviduct (**58350**), insertion of Heyman capsules for clinical brachytherapy (**58346**), thermal endometrial ablation (**58353**), and endometrial cryoablation with ultrasonic guidance (**58356**). Code **58353** involves insertion of a balloon catheter through the vagina into the uterus and inflation of the balloon, which can be heated to a high temperature to ablate the benign tissue associated with benign menorrhagia (eg, dysfunctional uterine bleeding). A similar procedure, which involves the use of a hysteroscope, reported as code **58563**, utilizes an electrode loop, roller ball, or laser to ablate the tissue.

The laparoscopy codes in this section are reported for supracervical hysterectomy, myomectomy, and vaginal hysterectomy procedures differentiated by size (> 250 gm or < 250 gm uterus) and inclusion of the salpingo-oophorectomy procedure. Codes **58541-58544** and **58548** describe various laparoscopic hysterectomy procedures. Codes **58541-58544** describe laparoscopic supracervical hysterectomy. The instructional parenthetical notes following codes **58542** and **58544** clarify that codes **58541-58544** should not be reported in addition to codes **49320**, **57000**, **57180**, **57410**, **58140-58146**, **58150**, **58545**, **58546**, **58561**, **58661**, **58670**, or **58671**. Code **58548** describes laparoscopic radical hysterectomy with bilateral total pelvic lymphadenectomy and para-aortic lymph node sampling. This code includes the removal of tubes and ovaries, if performed. An instructional parenthetical note following code **58548** clarifies that laparoscopic retroperitoneal lymph node biopsy (**38570-38572**), radical abdominal hysterectomy (**58210**), radical vaginal hysterectomy (**58285**), and laparoscopic vaginal hysterectomy (**58550-58554**) are all inclusive components of laparoscopic radical hysterectomy and should not be reported separately with code **58548**. Also, do not report codes **58550-58552** in conjunction with **49320**, **57000**, **57180**, **57140**, **58140-58146**, **58545**, **58546**, **58561**, **58661**, **58670**, or **58671**.

In addition to the procedure (**58563**) listed previously, many other procedures can be performed with the use of a hysteroscope, including code **58558**, which describes surgical hysteroscopy with sampling (biopsy) of the endometrium and/or polypectomy, with or without a D&C. A D&C is commonly performed with a hysteroscopy; thus, both of these procedures are described in a single code. The code is worded in this way to make it clear that when sampling (biopsy or curetting) of the endometrium and/or polypectomy is performed, the D&C should not be coded separately. Additionally, since a biopsy sample can be obtained by a D&C, the code also represents a hysteroscopy with biopsy. Two unlisted procedure codes are included within the Uterus series of codes to report unlisted laparoscopy and hysteroscopy procedures. (Refer to Chapter 2 for further discussion of unlisted codes.)

Within the series of codes describing procedures of the oviduct/ovary (**58600-58770**), codes are available for reporting ligation or transection of fallopian tube(s) (tubal ligation) and occlusion of fallopian tube(s) by device. Following is a review of the various codes for reporting these procedures.

Code **58600** describes tubal ligation or transection via abdominal or vaginal approach. This code is appropriate for reporting either a unilateral or a bilateral procedure. This code is not appropriate if the procedure is performed during the postpartum period during the same hospitalization as the delivery (see code **58605**). Also, this code is not used to report tubal ligation or transection when done at the time of a cesarean delivery or intra-abdominal surgery (see code **58611**).

Code **58605** describes a postpartum tubal ligation or transection performed during the same hospitalization as the delivery. This code is appropriate for procedures performed via either an abdominal or a vaginal approach, with unilateral or bilateral tubal ligation or transection. Do not report this code for tubal ligation or transection performed at the time of cesarean delivery or intra-abdominal surgery (see code **58611**). This code is designated as a separate procedure. (Refer to Chapter 4 for detailed discussion of the separate procedure designation.)

Code **58611** is an add-on code that describes tubal ligation or transection when done at the time of cesarean delivery or intra-abdominal surgery (during the same operative session). This code is to be reported separately, in addition to the code for the cesarean delivery or intra-abdominal surgery performed. Do not report this code if the tubal ligation or transection is performed at a separate operative session from the cesarean delivery or intra-abdominal surgery (see code **58600** or **58605**, as appropriate). (Refer to Chapter 4 for further discussion of CPT add-on codes.)

The occlusion of fallopian tube(s) by device (eg, band, clip, Falope ring) is reported with code **58615**. This code is appropriate whether a vaginal or a suprapubic approach is employed.

Laparoscopic procedures for fulguration or occlusion of oviducts are reported with codes **58670** and **58671**. Code **58670** describes laparoscopic fulguration of oviducts (with or without transection), and code **58671** is used to report laparoscopy with occlusion of oviducts by device (eg, band, clip, or Falope ring).

The excision and repair listing of the oviduct/ovary series of codes following the laparoscopy procedures describes open procedures without the use of a laparoscope. Codes **58700** and **58720** describe the partial or complete excisional removal of the fallopian tubes (**58700**) and the fallopian tubes with removal of the ovaries (**58720**). These two codes should not be reported when the procedures described are performed as part of a more major procedure (eg, hysterectomy, pelvic exenteration) (see previous discussion of codes in the Corpus Uteri subsection). Codes **58740-58770** describe procedures related to

**CODING TIP**

The use of modifier 50 with any of the codes describing tubal ligation or transection procedures is not appropriate. The codes inherently describe unilateral or bilateral procedures.

the repair of the fallopian tubes, including anastomosis procedures (**58740, 58750, 58752, 58770**) and lysis of adhesions occurring within the fallopian tubes or ovary(s).

The **58800-58960** series of codes describes procedures involving primarily the ovary(s), including biopsy (**58900**), resection (**58920, 58950-58952**), cyst removal (**58925**), and partial or total removal (**58940**) in cases of ovarian, tubal, or primary peritoneal malignancy. These codes describe both unilateral and bilateral procedures. Codes **58943** and **58950-58952** are reported for procedures involving the ovary(s) and other adnexal structures, including a total abdominal hysterectomy (**58951**) in cases of ovarian, tubal, or primary peritoneal malignancy. Code **58960** describes a staging or restaging procedure for ovarian, tubal, or peritoneal malignancies.

## Introduction Procedures

### Fitting and Insertion of Pessary
The fitting and insertion of a pessary or other intravaginal support device is reported with code **57160**.

The supply of the pessary is not included when code **57160** is reported. It is appropriate to separately report the supply item with CPT code **99070** or the appropriate HCPCS Level II code.

### Diaphragm or Cervical Cap Fitting
Diaphragm or cervical cap fitting is reported by means of CPT code **57170**. As indicated in the code descriptor, instructions to the patient regarding the use of the diaphragm or cervical cap are included when this code is reported.

The supply of the diaphragm or cervical cap is not included when code **57170** is reported. Separately report the supply item with CPT code **99070** or the appropriate HCPCS Level II code.

### Insertion and Removal of an Intrauterine Device (IUD)
CPT code **58300** is used to report the insertion of an IUD. This code is intended to be used to report only the insertion of an IUD. It does not include the supply of the IUD itself. CPT code **99070** or the appropriate HCPCS Level II code is reported separately to describe the supply of the IUD.

**CODING TIP**

HCPCS Level II code **A4560** may be used instead of CPT code 99070 to report the supply of a pessary.

**CODING TIP**

HCPCS Level II code **J7300** describes the supply of an intrauterine copper contraceptive. This code may be used instead of CPT code **99070** for the supply of an IUD.

# VIII. Maternity Care and Delivery

Codes for reporting maternity care and delivery services can be found in the **59000-59899** series. The following table indicates the specific services identified within this code series:

| Maternity Care and Delivery Services Code Series | |
|---|---|
| Procedure/Service Described | Code Range |
| Antepartum Services | 59000-59076 |
| Excision | 59100-59160 |
| Introduction | 59200 |
| Repair | 59300-59350 |
| Vaginal Delivery, Antepartum and Postpartum Care | 59400-59430 |
| Cesarean Delivery | 59510-59525 |
| Delivery After Previous Cesarean Delivery | 59610-59622 |
| Abortion | 59812-59857 |
| Other Procedures | 59866-59899 |

Following is a review some of the listings for maternity care and delivery procedures.

The codes for amniocentesis (**59000**), cordocentesis (**59012**), and chorionic villus sampling (**59015**) describe only the procedural portion of the service. The radiological S&I are reported separately with the appropriate **70000** series code from the Radiology section of the CPT codebook. (Refer to Chapter 7 for more on radiological S&I.)

Notice that codes **59050** and **59051**, used to report fetal monitoring during labor, are reported only when the service is performed by a consulting physician (ie, not the attending physician). Code **59050** describes the S&I of the monitoring, and code **59051** is reported when the only service provided is the interpretation of the fetal monitoring. This service is not reported separately when provided by the attending physician.

Codes **59070-59076** describe intrauterine fetal surgical procedures, including ultrasound guidance. Ultrasound guidance should not be separately reported. Code **59074** describes a procedure in which a needle is inserted into an organ to aspirate fluid. Code **59076** describes fluid drainage using a fetal shunt, which allows for continuous drainage of excessive fluid such as in the instances of hydronephrosis or hydrothorax. Fetal invasive procedures that are not listed in this series should be reported using code **59897**.

Codes for surgical treatment of an ectopic pregnancy are found in the **59120-59151** series. The appropriate code is selected on the basis of the site of the ectopic pregnancy and the specific procedure performed. Codes **59150** and **59151** are used to report laparoscopic treatment of an ectopic pregnancy. The appropriate code is selected according to whether the laparoscopic treatment was performed without salpingectomy and/or oophorectomy (**59150**) or with salpingectomy and/or oophorectomy (**59151**).

Episiotomy or vaginal repair performed by a physician other than the attending physician is reported with code **59300**. When episiotomy or vaginal repair is performed by the attending physician, this service is not reported separately, as it is included in the code reported for the vaginal delivery. For CPT Nomenclature coding purposes, small vaginal tears are not considered a complication of the delivery. If minor vaginal tearing occurs and the repair is minimal, it would be considered management of uncomplicated labor and delivery and would not be reported separately. If, however, an extensive laceration occurs, modifier 22, Unusual procedural service, may be appended to the code reported for the vaginal delivery to identify the additional effort involved in the repair. (Refer to Chapter 10 for further discussion of modifier 22.)

Cerclage of the cervix during pregnancy is reported by means of codes **59320** and **59325**. The appropriate code is selected on the basis of the approach used to perform the procedure. Code **59320** describes a vaginal approach, and code **59325**, an abdominal approach.

Subsequent removal of cerclage sutures at the time of delivery is considered part of the delivery and would not be reported separately. However, removal of the cerclage suture under anesthesia before the onset of labor, or at a time that extends beyond the global period of the placement procedure, is reported separately with code **59871**, provided the removal is performed under anesthesia (other than local).

The next sections focus on the various code series and associated guidelines for reporting services normally provided in uncomplicated maternity cases.

## The Obstetric Package

The services normally provided in uncomplicated maternity cases include routine antepartum care, delivery, and postpartum care. This is the global package for maternity care and delivery. The guidelines at the beginning of the Maternity Care and Delivery subsection define the services included when antepartum care, delivery services, and postpartum care are reported.

Antepartum care includes the following:
- The initial and subsequent history
- Physical examinations
- Recording of weight, blood pressures, and fetal heart tones
- Routine chemical urinalysis
- Monthly visits up to 28 weeks' gestation, biweekly visits to 36 weeks' gestation, and weekly visits until delivery

The E/M services (visits) provided with those services included in the provision of antepartum care are not separately reported. However, any other visits or services provided within the antepartum period other than those listed previously should be reported separately.

Medical complications of pregnancy (eg, cardiac problems, neurologic problems, diabetes, hypertension, toxemia, hyperemesis, preterm labor, premature rupture of membranes) may require the provision of additional E/M services and/or services described in the Medicine section of the CPT codebook. When medical complications require additional services beyond those specified in the maternity care and delivery guidelines, those services are reported separately in addition to the codes for maternity care.

For surgical complications of pregnancy (eg, appendectomy, hernia repair, ovarian cyst, Bartholin cyst), the appropriate code(s) from the Surgery section of the CPT codebook should be reported in addition to the codes for maternity care and delivery.

Delivery services include the following:

- Admission to the hospital
- The admission history and physical examination
- Management of uncomplicated labor
- Vaginal delivery (with or without episiotomy, with or without forceps) or cesarean delivery

Delivery of the placenta is considered to be an integral component of the total vaginal or cesarean delivery. Therefore, code **59414** is not reported in addition to the code for the delivery service. Code **59414** is appropriately reported for the delivery of placenta in situations in which the patient delivers vaginally before admission with subsequent delivery of the placenta by a physician.

As stated in the Maternity Care and Delivery guidelines, medical problems complicating labor and delivery management may require additional resources. These additional resources should be identified and reported separately, in addition to the codes for maternity care, by means of the codes in the Medicine and E/M sections, as appropriate.

Postpartum care includes hospital and office visits following vaginal or cesarean delivery.

Following is a review of the codes available for reporting routine obstetric care. Separate codes exist for reporting routine obstetric care associated with the following:

- Vaginal delivery
- Cesarean delivery
- Delivery after previous cesarean delivery

## Global Services for Routine Obstetric Care

When the same physician (solo practice) or same physician group (group practice) provides the global routine obstetric care (including antepartum care, delivery, and postpartum care), the appropriate global code is reported to describe the services rendered. Codes **59400**, **59510**, **59610**, and **59618** describe the global services for routine obstetric care. Following is a review of the differences in these code descriptors.

Code **59400** describes routine obstetric care including antepartum care, vaginal delivery (with or without episiotomy and/or forceps, vacuum), and postpartum care.

Code **59510** describes routine obstetric care including antepartum care, cesarean delivery, and postpartum care. This code is also used to report global care provided to patients who have had a previous cesarean delivery and return for elective repeat cesarean delivery.

**CODING TIP**

Artificial rupture of membranes before delivery is an inclusive component of the delivery code reported. Therefore, a separate code would not be reported.

Code **59610** describes the global care associated with vaginal birth after previous cesarean delivery. Included when this code is reported are antepartum care, vaginal delivery (with or without episiotomy and/or forceps), and postpartum care for a patient who has had a previous cesarean delivery.

Code **59618** describes the global care associated with cesarean delivery after attempted vaginal delivery after previous cesarean. If the attempt to deliver vaginally after a previous cesarean delivery is unsuccessful and another cesarean delivery is performed, then code **59618** is used to report the global service.

Notice that all of the codes for vaginal delivery include the parenthetical statement "with or without episiotomy and/or forceps." No separate reporting occurs for the performance of an episiotomy and/or the use of forceps during delivery. Also, when performed by the attending physician, the subsequent repair of the episiotomy is an inclusive component of the delivery service. As mentioned earlier, code **59300** is used to report episiotomy repair by other than the attending physician.

Under certain circumstances, the same physician (in a solo practice) or same physician group (group practice) does not provide the global maternity care and delivery services. Under these circumstances, the use of the global codes is not appropriate. Codes in the CPT Nomenclature exist for reporting the specific services provided when the global codes are not appropriate.

When the global care is not provided by the same physician or same physician group, the following codes and guidelines apply. Codes **59409**, **59514**, **59612**, and **59620** describe delivery services only. Codes **59410**, **59515**, **59614**, and **59622** describe delivery services including postpartum care. The following paragraphs highlight the differences in these code descriptors.

Code **59409** describes vaginal delivery only (with or without episiotomy and/or forceps). If the postpartum care is also provided by the same physician or the same physician group, then code **59410** is reported. These codes are not used to describe vaginal delivery after a previous cesarean delivery (refer to codes **59610-59612**).

Code **59514** describes cesarean delivery only. If the postpartum care is also provided by the same physician or same physician group, then code **59515** is reported.

Code **59612** describes vaginal delivery only (with or without episiotomy and/or forceps) after a previous cesarean delivery. If the postpartum care is also provided by the same physician or the same physician group, then code **59614** is reported.

Code **59620** describes an attempted vaginal delivery following a previous cesarean delivery that results in another cesarean delivery. If the postpartum care is also provided by the same physician or same physician group, then code **59622** is reported.

Codes **59425** and **59426** are available for reporting antepartum care only. If four to six antepartum visits are provided, then code **59425** is reported. Seven or more antepartum visits are reported with code **59426**. If the physician provides one to three antepartum visits, they are individually reported with the appropriate E/M codes. When filling out the *units* box on the claim form, indicate that "1" unit of service was provided when reporting code **59425** or **59426**.

The provision of outpatient postpartum care only is reported with code **59430**.

If the global care is provided by the same physician or same physician group, the appropriate global code is reported. Under these circumstances, it is not appropriate to separately report the antepartum, delivery, and postpartum care. Following are a few examples of when one should separately report the provision of antepartum, delivery, and postpartum care.

**EXAMPLE 1:** Termination of Pregnancy. A patient is seen by the physician for three antepartum visits and then experiences a miscarriage (abortion); the entire global maternity care service was not provided.

In this case, each of the three visits is coded as E/M services on the basis of the services provided. If the patient is new to the physician, a new patient office or other outpatient visit code (**99201-99205**) would be chosen for the initial visit; codes from the established patient office or other outpatient services (**99211-99215**) would be reported for the next two visits. If the patient is not new to the physician, the appropriate level of E/M service from the established patient office or other outpatient services would be reported for the initial and subsequent visits. (Refer to Chapter 3 for further discussion on appropriate selection of a level of E/M service.)

**EXAMPLE 2:** Relocation of the Patient. Dr Long provided Mrs Adams with eight antepartum visits before she relocated from Illinois to Texas. After her arrival in Texas, Mrs Adams resumed her prenatal care with Dr Short. Dr Short provided a total of five antepartum visits. In addition, he performed a vaginal delivery and provided all of her postpartum care. No complications occurred during maternity care and delivery.

In this example, Dr Long reports code **59426** for the antepartum care he provided. Dr Short reports code **59425** for the antepartum care he provided, in addition to code **59410** for the vaginal delivery and postpartum care.

**EXAMPLE 3:** Cesarean Delivery by Another Physician. Mrs Kay sees Dr Car for her entire pregnancy. While in labor, Mrs Kay develops a complication that requires the performance of a cesarean delivery. Dr Rose assists Dr Car with the cesarean delivery. After delivery, Dr Car provides Mrs Kay's postpartum care.

In this example, Dr Car reports code **59510** to describe his services. Dr Rose reports code **59514-80**. Modifier 80, Assistant surgeon, is appended to the cesarean delivery only code to indicate Dr Rose's services as assistant surgeon for the cesarean delivery.

> **CODING TIP**
>
> If the physician assists in a cesarean delivery but provides none of the antepartum or postpartum services, do not use a code for global obstetric care. Instead, use the appropriate code for the delivery only, and append modifier 80 to denote the surgical assistant services provided.

## Coding for Delivery of Twins

Coding for the delivery of twins requires careful consideration of the specific services provided. Recognize that third-party payer reporting requirements in these circumstances may vary from CPT coding guidelines. For successful coding results, become familiar with coding guidelines as well as payer reporting requirements.

The preferred method of reporting vaginal delivery of twins, when the global obstetric care is provided by the same physician or same physician group, is with code **59400** or **59610**, as appropriate, with modifier 22, Increased Procedural Service, appended. However, in some areas, an alternative reporting method is to use the global code for the delivery of the first twin (code **59400** or **59610**, as appropriate) and report the vaginal delivery only code (code **59409** or **59612**, as appropriate) for the second twin with modifier 51, Multiple procedures, appended. (Refer to Chapter 10 for further discussion of modifier 51.)

If one twin is delivered vaginally and the other by cesarean delivery, and the global obstetric care is provided by the same physician or same physician group, then report the global code (code **59510** or **59618**, as appropriate) for the cesarean delivery and the vaginal delivery only code (code **59409** or **59612**) with modifier 59, Distinct procedural service, appended to the vaginal delivery code. If both twins are delivered by cesarean, the appropriate cesarean code should be reported, appended by modifier 22.

## Coding for Treatment of "Abortions"

The definition of *abortion* is the premature expulsion from the uterus of the products of conception, the embryo, or a nonviable fetus. However, for the lay person, the coding or labeling of a medical record or report as "spontaneous abortion" may be somewhat problematic. The CPT codes properly use the medical term *abortion*. Appropriate coding for the treatment of abortions requires an understanding of how various types of abortions are defined. Next will be a review of the definitions of the various types of abortions and the related CPT codes.

On the basis of the cause, abortions may be categorized as either spontaneous or induced. A spontaneous abortion is the natural (with no active interference) termination of pregnancy before 20 weeks, 0 days of gestation. An induced abortion is one in which a deliberate attempt has been made to terminate the pregnancy.

A threatened abortion is diagnosed when vaginal bleeding occurs in the first 20 weeks of pregnancy. The differential diagnosis of this bleeding that occurs in early pregnancy in approximately 20% of all patients is usually included in the antepartum care component of "routine" obstetric care of the patient who successfully delivers. In the event that the patient being treated for a threatened abortion requires additional visits, these should be reported separately by means of E/M codes, according to the services provided by the physician.

Following is a review of the terms used in the CPT Nomenclature and their definitions as well as the various codes available for reporting the treatment of spontaneous abortions.

## Spontaneous Abortion (Miscarriage)

The types of spontaneous abortion include:
- Complete abortion
- Incomplete abortion
- Missed abortion
- Septic abortion
- Blighted ovum

When a spontaneous abortion that is complete (the uterus is entirely emptied of its contents) occurs (any trimester), and the physician manages the patient medically with no surgical intervention, the physician reports the appropriate level of E/M code. The category of E/M service is selected on the basis of the place where the patient is seen (eg, physician office, hospital, emergency department).

An incomplete abortion occurs when the uterus is not entirely emptied of its contents. Fragments of the products of conception may remain within the uterus, protrude from the external os of the cervix, or be found in the vagina. Some fragments of the products of conception may have spontaneously passed out of the vagina.

CPT code **59812** is used to report the D&C (either sharp or suction curettage) for the surgical management of an incomplete abortion. However, if the patient is septic and is diagnosed as having an incomplete abortion, do not use code **59812**. (See septic abortion.)

A *missed abortion* refers to the prolonged retention of a fetus that died in the first half of pregnancy. The evacuation of the uterus in these cases is coded according to the trimester in which the procedure is performed. Code **59820** is reported for procedures performed in the first trimester. Code **59821** is reported for procedures performed in the second trimester.

Septic abortions are those in which intrauterine infection is present. Most often this infection is confined to the uterus, but peritonitis and septicemia are not rare. Treatment of the infection involves, in addition to treatment with antibiotics, the prompt evacuation of the products of conception. Code **59830** is used to report these services.

A blighted ovum is a fertilized egg that fails to develop. The advances of diagnostic tools that aid in the very early detection of pregnancy, such as beta-subunit human chorionic gonadotropin (HCG) and ultrasound, have clouded the clinical coding picture as to when early abortion occurs. To positively diagnose a blighted ovum, there must be a positive pregnancy test and a blighted ovum (a pathologic ovum in which there is a degenerated or absent embryo) identified on an ultrasound.

Before the use of ultrasound and beta-subunit HCG testing, a blighted ovum may have gone undetected and not been considered a form of early abortion. Today, since it is possible to detect pregnancy at a very early stage (several days after conception), a blighted ovum diagnosis is more common.

In the instance of a positive pregnancy test with a blighted ovum identified on ultrasound, questions arise regarding appropriate code assignment for the treatment of a blighted ovum. Since no (viable) product of conception is present, should a code for treatment of abortion be selected or a code for nonobstetric D&C?

A blighted ovum is a fertilized egg and is considered obstetric rather than nonobstetric. If a pregnancy is diagnosed and terminates either by spontaneous or induced means, the abortion codes should be used to report the physician services related to the abortion.

A blighted ovum may result in one of the following treatments:

**Complete spontaneous abortion**—In this case, the physician manages the patient medically with no surgical intervention. The physician reports his or her service using the appropriate level of E/M code, based on where the service is provided.

**Incomplete abortion**—In this case, the uterus is not entirely emptied of the products of conception. The tissue may be found in the uterus, cervix, or vagina. The physician performs a D&C to remove all remaining tissue for the surgical management of an incomplete abortion. This is reported with code **59812**.

**Missed abortion**—A missed abortion refers to the prolonged retention of an embryo/fetus that died in the first half of pregnancy. The evacuation of the uterus in these cases is reported by means of code **59820** or **59821**, based on the trimester in which the procedure is performed.

When the treatment of a blighted ovum is reported, the use of CPT code **58120**, Dilation and curettage, diagnostic and/or therapeutic (nonobstetrical), is not appropriate. As stated previously, a blighted ovum is a fertilized egg and is considered obstetric rather than nonobstetric.

### Induced Abortion

Both therapeutic and elective abortions may be classified as induced abortions. Therapeutic abortion is the termination of pregnancy before the time of fetal viability for medical indications. Elective abortion is the interruption of pregnancy before viability at the request of the woman.

Coding for an induced abortion is based on the technique used. This may be done surgically by dilating the cervix and performing curettage or using vacuum aspiration. Medical induction may be performed by the administration of oxytocin or prostaglandins. Intra-amniotic injections of saline or urea are also used to induce abortions.

When an induced abortion is performed by dilating the cervix and performing sharp and/or suction curettage, code **59840** is reported.

If the cervix is dilated and the uterus mechanically evacuated, code **59841** is reported. In the event that a small amount of sharp curettage is needed to complete the dilation and evacuation, this is included when code **59841** is reported.

Abortions performed during the second trimester are sometimes performed with intra-amniotic hyperosmotic solutions (saline or urea). These solutions are injected to stimulate uterine contractions and cervical dilation to deliver the products of conception. This is reported with code **59850**. As indicated in the code descriptor, admission to a facility, necessary hospital visits, and follow-up care are included when this code is reported.

In the event that the intra-amniotic injections facilitate the evacuation of the uterus but curettage and/or dilation is necessary to complete the procedure, code **59851** is reported.

If other methods are not successful or if there are additional indications, an abdominal hysterotomy may be necessary to terminate pregnancy. This technique is similar to the technique of cesarean delivery except that the abdomen and uterus are generally smaller. In this case, code **59852** is reported and encompasses both the attempted intra-amniotic injections and the surgical hysterotomy.

# IX. Nervous System

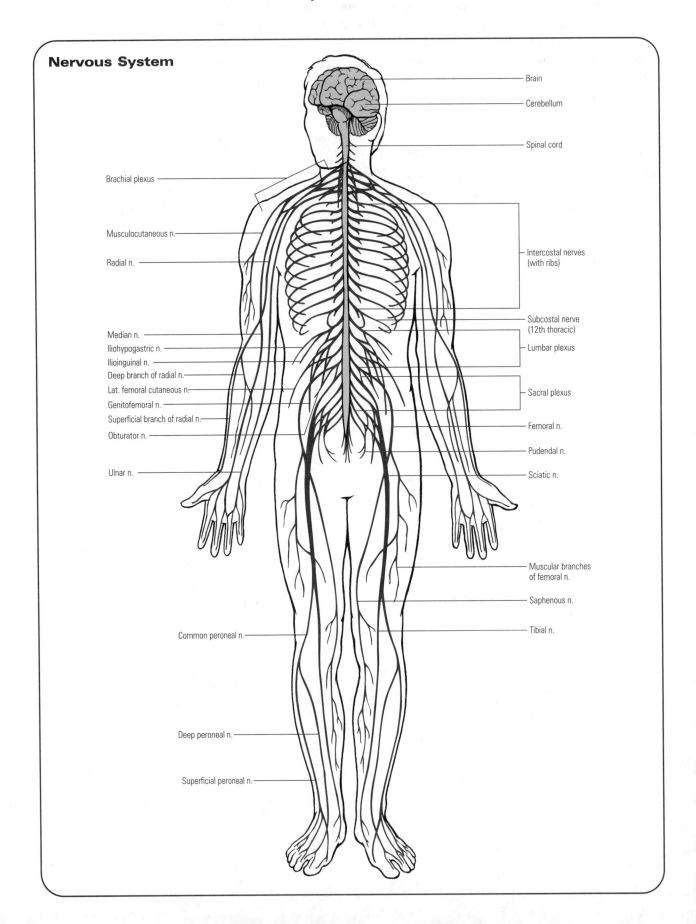

**Nervous System**

Brachial plexus

Musculocutaneous n.

Radial n.

Median n.
Iliohypogastric n.
Ilioinguinal n.
Deep branch of radial n.
Lat. femoral cutaneous n.
Genitofemoral n.
Superficial branch of radial n.
Obturator n.

Ulnar n.

Common peroneal n.

Deep peroneal n.

Superficial peroneal n.

Brain

Cerebellum

Spinal cord

Intercostal nerves
(with ribs)

Subcostal nerve
(12th thoracic)

Lumbar plexus

Sacral plexus

Femoral n.

Pudendal n.

Sciatic n.

Muscular branches
of femoral n.

Saphenous n.

Tibial n.

## Skull

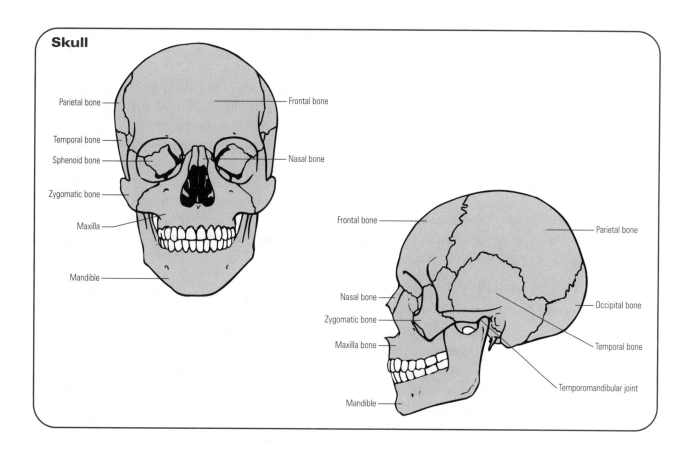

## Brain Anatomy & Sagittal Section of Brain and Brain Stem

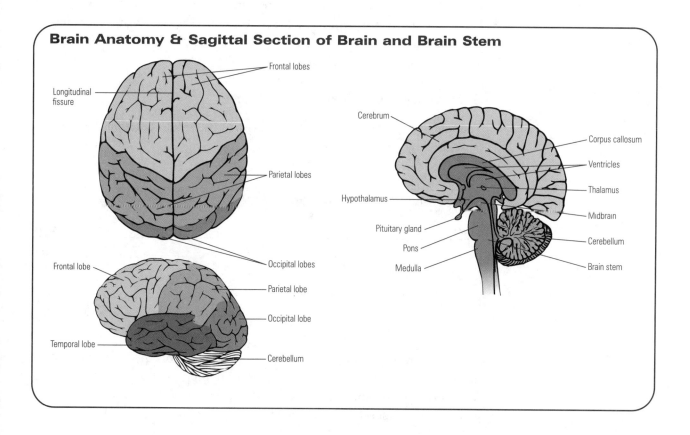

This Surgery section describes diagnostic and therapeutic procedures performed on the nervous system. The illustrations depict the nervous system anatomy, which consists of the following three main divisions:

- The central nervous system (CNS), comprising the brain and spinal cord
- The peripheral nervous system, controlling nerves that relay and receive messages connecting the CNS and other body parts
- The autonomic nervous system, controlling involuntary functions of internal organs

The intricacies of the nervous system occur at the unconscious level, where the autonomic nervous system (and its two antagonistic systems) control the involuntary physiologic regulatory functions (eg, digestion, respiration, cardiovascular function).

To maintain homeostasis, a physiologic balance is created by the sympathetic nervous system, which controls energy expenditure (especially during stress) by releasing the adrenergic catecholamine norepinephrine, and the parasympathetic nervous system, which helps conserve energy by releasing the cholinergic neurohormone acetylcholine.

At the conscious level (activated by will), homeostasis is maintained by the body's voluntary (somatic nervous system) functions (eg, the smallest, action or movement; the highest, mental processes, learning, communication, cognitive capacity, introspection, abstract thought, wonder, ideas, creativity) and the spinal cord, which receives and transmits messages to its attached 31 pairs of segmentally arranged spinal nerves to reach outlying areas of the peripheral nervous system. These fragile structures, threadlike fibers, and microscopic cell bodies are the neurochemical and electrochemical receptors and transmitters that work to control and regulate every mental and physical function.

## Section Layout—Nervous System

The following table indicates the categories of codes found within the Nervous System subsection of Surgery.

| Nervous System Categories and Range of Codes | |
| --- | --- |
| **Category** | **Range of Codes** |
| Skull, Meninges, and Brain | 61000-62258 |
| Spine and Spinal Cord | 62263-63746 |
| Extracranial Nerves, Peripheral Nerves, and Autonomic Nervous System | 64400-64999 |

Consistent with the communication network of the nervous system anatomy, the Nervous System subsection attempts to list procedures in an anatomic "head-to-toe" (ie, brain to peripheral nerves) format. However, from a procedural perspective, a strict anatomic separation is not entirely possible, as certain procedures inherently affect communication and coordination of information to and from the central nervous system (brain and spinal cord) and the peripheral nervous system (voluntary and autonomic systems). Familiarity with the medical terminology and differentiation of intracranial vs extracranial anatomy will help in the use of these codes.

## Skull, Meninges, and Brain

### Twist Drill, Burr Hole(s), or Trephine

Codes **61000-61070** describe diagnostic or therapeutic injection, drainage, or aspiration procedures. Codes **61000-61070** do not include imaging guidance. When performed, the appropriate imaging guidance code from the Radiology section should be additionally reported. For example, if a cisternal or lateral cervical (C1-C2) puncture is performed with injection of contrast material to ascertain placement for injection of a drug and/or for further radiological study, both codes **61055** and **70015** may be reported. Code **61050** describes C1-C2 puncture without injection and is designated as a separate procedure. Since for this example both puncture and injection(s) are performed, the puncture procedure is considered inclusive of code **61055**. Therefore, codes **61050**, **61055**, and **70015** are not reported.

Codes **61105-61253** describe several techniques used to enter the skull and brain for performance of diagnostic or therapeutic procedures. For example, code **61108** describes a therapeutic procedure performed by twist drill hole puncture into the subdural space to evacuate and/or drain a subdural hematoma. Code **61140** describes a diagnostic procedure performed by burr hole(s) or trephine technique for biopsy of brain tissue or an intracranial lesion.

Code **61210** describes implantation of ventricular catheter, reservoir, electroencephalogram electrode(s), or pressure recording device by burr hole technique and, because of its separate procedure designation, may not be reported when these procedures are considered inherent in the larger or major procedure performed. Neuroendoscopic placement or replacement of a ventricular catheter and attachment to a shunt system, performed at the same session as the implantation of the catheter, is reported separately with add-on code **62160**.

The **61105-61250** codes may be performed unilaterally or bilaterally, depending upon the involved anatomy. If a bilateral procedure is performed, append modifier 50. Note that the descriptor of code **61253** is an exception, as this code describes unilateral or bilateral infratentorial cranial access via burr hole(s) or trephine. Do not report codes **61250** or **61253** if burr hole(s) or trephine access is followed by a craniotomy at the same operative session.

### Craniectomy or Craniotomy

The **61304-61576** series of codes describes craniotomy and craniectomy procedures involving various surgical approaches through the skull to reach a specific area of the brain because of disease or trauma (eg, **61546**) or for reconstructive procedures related to congenital or acquired defect (eg, **61556**). Anatomic landmarks and approaches may assist in choosing the best codes. For example, excision of a cerebellopontine angle tumor of the infratentorial or posterior fossa is reported with code **61520**, as opposed to excision of a cerebellopontine angle tumor (ie, acoustic neuroma) involving a transtemporal craniectomy/bone flap craniotomy reported by code **61526**.

Harvest of graft material requiring separate incision should be additionally reported by means of the appropriate graft code. An example is a separate abdominal incision performed to obtain fat for grafting in conjunction with excision of an acoustic neuroma (code **61526**). In this instance, the graft code **20926** should be additionally reported. Also, if the operating microscope is required, code **69990** should also be reported. Implantation of a chemotherapeutic agent following excision of a brain tumor (as described by codes **61510** and **61518**) into the cavity of the excised tumor is reported with add-on code **61517**.

Some of the craniotomy procedures (**61340**, **61490**) may be performed unilaterally or bilaterally, depending on the involved anatomy. If a bilateral procedure is performed, append modifier 50. Depending on the region involved, reconstructive codes from the Musculoskeletal System subsection or a combination of craniectomy and musculoskeletal system reconstructive codes may more accurately describe the procedure performed. For example, for cranial reconstruction for orbital hypertelorism, codes **21260-21263** should be reported, as opposed to **61550-61552**. Other procedures involving the frontal bone (forehead) may require a combination of procedures such as codes **21172-21180** with codes **61552**, **61558**, and **61559**, as appropriate.

Codes **61533-61543**, **61566**, and **61567** are procedures performed for treatment of intractable epilepsy. Codes **61537-61540** describe lobectomy procedures differentiated by anatomy (temporal lobe, other than temporal lobe) and use or absence of electrocorticography during surgery. Electrocorticography is used to record the electrical activity of the brain directly from the exposed cerebral cortex and to map and identify abnormal brain tissue in the motor and sensory cortex during surgery.

The partial or subtotal (functional) hemispherectomy (code **61543**) consists of removal of temporal lobe, followed by a corpus callosotomy and disconnection of the frontal and occipital lobes, with preservation of blood supply to the remaining brain for intractable epilepsy originating from a single side of the brain. The more complete hemispherectomy described by code **61542** is the most radical focal brain excision, for a seizure focus localized to one hemisphere, performed for checking the disease process of progressive seizure conditions.

Codes **61566** and **61567** describe less invasive approaches than the partial/total lobectomies and hemispherectomies, for the removal of the hippocampus and amygdala. These structures are the focal sites of epileptic seizure origin. Removal of these sections has been demonstrated to completely eliminate seizures. Therefore, code **61566** describes a technique that does not involve electrocorticography and that requires removal of only a relatively small deep portion of the temporal lobe.

The multiple subpial transections described by code **61567** cut the horizontal intracortical fibers that contribute to the spread of epileptic seizures. This allows the preservation of the vascular supply to the vertical column structures in the cortex and preservation of the critical motor and speech functions, which are governed by vertical columns in the cortex. Code **61567** includes the electrocorticography procedure, which is not separately reported in addition to code **61567**, when performed.

## Surgery of Skull Base

This coding system of surgical procedures involves operating on a portion of the skull for lesions affecting the deep cranial structures that are adjacent to the undersurface of the cranium (ie, the base of the skull). To treat lesions found at the base of the skull, the expertise of head and neck surgeons, neurologists, neurological surgeons, and plastic and reconstructive surgeons is often required. The techniques described by codes **61580-61619** include single-stage tumor resections and defect reconstruction, use of one general anesthetic procedure, and complete, en bloc tumor resection.

The skull base surgery codes should not be confused with codes that describe a more standard approach for treating a midline tumor at the base of the skull (eg, code **61521**). This code should be reported when performed as a single procedure by one surgeon, compared to the skull base surgery codes. Code **61521** would not be listed in addition to a code from the **61580-61619** series.

Skull base surgery can be performed as the initial treatment for lesions of the base of the skull or to excise a lesion after the initial surgery to excise a lesion has failed because of recurrence of the initial tumor. Coding for skull base procedures requires a thorough understanding of anatomy of the brain and adjoining structures and access to a good anatomy and physiology text and medical dictionary.

## Guidelines for Use of Codes for Surgery of Skull Base

The format of the skull base procedures is based on the division of the cranium into anterior, middle, and posterior fossae. Within this format, any number of surgeons can use the appropriate codes for his or her specific role in the overall treatment of a patient with a cranial base lesion.

The surgical management of lesions involving the skull base often requires the skills of several surgeons of varying specialties working together or in tandem during the operative session. These operations are single-staged and require primary closure of the surgical defect to avoid life-threatening infectious complications such as meningitis and/or osteomyelitis. The procedures are categorized according to

- approach procedure necessary to obtain adequate exposure to the lesion,
- definitive procedure(s) necessary to biopsy, excise, or otherwise treat the lesion, or
- reconstruction/repair of the defect present after the definitive procedure(s).

The approach procedure is described according to the anatomic region involved (ie, anterior cranial fossa, middle cranial fossa, posterior cranial fossa, or any combination of these). The definitive procedures are transection, excision, ligation, or resection of various lesions of the skull base and, when appropriate, the primary closure of the dura, mucosal membranes, and skin. The reconstruction/repair procedure is reported separately if extensive dural grafting, cranioplasty, local or regional myocutaneous pedicle flaps, or extensive skin grafts are required.

Skull base surgery involves several variables such as the size of the tumor, whether this is the initial operation to treat the condition or a reoperation, and the anatomy of the individual patient. For these reasons, no hard and fast rules exist that indicate that all patients with the same diagnosis will receive the same treatment. Before the surgery, each case is studied to plan the surgery among the surgeons who will be involved with the patient. No "surgical team" exists as there might be for a heart transplant, where one surgeon generally is designated to perform one particular portion of each operation. For example, one physician may remove the diseased heart while another may implant the new heart nearly every time a heart transplantation is performed. Both surgeons performing the heart transplantation report the same code (eg, code **33945**) and both append modifier 66 to that code. In skull base surgery, there is no team that is involved in each operation. For this reason, modifier 66 is not reported with skull base surgery.

Several surgeons of different surgical specialties working together or in tandem during the operative session are often needed for skull base surgery. The entire operation may take as long as 32 continuous hours, depending on the extent and complexity of the lesion. In some cases, one physician may perform the approach procedure and the definitive procedure for a specific disease, while another patient with the same disease may have one physician perform the approach procedure while another performs the definitive procedure. Each surgeon reports the individual procedure(s) he or she performs related to skull base surgery. Generally, one physician performs the approach procedure, which exposes the lesion that is to be excised or treated. Another physician, usually of a different specialty, may then excise or otherwise treat the lesion. A third physician may then repair the defect created by tumor removal. If this were the case, each of the three physicians would code only the procedure he or she performed. When one surgeon performs the approach procedure, another performs the definitive procedure, and a third surgeon performs the reconstruction/repair procedure, each surgeon reports only the CPT code number and descriptor for the specific procedure performed. However, if one surgeon performs more than one procedure (ie, approach and definitive procedure), then both CPT codes are reported, with modifier 51 added to the secondary additional procedure(s). It should be noted, however, that the approach and repair add-on procedures cannot be reported if the basic procedure is not reported.

Certain procedures in the skull base, reported by codes **61609-61612**, are "add-on" procedures. They cannot be performed alone; another basic procedure must be performed (eg, code **61605**) and then the add-on (additional) procedure is performed. As with all other CPT add-on codes, these add-on procedures (codes **61609-61612**) are considered to be modifier 51-exempt and are reported without modifier 51. The reconstruction/repair procedure is reported separately if grafts, cranioplasty, or flaps are used to close the defect.

The appropriate codes from the integumentary system are reported, depending on the reconstruction/repair procedure(s) performed. These codes are used if a secondary procedure is required to reconstruct the defect at the time of the initial surgery.

*Secondary Repair of the Defect*

A serious postoperative complication of cerebrospinal fluid (CSF) leakage may occur after skull base surgical procedures. Code **61618** is used to report the secondary repair of a CSF leak that can be accomplished through primary grafting of the dura by means of free tissue grafts (eg, pericranium, fascia, tensor fascia lata, adipose tissue, or autologous or synthetic grafts). More extensive surgical defects with associated postoperative CSF fistula may require the use of local or regional vascularized pedicled grafts or myocutaneous flaps (galea, temporalis, frontalis, or occipitalis), in which case code **61619** is reported.

## Endovascular Therapy

Codes **61623-61642** are reported for intracranial transcatheter procedures. While codes **61624-61626** are intended to report permanent occlusion of the vascular supply to vascular lesions and malformations in the intracranial, head, and neck regions, code **61623** is reported for temporary percutaneous endovascular occlusion. This procedure includes continuous and repetitive neurological assessment throughout the procedure to allow assessment of the results of the temporary occlusion. The descriptor nomenclature of codes **61623** and **61624** is differentiated by the terms *temporary* and *permanent* endovascular balloon occlusion procedures. These codes represent different devices, procedural techniques, and intended outcomes. For code **61623**, the selective catheterization of the vessel to be occluded, positioning, and inflation of the occlusion balloon are inherent intraprocedural steps and not additionally reportable (eg, **36215**, **36216**, **36217**). However, additional codes should be reported in the event separate nonselective (eg, **36100, 36120, 36140, 36160, 36200**) or selective (eg, **36215, 36216, 36217, 36218**) catheterization is performed for angiography of arteries other than the cerebral artery to be occluded and for instances when diagnostic imaging of the artery to be occluded needs further examination outside of the imaging necessary to perform the occlusion. The radiologic imaging to facilitate the placement of an intravascular occlusion device is considered inherent in code **61623** and not separately reportable. However, radiological S&I may be additionally reported when performed for angiography of arteries other than the artery to be occluded (eg, **75650, 75660, 75665, 75671, 75676, 75680, 75685, 75774**).

Code **61624** represents endovascular therapy involving permanent occlusion of the target vessel (eg, for tumor destruction, to achieve hemostasis, to occlude a vascular malformation), as opposed to reversible occlusion specifically intended to not result in damage. Permanent endovascular vessel occlusion of the central nervous system involves traditional component coding conventions (ie, selective catheterization and all appropriate radiological supervision and interpretation are separately reportable).

**CODING TIP**

Modifier 59 must be appended to diagnostic angiography codes when reported in conjunction with a therapeutic radiological supervision and interpretation code on the same date of service.

**CODING TIP**

Embolotherapy performed in one operative field (even through multiple vessels) is reported only once. Multiple operative sites (eg, bilateral arteriovenous malformations, multiple tumors) are considered independent operative fields with treatment reported for each separate operative field. Modifier 59 is recommended to communicate that separate operative sites were treated.

Code **61626** describes the permanent occlusion or embolization of non-central nervous system of head or neck. The device(s) for *temporary* versus *permanent* occlusion are different in their behavior and usage. The procedure and intended outcome are completely different than that described by **61623**. Although **61623** departs from traditional interventional radiology component coding convention, codes **61624** and **61626** follow the component coding usage (refer to the Cardiovascular System section in this chapter for further information on component coding). Code **75894** should be reported in addition to codes **61624** and **61626**. Code **75898** should also be reported for postembolization arteriography.

The endovascular approach angioplasty codes **61630-61642** are distinguished according to diagnosis, in which one series of codes describes balloon angioplasty and/or stenting for recanalization of an intracranial vessel, and a second series of codes is reported for balloon angioplasty for stenosis due to vasospasm. Codes **61630** and **61635** include all selective vascular catheterization of the target vascular family, all diagnostic imaging for arteriography of the target vascular family, and all related radiological S&I. When diagnostic arteriogram (including imaging and selective catheterization) confirms the need for angioplasty or stent placement, **61630** and **61635** are inclusive of these services.

Codes **61640-61642** are reported for intracranial endovascular balloon dilatation for the treatment of the smooth muscle lining of the intracranial vessel. These procedures are most frequently necessary following subarachnoid hemorrhage, in which changes in the intima lining are detected, ultimately resulting in luminal narrowing and rigidity of the vessel wall. This family of codes delineates dilatation of the initial vessel (**61640**) and two add-on codes for dilatation of each additional vessel in the same vascular family (**+61641**) and each additional vessel in a different vascular family (**+61642**).

Codes **61640-61642** include all selective vascular catheterization of the target vessel, contrast injection(s), vessel measurement, roadmapping, post dilatation angiography, and fluoroscopic guidance for the balloon dilatation. Completion cerebral angiography (even if performed on the same day) may be reported separately.

*Surgery for Aneurysm, Arteriovenous Malformation, or Vascular Disease*
Codes **61697-61702** delineate the specific procedures related to the open approach surgical treatment of simple and complex intracranial aneurysms of the carotid and vertebrobasilar circulation aneurysms. The treatment planning, operative time, and use of intraoperative adjunctive treatment vary considerably on the basis of the size, configuration, location, and tissue characteristics of individual aneurysms in the carotid and vertebrobasilar circulation. When use of the operating microscope is required for these procedures, code **69990** is separately reported.

Stereotaxis
Codes **61720-61793** describe intracranial procedures utilizing stereotaxis, a unique type of radiologic guidance/localization method. Code **61751** may be

reported when the stereotactic biopsy, aspiration, or exclusion of an intracranial lesion is performed, requiring CT and/or MRI guidance for MRI or CT marker points of the desired target in the performance of the specific intracranial stereotactic procedure. Note that in certain cases, mounting of a stereotactic head frame is an integral part of the proposed procedure when performed. Therefore, do not additionally report the application/removal of the stereotactic frame code **20660** unless performed as a separate procedure on a date before the procedure by the same or a different physician. Codes **61750** and **61751** include only the procedure(s) that utilize stereotactic guidance. The appropriate radiological supervision and interpretation code should be additionally reported (by either the same or a different physician) when formal interpretation is performed separately from the guidance procedure. For example, CT code **70450**, **70460**, or **70470** may be additionally reported. Also, MRI code **70551**, **70552**, or **70553** may be additionally reported. Code **61751** should be reported only one time, regardless of the number of lesion aspirations performed. Although one specific trajectory path is calculated for insertion of the needle, it may be necessary to reposition the needle. The needle may be guided to either a deeper or more superficial location or along an entirely different trajectory in order to obtain sufficient tissue or fluid to determine the nature of the biopsied lesion.

Stereotactic radiosurgery/therapy (SRS/SRT) is a method of treating brain disorders with a precise delivery of a single high dose of radiation in a one-day session. Through the use of three-dimensional computer-aided planning and a degree of immobilization, the system can minimize the amount of radiation to healthy brain tissue. Treatment involves the use of focused radiation beams delivered to a specific area of the brain to treat cerebral arteriovenous malformations, benign or malignant primary brain tumors or other metastatic brain tumors, or functional disorders. Fractionated stereotactic radiation treatments (SRTs)—which are received over a period of days or weeks—may be administered to the brain with the assistance of removable masks and frames. The radiation source may come from a radioactive material (gamma ray photon), linear accelerator (X-ray photon), or cyclotron particle beam (eg, protons, neutrons).

Code **61770** includes the insertion of radiosurgical probes or catheters for the placement of a radiation source, which involves positioning the probe tip to the targeted coordinates within the needle track created for the radiation or within a needle track that has been enlarged after a previous biopsy. A stereotactic brain biopsy may also be performed. If the brain biopsy is performed, the track that is needed for insertion of brachytherapy seeds or a photon radiosurgery probe has already been established. In this instance, modifier 51 should be appended to the secondary procedure.

As indicated previously for codes **61750** and **61751**, any contrast-enhanced CT or MRI filming performed before treatment is separately reportable. Code **61795** is an add-on code that describes stereotactic computer-assisted volumetric (navigational) technology planning for stereotactic surgery. This planning may take approximately 1 to 2 hours and includes determination of the coordinates for the target, measurement of the anterior commissure-posterior commissure line, and angle calculation. Using a computer, various trajectories are determined to assist the physician in choosing the specific trajectory and calculating the entry point through the skull. The anatomic references within the descriptor direct the use of this code in addition to other intracranial, extracranial, or spinal stereotactic procedures.

Code **61793** represents placement (and removal) of the immobilization system (eg, stereotactic head frame, relocatable head frame or thermoplastic mask with localization system) participating in the scanning for target localization, identification of appropriate target and avoidance structure, and return to the radiation facility where the patient is placed on the table and the immobilization system is applied on the table and treatment is delivered. Code **61793** is used to identify stereotactic radiosurgery performed using any number of different devices.

Code **61795** may also be reported when this procedure is performed in conjunction with various "extracranial" procedures of the ear, nose, and throat (ENT), head and neck (including functional endoscopic sinus surgery [FESS]). Examples include those procedures described by codes **31254-31256**, **31267**, **31276**, **31287**, **31288**, **31290-31294**, and **61548**.

### Neurostimulators (Intracranial)

There are three neurostimulator code sections in the CPT codebook. These sections describe intracranial neurostimulators (**61850-61888**), spinal neurostimulators (**63650-63688**), and peripheral nerve neurostimulators (**64553-64595**).

The deep brain stimulation codes **61850-61886** describe procedures targeting sites where electrodes can be applied for stimulation, the radiologic technology (computer-guided MRI or CT stereotactic elements) necessary for placement of these electrode arrays, and the technique/approach used to implant the neurostimulator components (ie, electrodes or pulse generator). Deep brain stimulation is used in the treatment of functional disorders (eg, movement problems from Parkinson's disease, essential tremor, multiple sclerosis, head trauma, drug-induced hyperkinesias, vascular malformations, cerebral hemorrhage, intractable pain). The cranial neurostimulator series of codes in the CPT code set describes placement of an electrode into the brain tissues targeted for stimulation through an introducer needle. The electrodes are then tested for verification of appropriate placement. In deep brain stimulation, delivery of small electric shocks from the implanted electrodes inactivates the targeted area of the brain (eg, the overactive globus pallidus in the Parkinson's patient and the abnormal brain activity in the multiple sclerosis patient).

This series of codes in the Cranial Neurostimulator subsection is differentiated by the following:

- Inclusion of stereotactic guidance for implantation
- Approach (twist drill, burr hole, craniotomy/craniectomy)
- Site (subcortical, cortical, cerebral, cerebellar)
- Use of microelectrode recording

Codes **61850** and **61860** are reported for nonstereotactic implantation of neurostimulator electrodes in a cortical site. These codes are differentiated only by approach: by twist drill or burr hole technique (**61850**) or by craniectomy or craniotomy (**61860**).

The remaining codes describe stereotactically placed subcortical insertion of a multicontact (eg, quadripolar) deep brain stimulator lead (neurostimulator arrays) by twist drill, burr hole, craniotomy, or craniectomy technique. Various portions of the subcortical anatomy may be the target site, including the thalamus, globus pallidus, subthalamic nucleus, periventricular area, and periaqueductal gray matter. Codes **61863**, **61864**, **61867**, and **61868** are distinguished primarily by the absence (**61863**, **61864**) or use (**61867**, **61868**) of intraoperative microelectrode recording. Microelectrode recording is used during the targeting and repositioning of the electrode array to optimize the accuracy of placement for clinical effect while minimizing side effects of the stimulation. These codes are additionally distinguished by the number of neurostimular arrays implanted, one (**61863**, **61867**) or two (bilateral, **61864**, **61868**). These procedures include placement of a stereotactic frame, with determination of placement/alignment by CT or MRI. Therefore, the application/removal of the stereotactic frame, code **20660**, is not additionally reported unless performed as a separate procedure on a date before the procedure by the same or a different physician. The appropriate radiological S&I code (preoperative and postoperative MRI scan of brain [**70551**], CT scan of brain [**70450**]) should be additionally reported (by either the same or a different physician). Add-on code **61795** may not be reported when computer-assisted planning is performed in conjunction with these stereotactic implantation procedures. Placement of the neurostimulator pulse generator (code **61885**) is also separately reported.

Codes **61867** and **61868** are reported when microelectrode recording is performed as a service of the operating surgeon. If another physician (eg, neurologist) performs the neurophysiological mapping, the second physician should report codes **95961** and **95962**.

On the basis of the approach used (twist drill, burr hole, craniotomy, or craniectomy), the components of the frame are assembled and coordinates set, and the electrode array is marked for the appropriate depth of placement. The electrode array is passed into the predetermined site and is repositioned and restimulated as many times as necessary to obtain the best degree of tremor suppression and least side effects, and the electrode array is implanted.

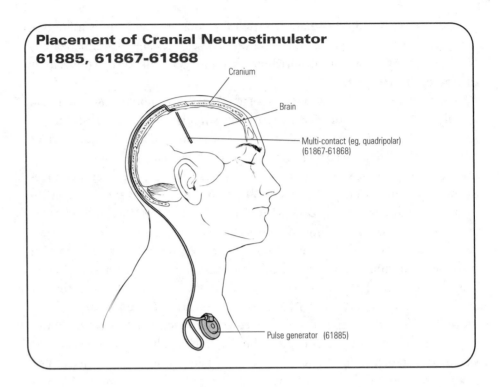

**Placement of Cranial Neurostimulator
61885, 61867-61868**

Cranium

Brain

Multi-contact (eg, quadripolar)
(61867-61868)

Pulse generator (61885)

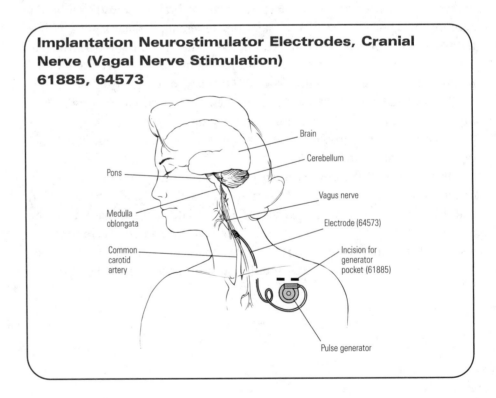

**Implantation Neurostimulator Electrodes, Cranial
Nerve (Vagal Nerve Stimulation)
61885, 64573**

Brain

Cerebellum

Pons

Vagus nerve

Medulla
oblongata

Electrode (64573)

Common
carotid
artery

Incision for
generator
pocket (61885)

Pulse generator

In certain cases, a trial implantation of one stereotactically guided deep brain stimulator electrode array is performed. If a one-stage operation is performed (ie, the stimulator generator is placed at the same operative setting), then the lead is coiled in a subgaleal pocket. Because of the nature of the disorders responding to deep brain stimulation (eg, Parkinson's disease, essential tremor, multiple sclerosis), bilateral symptoms and findings are now frequently treated. Therefore, sometimes one electrode array might be connected to one pulse generator or receiver. At other times, two electrode arrays (one on each side of the brain) may be required and might be connected to one generator or receiver (code **61886**). CPT codes **61885** and **61886** reflect the increased physician work and risk involved in the placement of a cranial neurostimulator pulse generator or receiver in the patient's subcutaneous tissue, creation of a pocket, and coupling with intracranial or cranial nerve (eg, vagal) electrode(s), as indicated. Insertion of a multicontact (eg, quadripolar) deep brain stimulator lead is separately reported by means of the appropriate code from the series **61863-61868**. If the cranial neurostimulator pulse generator or receiver requires connection to a single electrode array, code **61885** should be reported in addition to the electrode insertion code. If the cranial neurostimulator pulse generator or receiver requires connection to two or more electrode arrays, code **61886** should be reported.

For open insertion of a cranial nerve (eg, vagal) neurostimulator electrode, code **64573** should be reported in addition to code **61885**. For percutaneous insertion of a cranial nerve neurostimulator electrode, code **64553** should be reported in addition to code **61885**. If this is planned to be a two-stage operation (ie, the stimulator generator is placed at a later date), then the tail of the electrode is subcutaneously tunneled and exits the scalp at a separate site. The wound is closed, the stereotactic frame is removed, and the pin sites are dressed. If a trial implantation is successful in eliminating or decreasing the patient's tremor and a neurostimulator pulse generator is placed later, code **61885 58** should be reported at the time of the future placement of the neurostimulator pulse generator. Code **61886 58** would be reported for subcutaneous placement of a cranial neurostimulator pulse generator or receiver when the connection is to two or more electrode arrays.

Codes **61885** and **61886** involve internalization of the tail of the electrode array and placement and connection of a subcutaneous neurostimulator generator for long-term brain stimulation. These codes describe procedures that involve general anesthesia or local anesthesia with light sedation, recovery of the cranial lead from the subgaleal space, linear incision just below the clavicle, and creation of a subcutaneous pocket for placement of the pulse generator/transmitter.

Code **61886** differs in that the same insertion procedure is repeated for the electrode array on the other side, including tunneling of the tail of this electrode to the second limb of the bifurcated extension wire. The distal ends of both leads of the bifurcated extension wires are inserted into the generator and tightened, and the generator is sutured into place in the subcutaneous tissue. The neurostimulator pulse generator/transmitter is tested (see codes **95971-95973**, **95978**, **95979**) and the wounds and skin are closed. When the electrodes have been inserted for deep brain stimulation, the neurostimulator pulse genera-

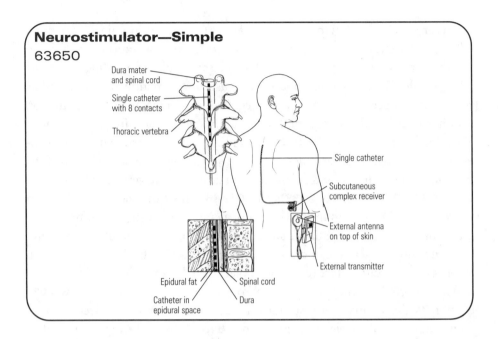

**Neurostimulator—Simple**
**63650**

Dura mater and spinal cord
Single catheter with 8 contacts
Thoracic vertebra
Single catheter
Subcutaneous complex receiver
External antenna on top of skin
External transmitter
Epidural fat
Spinal cord
Catheter in epidural space
Dura

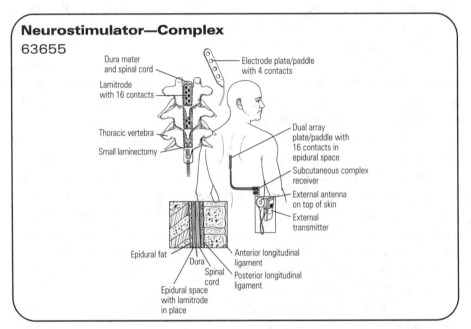

**Neurostimulator—Complex**
**63655**

Dura mater and spinal cord
Lamitrode with 16 contacts
Thoracic vertebra
Small laminectomy
Electrode plate/paddle with 4 contacts
Dual array plate/paddle with 16 contacts in epidural space
Subcutaneous complex receiver
External antenna on top of skin
External transmitter
Epidural fat
Dura
Spinal cord
Epidural space with lamitrode in place
Anterior longitudinal ligament
Posterior longitudinal ligament

tor/transmitter testing is reported with codes **95978** and **95979**, based upon the time required for the testing. For both codes **61885** and **61886**, the neurostimulator generator is sutured into place in the subcutaneous tissue. The neurostimulator is tested (see codes **95974** and **95975**) to determine the impedance of the connections and to rule out any electrical short.

The neurostimulator insertion/removal codes do not differentiate simple vs complex device components. Therefore, for revision or removal of either a simple or a complex neurostimulator pulse generator or receiver, see codes **61888**,

**63688**, and **64595**. For implantation of either simple or complex neurostimulator system electrodes, see codes **61850-61875**, **63650-63655**, and **64553-64581**. For revision or removal of either simple or complex neurostimulator electrodes, see codes **61880**, **63660**, and **64585**.

The series of codes **62000-62148** is reported for skull repair or cranioplasty procedures. The procedure reported by code **62148** is performed at the time of a primary surgical procedure for the treatment of intracranial hypertension (eg, decompressive craniotomy, lobectomy, or evacuation of intracranial hematoma) where immediate replacement of the cranial bone flap may aggravate intracranial hypertension from brain swelling. An incision is made into a suitable area of the abdominal wall and a subcutaneous pocket is created for placement and retention of the cranial bone flap. Subsequent to the completion of the cranioplasty, the area of the abdomen where the bone flap was previously implanted is incised through the scar, the pocket opened, and the bone flap retrieved from the subcutaneous tissues for replacement at the site of the cranioplasty. Notice that code **62148** is an add-on code, and modifier 51 should not be used when code **62148** is reported with the cranioplasty procedure codes **62140-62147**. (Refer to Chapter 4 for further discussion of add-on codes.)

## Neuroendoscopy

Neuroendoscopic placement or replacement of a ventricular catheter and attachment to a shunt system, performed at the same session as the implantation of the catheter, is reported separately with add-on code **62160**.

The series of neuroendoscopy codes **62161-62165** are intended to report the various intracranial procedures performed solely via the endoscopic approach. Since the procedures in this series that might require the placement of the ventricular catheter include this procedure, codes **62161**, **62162**, **62164**, and **62165** would not be reported in addition to code **62160**. Intracranial procedures performed via the open approach would be reported with the appropriate open procedure codes (ie, removal of intracranial foreign body or lesion; see codes **61333** and **61334**). Code **62161** is typically performed for opening intraventricular barriers to the free flow of CSF for the treatment of hydrocephalus. Codes **62164** and **62165** may be reported respectively for any type of brain or pituitary tumor.

Codes **62180-62258** involve procedures related to controlling or redirecting the circulation of CSF. This series of codes describes the various types of technology and insertional techniques used for noninvasive changes in the pressure settings of programmable CSF shunts.

The cross-reference following code **62201** for neuroendoscopic ventriculocisternostomy is intended to refer the user to other intracranial procedures performed via the neuroendoscopic method. Codes **62200** and **62201** may be used to describe third ventricle ventriculocisternostomy performed by: stereotactic method only, combined stereotactic and endoscopic methods, or endoscopic method only (with an endoscope but without the use of stereotactic method).

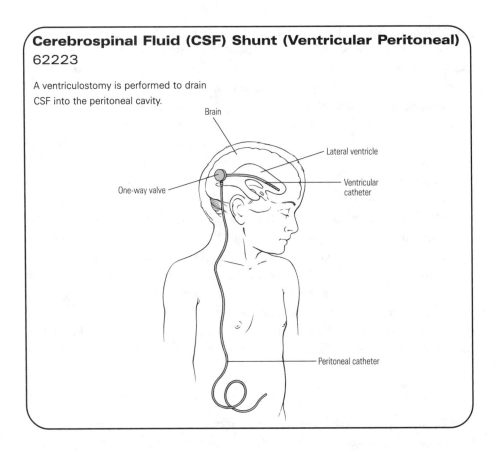

**Cerebrospinal Fluid (CSF) Shunt (Ventricular Peritoneal)**
62223

A ventriculostomy is performed to drain CSF into the peritoneal cavity.

Brain

One-way valve

Lateral ventricle

Ventricular catheter

Peritoneal catheter

Code **62252** describes the procedure used in the adjustment of previously inserted intracranial CSF shunts. Certain patients are prone to the incidence of overdrainage or underdrainage of CSF. Reprogramming is intended to treat shunts inserted for overdrainage and underdrainage of CSF in a hydrocephalus patient or underdrainage of a cyst or other fluid collection in the brain of the patient after initial implantation of a programmable shunt. Unless the decision for reprogramming has not yet been made, assessment of the patient during reprogramming includes the actual reprogramming of the shunt, along with confirmation of the changes made to the pressure setting. Reprogramming is required after a patient with a programmable CSF shunt undergoes an MRI. An X-ray must be performed to verify the proper setting of the valve mechanism of the shunt. Code **62252** is reported one time only for each encounter and is not reported separately for different settings during the same encounter.

## Spine and Spinal Cord

The Spinal Injection subsection reflects the systematic organization of this series of codes to differentiate the specific spinal anatomy (subarachnoid, epidural), levels (cervical, thoracic, lumbar, sacral), and types of substances injected (neurolytic, opioid, anesthetic, steroid, antispasmodic). Also clarified are the intent and use of this series of injection procedures, with particular differentiation related to the use of the corresponding radiology codes, namely, the use of the fluoroscopic guidance and localization code **77003**, epidurography code **72275**, sacroiliac joint arthrography code **73542**, and myelography codes **72240**, **72255**, **72265**, and **72270**. The spine injection procedures differentiate the following:

- Time and complexity between a single injection vs a continuous infusion (or multiple injections through the same catheter)
- Differences between subarachnoid and epidural routes of administration
- Time and complexity related to injections performed at the cervical, thoracic, lumbar, or sacral levels of the spine (eg, significant difference in complexity and time related to a cervical/thoracic injection as compared to a lumbar/sacral injection)
- Time and complexity related to injections of different substances (eg, opioid, steroid, neurolytic)

In certain instances, fluoroscopic assistance is required to visualize and identify specific spinal anatomy in the performance of either epidural or subarachnoid injection procedures **62270-62273**, **62280-62282**, and **62310-62319**. With the exception of the percutaneous lysis of adhesion codes **62263** and **62264**, none of the spinal injection codes include fluoroscopic guidance and localization for placement of the needle or catheter. Code **77003** identifies the fluoroscopic guidance to assist in accurately localizing specific spinal anatomy for placement of a needle or catheter tip for spine or paraspinous diagnostic or therapeutic injection procedures (epidural, transforaminal epidural, subarachnoid, paravertebral facet joint, paravertebral facet joint nerve, or sacroiliac joint) including neurolytic agent destruction. Therefore, code **77003** should be reported in conjunction with codes **62270-62273**, **62280-62282**, and **62310-62319**, when fluoroscopic guidance is required in the performance of these injection procedures.

Code **77003** does not represent a formal contrast study. Examples of formal contrast studies are myelography, epidurography, and sacroiliac joint arthrography. Therefore, code **77003** is considered an inclusive component of codes **72240**, **72255**, **72265**, **72270**, **72275**, and **73542**. However, for sacroiliac joint injection (code **27096**), if a formal arthrography (code **73542**) is not performed and recorded and a formal radiologic report is not issued, then it is appropriate to report code **77003** for the fluoroscopic guidance used to locate the specific anatomic site for needle insertion.

Although not specifically stated in the descriptor nomenclature, the introductory notes clarify that injection of contrast is inclusive of the injection procedures described by codes **62263**, **62264**, **62270-62273**, **62280-62282**, **62310-62319**, and **0027T**. For codes **62270-62273**, **62280-62282**, **62310-62319**, and **0027T**, the guidance, localization, and interpretation of the filming should be additionally reported by means of code **72275** or **77003**. Codes **62263** and **62264** include guidance, localization, epidurography, and interpretation of the filming. Therefore, codes **72275** and **77003** should not be reported in addition to **62263** and **62264**. If injections are performed at different spinal levels, the spinal injection codes should be reported for each level of the involved spinal region. For example, epidurography at the cervical and lumbar region would be reported by means of codes **62310** and **72275** (cervical) plus **62311** and **72275 59** (lumbar).

> **CODING TIP**
>
> Code **72275** is to be used only when an epidurogram is performed, images are documented, and a formal radiologic report is issued.

The descriptor of code **62263** refers to a percutaneous catheter-based treatment involving the targeted injection of various substances via an indwelling epidural catheter for the administration of multiple neurolytic injections for serial treatment sessions spanning two or more treatment days. Code **62263** should not be reported for each substance injected, since there is no added physician work in adding multiple liquid drugs to the solution injected, including an anesthetic agent. Because the treatment goal involves a concerted effort to break down scar formation (adhesions), reduce edema, reduce inflammation, and block propagation of nociception (pain transmission) to the central nervous system, several separate treatments are frequently required. Code **62263** is reported once, even though the treatment occurs over several days and may address several specific area(s) of scarring and inflammation in the epidural space. Code **62264** describes multiple catheter adhesiolysis treatment sessions performed during the same day via neurolytic injections or infusions. Each of these codes includes any mechanical lysis of adhesions or scarring using a percutaneously deployed catheter.

Codes **62263** and **62264** have no limits on the number of needle passes necessary to break up the adhesions. Both codes **62263** and **62264** should be reported only one time for the entire series of injections/infusions or mechanical lysis procedures performed, not per adhesiolysis treatment. For code **62263**, this treatment series will span two or more treatment days but the code would still be reported only one time. Before initiation of percutaneous lysis of epidural adhesions, epidurography is performed to identify the areas of scarring, nerve constriction, possible nerve inflammation, and degree of fluid flow (or lack thereof) in the epidural space. This radiological multiplanar imaging of a specific anatomic region (ie, cervical, thoracic, lumbar) is performed at the same session as the initiation of percutaneous epidural adhesiolysis. In essence, after fluoroscopic confirmation of the accurate needle location in the epidural space, a catheter is percutaneously threaded through the needle and placed in the epidural space.

Codes **62263** and **62264** include the procedure of injections of contrast for epidurography (**72275**) and fluoroscopic guidance and localization (**77003**) during initial or subsequent sessions. Mechanical adhesion lysis that uses an epiduroscope is reported with Category III code **0027T**. The physician uses an epiduroscope as an adjunctive mechanical-based technique performed in addition to the administration of neurolytic substance(s) via the initially or previously placed epidural catheter. Intentional mechanical adhesion lysis is achieved by maneuvering the epiduroscope with direct visualization. Alternatively, the epiduroscope may be used to deploy a type of mechanical device specifically for mechanical adhesiolysis.

The unlisted nervous system code **64999** should be reported to describe placement of an endoscope in the epidural space for diagnostic epiduroscopy. When required, epidurography (**72275**) performed at multiple spinal levels should be reported only once for each spinal region examined (eg, once for the thoracic region and once for the lumbar region). Code **72275** includes a formally interpreted contrast study involving multiplanar imaging generating hardcopy images, fluoroscopic guidance, and localization. Therefore, code **77003** should not be reported in addition to code **72275**. The performance of radiologic multiplanar imaging is included in codes **62263** and **62264**, as is the fluoroscopic guidance and injection of contrast; therefore, codes **77003** and **72275** are not reported in addition to these codes during initial or subsequent sessions. The daily hospital management performed in conjunction with these services is separately reported with the appropriate E/M codes.

Code **62273** is used for epidural injection of blood or blood clot performed in either the cervical, thoracic, or lumbar region. Ongoing CSF fluid leak can occur at any level of the spinal column. A CSF leak, for example, may be present in post-lumbar puncture headache, CSF hygroma, posttraumatic CSF leakage, or actual CSF leakage outside the skin.

Codes **62280-62282** describe neurolytic injections performed when ablation of a nerve, nerve root, or portion of the spinal cord is desired. This clinical need often occurs because of intractable pain from malignancy, tumor, radiation therapy effects, and/or surgical scarring. Neurolytic injections can also be performed where ablation of a primarily sensory nerve root, nerve, or a specific spinal cord dermatome level is desired without causing significant functional impairment to the patient (eg, prior trauma that eliminated motor function from the target site). Because the site of the pain could be at the cervical, thoracic, lumbar, or caudal vertebral levels, codes **62280-62282** specify either the subarachnoid or epidural spaces of the spinal column, and codes **62281** and **62282** differentiate upper vs lower spinal regions. From a procedural standpoint, the same procedure is performed. The difference is that after the needle is initially placed but before the neurolytic injection, an epidural contrast injection (epidurography) is performed. Again as with other neurolytic injections, it is important to determine and confirm the exact level for injection to affect the desired nerve, nerve root, or level of spinal cord.

Code **62287** describes various percutaneous methods for decompressing a lumbar intervertebral disc and states examples for each method to clarify appropriate application of this code, including percutaneous aspiration or decompression of an intervertebral disc by means of a laser. A cross-reference directs users to the fluoroscopic localization code **77002** (for fine needle biopsy or aspiration), as fluoroscopic imaging guidance is not inclusive of code **62287**.

Codes **62310** and **62311** describe epidural or subarachnoid injection of nonneurolytic substances including opioids, steroids, antispasmodic, and anesthetic substances. Code **62310** should be reported to describe cervical or thoracic injection of substances other than neurolytics, while code **62311** is reported for lumbar or caudal epidural or subarachnoid injections. If injections are performed at different spinal levels, the spinal injection codes should be reported for each level of the involved spinal region. For example, epidurography at the cervical and lumbar region would be reported by means of codes **62310** and **72275** (cervical) plus **62311** and **72275 59** (lumbar).

Codes **62310-62319** describe the epidural (interlaminar) injection performed when analgesia is desired for spine or nerve root pain. This clinical need occurs in both cancer and noncancer patients with intractable pain. This injection can also be used for diagnostic purposes or for testing a patient's sensitivity to narcotic prior to a long-term spinal infusion using an external or implanted

**CODING TIP**

The services for refilling and maintenance of an implantable reservoir or infusion pump (intrathecal, epidural, or intraventricular) should be additionally reported by code **95990** or **95991**. The refilling and maintenance of an external pump is not reportable by the CPT code set.

**CODING TIP**

Although not specifically stated in the descriptor nomenclature, injection of contrast material is considered an inclusive component of codes **62280-62282**.

**CODING TIP**

Codes **62310-62319** do not differentiate the type of agent(s) (eg, narcotic, anesthetic, steroid, antispasmodic) injected but focus upon the route of injection. They do exclude injection of a neurolytic substance, since that procedure is represented by codes **62280-62282**.

infusion pump. The choice of an epidural or subarachnoid route for such diagnostic testing is variable and based upon the physician's personal preference. Codes **62310-62319** are reported once per level, regardless of the number or type of injections performed per level. Therefore, it is inappropriate to report the spinal injection code(s) for each injection performed at a particular level. If injections are performed at different spinal levels, the spinal injection codes should be reported for each level of the involved spinal region. For example, epidurography at the cervical and lumbar region would be reported by means of codes **62310** and **72275** (cervical) plus **62311** and **72275 59** (lumbar).

For codes **62318** and **62319**, a catheter is threaded through the needle and placed in the epidural space. Through this catheter a continuous infusion is started for several hours or several days. Occasionally, as part of a detailed diagnostic or treatment regimen, multiple (three or more) injections might be given through this catheter over a period of hours or one to two days. These multiple injections often involve different substances, such as placebo injection or varying amounts of narcotic. Insertion of the catheter at the cervical/thoracic levels involves risk related to possible damage to the spinal cord and delayed respiratory side effects from a cervical/thoracic opioid infusion as compared to a similar infusion in the lumbar/sacral region (**62319**). The descriptor for codes **62318** and **62319** specifies the inclusion of a contrast injection and clarifies the type of administration performed, the substances injected, and the involved spinal anatomy. Subsequent daily management is not included in codes **62318** and **62319** and is separately reportable.

### Catheter Implantation

Codes **62350** and **62351** are differentiated by the insertional technique that requires (**62351**) or does not require (**62350**) laminectomy. Code **62350** is reported when an intrathecal or epidural catheter is connected to an external pump, an implantable reservoir, or an implantable infusion pump not requiring laminectomy. Code **62351** is reported when the catheter placement requires laminectomy. Both codes **62350** and **62351** are intended to describe medication administration performed not only for long-term pain management, but for other indications such as administration of chemotherapeutic agents, antibiotics, antispasmodic agents, etc.

### Posterior Extradural Laminotomy or Laminectomy for Exploration/Decompression of Neural Elements or Excision of Herniated Intervertebral Discs

Code **63020** describes an open posterior approach to decompress nerve roots with/without excision of a herniated disc. However, in certain instances, the endoscope may also be used for lumbar nerve root decompression to improve illumination and visualization. Nerve root decompression with excision of a herniated disc uses a similar but "minimally open" approach to that described by **63020** in the cervical spine. Code **63030** is reported when laminotomy for discectomy is performed with endoscopic assistance in the lumbar spine.

Codes **63040-63044** are the only codes that may be reported for procedures performed on a recurrent herniated nucleus pulposus at previously explored

**CODING TIP**

No CPT codes exist for reexploration procedures of the thoracic region of the spine, as this procedure is rarely performed.

**CODING TIP**

If the operating microscope is used, report code **69990**.

cervical or lumbar interspaces. The term *reexploration* simply relates to the repeat surgical exposure of a previous surgical tract and target at the same site on the same patient at a time after an initial surgical procedure(s) was performed. The time frame associated with the reexploration procedures is not specifically stated. Should reexploration be required within the operative period of an initial procedure, then the appropriate reexploration code(s) should be reported with modifier 78 appended. The **63040-63044** code series delineates that reexploration laminotomy or hemilaminectomy is considered a unilateral (vs a bilateral) procedure and that the reexploration procedure involves a single interspace (as opposed to an entire region of the spine (ie, cervical, lumbar)

Codes **63040-63044** are performed at each vertebral interspace. Codes **63043** and **63044** describe reexploration procedures performed at each additional cervical and lumbar interspace. For coding purposes, a vertebral interspace is defined as "the non-bony compartment between two adjacent vertebral bodies, which contains the intervertebral disk, and includes the nucleus pulposus, annulus fibrosus, and two cartilaginous endplates."

Anatomically, either right and/or left lamina or disc material may be excised. Therefore, if a right and left hemilaminectomy are performed at a cervical or lumbar interspace, then codes **63040-63044**, as appropriate, should be reported with modifier 50 appended.

In certain instances, other spinal procedures may be performed at the time of the reexploration procedure(s), involving vertebral segment(s) or interspace(s) not previously explored. Therefore, the appropriate bone graft, arthrodesis, and/or spinal instrumentation codes should be additionally reported. In this circumstance, modifier 51 should be appended to code **63040** or **63042**. It is not appropriate to append modifier 51 to add-on codes **63043** or **63044**. (Refer to Chapter 4 for further discussion of add-on codes.) However, if a laminectomy, facetectomy, and foraminotomy are performed concurrently, unilaterally or bilaterally, with decompression of the spinal cord, cauda equina, and/or nerve roots, on a single vertebral segment at the lumbar level and this segment has not been previously explored, then report code **63047**. Code **63048** is an add-on code that may be reported only when code **63047** has been reported for the first lumbar vertebral segment procedure and it is necessary to report procedures for one or more additional segments. For coding purposes, a segment is defined as "a single complete vertebral bone with associated articular processes and laminae."

The cervical laminoplasty codes (**63050**, **63051**) describe the surgical decompression and reconstruction of the posterior elements of the cervical spine. In contrast to the cervical decompression procedures **63001** and **63015**, which describe complete removal of the posterior spine elements, code **63050** describes the performance of a unilateral osteotomy between the facet joint and the lamina and a partial osteotomy on the contralateral side, to create a "swinging door" to allow expansion of the stenotic spinal canal. Bone graft and/or nonsegmental fixation should be reported with code **63051**, when performed. Cervical arthrodesis (**22600-22614**), spinal fixation and instrumentation (**22840-22842**), and laminectomy (**63045**, **63048**) are included in these procedures and not separately reported.

### Transpedicular or Costovertebral Approach for Posterolateral Extradural Exploration/Decompression

Certain far lateral disc herniations are excised via a posterior or posterolateral approach that does not involve a laminotomy/laminectomy (ie, does not require the removal of laminar bone), which is intrinsic to code **63030**. Code **63056** should be reported when an extralaminar transfacet or lateral extraforaminal approach is required. These types of approaches are similar to those described by code **63055** (but not described by code **63030**) in the treatment of far lateral disc herniations.

### Anterior or Anterolateral Approach for Extradural Exploration/Decompression

The series of codes **63081-63103** describes vertebral corpectomy procedures performed for treatment of several types of spinal pathology, including fracture, tumor, and infection, for relief of spinal stenosis. Vertebral corpectomy procedures involve removal of the damaged vertebral body, arthrodesis, and spinal instrumentation for stabilization of the bone graft. The vertebral corpectomy codes, reported per segment, are differentiated according to approach (anterior/anterolateral, lateral extracavitary), spinal region (cervical, thoracic, lumbar), and initial segment vs additional segments. The lateral extracavitary procedures do not describe corpectomy of the cervical region.

As these procedures commonly require surgeons of different surgical specialties working together, each surgeon reports the individual procedure(s) he or she performs related to vertebral corpectomy surgery. When two surgeons work together as primary surgeons performing distinct part(s) of a spinal cord exploration/decompression operation, each surgeon should report his or her distinct operative work by appending modifier 62 to the procedure code (and any associated add-on codes for that procedure code as long as both surgeons continue to work together as primary surgeons). In this situation, modifier 62 may be appended to the definitive procedure code(s) **63081**, **63085**, **63087**, **63090**, **63101**, and **63102** and, as appropriate, to additional segment add-on code(s) **63082**, **63086**, **63088**, **63091**, and **63103**, as long as both surgeons continue to work together as primary surgeons. However, if one surgeon performs more than one procedure (ie, approach and definitive procedure), then both CPT codes are reported, with modifier 51 added to the secondary additional procedure(s) (eg, arthrodesis). The add-on code(s) **63082**, **63086**, **63088**, **63091**, and **63103** are modifier 51-exempt.

## Neurostimulators (Spinal)

Codes **63650**, **63655**, and **63660** all relate to the operative placement, revision, or removal of the neurostimulator for patients with chronic, intractable pain in the trunk or limbs either as the sole mitigating agent or as an adjunct to other modes of therapy (eg, used in a multidisciplinary approach). It is used for numerous neuropathic pain disorders that require either simple or complex treatment (eg, management of postamputation neuralgia [stump pain], intractable neuralgia, unilateral cervical, or lumbosacral radiculopathies, postherpetic neuralgia, vasculopathic [peripheral ischemic] pain). Pain of neurologic origin may be due to peripheral nerve injuries, which are unilateral, afflict only one or a few dermatomes, and involve appendicular rather than axial regions of the body. Bilateral pain is among the more complicated indications because stimulation must also be bilateral. The choice of the type of device depends on the diagnostic indication for spinal stimulation.

Codes **63650**, **63655**, and **63660** describe the operative placement, revision, or removal of the spinal neurostimulator system components to provide spinal electrical stimulation. A neurostimulator system includes an implanted neurostimulator, external controller, extension, and collection of contacts. Multiple contacts or electrodes (4 or more) provide the actual electrical stimulation in the epidural space. For percutaneously placed neurostimulator systems (**63650**, **63660**), the contacts are on a catheter-like lead. An array is the collection of contacts that are on one catheter or the plate-paddle surface. The contacts are permanently attached to the catheter or the plate-paddle surface. After placement of the stimulation system, the catheter or plate-paddle is left permanently implanted. CPT Nomenclature makes no distinctions as to the number of sites required for the placement of electrode catheters. Code **63650** is reported for the placement of the initial neurostimulator electrode catheter. Percutaneous placement of additional catheters is reported using code **63650** with modifier 51 appended. Fluoroscopy to position the catheter or plate-paddle containing the electrode array is considered an inclusive component of code **63655** and not separately reportable (eg, **76000**, **77002**, **77003**).

Code **63685** should not be reported in addition to **63688** for the same pulse generator or receiver. This instruction refers to the circumstance where a pulse generator is removed and the same generator is reinserted. For example, the pulse generator is removed because of disconnection of the lead(s), the lead(s) are reconnected and the same generator is reinserted. Another example is in the event the generator is resting on the pelvic rim and is moved due to pain. In these two specific circumstances, the work is considered revision of an existing generator, so only code **63688** should be reported. It would not be appropriate to report code **63688** for removal of the generator in addition to code **63685** to describe reinsertion of the same generator. To further clarify, code **63688** may also be reported independently, for example, in the event of infection or because a satisfactory response to treatment has not been achieved. In this circumstance, for removal of the lead array, code **63660** should also be reported.

## Extracranial Nerves, Peripheral Nerves, and Autonomic Nervous System

### Introduction/Injection of Anesthetic Agent (Nerve Block), Diagnostic or Therapeutic

The **64400-64484** code series describes spine injection procedures to various portions of the spinal anatomy, for example, the cervical and thoracic regions of the spine.

---

**CODING TIP**

Test stimulation via the implanted electrode is inherent in code **63655**. However, for initial programming of generator or transmitter-receiver during and/or immediately at the end of the implantation operation, use **95970-95973**.

---

**CODING TIP**

Third-party payers may have specific reporting guidelines for ICD-9-CM diagnosis reporting associated with facet joint nerve and facet joint injection procedures. Therefore, it is best to check with third-party payers for their individual policies.

---

**CODING TIP**

Code **64435 47** would be reported for the administration of general or regional anesthesia when a paracervical uterine nerve injection is given by the surgeon as an anesthetic agent for a conization of the cervix, reported with code **57522**. Since code **57522** describes a loop electrode excision of the cervix under a local anesthetic, general or regional anesthesia is separately reported in addition to the surgical procedure.

Codes **64400-64450** are differentiated by single injections, multiple injections, or continuous infusion, with codes **64416**, **64446**, and **64448** describing continuous catheter infusions to the brachial plexus and sciatic and the femoral nerves following the insertion of an infusion catheter into the sheaths of nerves. The services provided for the daily management of the anesthetic administration to the brachial plexus and sciatic and femoral nerves are included in these codes and therefore are not separately reported.

Code **64415** is reported for brachial plexus blocks (if the block is to provide regional anesthesia, the appropriate code from **00100-01999** is reported. If the block is done to provide postoperative pain relief and not to deliver anesthesia for a surgical procedure, the anesthesiologist reports both the anesthesia code and the block appended by modifier 59) or occasionally for treatment of reflex sympathetic dystrophy (complex regional pain syndrome), or other painful conditions of the upper extremity. Alternatively, code **64416** describes continuous administration of local anesthetic to the brachial plexus via a catheter for postoperative pain control and chemical sympathectomy. Such procedures are used to provide pain relief or a reversible sympathectomy to provide increased blood supply to the upper extremity for several days; for ischemia of the extremity, replanted digits, postoperative pain control, and occasionally for reflex sympathetic dystrophy and chronic pain.

The paravertebral facet joint or facet joint nerve codes (codes **64470-64476**) specify the spinal anatomy, the substances injected, and the spinal level or levels involved. Codes **64470-64476** are considered unilateral procedures. When injections are performed at both the right and left paravertebral facet joints or paravertebral facet joint nerves, append the bilateral procedure modifier 50 to the appropriate code.

The technical goal of paravertebral facet joint or facet joint nerve injection(s) is directed at temporarily interrupting pain of facet joint origin from reaching the spinal cord. The presumptive purpose of steroid injection is to reduce inflammation and/or swelling of tissue in or around the joint space, which may in turn reduce pain and other symptoms caused by inflammation/irritation of the joint and surrounding structures. Temporary relief of pain following selective facet joint or facet nerve injections can assist the treating physician in confirming or negating the specific diagnosis of facet pain.

## Paravertebral Facet Joints L3-S1

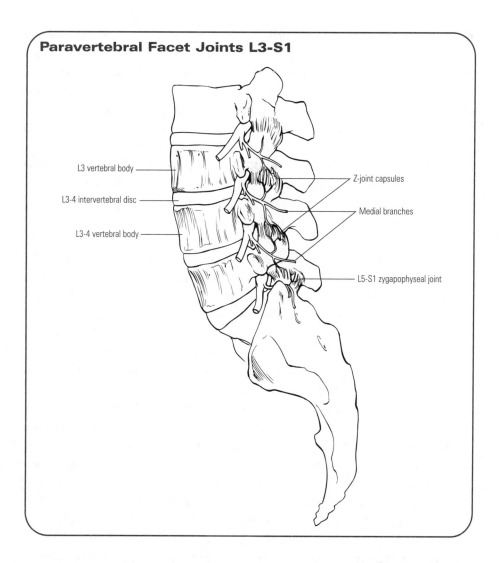

L3 vertebral body

L3-4 intervertebral disc

L3-4 vertebral body

Z-joint capsules

Medial branches

L5-S1 zygapophyseal joint

**CODING TIP**

Codes **64480** and **64484** are reported once, regardless of the number of injections performed at a particular spinal level. Although not specifically stated in the descriptor nomenclature, injection of contrast material is considered an inclusive component of codes **64479-64484**.

To choose the appropriate facet injection code, it is helpful to identify whether the following conditions exist:

- Different terminology is used (eg, facet injection, facet joint nerve).
- The approach technique (ie, transforaminal, interlaminar) to access the spinal anatomy requires the use of a different series of codes (ie, **62310-62311**, **64479-64484**).
- Injection(s) targeted the paravertebral facet joints at one or both sides at a given spinal level.
- The facet injection(s) occurred at single or multiple vertebral level(s)
- Injections were performed at differing spinal regions (eg, cervical/thoracic or lumbar).
- The injections were performed within the facet joint(s) or over facet joint nerve(s).
- The injections were performed unilaterally or bilaterally at a given level.

Codes **64470-64476** describe an injection procedure that involves insertion of the needle in the medial branch nerve or a cervical or thoracic facet joint (which is much smaller than a lumbar facet joint). The cervical and thoracic facets are located closer to more delicate neural and vascular structures, making it a higher-risk procedure than when it is performed at the lumbar facet joint(s). For this reason, it is critical that the needle be directed into the facet joints or over the facet joint nerves at the proper vertebral level with X-ray fluoroscopic guidance to prevent complications should any medication be injected into the vascular structures or too close to a nerve root. When fluoroscopic guidance and localization for needle placement and injection are performed in conjunction with codes **64470-64476**, code **76005** should be additionally reported. Code **76005** is reported by region and not per level. To determine whether the needle is in the joint, contrast is then injected. Although not specifically stated in the descriptor, injection of contrast material is considered an inclusive component of codes **64470-64476** and is not separately reported.

The paravertebral facet joint injection codes **64470-64476** should be reported per spinal level. Each vertebra in the spine is joined to the one above and the one below it by articular facet joints. There are four facet joints associated with each single vertebra in the spine below the level of C2 and above the level of S1. For example, at the L4 vertebral level, there is an L3-L4 facet joint at the upper end and also an L4-L5 facet joint at the inferior end.

Generally, each facet joint has dual innervation: one from the dorsal rami at the same level and one from the level above (eg, the L4-L5 lumbar facet joint is innervated by the medial branches of the dorsal rami from L3 and L4). Multiple injection levels are frequently performed when treating neck and upper back pain, as it is often difficult to isolate the exact joint level, and two to three level injections may be performed at one sitting. Therefore, depending on the involved pathology, multiple-level facet joint and facet joint nerve blocks may be necessary for proper E/M of chronic pain in a given patient.

The lumbar facet injection codes (**64475** and **64476**) and cervical/thoracic facet joint injection codes (**64479** and **64480**) are reported once when the injection procedure is performed, irrespective of whether a single or multiple puncture is required to anesthetize the target joint at a given level and side. Commonly, physicians use a technique that involves insertion of the needle once, with attachment of a short piece of extension tubing through which the first drug is injected. The syringe is then changed, and the next drug is injected through the same tubing/needle. Should the physician choose to perform separate needle punctures, this multiple needle technique does not alter reporting. To clarify, only one facet injection code should be reported at a specified level and side injected (eg, right L4-5 facet joint), regardless of the number of needles inserted or number of drugs injected at that specific level.

It should be further emphasized that codes **64475**, **64476**, **64479**, and **64480** refer to the injection of a facet joint either by injection into the joint with one needle puncture or by anesthetizing the two medial branch nerves that supply each joint (two needle punctures). For example, a left-sided L4-L5 intra-articular injection performed with a single needle puncture would be coded as **64475**. Injection of the L3 and L4 medial branch nerves supplying the L4-L5 facet joint would also be coded as **64475**, even though two separate injections are performed to effect the same result.

If there is a favorable response to facet joint or facet joint nerve (ie, medial branch) injections, then more permanent techniques for the treatment of facet pain may be considered. In this instance, a destructive lesion of the medial branch nerve is performed, blocking the passage of painful messages from the affected facet joint to the rest of the central nervous system. The **64470-64476** series of codes should not be reported to describe denervation procedures.

Fluoroscopic guidance is required to perform paravertebral facet joint and paravertebral facet joint nerve or sacroiliac joint injections; code **77003** should be additionally reported with codes **64470-64476**, **64479-64484**, and **64622-64627**, and in certain circumstances, with code **27096**. Code **77003** is reported by region and not per level. Codes **64470-64484** and **64622-64627** are not reported for each substance injected on one side at a particular spinal level. The paravertebral facet joint and facet joint nerve injection procedure codes **64470-64476** and the transforaminal epidural injection codes **64479-64484** are considered unilateral procedures. Therefore, these codes are reported once per level, per side (right or left) regardless of the number or types of injections performed on the right or left side at a specific spinal level. If both sides are injected at a specific spinal level, then the appropriate injection code should be reported with modifier 50 appended.

Transforaminal epidural spinal injection (**64479-64484**) technique is a technically different approach from central epidural injection (**62310-62311**) and the facet joint nerve injection technique (**64470-64476**). Because the vertebral artery as well as the spinal cord is close to the nerve root, this procedural technique is more difficult than a central epidural injection. Codes **64479-64484** identify the spinal anatomy, the substances injected, and the spinal level or levels involved. Codes **64480** and **64484** represent add-on codes for each additional spinal level injected.

Codes **64479-64484** describe both diagnostic and therapeutic nerve root injections that enter the epidural space through the intervertebral foramen requiring separate needle insertions at several unilateral spinal levels. This technique differs from transforaminal epidural injection technique (**62310-62311**) and the facet joint nerve injection technique (**64470-64476**). Fluoroscopic guidance and contrast material is used to localize the flow pattern (eg, either in the foramen and into the epidural space or in a fascial plane, or in an epidural vein). The needle is moved until contrast outlines the selected spinal nerve and flows into the foramen and then into the epidural space. Since the vertebral artery (in the cervical spine), radiculomedullary arteries, as well as the spinal cord are in close proximity to the nerve root, this procedure involves a much higher risk with more work than an interlaminar epidural injection.

Depending on the treatment required, multiple spinal levels may require injection (eg, foraminal stenosis from a variety of disorders, cervical spondylosis, lumbar spinal stenosis, postoperative back and leg pain, herniated discs in the far lateral or neuroforaminal position). Previous cervical or lumbar fusions make this procedure more difficult. In the case of a previous lumbar or cervical fusion, sometimes the only way to access the injured nerve root is through the transforaminal approach.

**CODING TIP**

Code **77003** is intended to be reported per spinal region (eg, cervical, lumbar) and not per level.

**CODING TIP**

Code **77003** is intended to be reported per spinal region (eg, cervical, lumbar) and not per level.

Since there can be multiple levels of pathology, which may require more than one injection site for diagnostic and therapeutic reasons, codes **64480** and **64484** were established. When performing transforaminal epidural injections at different levels, the patient's position does not change but a new injection at the different level is performed. Each level is a separate injection with more physician work needed. Multiplanar real-time fluoroscopic imaging is mandatory for any transforaminal injection. When a transforaminal injection is performed on the opposite side, the work may involve redraping and positioning of the patient. Therefore, when performing bilateral transforaminal epidural injections at a single spinal level, modifier 50 is appended to the appropriate code(s).

Transforaminal epidural spinal injections are performed under fluoroscopic guidance for precise anatomic localization to avoid potential intrusion of the vertebral artery or damage to the spinal cord or surrounding nerve roots. Code **77003** for fluoroscopic guidance and localization is not an inclusive component of codes **64479-64484** and should be additionally reported.

Code **64479** describes both diagnostic and therapeutic nerve root injections that enter the cervical or thoracic epidural space through the intervertebral foramen. This is important when treating patients who have foraminal stenosis from a variety of disorders including foraminal spinal stenosis and disc herniations.

Code **64480** represents the add-on code for each additional cervical or thoracic level injected by the transforaminal epidural technique. Because certain spinal pathology occurs at multiple levels (eg, cervical spondylosis), it is necessary to separately inject multiple levels. Each level injected is reported separately.

Code **64483** describes lumbar or sacral transforaminal injections for the cervical or thoracic levels. This code represents nerve root injections performed, for example, for lumbar spinal stenosis, postoperative back and leg pain, and herniated discs in the far lateral or neuroforaminal position.

Code **64484** represents the add-on code for each additional cervical or thoracic level injected by the transforaminal epidural technique. Multiple levels of pathology may exist that may require more than one injection site for diagnostic and therapeutic reasons. Each level injected is reported separately.

## Destruction by Neurolytic Agent (eg, Chemical, Thermal, Electrical, Radiofrequency, or Chemodenervation)

### Somatic Nerves

The term *destruction* does not apply to all of the **64600-64640** series of codes. Destruction does not apply to codes **64612-64614**, as the nerve is technically not destroyed but is chemodenervated—meaning that the effect of the drug injection (eg, type A botulinum toxin) is largely or completely reversible. To innervate muscles of the limb or trunk muscles, botulinum toxin is injected directly into the muscle through an electrode to treat dystonia, spasticity, cerebral palsy, multiple sclerosis, muscle spasms, spinal cord injuries, and multiple sclerosis. Codes **64612-64614** are reported once, even though multiple injections are performed in sites along a particular muscle (several muscles are typically injected). Use code **64999** if the botulinum toxin injection is performed on a muscle(s) not specified in these codes.

The codes for destruction by neurolytic agent (eg, chemical, thermal, electrical, radiofrequency) (**64622-64627**) refer to paravertebral facet joint nerve destruction at the cervical, thoracic, lumbar, or sacral region(s). Unlike facet joint nerve (medial branch) codes used to describe facet joint injection (**64470-64480**), facet nerve destruction codes **64622-64627** refer to individual nerve level destruction. Thus, although injection of the left L3 and L4 medial (facet joint) nerve would be coded as **64475**, destruction of the L3 and L4 medial branch nerves would be coded as **64622** and **64623**.

Paravertebral facet joint nerve "destruction" by a neurolytic agent (eg, phenol injection, radiofrequency) (**64626, 64627**) at the cervical/thoracic, lumbar, or sacral regions of the spine differentiates the more intense cervical/thoracic levels from the lumbar/sacral region injections (**64622, 64623**). Codes **64623** and **64627** are add-on codes delineating the neurolytic destruction technique performed at each additional single spinal level.

Codes **64622-64627** are considered unilateral procedures. When both right and left transforaminal epidural injections are performed, append the bilateral procedure modifier 50 to the appropriate code to indicate that a bilateral procedure was performed.

Fluoroscopic guidance and localization are performed to assist in accurately localizing specific spinal anatomy for placement of a needle or catheter tip for spinal or paraspinous diagnostic or therapeutic injection procedures. Although not specifically stated in the descriptor nomenclature, injection of contrast material is an inclusive component of codes **64622-64627**. Code **77003** for fluoroscopic guidance and localization is not an inclusive component of codes **64622-64627** and should be additionally reported.

# X. Eye and Ocular Adnexa

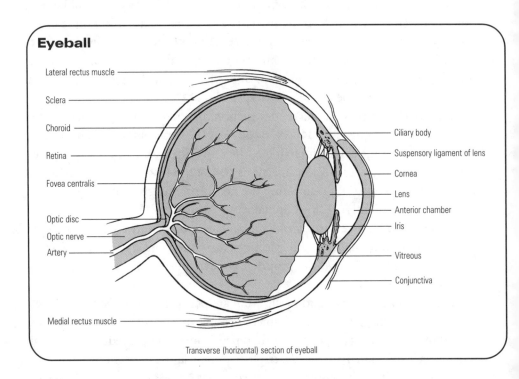

**Eyeball**

Lateral rectus muscle
Sclera
Choroid
Retina
Fovea centralis
Optic disc
Optic nerve
Artery
Medial rectus muscle

Ciliary body
Suspensory ligament of lens
Cornea
Lens
Anterior chamber
Iris
Vitreous
Conjunctiva

Transverse (horizontal) section of eyeball

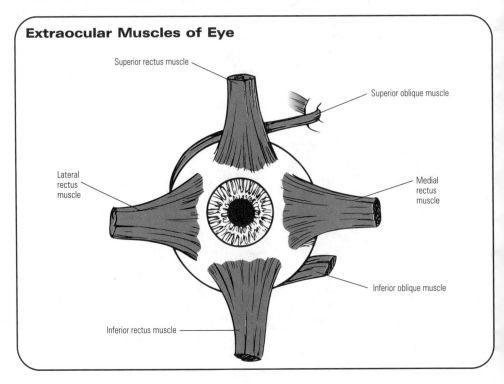

**Extraocular Muscles of Eye**

Superior rectus muscle
Superior oblique muscle
Lateral rectus muscle
Medial rectus muscle
Inferior oblique muscle
Inferior rectus muscle

Coding for surgical procedures on the eye and its surrounding tissues can be complex because of the numerous anatomic structures in the ocular system. Before reviewing the related codes, here is a study of the fundamental anatomy of the eye.

Almost the entire eyeball (globe) is recessed into the orbit. The bony orbit of the eye is made up of seven cranial bones including the ethmoid, frontal, lacrimal, palatine, sphenoid, zygomatic, and maxillary. This bony encasement protects the globe and its blood and nerve supply. Only about one sixth of the eye is exposed.

Three layers of tissue make up the eyeball. The outermost layer consists of the sclera posteriorly and cornea anteriorly. The middle layer is called the *uvea*. The innermost layer is the retina.

The sclera is composed of tough white opaque fibrous tissue. The clear, most anterior portion of the eye, which is continuous with the sclera, is called the *cornea*. The cornea overlies the iris, the colored portion of the eye, and the pupil. The cornea, along with the lens, focuses the object being viewed by the eye on the retina.

The uveal layer is divided into its anterior structures (iris and ciliary body) and its posterior structure (choroid). The anterior extension of the uvea is the iris (colored portion of the eye). The opening in the center of the iris is the pupil. The iris contains muscle fibers arranged in a circular and radial fashion. The iris also attaches to the ciliary body. The ciliary body contains the ciliary processes that produce the aqueous humor, a fluid that is responsible for maintaining intraocular pressure. The ciliary body also contains the ciliary muscle that is responsible for accommodation (changing the focus of the lens of the eye from distance to a near object). The zonules are fiber-like structures that extend from the ciliary processes to the lens and suspend it between the anterior and posterior segments of the eye.

The choroid is the posterior portion of the uvea. One layer of the choroid is the choriocapillaris, which is a vascular network that supplies nourishment to the retina anterior to it and the sclera behind it. The vascular choriocapillaris is responsible for the "red-eye" seen in flash photographs.

The retina is the innermost portion of the three layers of the eye. It is a transparent structure consisting of 10 individual layers. Light entering the eye must travel through all 10 layers before striking the rods and cones, which are positioned in the outer layer of the retina. The retinal impulse must then travel back through the inner retinal layers, which form a complex network of axons that converge to form the optic nerve. All of these neurons converge on a small area in the posterior portion of the eye. This is called the *optic nerve head* or *optic nerve disc*. The nerve fibers exit the eye from this portion of the disc and form the optic nerve, also known as the *second cranial nerve*.

The inside of the eye is divided by the lens into two segments, anterior and posterior. The anterior segment is further divided into two chambers, the anterior and posterior chambers. The anterior chamber is located behind the cornea and in front of the iris. The anterior chamber is filled with aqueous humor. The posterior chamber is behind the iris and in front of the lens. It is also filled with

**CODING TIP**

When coding for removal of an intraocular foreign body from the eye, check the patient's record to see if any imaging procedures were performed. If so, remember to code the echography procedure (code **76529**) when appropriate.

aqueous humor. The posterior segment is the portion of the eye behind the lens. It contains the vitreous humor, a clear tissue filling much of the eye.

Muscles of the eye are classified as two types: intraocular and extraocular. Intraocular muscles are inside the globe. These muscles include the ciliary muscle and the sphincter and dilator muscles of the iris. They are generally involuntary muscles.

The extraocular muscles are part of the ocular adnexa. They are on the outside of the eyeball and attach to the bones of the orbit. These muscles, which are under voluntary control, move the eye in various directions. Four of the muscles follow a course from the back of the eye socket to the eye, while two follow a more oblique course. The extraocular muscles are named for their anatomic positions on the eye: superior, inferior, medial, and lateral rectus, and the superior and inferior oblique muscles.

Other accessory structures of the visual system include the eyelids, the lacrimal apparatus, the eyebrows, and the eyelashes.

The eyelids are made up of muscle, skin, connective tissue, and conjunctiva. The tarsal plate (tarsus) is responsible for the form and shape of each eyelid. This 1-mm thick connective tissue structure contains the meibomian glands, which contribute the oily (sebaceous) layer to the three-layer tear film. The posterior surface of the eyelids is lined with a mucous membrane called the *conjunctiva*. The conjunctiva that lines the eyelid is called the *palpebral conjunctiva*. The conjunctiva over the anterior surface of the sclera is called the *bulbar conjunctiva*. The bulbar and palpebral conjunctivae join superiorly and inferiorly in areas referred to as the *superior fornix* and *inferior fornix*, respectively. The conjunctiva is transparent and is vascular. The angle or corner where the upper and lower eyelids join is called the *canthus*. There is an inner or medial canthus (closer to the nose) and an outer or lateral canthus (away from the nose).

The main and accessory lacrimal glands produce tears, which lubricate the eye. The nasolacrimal duct system provides drainage from the surface of the eye into the nose.

The lacrimal gland is located in a small depression in the frontal bone in the upper outer quadrant of the anterior orbit. Several ducts lead from each gland to the surface of the conjunctiva in the outer corner of the superior fornix of each eye. The openings of the nasolacrimal duct system are called the *puncta*. There is one punctum in each eyelid, which is located in the medial aspect of each eyelid margin. These open into small channels (canaliculi) that lead to the lacrimal sac. The lacrimal sac is located in a depression, or fossa, in the lacrimal bone. Tears fill the lacrimal sac as the eyelids blink and pump the tears into the lacrimal sac. The nasolacrimal duct drains the tears from the lacrimal sac to the nose through a small opening under the inferior turbinate.

## Section Layout—Eye and Ocular Adnexa

Now that eye anatomy essentials have been reviewed, it will be evident how these terms are critical to one's understanding of operative procedures performed on the eye and the CPT codes that describe them. Next, read through the listings in the eye and ocular adnexa series and review the guidelines and codes for reporting procedures of the eye and ocular adnexa.

First, notice that diagnostic and noninvasive tests of the eye are not coded in this section. They are listed in the Medicine section of the CPT codebook under the Ophthalmology subheading or the appropriate section, such as Diagnostic Ultrasound. Although not explicitly stated here, the E/M codes and some Radiology codes are applicable to those practitioners treating eye diseases or conditions.

It is also important to note that the add-on code **69990** that describes the use of the operating microscope is not applicable to any of the codes in the Eye and Ocular Adnexa subsection. Any use of the operating microscope is not reported separately, because it is an essential part of many of the procedures described.

The codes in this section are divided between the eyeball (the globe) and the ocular adnexa. Within the portion of the codes describing procedures performed on the globe, these are generally divided between the globe in its entirety, the anterior segment, and the posterior segment. The further subheadings are anatomically based and then broken into procedure categories.

The ocular adnexa codes are divided anatomically by the extraocular muscles, the eyelids, the conjunctiva, and the orbit. The orbital bones are ordinarily considered part of the musculoskeletal system, but incisions and excisions of bone of the orbit are described here for convenience of the user of the CPT codebook. Treatments of fractures of the orbital bones are described and coded in the Musculoskeletal subsection.

## Eyeball

Codes **65091-65114** describe removal of the eye, contents of the eye, or the eye and surrounding adnexa. The codes describing the eyeball in its entirety begin with removal of the entire globe. The following three important terms are referred to here that must be distinguished to accurately code these procedures:

- **Evisceration**—removing the intraocular contents of the eyeball while leaving the sclera (a scleral "shell") intact. An implant may be placed inside this scleral shell to maintain the shape of the eye.
- **Enucleation**—removing the entire eyeball (intraocular contents and scleral shell), typically leaving the extraocular structures (eg, extraocular muscles, orbital fat) intact.
- **Exenteration**—extensive removal of the entire contents of the orbit, including the eyeball and all of the extraocular adnexa (eg, extraocular muscles, orbital fat, nerves, eyelids).

Codes **65125-65175** describe secondary implant procedures. Ocular and orbital implants are used to replace the volume loss created by removing the eye and/or orbital contents. When implants are placed in the orbit at a time after the initial surgery to enucleate or eviscerate the eye, they are called *secondary implant procedures*. An ocular implant may be located inside the cone formed by the extraocular muscles or placed posterior to the posterior layers of Tenon's capsule within the fatty tissue of the muscle cone.

An orbital implant is one that is placed outside of these muscles (extraconal). The codes in this section describe the insertion, reinsertion (replacement), and removal of the implants as well as modification of the implant.

**EXAMPLE:** Evisceration with implant and placement of a regional orbital block catheter. In this instance, Code **65093** should be reported. The placement of the pain pump/catheter during other surgery in the operative site is not separately reported. When the pump/catheter is placed during a surgical procedure in the same site for pain management, only the surgical code identifying the definitive/main procedure for that surgical site should be used. (No additional codes should be used to identify the placement of the catheter or pump device when other surgery is performed for that site.)

Codes **65205-65265** describe various procedures for removal of foreign bodies. These codes apply to the globe and the conjunctiva. Cross-references are provided to direct reporting for removal of foreign bodies from the orbit, eyelid, and lacrimal system, under their respective anatomic subheadings. Although the conjunctiva does have its own subheading, removal of foreign bodies from the external surfaces of the eye (conjunctiva and cornea) and from the inside of the eye (anterior chamber, posterior chamber, posterior segment, or lens) are reported with this series of codes.

Codes in the **65270- 65286** series describe repair of lacerations of the conjunctiva, cornea, and sclera. Separate wound repair of the iris or ciliary body is referred to code **66680**. Repair of wounds of the eyelid and the skin of the face surrounding the orbit are coded in the integumentary system (**12011-12018**).

One of the key differences in reporting laceration repair in this section as compared with the Integumentary subsection is that the repair is described by location of the laceration and the type of repair performed. The sum of the lengths of the lacerations is not a feature of this coding structure, although these lengths may sometimes be found in the operative report.

## Anterior Segment

The anterior segment contains the cornea, anterior chamber, limbus, iris and ciliary body, and lens. This section of the CPT codebook on the anterior segment begins with the cornea and follows a template of excision and removal or destruction. Here, the typical categories are replaced with the specialized keratoplasty (corneal transplant), followed by other procedures.

Corneal excision procedures, described by codes **65400-65426**, include biopsies and lesion excision. There is a special term mentioned in this area, *pterygium.* This is a degenerative and hyperplastic process of the ocular surface, which is typically made up of a small triangular fold of tissue that extends from the conjunctiva over the cornea. If left untreated, this membrane may grow to

**CODING TIP**

When destroying noncontiguous lesions in a small anatomical area such as the cornea, if multiple lesions are destroyed unilaterally, remember to use modifier 59 to indicate a separate lesion in the same eye. (Refer to Chapter 10 for further discussion of modifier 59.)

**CODING TIP**

For removal of foreign body from the eyelid (embedded) use **67938**. For removal of a foreign body from the lacrimal system, use **68530**. For removal of foreign body from the orbit; frontal approach, use **67413**; lateral approach, use **67430**, transcranial approach, use **61334**.

**CODING TIP**

Repairs of wounds of the eyelid, skin, can be reported with the code series beginning with codes **12011** (simple), **12051** (intermediate layered closure), and **13150** (linear, complex), as appropriate. Other, see **67930, 67935**.

cover most of the cornea. The treatment is surgical excision, although antineo-plastic drugs, radiation, and tissue transplants are also used.

Within the **65430-65600** code series, there are codes for reporting removal or destruction of tissues in the anterior segment, including the procedures of obtaining cells for diagnostic smears or cultures and destruction of lesions by means of cryotherapy, photocoagulation, or thermocoagulation.

Codes **65710-65755** are used to report keratoplasty. The term *keratoplasty* is generally defined as a repair of the cornea. Here, the term specifically refers to corneal transplants. All of the codes in this section may be applied whether the transplanted tissues are directly from the donor ("fresh") or from a tissue/organ or eye bank. Included in the codes is all preparation or sizing of the donor graft corneal tissue done by the surgeon.

The following two special terms are used to describe these procedures: *lamellar* is a transplant method that removes the anterior layer of the diseased cornea and replaces it with a piece of donor cornea cut to the same size and shape; *penetrating* refers to the full-thickness replacement of the cornea. The transplant involves removal of the diseased corneal tissue ("penetrating" through the entire thickness of the corneal tissue) and replaces the tissue with a piece of donor cornea cut to the same size and shape.

Codes in the **65800-66030** series describe procedures in the anterior chamber. The anterior chamber codes are limited to subsections of incision and other procedures. A coder for a medical practice that performs these procedures should refer to a more detailed anatomical text that describes the specialized structures of the anterior segment. In addition, an understanding of the disease processes affecting the anterior chamber will enable one to accurately code the operation performed.

A key concept used throughout this section is that of *separate procedure*. (Refer to Chapter 4 for further discussion of separate procedure.) As discussed earlier in this chapter, because of the complex nature of the visual system, this designation is often misunderstood. For example, code **65860** for severing adhesions of the anterior segment by laser technique may be an integral part of another procedure on the anterior segment; however, it is not a part of surgical procedures on the sclera. Unfortunately, some users of the CPT Nomenclature mistake the separate procedure designation to include any procedure performed on the eye or its component parts. This misconception causes many procedures that should be reported separately to be inappropriately bundled, or combined with other procedures, and not individually identified.

Codes in the **66130-66250** series describe procedures of the anterior sclera. The anterior sclera codes are limited to excision and repair or revision subsections. Although removal of foreign bodies from the anterior sclera could be considered a type of excision, these procedures are coded in the more specific subsection of removal of foreign body.

The iris and ciliary body codes, **66500-66770**, are divided among incision, excision, repair, and destruction. Be certain to read the parenthetical notes in this section, which instruct coders to see other sections that relate to procedures performed on or adjacent to the iris. These notes are critical for correct coding, as it is easy to mistakenly choose the code for one procedure instead of

**CODING TIP**

When coding for an intraocular lens (IOL) implantation, remember that the provision of the IOL itself is not included in the CPT description. If the surgeon provided the IOL, CPT code **99070** should be used to report the supply of the lens. Alternatively, depending on the reporting circumstances, the appropriate HCPCS Level II code may be reported for the supply of the IOL.

a more precise procedure, especially when using the operative report as the basis for selection.

Codes for procedures on the lens, **66820-66986**, can be described as incisions and removal of cataracts. The incision procedures on the lens, however, are all related to postcataract surgical procedures, including repositioning of an intraocular lens prosthesis that requires incision. Other, nonsurgical repositionings are included in the routine postoperative follow-up for cataract procedures and are not coded separately.

Code **66990** describes the use of the ophthalmic endoscope for visualization of elements of the ocular anatomy not visible with the operating microscope, and is reported in addition to those anterior and posterior segment procedures in which it is not considered a component. Code **66990** is an add-on code. This code is reported separately, in addition to the appropriate code(s) for the primary procedure performed, to represent the additional physician work necessary to use the ophthalmic endoscope in the performance of various ophthalmic surgeries, including pars plana approach vitrectomies, removal of implanted materials from the anterior eye segment, and intraocular lens exchanges. The cross-reference parenthetical instruction that follows the codes provides the list of procedures with which code **66990** may be reported. As discussed in Chapter 4, add-on codes do not stand alone; modifier 51 is not appended to these add-on codes, since they are not independent procedures. (Refer to Chapter 4 for further discussion of add-on codes.)

The anterior segment of the eye includes an unlisted procedure code, **66999**.

## Posterior Segment

The Posterior Segment subsection, codes **67005-67299**, includes procedures performed on the vitreous, the retina or choroid, and the posterior sclera. The section on the vitreous, **67005-67040**, currently has no subheadings. This section includes removal and aspiration of vitreous or other posterior segment fluids, fluid-gas exchange, implantation of intravitreal drug delivery systems, vitrectomy, and excision or destruction of adhesions. Again, the parenthetical notes are key for referral to other codes that are closely related to these vitreous procedures.

The Retina (Choroid) subsection, codes **67101-67228**, includes the subheadings of repair, prophylaxis, and destruction. *Repair* refers to treatment of retinal detachments. The retina becomes detached when the sensory layers of the retina become separated from their underlying pigment epithelial layer. This can occur after the formation of a break in the retina or from leakage beneath the retina.

The goal of repairing the retinal detachment is to seal any tears that are present and to prevent further detachment from developing. This preventive treatment is called *prophylaxis*. When repair of retinal detachments is coded, the codes refer to the series of treatments needed to close or repair the holes or tears that are present. This treatment series may be accomplished at one or more treatment sessions on the same or different days. (Refer to the discussion at the end of this section regarding reporting codes with the phrase "one or more sessions" in the descriptor.)

If more than one method is used to treat the holes, tears, or detachment, such as diathermy, cryotherapy, and/or photocoagulation, select the code that corresponds to the principal modality that the physician uses. For example, if retinal tears are treated by both cryotherapy and photocoagulation but the predominant therapy was photocoagulation, code **67105** should be selected.

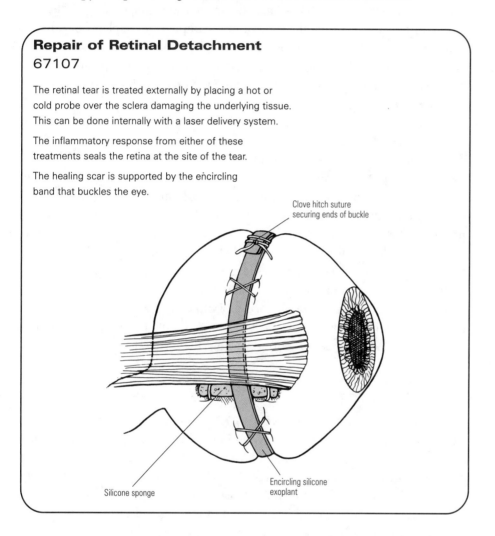

**Repair of Retinal Detachment**
67107

The retinal tear is treated externally by placing a hot or cold probe over the sclera damaging the underlying tissue. This can be done internally with a laser delivery system.

The inflammatory response from either of these treatments seals the retina at the site of the tear.

The healing scar is supported by the encircling band that buckles the eye.

Clove hitch suture securing ends of buckle

Silicone sponge

Encircling silicone exoplant

The retinal tear is treated externally by placing a hot or cold probe over the sclera, damaging the underlying tissue. This can also be done internally with a laser delivery system. The resulting inflammatory response from either of these treatments seals the retina at the site of the tear. The healing scar is supported by the encircling band that buckles the eye.

Scleral buckling is a widely used treatment for retinal detachment. Once subretinal fluid has accumulated beneath the retina, it is difficult to treat the detachment with cryotherapy or photocoagulation, and it is typically treated with scleral buckling. The scleral buckling procedure has many variations. The holes or tears are localized and are marked by indenting the sclera and then

**CODING TIP**

Do not append modifier 50 to code **67221**. Use add-on code **67225** when photodynamic therapy is performed on the second eye at a single session.

applying cryotherapy, diathermy, or photocoagulation. This will cause the retina to adhere to the retinal pigment epithelium and choroid. Once this portion of the procedure has been done, an explant (material sutured to the sclera on the outside of the eye) or an implant (material placed under a scleral flap) is placed. Subretinal fluid is then drained and the implant or explant material is tightened and sutured. This causes the sclera and treated areas to indent or "buckle" inward and helps in closing the tears or holes. Implants or explants of different materials are used, most often solid silicone rubber. Air or other gases may also be injected into the vitreous to restore vitreous volume and to push the tear or hole against the area of indentation to close the break and allow the scar from choroids to retina to form.

Code **67221** describes ocular photodynamic therapy, a noninvasive treatment for age-related macular degeneration. Code **67221** separates this procedure from laser photocoagulation of the choroid, which is reported by code **67220**. Laser photocoagulation (**67220**) relies on the laser to ablate the abnormal tissue by heating, which involves greater work intensity because of the risk of complications and usually requires more than one treatment session and postoperative office visits. On the other hand, photodynamic therapy is a procedure that relies on the ability of the photoactive drug activated by laser light to destroy the cells the laser light has targeted.

Ocular photodynamic therapy usually requires a single session. However, this procedure may also be performed on both eyes at a single session. In that instance, a special bilateral add-on code, **67225**, should be reported in addition to code **67221**. This code is reported without the bilateral modifier.

## Ocular Adnexa

The Ocular Adnexa subsection, codes **67311-67999**, is dominated by codes describing strabismus surgery. The section on the orbit, codes **67400-67599**, includes exploration, excision, and decompression procedures as well as injections and orbital implants. Although the orbit is made up of bony structures that may also be classified under the Musculoskeletal System subsection, nonfracture treatments of the orbit are coded in the Eye and Ocular Adnexa subsection. For treatment of fractures of the bones of the orbit (frontal, sphenoid, zygomatic, maxilla, ethmoid, and lacrimal bones), see the Musculoskeletal System, Head subsection, fracture, and/or dislocation subsection.

Procedures involving the eyelids, described by codes in the **67700-67999** series, include incision, excision of lesions involving more than skin, and correction of trichiasis (ingrown or misdirected eyelashes). Repairs of the eyelid area also include repair of brow ptosis, lid retractions, entropion, and ectropion.

### Strabismus Surgery

Strabismus surgery is an operation on the extraocular muscles. This surgery is performed to realign the eyes so that they are both aimed in the same direction. The correction of extraocular muscle misalignment may allow restoration of depth perception, single binocular vision, and expansion of the visual field.

The position of each eye is controlled by the six extraocular muscles. These muscles and the eye are contained in the orbit. Each of these muscles is controlled by one of three cranial nerves. There are two horizontal muscles, the lateral rectus muscle and the medial rectus muscle, on each eye. There are four vertical muscles: the superior and inferior rectus muscles, and the superior and inferior oblique muscles. A surgeon may elect to operate on one or more muscles in one or both eyes to attempt to correct the ocular misalignment.

The coding of modern strabismus surgery often requires the use of multiple procedural codes. CPT codes for strabismus surgery refer to each eye individually. If the same operation is performed in both eyes, the physician should use the muscle code for the first eye with the appropriate bilateral modifier. If horizontal and vertical surgeries are performed in the same eye, the appropriate codes are reported with modifier 51 appended to the additional procedure(s) reported.

Codes **67311-67318** describe the specific type of muscle (eg, horizontal, vertical, oblique) and the number of muscles operated on in each eye. To appropriately use these codes, the specific type of muscle operated on in each eye must be indicated in the operative report and in the procedural codes. If the physician operates on the same type of muscle in both eyes, modifier 50 should be appended to indicate that the procedure was performed bilaterally. (Refer to Chapter 10 for further discussion of modifier 50.) Modifier 50 is used only when exactly the same service is to be reported for each eye.

Consider the following three examples:

**EXAMPLE 1:** One horizontal muscle in each eye is operated on for the first time.

In this case, CPT code **67311 50** is reported to indicate that one horizontal muscle in each eye was operated on.

**EXAMPLE 2:** Two horizontal muscles in both eyes are operated on for the first time.

In this case, CPT code **67311 50** is reported to indicate that the same two muscles in both eyes were operated on.

**EXAMPLE 3:** One horizontal muscle of the right eye is operated on for the first time, and the superior oblique muscle of the left eye is operated on.

In this case, modifier 50, Bilateral Procedure, is not used. The individual codes for these specific services are reported (**67311** and **67318**). Modifier 51, Multiple Procedures, is appended to code **67311**. Code **67318** is listed first on the claim form, without any modifier.

Strabismus surgery can be performed with the patient under general or local anesthesia, depending on the age and temperament of the patient. Usually no surgery is performed on the eyelid skin, and the eyes are not removed from the eye socket. The eyes are simply rolled into one position or another to allow the surgeon to gain access to the eye muscles. The eye muscles are approached by making incisions through the conjunctiva overlying the sclera.

Although there are six eye muscles affecting each eye that may undergo surgery, there are basically only two methods of adjusting the effectiveness of any muscle. The surgeon will either decrease the effectiveness of the muscle by lengthening it (recession) or enhance the performance of the muscle by shortening it (resection).

## Recession and Resection Procedures

In the recession operation, the muscle is detached from its insertion site on the surface of the eyeball and reattached at a fixed distance posterior to the original insertion site along the surface of the eye. In a resection operation, a small portion of the muscle is removed and the eye muscle is then reattached to the original insertion site.

CPT Nomenclature does not differentiate between recession and resection procedures. CPT strabismus surgery codes do, however, specify other important characteristics of the surgery. The selection of a code demands attention to the patient's clinical history as well as the operative report. The following questions need to be answered for appropriate code selection to occur:

- Has the patient previously had surgery to correct strabismus with scarring around the eye muscle?
- Has the patient previously had surgery on the eye or ocular disease that affects eye movements, like retinal detachment surgery or thyroid disease?
- Is the surgery being performed on horizontally or vertically acting muscles?
- Was surgery performed on the superior oblique muscle?
- Which muscles were operated on in each eye?

It is common to operate on at least two and often four muscles during the same operative session. Thus, it is usually necessary to report two or more codes for any strabismus operation. The CPT Nomenclature does not differentiate coding for the right or left eye, but the surgery for each eye is coded separately. However, one must clearly identify the muscles in each eye on which the physician operated. The operative report will assist in identifying the correct code(s) to report for each eye.

## Conjunctiva

Surgical procedures performed on the conjunctiva, described by codes **68020-68399**, include incision and drainage and excision and/or destruction. This latter section excludes removal of foreign bodies, which are coded in the Removal of Foreign Body subsection, located at the beginning of the Eye and Ocular Adnexa subsection of Surgery. (See discussion earlier in this chapter regarding removal of foreign bodies.)

Also included are procedures of subconjunctival injections, conjunctivoplasty, and conjunctival flaps. An unlisted procedure specifically for the use for conjunctival procedures is also included (code **68399**).

## Lacrimal System

Coding for procedures on the lacrimal system, described by codes **68400-68899**, include incision, excision repairs, and probing or related procedures. The incisional procedures typically involve drainage-type procedures. The excisional procedures include biopsies of the lacrimal gland and lacrimal sac. This category of biopsy would include so-called incisional biopsies, in which only a small tissue sample is removed and the remainder of the sac or gland is left intact.

As mentioned, removal of foreign bodies from the conjunctiva is not coded in the Conjunctival subsection but is coded in the Removal of Foreign Body subsection. In coding for procedures on the lacrimal system, removal of foreign bodies or a dacryolith is coded in the Anatomic subsection rather than in the more general Removal of Foreign Body subsection.

One of the most common procedures performed that is described in the repair subsection of the lacrimal system involves the closure of the lacrimal puncta. Code **68760** describes closure of the lacrimal punctum by thermocauterization, ligation, or laser surgery. Code **68761** is reported if the closure is performed by punctal plug.

In code **68761**, the word *each* refers to each plug that is placed in a punctum. The punctum (puncta, plural) is an opening in the lacrimal canaliculi, located on the upper and lower eyelid margin near the nose. This is the entrance to the tear drainage system from the eye surface to the nose. Since there is one punctum in each eyelid, if both puncta of one side are occluded, then code **68761** would be reported twice. If both eyes are treated (all four puncta), then code **68761** is reported four times.

The occlusion of lacrimal puncta by collagen plugs is used for the diagnosis (and temporary treatment) of dry eye syndrome. With dry eye syndrome, patients may have many differing complaints that mimic other ocular conditions, such as chronic infectious conjunctivitis, allergic conditions, blepharoconjunctivitis, and ocular manifestations of systemic collagen and/or immunologic disorders. The collagen plugs dissolve in 4 to 6 days. If these plugs are inserted and the patient has dry eye syndrome, the patient may experience relief during the period of occlusion. Patients may experience epiphora (overflow tearing). This can occur if the eyes are indeed producing a sufficient quantity of tears that under the influence of the punctal plugs, have nowhere to go except over the eyelid margin and down the cheek. Since the collagen plugs dissolve in a matter of days, the tear overflow will resolve.

Silicone plugs are both diagnostic and therapeutic (semipermanent). After the silicone plugs are inserted, the patient intermittently returns to the physician so that integrity of the plugs may be ensured.

Code **68761** does not differentiate between silicone and collagen plugs. The HCPCS Level II codes **A4262** and **A4263** are used to differentiate between the collagen and silicone plugs, respectively. The same procedure code is used for either type. Consequently, both a diagnostic occlusion of the puncta and a therapeutic occlusion may be done on the same patient in a short time frame. Modifier 76, Repeat Procedure or Service by Same Physician, is not reported, because the

**CODING TIP**

Closure of the lacrimal punctum by plug typically involves the use of two types of plugs. The first type is a collagen plug that is temporary to test whether the occlusion will work. These collagen plugs typically dissolve in the puncta. If the treatment is effective, permanent plugs are placed. The use of HCPCS Level II codes may be necessary to distinguish between these procedures. These may vary by payer.

**CODING TIP**

Nasolacrimal duct probing is included in the descriptor for code **68815**. It would not be appropriate to separately report codes **68810** and **68811** for probing the nasolacrimal duct and insertion of a tube or stent.

two services, although coded the same, are performed for different purposes and are not repeat in nature. (Refer to Chapter 10 for further discussion regarding the use of modifier 76.)

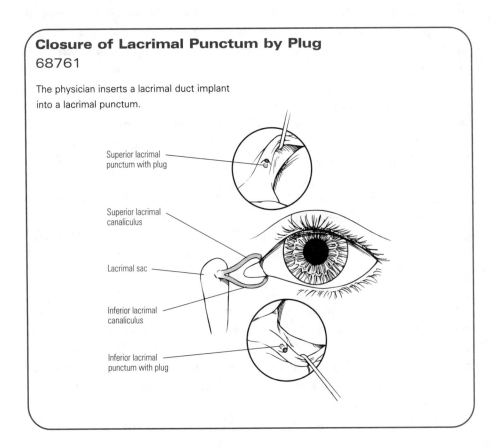

**Closure of Lacrimal Punctum by Plug**
68761

The physician inserts a lacrimal duct implant into a lacrimal punctum.

Superior lacrimal punctum with plug

Superior lacrimal canaliculus

Lacrimal sac

Inferior lacrimal canaliculus

Inferior lacrimal punctum with plug

## One or More Sessions

A number of codes (**67141**, **67145**, **67208-67220**, **67227**, **67228**, **67229**) in the Eye and Ocular Adnexa subsection contain the phrase "one or more sessions" in their descriptor. When this phrase appears in a code descriptor, the code should be reported only once for the entire defined treatment period, regardless of the number of sessions necessary to complete the treatment. In other words, the code would not be reported for each session the patient presented if it was a visit included in a defined treatment period. The defined treatment period is determined by the physician and varies depending on the patient, diagnosis, and, often, the area to be treated.

If the patient experiences a recurrence of the condition and retreatment is necessary, these subsequent retreatment sessions would not be considered to be included in the first treatment series. This retreatment would be reported with the appropriate code, as it represents a new defined treatment period of one or more sessions performed to treat the problem. If the retreatment is of greater complexity, it may be necessary to append modifier 22 to identify greater complexity. Likewise, if the retreatment is of lesser complexity, modifier 52 may be appended to identify this situation. (Refer to Chapter 10 for further discussion of modifiers 22 and 52.)

# XI. Auditory System

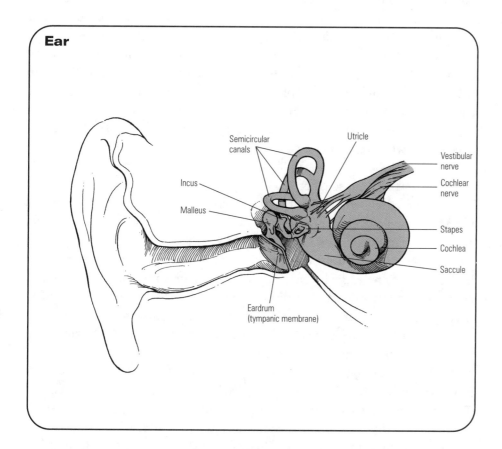

**Ear**

Semicircular canals

Utricle

Incus

Malleus

Vestibular nerve

Cochlear nerve

Stapes

Cochlea

Saccule

Eardrum (tympanic membrane)

## Section Layout—Auditory System

The auditory system subsection of the CPT codebook is further divided into code ranges for reporting procedures of the following:

1   External Ear (**69000-69399**)

2   Middle Ear (**69400-69799**)

3   Inner Ear (**69801-69949**)

4   Temporal Bone, Middle Fossa Approach (**69950-69979**)

Read the parenthetical note at the beginning of this subsection that provides direction for reporting diagnostic services of the auditory system. Those services are not described here but rather are reported with codes from the Special Otorhinolaryngologic Services subsection in the Medicine section of the CPT codebook (**92502** et seq).

In the section for procedures of the external ear (**69000-69399**), separate headings indicate incision, excision, removal repair, and other procedures. The external ear consists of the portion on the side of the head called the *auricle* or *pinna* and the tube that connects the auricle to the temporal bone, called the *external auditory meatus* or *ear canal*. The tympanic membrane stretches across the inside end of the canal to separate it from the inner ear.

Code **69399** is used to report unlisted procedures of the external ear. Use of this code is appropriate when a procedure is performed on the external ear that is not described with a more specific code from the external ear section. (Refer to Chapter 2 for further discussion regarding the use of unlisted codes.)

Code **69150** is used to report radical excision for external auditory canal lesion, which can be performed without neck dissection or with neck dissection (**69155**). These procedures involve the removal of the entire tympanic bone and the tympanic membrane. However, if a separate skin graft or flap is performed, then separately report the surgical preparation codes **15004-15261**. Specifically, when reporting for the graft repair of the external auditory canal, report code **15004**. (Refer to the Skin Replacement Surgery and Skin Substitute guideline for further discussion.)

The subsection Removal listed in the External Ear (**69200-69222**) section is intended to include those procedures in which removal is performed for materials other than foreign bodies.

Code **69210** is used to report removal of impacted cerumen from one or both ears. This procedure involves direct visualization with removal of impacted cerumen by means of suction, a cerumen spoon, or delicate forceps. If no infection is present, the ear canal may also be irrigated. If the use of an operating microscope is necessary during this procedure, separately code **69990** to report the use of the operating microscope.

In the section of procedures of the middle ear (**69400-69799**), separate headings indicate introduction, incision, excision, repair, and other procedures. The middle ear consists of several parts: the malleus, incus, stapes, and tympanic cavity. This cavity has several openings including the oval window, the round window, and the eustachian tube. One will notice these terms throughout the middle ear section. Review the illustrations and an anatomy text to become familiar with these sense organs. This section of codes also contains an unlisted code, **69799**, that is used to report unlisted procedures of the middle ear.

Codes **69714, 69715, 69717,** and **69718** are used to report procedures related to atraumatic preparation of the implant site and placement of an osseointegrated implant for restoring hearing sensitivity and speech comprehension. The introduction of a mastoid-integrated implant offers a direct and effective alternative for restoring hearing under conditions of chronic infection, anomalies of the ear canal, and bone or nerve degeneration. This concept is based on a specific type of metal, titanium, which has the capability of directly integrating with bone to form a biologic and mechanical attachment. The implant activates the cochlea by an externally worn speech attachment. The speech processor-stimulator is fitted onto the implanted platform.

Codes **69710** and **69711** procedurally differ from codes **69714-69718** and describe placement (and removal) of a magnet within the temporal bone. The magnet is covered with skin and interfaced with a processor worn on the skin surface.

Osseointegrated temporal bone implant is performed to reestablish hearing when hearing loss results from disease of the middle ear and cochlea. Although there are many etiologies for middle ear and cochlear pathology, most disorders are related to chronic (infectious) disease, trauma, otosclerosis, and congenital malformation. This procedure is indicated in patients who are unable to use conventional amplification (ie, a hearing aid) because of aggravation of ongoing infection, or a nonpatent (stenotic) ear canal.

In the section of procedures of the inner ear (**69801-69949**), separate headings indicate incision and/or destruction, excision, introduction (**69930**), and other procedures (**69949**).

Procedure code **69930** involves an internal coil being attached to the temporal bone and the ground wire attached to the internal coil, which is connected to the temporalis muscle. This procedure is intended to stimulate nerve fibers and to capture and amplify sound. Consider the following illustration to further clarify:

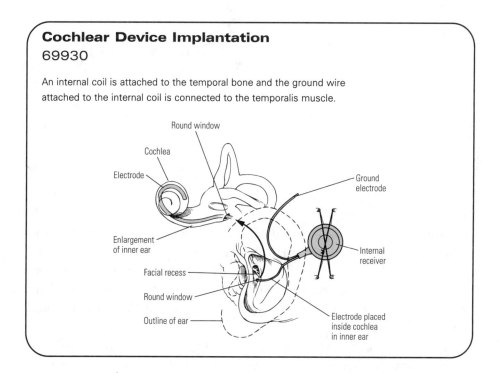

**Cochlear Device Implantation**
69930

An internal coil is attached to the temporal bone and the ground wire attached to the internal coil is connected to the temporalis muscle.

The inner ear is also called the *labyrinth* and is further divided into a bony and a membranous labyrinth. The primary terms used in the CPT Nomenclature to describe the inner ear are the *cochlea, vestibule,* and *semicircular canal.* Code **69949** is available for reporting unlisted procedures of the inner ear.

Codes **69950-69979** are used to report procedures of the temporal bone via the middle fossa approach. The parenthetical note at the beginning of this code series directs the user to code **69535** for procedures of the temporal bone performed via an external approach.

Codes **69433** and **69436** are used to report tympanostomy requiring the insertion of a ventilating tube. The appropriate code is selected on the basis of whether the procedure is performed with local or topical anesthesia (**69433**), or under general anesthesia (**69436**). As indicated by the parenthetical notes following each of these codes, both codes represent unilateral procedures. Therefore, if a bilateral procedure is performed, then modifier 50, Bilateral Procedure, should be appended to the code reported. (Refer to Chapter 10 for further discussion of the use of modifier 50.)

**Tympanostomy**
69433-69436

A ventilating tube is inserted into the opening of the tympanum.

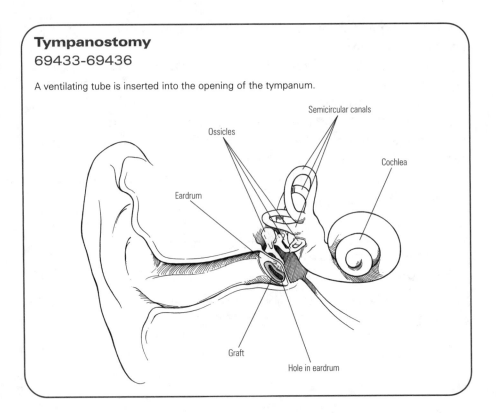

### Removal of Tubes

The subsequent removal of ventilating tubes, when performed by the same physician who performed the original placement procedure, is not a separately reportable service. This would be considered included in the normal, uncomplicated follow-up care associated with the placement procedure. When ventilating tubes are removed by a physician with the patient under general anesthesia, code **69424** is used to report this procedure. Ventilating tube removal may be performed in those instances where the tympanostomy tube has failed or is causing problems (ie, local infection, granulation, cholesteatoma formation). Code **69424** is considered a unilateral procedure. Therefore, if tubes are removed from both ears, then modifier 50 should be appended to procedure code **69424**.

## CHAPTER 5

# EXERCISES

1   Assign the appropriate codes for the following procedures:
    **a**  Fine needle aspiration of a lesion of foreleg without imaging guidance
    **b**  Fine needle aspiration of a lesion of foreleg requiring CT imaging guidance

2   True or False: Fine needle aspiration codes are anatomy-specific.

3   True or False: Benign or malignant designation is a factor in selecting a code for shaving of lesions.

4   For wound repair involving more than one method of repair, how is the code chosen?

5   True or False: One benign lesion measuring 0.5 cm is removed from the hand, and another benign lesion measuring 0.5 cm is removed from the foot. Since multiple lesions were excised and both anatomic areas are grouped into the same code descriptor, the diameters of the lesions are added together. The appropriate code for these excisions would be **11421** (lesion diameter 0.6 cm to 1.0 cm).

What are the correct codes used to describe the following procedures?

6   Initial escharotomy of two different anatomic areas.

7   Fourteen premalignant lesions are removed by cryosurgical destruction from the back.

8   A split thickness graft measuring 230 sq cm is applied to a defect on the leg.

9   Image-guided stereotactic percutaneous needle core biopsy of breast.

10  Image-guided mammographic percutaneous biopsy utilizing automated vacuum-assisted or rotating device.

11  Anterior arthrodesis L2-L4 utilizing morselized autogenous iliac bone graft harvested through a separate fascial incision with anterior instrumentation.

12  Vertebroplasty of L1 and L2.

13  Reexploration of recurrent herniated nucleus pulposus at a single, previously explored lumbar interspace.

14  Diagnostic bronchoscopy with transbronchial lung biopsy of single lobe.

15  Bronchoscopy with bronchial alveolar lavage.

16  Sleeve pneumonectomy (that includes reservoir of the tracheal carina with end-to-end anastomosis of the trachea and contralateral mainstem bronchus).

17  Sleeve lobectomy (includes removal of a portion of bronchus to other lung).

18 Direct laryngoscopy with injection of vocal cords, requiring the use of an operating microscope or telescope.

19 Diagnostic laryngoscopy performed using a mirror.

20 Transmyocardial laser revascularization by thoracotomy performed at the time of other open cardiac procedure.

21 Replacement of a dual-chamber permanent pacemaker and transvenous electrodes with a new dual-chamber permanent pacemaker and electrodes.

22 Radial artery harvesting for coronary artery bypass procedure.

23 Redo CABG × 2, original procedure 2 years ago. Current procedure involves left internal mammary artery (LIMA) to left anterior descending (LAD) artery and saphenous vein graft (SVG) to right coronary artery (RCA).

24 Bilateral open surgical exposure of the femoral arteries for passage of endovascular sheath to repair an abdominal aortic aneurysm.

25 Thrombectomy of autogenous or nonautogenous dialysis graft
   a performed by open technique with or without revision.
   b performed by percutaneous technique.
   c performed on external types of dialysis devices.

26 Therapeutic occlusion of an artery by means of imaging guidance.

27 Repositioning of left ventricular pacing electrode two days after initial placement.

28 Replacement of the catheter portions only of a dual-catheter subcutaneous pump involving two separate access sites.

29 Resection of a segment of small intestine to correct a congenital atresia with tapering of the intestine.

30 EGD with biopsy of esophagus and stomach.

31 Percutaneous placement of a gastrostomy tube that requires radiological guidance performed by the same physician.

32 Proctosigmoidoscopy with removal of two polyps by snare technique.

33 Colonoscopy with removal of a polyp from the transverse colon by hot biopsy forceps and polyp removal from ascending colon by snare technique.

34 Repair of initial incisional hernia, incarcerated, with implantation of mesh.

35 Cystourethroscopy with ureteral meatotomy.

36 Transurethral destruction of prostate tissue by water-induced thermotherapy.

37 Laser coagulation of prostate with small amount of laser vaporization.

38 Incision and drainage of vaginal hematoma unrelated to delivery.

39 Insertion of Heyman capsules into uterus for clinical brachytherapy.

**40**  Thermal endometrial ablation (nonhysteroscopic).

**41**  Vulvectomy with removal of 50% of the skin and deep subcutaneous tissue of vulva.

**42**  Total abdominal hysterectomy with right salpingo-oophorectomy.

**43**  Patient visit for fitting and insertion of pessary.

**44**  A patient delivers a baby vaginally before admission. The physician delivers the placenta and provides postpartum care but not antepartum care.

**45**  Secondary repair of CSF leakage following skull base surgery "by free tissue graft."

**46**  Lumbosacral transforaminal epidural injection bilateral, multiple levels, left and right L4-L5 foramen, L4 spinal nerves and left and right L5-S1 foramen, L5 spinal nerves using fluoroscopic guidance.

**47**  Lumbar facet joint nerve injection unilateral, multiple levels, L3 and L4 medial branch nerves/facet joint nerves and L5 dorsal ramus for the L4-L5 and L5-S1 joints using fluoroscopic guidance.

**48**  Iridectomy with extracapsular removal of cataract by phacoemulsification technique. An intraocular lens is also inserted at this time.

**49**  Removal of intraocular foreign body from anterior chamber of right eye.

**50**  Strabismus surgery on one horizontal muscle of the right eye and one horizontal muscle in the left eye.

**51**  Bilateral tympanostomy with insertion of ventilating tubes under general anesthesia.

**52**  Removal and replacement of an osseointegrated implant to the temporal bone (with mastoidectomy) and attachment to external speech processor-stimulator.

**53**  If a frozen section pathology report comes back during the same operative session showing the margins of excision are not adequate and an additional excision is performed to remove the entire tumor, should two excision of lesion codes be used?

**54**  True or False: A tissue block in Mohs surgery is defined as an individual tissue piece embedded in a mounting medium for sectioning.

**55**  An approach surgeon opens and closes the operative site. To which procedure(s) should modifier 62 be appended? When may modifier 80 be used by the approach surgeon?

**56**  True or False: modifier 62 may not be appended to bone graft codes.

**57**  True or False: Synovial biopsy, when performed at the first MTP joint in conjunction with a bunion correction procedure, is reported separately.

**58**  Patient L presents to the emergency department after falling off a ladder. The emergency department physician determines that her left forearm is fractured. He applies a short arm cast and instructs her to follow up with an orthopedic surgeon. Code for the emergency department physician's services.

**59**  Surgical treatment is performed for a patient who has sustained a humeral shaft fracture. The orthopedic surgeon performs open treatment of the fracture by using an intramedullary implant and locking screws. After the surgical procedure, a cast is applied. Assign the appropriate code(s).

**60**  How many times should code **20550** be reported when multiple injections are administered to the same tendon?

**61**  True or False: Codes **20552** and **20553** should be reported once per session, regardless of the number of trigger points injected.

**62**  True or False: Removal of an existing pacing cardioverter-defibrillator device is not included in the replacement code and should be separately reported.

**63**  True or False: Code **93640** or **93641** may be reported in addition to code **33240**.

**64**  True or False: Procurement of an upper extremity vein is included when a coronary artery or lower extremity bypass procedure is reported.

**65**  True or False: If a laparoscopic procedure is performed, but there is not a CPT code that accurately describes the laparoscopic procedure, the open procedure code should be reported.

**66**  True or False: Diagnostic laparoscopy or laparoscopic lysis of adhesions is separately reportable when a laparoscopically assisted small bowel resection is performed.

**67**  True or False: A separate code is usually not reported when an incidental appendectomy is performed during intra-abdominal surgery.

**68**  True or False: Transendoscopic ultrasound guidance is included in transendoscopic biopsy through or across the esophagus.

**69**  True or False: Placement of an anal seton may be reported in addition to surgical treatment of anal fistula.

**70**  True or False: Code **43201** should be reported one time, regardless of the number of injections performed.

**71**  Assign the appropriate code(s) for the following procedures:
  **a**  Bilateral initial inguinal hernia repair, strangulated, 55-year-old patient
  **b**  Right recurrent inguinal incarcerated hernia
  **c**  Left recurrent inguinal hernia, reducible
  **d**  Right hydrocelectomy

**72**  Assign the appropriate code(s) for the following procedures:
  **a**  Bilateral extracorporeal shockwave lithotripsy of the kidneys
  **b**  Insertion of a nonindwelling bladder catheter to obtain postvoid residual urine

**73** Assign the appropriate code(s) for the following procedures:
   **a** Cystourethroscopy with removal of ureteral calculus
   **b** Cystourethroscopy with insertion of indwelling right ureteral stent

**74** Assign the appropriate code(s) for the following procedures:
   **a** Vaginal delivery after previous cesarean delivery, including provision of antepartum and postpartum care
   **b** Postpartum bilateral tubal ligation during same hospitalization

**75** True or False: Burr hole(s) or trephine procedures (codes **61250**, **61253**) may not be reported if followed by a craniotomy at the same operative session.

**76** True or False: Craniotomy procedures **61340** and **61490** may be performed unilaterally or bilaterally, depending on the involved anatomy.

**77** List the skull base surgery add-on codes.

**78** True or False: The mounting of a stereotactic head frame is reported by code **20660** when performed by the same physician at the time of stereotactic biopsy of an intracranial lesion.

**79** List the radiological supervision and interpretation code separately reportable in addition to codes **61750** and **61751**.

**80** True or False: The neurostimulator insertion/removal code **63660** does not include evaluative testing, programming, or reprogramming.

**81** Assign the appropriate code(s) for the following procedures:
   **a** Catheter implantation of an intrathecal or epidural catheter, connected to an external pump, implantable reservoir, or implantable infusion pump, not requiring laminectomy
   **b** Catheter implantation of an intrathecal or epidural catheter, connected to an external pump, implantable reservoir, or implantable infusion pump, requiring laminectomy

**82** True or False: Code **62350** is only intended to describe medication administration for long-term pain management.

**83** Code for refilling and maintenance of an implantable pump or reservoir for systemic drug delivery.

**84** Code for laminotomy for endoscopic discectomy.

**85** True or False: The phrase "reexploration of a previously explored cervical or lumbar interspace" is associated with a specific time frame from the initial procedure.

**86** Botulinum toxin injection into lumbar trunk muscles results in what effect: destruction or chemodenervation?

**87** True or False: Codes **64612-64614** are reported once, even though multiple injections are performed.

**88** Is facet joint nerve destruction by a neurolytic agent considered a unilateral or a bilateral procedure?

**89** Assign the appropriate code(s) for the following procedures:
  **a** Ocular photodynamic therapy of the right eye
  **b** Ocular photodynamic therapy of both the right and left eyes at the same session

**90** True or False: Renal pelvic stent procedures are usually performed for the treatment of ureteral strictures and obstructions.

**91** Assign the appropriate code for supracervical hysterectomy, 300 g uterus, with removal of ovaries.

**92** True or False: For endovascular temporary balloon arterial occlusion head/neck (extra- or intracranial), (code **61623**), the selective catheterization of the vessel to be occluded, positioning, and inflation of the occlusion balloon are inherent intraprocedural steps and not additionally reported.

**93** Code **61626** describes the permanent occlusion of one or more extracranial vessels (eg, arteriovenous malformation, tumor destruction of the head or neck (non-central nervous system)). May codes **75894** (transcatheter therapy, embolization) and code **75898** (postembolization arteriograph) be reported in addition to **61624**?

**94** True or False: Codes **62200** and **62201** may be used to describe third ventricle ventriculocisternostomy performed by stereotactic method only.

**95** True or False: None of the spinal injection codes (**62263, 62264, 62270-62273, 62280-62282**, and **62310-62319**) include fluoroscopic guidance and localization for placement of the needle or catheter.

**96** Assign the appropriate code(s) for epidurography at the cervical and lumbar region.

**97** Iridectomy with extracapsular removal of cataract by phacoemulsification technique. An intraocular lens is also inserted at this time.

**98** Removal of intraocular foreign body from anterior chamber of right eye.

**99** Strabismus surgery on one horizontal muscle of the right eye and one horizontal muscle of the left eye.

**100** What are the key differences in reporting laceration or wound repair of the conjunctiva, cornea, or sclera compared to the repair codes in the Integumentary System section?

**101** True or False: Placement of a regional orbital block catheter may be separately reported when performed at the time of an evisceration with implant.

**102** True or False: Mohs micrographic surgery of the eyelid is reported using code(s) **17311-17315**.

# CHAPTER 6

# Anesthesia

Coding for the administration of anesthesia and any additional procedures/services may appear to be straightforward; however, widely varying payer reporting requirements can add complexity to coding for both categories of services. In particular, claims for separate procedures/services may be denied, bundled into anesthesia administration, require special payer-specific modifiers, or be misinterpreted by those who are not familiar with anesthesia services. This chapter looks at the Anesthesia section of the Current Procedural Terminology (CPT®) codebook.

The first step toward understanding how to code for anesthesia services and for any additional procedures/services provided is to develop an understanding of the Anesthesia Guidelines. In this chapter, we will do the following:

- Review the subsections within the Anesthesia section of the CPT codebook
- Review the services included in basic anesthesia administration services
- Discuss time reporting for anesthesia services
- Discuss the use of modifiers with anesthesia codes
- Review the use of codes for reporting qualifying circumstances for anesthesia services

## Subsections Within the Anesthesia Section

The primary anatomical subsections in the Anesthesia section relate to the therapeutic or diagnostic procedure being performed. The following table provides a listing of the subsections in the Anesthesia section of the CPT codebook and corresponding code ranges.

### Anesthesia Subsections and Code Ranges

| Subsection | Code Range |
|---|---|
| Head | 00100-00222 |
| Neck | 00300-00352 |
| Thorax (Chest Wall and Shoulder Girdle) | 00400-00474 |
| Intrathoracic | 00500-00580 |
| Spine and Spinal Cord | 00600-00670 |
| Upper Abdomen | 00700-00797 |
| Lower Abdomen | 00800-00882 |
| Perineum | 00902-00952 |
| Pelvis (Except Hip) | 01112-01190 |
| Upper Leg (Except Knee) | 01200-01274 |
| Knee and Popliteal Area | 01320-01444 |
| Lower Leg (Below Knee, Includes Ankle and Foot) | 01462-01522 |
| Shoulder and Axilla | 01610-01682 |
| Upper Arm and Elbow | 01710-01782 |
| Forearm, Wrist, and Hand | 01810-01860 |
| Radiological Procedures | 01916-01936 |
| Burn Excision or Debridement | 01951-01953 |
| Obstetric | 01958-01969 |
| Other Procedures | 01990-01999 |

**CODING TIP**

The moderate (conscious) sedation codes **99143-99145** should be reported only when the same physician who will be performing the procedure administers the sedation. If the moderate (conscious) sedation is provided by a physician other than the health care professional performing the procedure, codes **99148-99150** should be reported, as appropriate.

# Reporting Basic Anesthesia Administration Services

Basic anesthesia administration services are those services provided by or under the responsible supervision of a physician and include the following:

- Routine preoperative and postoperative visits to evaluate the patient for the planned anesthesia and monitor the patient's postsurgery recovery from anesthesia
- Administration of fluids and/or blood during the period of anesthesia care
- Interpretation of noninvasive monitoring such as electrocardiography, body temperature, blood pressure, oximetry (blood oxygen concentration), capnography (blood carbon dioxide concentration), and mass spectrometry

Invasive forms of monitoring (such as intra-arterial, central venous, and pulmonary artery catheters and transesophageal echocardiography) are not included in basic anesthesia administration services. When these procedures are performed, they should be reported separately according to standard CPT coding guidelines applicable to the given code and the respective CPT section in which they are listed.

Anesthesia administration services may be reported using the appropriate code in the Anesthesia section of the CPT codebook (**00100-01999**), the appropriate anesthesia modifier, and qualifying circumstances codes, as appropriate. However, some payers do not accept CPT anesthesia codes and instead require the use of codes from the Surgery section of the CPT codebook for reporting anesthesia services. This practice may cause problems, because the anesthesia services often cannot be distinguished from any additional procedures/services provided by the anesthesiologist. It is critical to develop an understanding of CPT coding guidelines and payer-specific guidelines for reporting anesthesia services. One must be able to make a clear distinction between services provided when coding.

Generally, a single code is reported for anesthesia administration, whether the operating physician performs one or multiple procedures. When multiple procedures are performed during a single anesthetic administration, usually only the anesthesia procedure code for the most complex service and the total time for all procedures are reported. Anesthesia add-on codes are an exception. Codes **01953**, **01968**, and **01969** describe anesthesia add-on procedures, which are reported in addition to the primary anesthesia code.

**EXAMPLE:** Neuraxial labor anesthesia services are provided to a 30-year-old patient who had planned a vaginal delivery; however, circumstances resulted in a cesarean delivery.

In this case, the physician reports the anesthesia service for the planned vaginal delivery (**01967**). Then on a separate line, the physician reports the code for the anesthesia for the cesarean delivery that followed (**01968**). Modifier 51 should not be appended to the add-on code **01968**. (Refer to Chapter 10 for further discussion of modifiers.)

**EXAMPLE:** An anesthesiologist percutaneously inserts an arterial line for monitoring in addition to providing the basic anesthesia administration service for the operation.

In this case, the physician reports the anesthesia services on one or more lines of the claim form (as appropriate and required by the payer). Then on a separate line, the physician reports the code for the percutaneous insertion of the arterial line (**36620**). On the basis of CPT coding guidelines, no modifier is appended to code **36620**.

It should be noted that there are certain CPT code descriptors in the CPT codebook that include the phrases "with anesthesia" or "requiring anesthesia." These phrases indicate that the work involved in performing that procedure requires anesthesia, whether it is general anesthesia, regional anesthesia, or monitored anesthesia care (MAC). The appropriate anesthesia code is separately reported. Moderate (conscious) sedation is not an anesthesia service.

Codes **99143-99145** are reported when the physician performing the procedure also provides the sedation. When a second physician other than the health care professional performing the diagnostic or therapeutic service provides moderate (conscious) sedation, separate codes may be reported dependent on whether the procedure/service was performed in a facility (eg, hospital, outpatient hospital/ambulatory surgery center, skilled nursing facility) or nonfacility (eg, physician office, freestanding imaging center). (These codes and the guidelines for reporting moderate [conscious] sedation will be discussed further in Chapter 9.)

Regional or general anesthesia provided by a physician who also performs the services for which the anesthesia is provided is reported using modifier 47, Anesthesia by surgeon, appended to the surgical procedure code, instead of the anesthesia code. (The use of modifier 47 will be discussed further in Chapter 10.)

# Monitored Anesthesia Care

MAC is a specific anesthesia service for a diagnostic or therapeutic procedure. Indications for MAC include the nature of the procedure, the patient's clinical condition, and/or the potential need to convert to a general or regional anesthetic.

MAC includes all aspects of anesthesia care: a preprocedure visit, intraprocedure care, and postprocedure anesthesia management. During MAC, the anesthesiologist provides or medically directs a number of specific services including but not limited to the following:

- Diagnosis and treatment of clinical problems that occur during the procedure
- Support of vital functions
- Administration of sedatives, analgesics, hypnotics, anesthetic agents, or other medications as necessary for patient safety
- Psychological support and physical comfort
- Provision of other medical services as needed to complete the procedure safely

# Time Reporting

Time spent providing the anesthesia service is reported separately when anesthesia services are coded. Anesthesia time begins when the anesthesia provider starts preparing the patient for anesthesia in the operating room or a similar location. Time ends when the patient is safely placed under postoperative supervision.

# Anesthesia Modifiers

All anesthesia services are reported with the five-digit anesthesia procedure code (**00100-01999**) and two-digit physical status modifier, as appropriate. The use of other CPT modifiers may also be appropriate, but first, let us discuss the physical status modifiers.

The physical status modifiers are found in the anesthesia guidelines. They are identified with the initial letter *P* followed by a single digit from 1 to 6 and defined as follows:

- P1—A normal, healthy patient
- P2—A patient with mild systemic disease
- P3—A patient with severe systemic disease
- P4—A patient with severe systemic disease that is a constant threat to life
- P5—A moribund patient who is not expected to survive without the operation
- P6—A declared brain-dead patient whose organs are being removed for donor purposes

The six levels of physical status modifiers indicated are consistent with the American Society of Anesthesiologists' ranking of a patient's physical status. Physical status is included in the CPT codebook to distinguish the various levels of complexity of the anesthesia service provided.

# Reporting Multiple Surgical Procedures

When multiple surgical procedures are performed during a single anesthetic administration, the anesthesia code representing the most complex procedure is reported. The time reported is the combined total for all procedures. Add-on anesthesia codes are an exception. They are reported in addition to the code for the primary anesthesia service. There are three add-on anesthesia codes as follows:

**+01953**    Anesthesia for second and third degree burn excision or debridement with or without skin grafting, any site, for total body surface area (TBSA) treated during anesthesia and surgery; each additional one percent total body surface area or part thereof

**+01968**    Anesthesia for cesarean delivery following neuraxial labor analgesia/anesthesia

**+01969**    Anesthesia for cesarean hysterectomy following neuraxial labor
analgesia/anesthesia

When the secondary anesthesia service is designated as an add-on procedure in the CPT coding system, it should be reported in conjunction with the primary procedure.

## Separately Reportable Services

Placement of invasive monitoring devices and the use of transesophageal echocardiography may be reported separately in addition to basic anesthesia service/procedure. Procedures performed to provide for postoperative pain management are also separately reportable.

**EXAMPLE:** An anesthesiologist places a centrally inserted nontunneled central venous catheter in addition to providing the anesthesia service for a diagnostic or therapeutic surgical procedure. The anesthesiologist also inserts an epidural catheter into the lumbar spinal region to induce continuous postoperative analgesia for therapeutic pain management.

The anesthesiologist reports the appropriate anesthesia code for the surgical procedure (**00100-01999**) as well as the codes for the central venous line (**36556**) and the epidural that was placed for postoperative pain management (**62319**). Some payers will require that modifier 59, Distinct procedural service, be appended to the code for the epidural.

Codes **36556**, **36620**, and **93503** are other examples of adjunctive invasive monitoring procedures that may be performed at the same time as anesthesia services. While the interpretation of the data obtained from these devices is included in the base unit value assigned to an anesthesia code, the placement of these devices is not. Therefore, the placement should be reported separately.

## Reporting Other CPT Modifiers

In addition to the physical status modifiers, it may also be appropriate to report other CPT modifiers when codes for procedural services are reported in addition to the basic anesthesia service. Remember, if the anesthesiologist performs other additional procedures, each is separately reportable.

**EXAMPLE:** An anesthesiologist places a centrally inserted nontunneled central venous catheter in addition to providing the anesthesia administration service for the operation. The anesthesiologist also inserts an epidural catheter into the lumbar spinal region to induce continuous postoperative analgesia for therapeutic pain management.

In this case, the physician reports the anesthesia service on one or more lines of the claim form (as appropriate and required by the payer). On separate lines of the claim form, the physician reports the following codes for the additional procedures performed:

**36556**     Placement of the central venous catheter; age 5 years or older (report code 36555 for patients under age 5)

**62319**     Insertion of the lumbar epidural catheter

Code **36556** is an example of a service that might be reported separately for invasive monitoring procedures when performed at the same time as anesthesia services. Code **36555** should be reported for patients under age five. Modifier 51 is appended to **36556**, as this is a procedure that is not designated as modifier 51-exempt. Modifier 59 is appended to the epidural catheter pain procedure to indicate that it is distinct and independent of the anesthesia service.

Codes **36620** and **93503** are other examples of adjunctive invasive monitoring procedures that might be performed at the same time as anesthesia services. As these codes are designated as modifier 51-exempt, modifier 51 would not be appended to these procedure codes when reported in addition to the anesthesia service codes. (Refer to Chapter 2 for further discussion regarding codes exempt from the use of modifier 51.)

**EXAMPLE:** A patient undergoing a thoracotomy receives an epidural injection of a local anesthetic for postoperative pain control in addition to the general anesthetic administered through an endotracheal tube.

In this case, the epidural (**62318**) is not the surgical anesthetic (**00540**) and it would be reported separately as an independent procedure. When general anesthesia is administered and epidural or nerve block injections are performed to provide postoperative analgesia, they are separate and distinct services and are reported in addition to the anesthesia code. Whether the block procedure (insertion of catheter; injection of narcotic or local anesthetic agent) occurs preoperatively, postoperatively, or during the procedure is immaterial.

**EXAMPLE:** A patient undergoes a total knee replacement surgery receiving a regional anesthetic and a postoperative pain management agent through the same epidural catheter.

When the block procedure is used primarily for the anesthesia itself, the service should be reported using the anesthesia code alone (**01402**). In a combined epidural/general anesthetic, the block cannot be reported separately.

## Qualifying Circumstances

Many anesthesia services are provided under particularly difficult circumstances, depending on factors such as the following:

- Extraordinary condition of the patient

- Notable operative conditions
- Unusual risk factors

Four codes (see list below) are available for reporting qualifying circumstances that have a significant impact on the anesthesia service provided. These codes can be found at the end of the Anesthesia Guidelines, as well as in their appropriate numeric sequence in the Medicine section of the CPT codebook. These codes are designated as add-on procedures and may be reported in addition to the primary anesthesia procedure/service, with the exception of code **99100**, which should not be reported in addition to an anesthesia code that is specific to the very young patient.

**+99100**    Anesthesia for patient of extreme age, under one year and over seventy (List separately in addition to code for primary anesthesia procedure)

**+99116**    Anesthesia complicated by utilization of total body hypothermia (List separately in addition to code for primary anesthesia procedure)

**+99135**    Anesthesia complicated by utilization of controlled hypotension (List separately in addition to code for primary anesthesia procedure)

**+99140**    Anesthesia complicated by emergency conditions (specify) (List separately in addition to code for primary anesthesia procedure)

Note that it is not appropriate to use code **99100**, Anesthesia for patient of extreme age, with the anesthesia codes that apply to specific procedures performed on young infants (codes **00834-00836**, which are for reporting anesthesia for hernia repairs; code **00326**, used to report anesthesia for procedures on the larynx and trachea; and code **00561**, which describes on-pump cardiac procedures on patients under one year of age).

For the purposes of reporting code **99140**, an emergency is defined as existing when delay in treatment of the patient would lead to a significant increase in threat to life or body part. This does not refer to a procedure merely because it is done outside of the normal, weekday schedule. If an elective procedure is delayed into evening hours, it is not considered an emergency.

Each of the codes above is considered an add-on code and is reported as an additional procedure number along with the code for the anesthesia service provided. It is not appropriate to report these codes alone. Remember that they are to be used only with anesthesia codes and not with other procedure codes in the CPT codebook. As with all add-on codes, these codes are exempt from the use of modifier 51. More than one qualifying circumstances code may be selected and reported, as appropriate.

## CHAPTER 6

# EXERCISES

1 Which physical status modifier is used to designate a patient with severe systemic disease that is a constant threat to life?

2 True or False: All anesthesia services are reported with the five-digit anesthesia procedure code (**00100-01999**).

3 How is anesthesia care reported when multiple surgical procedures are performed under a single anesthetic?

4 True or False: Only one qualifying circumstances code may be selected and reported per session.

5 The six levels of physical status modifiers (P1-P6) are consistent with which specialty society's ranking of patient physical status?

6 What codes are used to report moderate (conscious) sedation provided by a physician also performing the procedure/service for which the sedation is provided?

7 Regional or general anesthesia provided by the surgeon also performing the procedure is reported using which CPT modifier?

8 When does anesthesia time begin? When does it end?

9 Anesthesia for procedures of the ankle and foot is reported using which series of codes?

10 What is the appropriate code for reporting anesthesia for a total elbow replacement?

11 Which anesthesia codes may be reported in addition to the primary anesthesia service?

12 Anesthesia for therapeutic interventional radiology procedures is reported using which codes?

13 Anesthesia for obstetrical procedures is reported using which series of codes?

14 True or False: Basic anesthesia administration services include the placement of invasive monitoring lines.

15 True or False: When reporting anesthesia for pediatric hernia repairs codes **00834** and **00836**, the add-on code **99100** for anesthesia for patient of extreme age, younger than one year and older than 70, should also be reported.

16 True or False: Following an anesthesia service, if an anesthesiologist inserts an epidural catheter into the lumbar spinal region for therapeutic pain management, code **62319** may be reported separately.

**17** True or False: Generally, a single code is reported for anesthesia administration, whether the operating physician performs one or multiple procedures.

**18** True or False: Moderate (conscious) sedation is an anesthesia service.

# Radiology

In this chapter is a review of some of the basic guidelines for reporting codes from the Radiology section of the Current Procedural Terminology (CPT®) codebook, including the following:

- Introduction to Radiology

- Supervision and Interpretation

- Professional versus Technical Procedural Component

- Administration and Supply of Contrast Materials

- Written Reports

- Diagnostic Radiology (Diagnostic Imaging), including Interventional Radiology

- Diagnostic Ultrasound

- Radiologic Guidance

- Mammography, Breast

- Radiation Oncology

- Nuclear Medicine

# Introduction to Radiology

A fundamental understanding of the Radiology section structure and its instructional features is key to coding radiologic services. The CPT code set lists both diagnostic and therapeutic procedures according to the various types of imaging modalities. The structure and features of the Radiology section extend reporting functionality, as these codes may do the following:

- Describe the total service
- Describe a portion of a procedure performed
- Require reporting of procedure codes outside the **70000** series (eg, surgical procedure code)
- Allow reporting of the same radiology code for different procedures outside the **70000** series
- Require reporting of multiple radiology codes
- Require use of modifiers
- Disallow reporting of additional radiology codes

The Radiology section structure includes the following seven imaging modality subsections:

- Diagnostic Radiology (Diagnostic)
- Diagnostic Ultrasound
- Radiologic Guidance
- Breast, Mammography
- Bone/Joint Studies
- Radiation Oncology
- Nuclear Medicine

Each subsection lists procedures according to organ or anatomic site (ie, head and neck, chest, spine and pelvis, heart, vascular, etc.). Typically, the imaging technique is delineated either by the subheading title or specified in the code descriptor. Careful review of each descriptor is recommended, as the imaging modality (eg, conventional X-ray imaging, computed tomography [CT], magnetic resonance [MR], ultrasound, stereotaxis, mammography, fluoroscopy) may or may not be specified. For example, codes **70030-70330** are listed in the Diagnostic Radiology (Diagnostic Imaging) subsection under the Head and Neck anatomic heading. Although not specifically stated in the descriptor nomenclature, this series of codes represents radiologic examinations using conventional X-ray imaging. To differentiate, codes **70450-70498** are also listed in this subsection and anatomic heading, but the descriptor nomenclature specifies CT as the imaging modality used.

To further clarify, the type of imaging supervision and interpretation provided may change while the procedure remains the same. For example, a physician may perform a percutaneous needle biopsy of the liver (**47000**). However, this procedure may be performed under fluoroscopic, ultrasound, MR imaging (MRI), or CT guidance. Therefore, depending on the imaging service performed, code **76942**, **77002**, **77012**, or **77021** would be reported in addition to code **47000**.

**CODING TIP**

The codes listed in the Radiology section of the CPT codebook apply when radiological services are performed either by the physician or under physician supervision.

## Introductory Notes

To better understand certain types of imaging modality(s), introductory or instructional notes provide information such as definitions of procedural elements, specific reporting instruction, and requirements related to image documentation and final written report. An example of introductory notes can be found in the Diagnostic Radiology (Diagnostic Imaging) subsection following the Vascular Procedures/Aorta and Arteries heading.

## Parenthetical Notes/Cross-References

Throughout the Radiology section, parenthetical notes also provide instructional reporting information when combinations of imaging modality(s) are performed. The following is an example of the instructional notes pertaining to the use of fluoroscopy following code **77002**:

**77002**   Fluoroscopic guidance for needle placement (eg, biopsy, aspiration, injection, localization device)

(See appropriate surgical code for procedure and anatomic location.)

## Descriptor Phraseology

Besides specifying the involved anatomy, the descriptor nomenclature of the Radiology codes includes references to the number (eg, **73140**-finger(s), minimum two views) and/or type of views (eg, **74010**-abdomen, anteroposterior and additional oblique and cone views) performed. In order to assign and report appropriate CPT codes, the documentation should reflect the number/type of views taken and the method of examination performed and interpreted. If the number of views is not mentioned in the report, the coder should not assume the procedure performed. Instead, the coder should work closely with the interpreting physician to clarify and obtain the appropriate information. This will help ensure that all pertinent information has been captured, allowing for submission of the correct procedural CPT code, which reflects the level of work performed.

**EXAMPLE:** Views included in a spine survey study (**72010**) of an adult.

CPT code **72010** Radiologic examination, spine, entire, survey study, anteroposterior and lateral, is intended to be used to report a survey study of the entire spine. A survey study is commonly performed to obtain scoliosis measurements or evaluate for spine metastasis. This radiologic examination involves obtaining anteroposterior (AP) and lateral views of the entire spine. The number of films required will vary depending on the size of the film available and the size of the patient examined. For an adult patient, the study may require six films (the AP and lateral views of the cervical, thoracic, and lumbar spine). For smaller patients (eg, a pediatric patient), it may be possible to obtain the AP and lateral views of the entire spine with fewer films. These films are then interpreted as a single study (ie, one study is reported regardless of the number of films taken).

The terms *complete* (eg, **76700**) and *limited* (eg, **76705**) are found in certain code descriptors and refer to the elements comprising the examination for that anatomic region. The written report should contain a description of these elements or the reason that an element could not be visualized. If less than required elements for a complete exam are reported (eg, limited number of organs or limited portion of region evaluated), the "limited" code for that anatomic region should be used once per patient exam session. A "limited" exam of an anatomic region should not be reported for the same exam session as a "complete" exam of that same region.

> **CODING TIP**
>
> In order to assign and report appropriate CPT code(s), the documentation should reflect the number/type of views taken and the method of examination performed and interpreted.

**EXAMPLE:** A three-view X ray of the hand with a three-view X ray of the wrist when obtained on three films vs six films.

When three views of the hand and three views of the wrist are performed, it is appropriate to code **73130**, Radiologic examination, hand; minimum of three views, and **73110**, Radiologic examination, wrist; complete, minimum of three views, for the professional component, irrespective of whether these studies are performed together on three films or separately on six films. Both procedures should be coded if the physician performed a full and complete interpretation of both anatomic sites. For the technical component, however, if both studies are performed at the same time on three films, only a single charge should be reported.

## Supervision and Interpretation

> **CODING TIP**
>
> If the technical and professional components of the service are performed by the same provider, it is not appropriate or necessary to report the components of the service separately.

When a procedure that is a combination of an interventional (surgical) procedure and imaging is performed, the imaging portion of the procedure is designated as "radiological supervision and interpretation." When a physician performs both the procedure and provides radiological imaging supervision and interpretation, a combination of procedure codes outside the **70000** series and imaging (supervision and interpretation) codes are necessary to completely report the procedure(s) performed.

Before 1992, the Current Procedural Terminology (CPT®) nomenclature referred to many of these services as *complete procedures*. Revisions to the CPT Nomenclature in 1992 resulted in the deletion of complete procedure codes from the Radiology section of the CPT codebook. With the deletion of complete procedure codes, the codes for reporting radiological supervision and interpretation were revised, and several new supervision and interpretation codes were added. Also, codes found in other sections of the CPT codebook were added and revised to describe the procedures performed. Refer to the section on interventional radiology found later in this chapter for further discussion of radiological supervision and interpretation.

### Professional versus Technical Procedural Components

Certain procedures described by the CPT code set are a combination of a professional (physician) component (eg, diagnostic tests that involve a physician's interpretation, such as X rays) and a technical component. For diagnostic or therapeutic radiologic services, the professional component includes the physician work and associated overhead and professional liability insurance costs involved in the diagnostic or therapeutic radiologic service. The technical component of a service includes the cost of equipment, supplies, technician salaries, etc. The global charge refers to both components when billed together.

Since CPT codes are intended to represent physician and other health care practitioner services, CPT Nomenclature does not contain a coding convention to designate the technical component for a procedure or service. CPT coding does provide modifier 26, Professional Component, for separately reporting the professional (or physician) component of a procedure or service. This is because a hospital or other facility may be reporting the technical component of the procedure. Unmodified CPT codes are intended to describe both the technical and professional components of a service.

When reporting the technical component of a procedure or service, become familiar with the various reporting requirements of individual insurance companies. For example, the Health Care Common Procedure Coding System (HCPCS) Level II "TC" modifier is not one of the CPT modifiers but rather is required for Medicare reporting purposes to differentiate the professional versus technical components of the service provided (radiologic in this instance).

### Unlisted Service or Procedure

There are times when a physician performs a service or procedure that is not described with existing CPT codes. When reporting such a service, the appropriate "unlisted procedure" code may be used to indicate the service. A listing of these "unlisted" radiological procedure codes (including nuclear medicine and diagnostic ultrasound) can be found in the *CPT 2008* codebook, in the introduction guidelines prior to the **70000** series codes.

## Administration of Contrast Materials

Contrast material is commonly used for imaging enhancement. Contrast material improves visualization and evaluation of the body structure or organ studied. Some of the procedures listed in the Radiology section of the CPT codebook may be performed with or without the use of contrast material for imaging enhancement. The phrase "with contrast" used in the codes for procedures performed using contrast for imaging enhancement represents contrast material administered intravascularly, intra-articularly, or intrathecally.

For example, brain CT may be done with intravenous contrast (**70460**), without contrast (**70450**), or without contrast followed by injection of intravenous contrast (**70470**). In procedures where contrast material is always used, the CPT descriptor will not indicate that contrast material is used. For instance, intravenous pyelogram and abdominal aortogram do not list "with contrast," since contrast is an intrinsic part of the procedure. When contrast materials are administered only orally and/or rectally, the study does not qualify as "with contrast" and should be coded "without contrast." A CT scan of the abdomen with oral contrast should be coded as a CT of the abdomen without contrast (**74150**).

For intra-articular injection, use the appropriate joint injection code. If radiographic arthrography is also performed, also use the arthrography supervision and interpretation code for the appropriate joint (which includes fluoroscopy). If CT or MR arthrography is performed without radiographic arthrography, use the appropriate joint injection code, the appropriate CT or MR code ("with contrast" or "without followed by contrast"), and the appropriate imaging guidance code for needle placement for contrast injection.

Spine examinations using CT, MRI, or MR angiography (MRA) "with contrast" may be performed with intrathecal (within either the subarachnoid or the subdural space) or intravascular contrast injection. However, for intrathecal injection of contrast material, the injection procedure is separately reported with either code **61055** or **62284**, as appropriate.

Injection of intravascular contrast material is part of the "with contrast" CT, CT angiography (CTA), MRI, or MRA procedure.

Similarly, when an MRI of the knee is performed in which administration of contrast is performed through an intra-articular injection, code **73722**, Magnetic resonance (eg, proton) imaging, any joint of a lower extremity, would describe the imaging portion of the study. While code **73722** describes the imaging performed, this code would be reported in addition to code **27370**, Injection procedure for knee arthrography, to describe the intra-articular contrast administration. As stated later, the supply of contrast material is separately reported.

# Supply of Contrast Materials and Radiopharmaceuticals

It is appropriate to separately report the supply of the contrast material(s) with CPT code **99070**.

Medicare and some third-party payers require the use of HCPCS Level II codes to report the supply of contrast materials and radiopharmaceuticals. A number of HCPCS Level II codes (eg, **Q9945**, **Q9952**, **A9512**) are available for reporting the supply of contrast materials and radiopharmaceuticals. The HCPCS Level II codes are more specific to the type of contrast or radiopharmaceutical supplied (eg, low-osmolar contrast material, technetium Tc 99m, gadolinium) and the dosage administered. Third-party payers may have other specific reporting and reimbursement policies related to the reporting and reimbursement of the supply of radiopharmaceuticals and contrast materials. One should become familiar with individual third-party payer reporting and reimbursement policies and the CPT and HCPCS Level II codes available so that coding will be accurate.

---

**CODING TIP**

The following codes are provided as examples of HCPCS Level II codes used for reporting the supplies for radiologic procedures:

**A4641** Radiopharmaceutical, diagnostic, not otherwise classified

**A9500** Technetium Tc 99m sestamibi, diagnostic, per study dose, up to 40 millicuries

**A9600** Strontium Sr-89 chloride, therapeutic, per miillicurie

---

**CODING TIP**

In *CPT 2003*, the term *axial* was removed from many of the CT code descriptors. Typically, direct acquisition images are obtained in the axial plane for CT studies, but in certain instances, direct acquisition may be obtained in other planes (eg, coronal plane for sinus studies). Elimination of the term *axial* clarifies that the CT codes are appropriate for reporting CT direct acquisition imaging performed in any plane (ie, axial, coronal, sagittal, or multiplanar).

# Written Reports

A written report, signed by the interpreting physician, is an integral part of a radiological procedure or interpretation.

Although CPT coding guidelines do not specify the requirements for the content or format of the written report, this guideline indicates that a separate, distinctly identifiable, signed written report prepared by the interpreting physician is considered key to the radiological procedure or interpretation.

# Interpretation of Outside Films

When a physician's opinion or advice regarding a specific film is requested by another physician and, upon examination of the film, the consulting physician provides his or her opinion or advice to the requesting physician in a written report, the specific procedure code appended with modifier 26, Professional Component, should be reported. By using the specific procedure code to identify the service provided, statistics on usage are obtained and the proper relative value units are assigned.

Some Medicare carriers require that modifier 77, Repeat Procedure by Another Physician, also be used to indicate that a basic procedure or service performed by another physician had to be repeated. Check with your local Medicare carrier and other third-party payers for their guidelines. Other carriers may have different guidelines and recommend the use of CPT code **76140**, Consultation on X-ray examination made elsewhere, written report.

If a patient comes to an office for a new or established patient visit and brings the physician his or her medical records including X-rays, the review or reread of the X-rays would be considered part of the face-to-face evaluation and management (E/M) service provided to the patient and not reported separately.

# Diagnostic Radiology (Diagnostic Imaging)

Codes for reporting a number of diagnostic imaging techniques are described in this subsection. Some examples of the various techniques included in this section are conventional X-ray imaging, CT scan, CTA, MRI, MRA, angiography, venography, fluoroscopy, and various imaging-guided procedures. There are no individual subheadings for CT, CTA, MRI, MRA, angiography, venography, and fluoroscopy. Specific codes for the various diagnostic imaging techniques are distributed throughout the anatomic series of codes.

Conventional X-ray imaging consists of a high-voltage generator, an X-ray tube, an Al filter, a collimator, a grid, an intensifying screen, and a film (or solid state digital detector); ultimately, an image, which is a "shadow'" of the anatomy of the body, is generated. Conventional and digital systems provide the capability for a wide range of applications from examinations of the skull, spinal column, abdomen, and the extremities. These procedures can be performed on patients in a lying, sitting, or standing position. For example, code **73565**, Radiologic examination, knee; both knees, standing, anteroposterior, describes the anatomy, position, and type of views performed. Some of the codes representing diagnostic imaging using conventional X-ray imaging include **70030-70160**, **70190-70328**, **70360-70370**, **70380**, **71010-71035**, **71100-71130**, **72010-72120**, **72170-72190**, **72220**, **73000-73030**, **73050-73140**, **73500-73520**.

CT imaging, once known as "CAT scanning" (computed axial tomography), combines the use of a digital computer together with a rotating X-ray device to obtain image data from different angles around the body. Computer processing of the image data is then performed to show a cross-section of body tissue, bone, and organs. CT imaging is particularly useful because it can show several types of tissue with great clarity, including organs like the liver, spleen, pancreas, and kidneys. In addition, CT is a very useful diagnostic method because it can display and distinguish many different types of tissue in the same region, including bone, muscle, soft tissue, and blood vessels. CTA is a noninvasive technique for imaging vessels. The information obtained from the CTA is used in the evaluation of vascular anatomy (eg, renal or liver transplant donors, congenital anomalies), vascular disorders (eg, aortic or intracranial aneurysms, renal artery or carotid stenosis), vascular trauma (eg, aortic laceration), and in the follow-up of organ transplantation.

The key distinction between CTA and CT is that CTA includes three-dimensional reformatting of angiographic images and interpretation. If three-dimensional reformatting is not done, it is not a CTA study. Injection of contrast material is part of the "with contrast" CTA procedure; therefore, it is not appropriate to separately report the code for the administration of contrast.

MRI views internal structures of the body using magnetism, radio waves, and a computer to produce the images of body structures particularly in the soft tissue, brain and spinal cord, abdomen, and joints.

The existing CPT codes for MRI are silent with regard to patient positioning. Some MRI studies require more images and positioning and some require less. It may be appropriate to append modifier 22 to these studies to indicate more work, but only if one routinely appends modifier 52 to easier studies. For example, the coding of MRI with flexion and extension views is appropriately coded based on the anatomy studied (eg, MRI of the spine), not the type of views acquired or the type of equipment used. If a few additional pulsing sequences are acquired or dynamic positional changes made in a given anatomic region, they are included in the base procedure code and not coded separately. If the work for these additional dynamic position changes is greater than that usually provided, then this may be a case to use modifier 22.

**CODING TIP**

It is not appropriate to report **76376** or **76377** in conjunction with CTA (**70496**, **70498**, **71275**, **72191**, **73206**, **73706**, **74175**, **75635**), MRA (**70544-70549**, **71555**, **72159**, **72198**, **73225**, **73725**, **74185**), or nuclear medicine (**78000-78999**) procedure codes, or with Category III codes for CT colonography (**0066T**, **0067T**) or cardiac CT and coronary CTA (**0144T-0151T**).

**CODING TIP**

Functional MRI involves identification and mapping of stimulation of brain function. When neurofunctional tests are administered by a technologist or other nonphysician or nonpsychologist, see code **70554**. When neurofunctional tests are entirely administered by a physician or psychologist, use code **70555**.

MRA is a noninvasive diagnostic study used to evaluate disorders of the arterial and venous structures. Currently, the MRA procedure entails two- or three-dimensional, time-of-flight or phase contrast gradient echo sequences sensitive to blood flow covering the anatomic region of interest.

**EXAMPLE:** The patient is a 45-year-old man with severe headache and altered mental status. Noncontrast CT exam shows intracranial bleeding. The patient is allergic to iodinated contrast media. MRA is requested to look for a source of bleeding, such as aneurysm.

This example illustrates an MRA (**70544**) used to evaluate the anterior and posterior circulation vessels within the cranial vault for aneurysms. Cranial MRA is also used for the evaluation of atherosclerotic occlusive disease, acute thrombosis, dissection, vascular malformations, vascular loop syndromes, arterial causes of pulsatile tinnitus, and arteriovenous malformations and to assess the vascularity of tumors. The examination can also be tailored to assess the intracranial venous structures to exclude sinovenous thrombosis or to evaluate venous malformations or fistulae.

Fluoroscopy is an imaging technique commonly used by physicians to obtain real-time images of the internal structures of a patient through the use of a fluoroscope. A fluoroscope consists of an X-ray source and fluorescent screen between which the patient is positioned. The fluorescent screen is electronically and optically coupled to an image intensification system and television camera, allowing the images to be seen on a monitor, recorded, and stored. Fluoroscopy (**76000**) may be considered inclusive of the surgical portion of the procedure (**50590**) or radiographic service (**74300**) performed. See the appropriate surgical code for procedure and anatomic location for instruction regarding the additional reporting of fluoroscopy. (Refer to the Radiologic Guidance subsection for further discussion of fluoroscopic guidance codes **77001-77003**.)

Take time to review this subsection of radiology and become familiar with the specific code listings and the layout. Subheadings are found based on anatomic sites (eg, head and neck, chest, spine, and pelvis). Specific codes for the various diagnostic imaging techniques are distributed throughout the anatomic series of codes.

The following tables are provided as a summary reference for the specific codes available for reporting MRI, MRA, CT, and CTA scan procedures.

## Magnetic Resonance Imaging (MRI)

| | |
|---|---|
| Abdomen | 74181-74183 |
| Bone Marrow Blood Supply | 77084 |
| Brain | 70551-70553, 70557-70559 |
| Functional MRI | 70554, 70555 |
| Breast | 77058, 77059 |
| Cardiac, for Function/Morphology | 75557, 75561 |
| Cardiac, for Velocity Flow | 75558, 75560, 75562, 75564 |
| Cardiac, for Stress Imaging | 75559, 75560, 75563, 75564 |
| Chest | 71550-71552 |
| Extremity, Lower, Other than Joint | 73718-73720 |
| Extremity, Upper, Other than Joint | 73218-73220 |
| Joint, Lower Extremity | 73721-73723 |
| Joint, Upper Extremity | 73221-73223 |
| Orbit, Face, and Neck | 70540-70543 |
| Pelvis | 72195-72197 |
| Spinal Canal and Contents, Cervical | 72141, 72142, 72156 |
| Spinal Canal and Contents, Lumbar | 72148, 72149, 72158 |
| Spinal Canal and Contents, Thoracic | 72146, 72147, 72157 |
| Temporomandibular Joint | 70336 |
| Unlisted magnetic resonance procedure | 76498 |

## Magnetic Resonance Angiography (MRA)

| | |
|---|---|
| Abdomen | 74185 |
| Chest (Excluding Myocardium) | 71555 |
| Extremity, Lower | 73725 |
| Extremity, Upper | 73225 |
| Head | 70544-70546 |
| Neck | 70547-70549 |
| Pelvis | 72198 |
| Spinal Canal and Contents | 72159 |

## Computed Tomographic (CT) Scan

| | |
|---|---|
| Abdomen | 74150-74170 |
| Extremity, Lower | 73700-73702 |
| Extremity, Upper | 73200-73202 |
| Head or Brain | 70450-70470 |
| Maxillofacial Area | 70486-70488 |
| Neck, Soft Tissue | 70490-70492 |
| Orbit, Sella, or Posterior Fossa or Outer, Middle, or Inner Ear | 70480-70482 |
| Pelvis | 72192-72194 |
| Spine, Cervical | 72125-72127 |
| Spine, Lumbar | 72131-72133 |
| Spine, Thoracic | 72128-72130 |
| Thorax | 71250-71270 |
| Unlisted computed tomography procedure | 76497 |

| Computed Tomographic Angiography (CTA) | |
|---|---|
| Abdomen | 74175 |
| Chest | 71275 |
| Extremity, Upper | 73206 |
| Extremity, Lower | 73706 |
| Head | 70496 |
| Neck | 70498 |
| Pelvis | 72191 |

In addition to the CT scan studies indicated in the previous table, there are specific codes for reporting a limited or localized follow-up CT study (**76380**) and a CT bone mineral density study (**77078**, **77079**). A number of codes are also available in the **77011-77014** series for reporting the radiological supervision and interpretation portion of CT guidance procedures. Further discussion of coding for CT guidance procedures can be found later in this chapter under the Interventional Radiology heading.

Because there are numerous anatomic sites and related cross-references associated with arthrography procedures, a quick reference to help one appropriately report these procedures/services has been provided.

The following table, which reviews the procedures for radiography and CT/MRA, can be used as a quick reference to help one appropriately report these procedures/services.

| Procedures for Radiography and CT/MR Arthrography | | | | |
|---|---|---|---|---|
| Joint | Injection Code | Radiographic Arthrogram | CT Arthrogram | MR Arthrogram |
| Shoulder | 23350 | 73040 | 73201/73202 | 73222/73223 |
| Elbow | 24220 | 73085 | 73201/73202 | 73222/73223 |
| Wrist | 25246 | 73115 | 73201/73202 | 73222/73223 |
| Hip | 27093/27095 | 73525 | 73701/73702 | 73722/73723 |
| Knee | 27370 | 73580 | 73701/73702 | 73722/73723 |
| Ankle | 27648 | 73615 | 73701/73702 | 73722/73723 |

Note: If a combination study is performed, this table would still apply because only one injection procedure is being performed (eg, combined radiographic arthrography and CT arthrography of the shoulder would be coded **23350**, **73040**, and **73201** [presuming no precontrast shoulder CT was performed]).

# Interventional Radiology

Interventional radiology is the branch of medicine that diagnoses and/or treats a wide range of diseases using percutaneous or minimally invasive techniques with imaging guidance. Understanding how to code for interventional radiology services requires a thorough knowledge of anatomy and physiology as well as an in-depth knowledge of the use of CPT codes unique to this specialty.

Often, diagnostic and therapeutic services are delivered in a variety of combinations and permutations determined by the underlying disease process, the clinical evaluation of the patient, and the intraprocedural interpretation of the diagnostic portion of the service (including physiologic data and images obtained). These contingencies may result in several coding possibilities.

In recognition of the complexity of interventional radiology services and their proper description, complete procedure codes were deleted from the CPT Nomenclature in 1992 and "component" coding was introduced. Component coding facilitates more accurate coding by helping to completely describe the various procedures performed.

It allows for the following:
- Accurate tracking of professional services for outcome analysis, utilization review, and billing purposes
- Accurate service reporting whether one provider performs all the services or multiple providers work in concert to perform the services (eg, one physician performs the procedure and another physician provides imaging supervision and interpretation)
- Tracking and reporting of interventional radiological hospital services in a manner exactly the same as other surgical and radiological services
- Fair relative valuation of similar types of services without regard to the specialty of the provider

The following will give a clearer understanding of the deleted complete procedure codes and compare them with component codes.

The following is an example of the *CPT 1991* code entries:

**70332**    Temporomandibular joint arthrography; supervision and interpretation only

**70333**    complete procedure
             (For injection procedure only for arthrography, see **21116**)

**21116**    Injection procedure for temporomandibular joint arthrography
             (For temporomandibular arthrography, use **70332**)

Following are the same code entries as they appear in *CPT 2002*:

**70332**    Temporomandibular joint arthrography, radiological supervision and interpretation
             (Do not report **76003** [changed to **77002** in 2007] in addition to **70332**)
             (**70333** [complete procedure] has been deleted, see **21116**, **70332**)

> **CODING TIP**
>
> Component coding allows for the flexibility of combining diagnostic and therapeutic services on the same occasion without overstating or understating the services provided.

> **CODING TIP**
>
> When coding for interventional radiology procedures and services, a one-to-one relationship may not exist between the number of procedure codes and the number of radiological supervision and interpretation codes reported to describe the service provided.

**21116**   Injection procedure for temporomandibular joint arthrography
(For radiological supervision and interpretation, use **70332**)
(Do not report **76003** [changed to **77002** in 2007] in conjunction
with **70332**)

Review the code descriptors provided in these examples. If a single physician performs the injection procedure for temporomandibular joint arthrography (**21116**) and the radiological supervision and interpretation of the procedure (**70332**), the physician should report both components of the procedure (**21116** and **70332**) to completely describe the services rendered.

In some instances, one physician performs the injection procedure and another physician is responsible for its radiological supervision and interpretation. If Physician A performs the procedure and Physician B is responsible for the radiological supervision and interpretation of the study, Physician A would report his or her services with the appropriate procedure code outside the **70000** series. Physician B would report the appropriate code for the radiological supervision and interpretation.

Furthermore, when reporting only the professional component of the service, modifier 26 should be appended to the radiological supervision and interpretation code reported (eg, if the procedure is performed on hospital or facility-owned equipment). (Refer to Chapter 10 for further discussion regarding the use of modifier 26.)

When relatively straightforward services are provided, there may be a one-to-one correlation between a procedural service and an imaging supervision and interpretation service. However, when more extensive services are provided, the relationship of the procedural services to the imaging supervision and interpretation services may not be so obvious. Often, no one-to-one relationship exists between the number of codes reported for the procedural service and the number of codes reported from the **70000** series for the radiological supervision and interpretation portion of the service.

For example, introduction of a catheter into the aorta with injection procedures for an arch aortography, thoracic aortography, and abdominal aortography would be reported with the following codes:

**36200**   Introduction of catheter, aorta

**75650**   Angiography, cervicocerebral, catheter, including vessel origin, radiological supervision and interpretation

**75605**   Aortography, thoracic, by serialography, radiological supervision and interpretation

**75625**   Aortography, abdominal, by serialography, radiological supervision and interpretation

Only one code is reported for the catheter placement in the aorta. However, three separate codes are necessary to completely report the radiological supervision and interpretation portion of the service. Code **75650** is reported for the arch aortography, code **75605** for the thoracic aortography, and code **75625** for the abdominal aortography.

The rest of the discussion of interventional radiology is a review of various coding scenarios.

# Nonvascular Interventional Radiology

Let us begin by coding a nonvascular interventional service in which the imaging supervision and interpretation code correlates with the procedural code one-to-one.

**EXAMPLE:** A 67-year-old man with a clinical history of colon carcinoma treated by resection three years ago is now found to have an elevated carcinoembryonic antigen (CEA) level and a liver lesion noted on a recent ultrasound evaluation. The patient is referred for an ultrasound-guided liver biopsy. The interventional radiologist performs a needle biopsy of the liver with a report of the procedural aspect of the service and provides the imaging supervision and interpretation report.

This service would be described by the following CPT codes:

**47000**   Biopsy of liver, needle; percutaneous

(If imaging guidance is performed, see **76942**, **77002**, **77012**, **77021**)

**76942**   Ultrasound guidance for needle placement (eg, biopsy, aspiration, injection, localization device), imaging supervision and interpretation

This example clearly demonstrates the flexibility provided by component coding. If this biopsy had been done under CT guidance, the procedure code (**47000**) would not have changed. However, the radiological supervision and interpretation code would have been **77012** instead of the ultrasound guidance code.

The type of imaging supervision and interpretation provided may change while the procedure remains the same, thus requiring great flexibility in coding. Conversely, different procedures may be performed with the same imaging supervision and interpretation code. For example, a physician can perform a needle biopsy of the liver (**47000**), the kidney (**50200**), or a retroperitoneal/abdominal mass (**49180**). Each of these can be performed under fluoroscopic, ultrasound, MRI, or CT guidance. Component coding allows for the specific description of each of these guidance services with the same procedure code.

The number of codes reported changes when the clinical scenario is modified. Consider the following similar nonvascular example:

**EXAMPLE:** The patient's oncologist requests a diagnostic ultrasound examination for a 67-year-old man with an elevated CEA level three years after resection of colon carcinoma. The ultrasound examination reveals a solitary liver lesion. After calling and discussing the findings of the diagnostic ultrasound with the patient's referring oncologist, the interventional radiologist performs a needle biopsy of the liver lesion under ultrasound guidance.

**CODING TIP**

Unless otherwise stated in the code descriptor, the codes for imaging guidance include only the imaging guidance; they do not include a full examination of the area. If a separate radiological examination of the area is performed, it would be necessary to separately report the imaging guidance and the specific radiological examination performed.

In this case, the physician reports the diagnostic ultrasound examination and the ultrasound-guided needle biopsy of the liver. In addition to codes **47000** and **76942**, the correct diagnostic ultrasound code is reported. Which code (**76700** or **76705**) is reported depends upon the extent of the ultrasound examination performed as a diagnostic study (ie, limited or complete).

**76700**   ultrasound, abdominal B-scan and for needle time with image drumentation; complete

**76705**   limited (eg, single organ, quadrant, follow-up)

From this example, one can see that component coding allows for the flexibility of combining a diagnostic and a therapeutic examination on the same occasion without overstating or understating the services provided.

# Vascular Interventional Radiology

## Anatomy

Before discussing vascular interventional radiology, let us review some arterial system anatomy.

### Brachiocephalic/Thoracic Arterial System

**Selective Vessel Ordering**

| First Order (Vascular Family) | Second Order | Third Order and Higher |
|---|---|---|
| Innominate or Brachiocephalic | Right Common Carotid | Right Internal Carotid Right External Carotid |
| | Right Subclavian/Axillary | Right Vertebral Right Internal Mammary |
| Left Common Carotid | Left Internal Carotid | Right or Left Anterior Cerebral Right or Left Middle Cerebral |
| | Left External Carotid | Right or Left Maxillary Right or Left Middle Meningeal Right or Left Facial Right or Left Occipital |
| Left Subclavian/Axillary | Left Vertebral | Right or Left Posterior Cerebral Basilar |

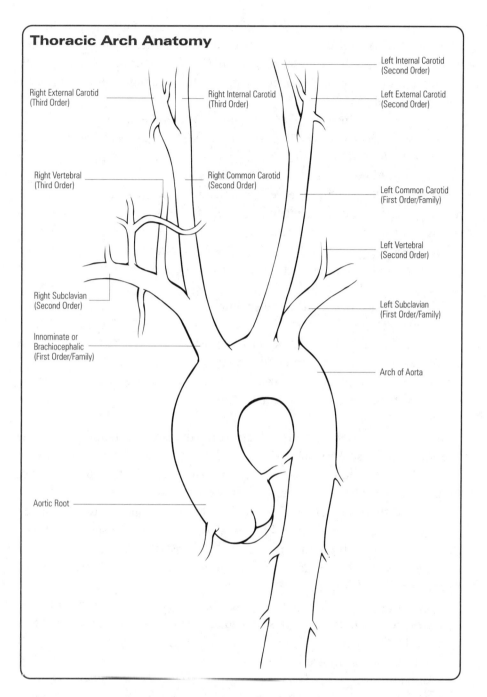

**Thoracic Arch Anatomy**

Right External Carotid (Third Order)

Right Internal Carotid (Third Order)

Left Internal Carotid (Second Order)

Left External Carotid (Second Order)

Right Vertebral (Third Order)

Right Common Carotid (Second Order)

Left Common Carotid (First Order/Family)

Left Vertebral (Second Order)

Right Subclavian (Second Order)

Left Subclavian (First Order/Family)

Innominate or Brachiocephalic (First Order/Family)

Arch of Aorta

Aortic Root

In the previous illustration, one can see how the vessels branch off of the arch of the aorta when the femoral artery is the site of access. The left subclavian, left common carotid, and innominate or brachiocephalic arteries are all first order vessels. Each of these vessels is in a separate vascular family.

This brief anatomy review will help in the discussion about some of the coding conventions associated with coding vascular interventional procedures.

## Coding Conventions for Vascular Interventional Procedures

Before considering an example of component coding in the vascular system, first some of the coding conventions associated with coding vascular interventional procedures must be explained. However, it is impossible to discuss all aspects of vascular service reporting in this one chapter. Instead, this is a review of some of the fundamentals for coding vascular interventional procedures. Afterward, there is a specific example that illustrates the use of the codes in combination. An Appendix of Resources is provided in the back of this text with information on a more comprehensive guide for coding interventional radiology services and procedures.

All vascular procedures, whether diagnostic or therapeutic, begin with establishing vascular access (vascular catheterization). The codes available for reporting the catheterization portion of the procedure are found in the vascular injection procedures series of codes (**36000** series).

Vascular catheterization procedures are either selective or nonselective. Use of the nonselective codes depends on the type of access (translumbar aortogram, nonselective aortic catheter placement, or nonselective extremity catheter/needle placement). Use of the nonselective codes is appropriate when the catheter is placed in the aorta, vena cava, or the vessel punctured and is not moved or manipulated further.

Selective catheterization is catheterization of a first, second, third, or higher order vessel. Selective vascular catheterization should be coded to include introduction of the catheter and all lesser-order selective catheterization positions within each vascular family accessed through the same approach. If a nonselective catheterization procedure is used for part of a service and the same access is then converted to a selective catheter placement, only the selective catheter placement is reported.

To code catheterization procedures correctly, become familiar with the anatomy of the vascular system. One must know to which vascular family each vessel belongs, the puncture site (or the approach), and the final position(s) of the catheter. Primary vessels branch off the aorta. When the primary vessels branch out, these branches are secondary branches, and as the secondary branches split, there are tertiary branches, etc. In the arterial system, catheter placement in a primary branch is described as a first order catheterization. The first order vessel is defined as selective catheterization of the first major branch off the main vessel (aorta).

Selective catheterization of a secondary branch is a second order catheterization, etc. A second order vessel is defined as a catheterization of the first major branch off a first order vessel. Likewise, a third order branch is the catheterization of a first major branch off a second order vessel. Each artery belongs to a vascular family, which is defined as a group of vessels (arteries) fed by a primary branch of the aorta or a primary branch of the vessel punctured. The five vascular systems considered for component coding are as follows:

- Systemic arterial
- Systemic venous
- Pulmonary
- Portal
- Lymphatic

Noncoronary vascular catheterization procedures are reported either using selective or nonselective catheter placement codes. Selective catheter placement involves more physician work and effort than nonselective catheterizations and increases complication risk to the target vessels. Selective catheterization typically involves the exchange of the catheter to a more flexible device that can be moved, manipulated, or guided into a part of the arterial system other than the aorta or the vessel punctured (usually under fluoroscopic guidance), most often using a guide wire. Nonselective catheter placement means the catheter or needle is placed directly into the major arterial conduit (not moved or manipulated further into a branch) or is delivered only into the aorta (thoracic and abdominal) from any approach (puncture site).

A nonselective catheter placement is not coded in addition to a selective catheter placement when a single access (puncture) is used. Even if a nonselective catheter placement is performed first, the highest selective placement with each vascular family is the determining factor for the level of coding. This vessel may or may not be the most distal in absolute distance from the puncture site or the origin of the primary vessel. All lesser order catheter placements in the same vascular family performed in order for the most selective catheter position to be achieved are included in the higher order catheterization code.

When coding selective vascular procedures from a single puncture site, each vascular family catheterized is coded according to the most selective position attained. Within each vascular family, the highest order catheterization is coded. If more than one vascular family is catheterized, one should code the highest order vessel catheterized within each vascular family.

If the same access site is used for both a diagnostic and a therapeutic service on the same occasion, the final catheter placement is coded only once. If multiple access sites are necessary, each catheterization is coded separately.

If two separate access procedures (two different punctures) are performed, each is treated separately for coding purposes. For example, if a nonselective catheter placement from one femoral artery puncture (ie, for an abdominal aortogram), and then a third order selective catheterization from the contralateral femoral artery puncture is performed, the nonselective code **36200** should be reported for the aortic catheter and **36247** for the third order abdominal selective catheterization from the other puncture. (The second puncture should be clearly documented.) It is appropriate to add a modifier (eg, 59) to **36200** to indicate that a separate access/distinct procedure was performed.

Venous catheterizations can be described as selective (requiring additional movement or manipulation of the catheter) or nonselective (direct placement of a catheter). The same vascular family concept as arterial procedures is used to describe venous catheterizations. Determination of first or second order is dependent upon the vein punctured. A venous vascular family includes a first order vein and all of its secondary branches. There are no codes for each additional second, third, or higher order catheterization in the venous system. Therefore, the codes may be reported again to describe the total number of separate catheterizations performed (eg, **36011** with two units). (For further information, refer to the Cardiovascular System subsection, Chapter 5.)

**CODING TIP**

Even if a nonselective catheter placement is performed first, the highest selective placement with each vascular family is the determining factor for the level of coding.

**CODING TIP**

Additional second, third, and higher order arterial catheterizations within the same vascular family include: **+36218**, **+36248**.

Next is an example of component coding in the arterial vascular system.

**EXAMPLE:** A 56-year-old woman with intracerebral hemorrhage is medically evaluated to rule out aneurysm. The patient undergoes cerebral arteriography. A catheter is placed from the right femoral artery approach. Via this single vascular access, selective catheterizations of the right common carotid artery, left common carotid artery, and the left vertebral artery are performed. Bilateral extracranial carotid, bilateral intracranial (cerebral) carotid, and left vertebral angiography is performed.

From the procedure description provided, it is known that the approach was performed from the right femoral artery. As coding for the selective catheterization procedures performed are discussed, refer to the table and illustration provided at the beginning of this section.

The subsequent selective catheterization procedures would then be reported as follows:

**EXAMPLE:** The right common carotid artery is a second order vessel. This catheterization procedure would be reported with code **36216**, Selective catheter placement, arterial system; initial second order thoracic or brachiocephalic branch, within a vascular family.

The left common carotid artery is a first order vessel within a vascular family separate from the right common carotid artery. Therefore, code **36215**, Selective catheter placement, arterial system; each first order thoracic or brachiocephalic branch, within a vascular family, would be reported for the selective catheterization of the left common carotid artery.

The left vertebral artery is a second order vessel within a different separate vascular family than the right common carotid and the left common carotid. Remember, within each vascular family, the highest order catheterization is reported. Therefore, code **36216**, Selective catheter placement, arterial system; initial second order thoracic or brachiocephalic branch, within a vascular family, would be reported a second time to describe the selective catheterization of the left vertebral artery.

In addition to the codes for the catheterization procedures, codes from the **70000** series are then selected to describe the radiological portion of the procedure (angiography). The bilateral selective common carotid angiography is reported with code **75680**, Angiography, carotid, cervical, bilateral, radiological supervision and interpretation.

A separate code, **75671**, Angiography, carotid, cerebral, bilateral, radiological supervision and interpretation, is reported for the bilateral internal (cerebral) carotid angiography. Finally, code **75685**, Angiography, vertebral, cervical, and/or intracranial, radiological supervision and interpretation is reported to describe the left vertebral angiography.

To summarize, the previous procedure is reported with the following codes:

**36216-RT**   (right common carotid artery)

**36215-LT**   (left common carotid artery)

**36216–59**   (left vertebral artery)

**75680**   (bilateral common carotid angiography, cervical)

**75671**   (bilateral internal carotid angiography, cerebral)

**75685**   (left vertebral angiography)

Note that the use of modifier 59 (or HCPCS Level II, RT and LT modifiers) is necessary to indicate catheterization of separate vascular families.

Coding for vascular interventional procedures requires a precise knowledge of the exact procedure performed and knowledge of vascular anatomy, interventional radiology procedures, and the coding conventions associated with reporting these services.

Some fundamental elements critical to the application of the vascular interventional reporting lie in the ability to recognize the circumstances under which a provider should report both a diagnostic angiogram/venogram radiological supervision and interpretation service and an interventional therapeutic vascular radiological supervision and interpretation service.

The following guidelines clarify the conditions under which it is appropriate for a provider to report both a diagnostic angiogram/venogram radiological supervision and interpretation service and an interventional therapeutic vascular radiological supervision and interpretation service:

- For angiography/venography performed in conjunction with therapeutic transcatheter radiological supervision and interpretation services, see the Radiology Transcatheter Procedures guidelines.
- Diagnostic angiography/venography (radiological supervision and interpretation) codes should not be used with interventional procedures for
  - contrast injections, angiography/venography, roadmapping, and/or fluoroscopic guidance for the intervention,
  - vessel measurement, and
  - post-angioplasty/stent angiography/venography, as this work is captured in the interventional procedure code(s).
- Diagnostic angiography/venography performed at the time of an interventional procedure is separately reportable if
  - no prior catheter-based angiographic/venographic study is available and a full diagnostic study is performed, and the decision to intervene is based on the diagnostic study,

  *or*

  - a prior study is available but as documented in the medical record,
    a) the patient's condition with respect to the clinical indication has changed since the prior study,
    b) there is inadequate visualization of the anatomy and/or pathology, or
    c) there is a clinical change during the procedure that requires new evaluation outside the target area of intervention.
- Diagnostic angiography/venography performed at a separate setting from an interventional procedure is separately reported.

- Diagnostic angiography/venography performed at the time of an interventional procedure is not separately reportable if it is specifically included in the interventional code descriptor.

Additionally, open communication must exist between the physician and the coder to resolve any coding uncertainties. Furthermore, it is imperative that the physician precisely report the procedures performed and angiographic areas studied for coding accuracy.

# Diagnostic Ultrasound

Codes for reporting diagnostic ultrasound are located in the **76506-76999** series. The following guidelines and definitions can be found preceding this series of codes for the various types of ultrasound procedures and are critical applications to consider.

- All diagnostic ultrasound examinations require permanently recorded images with measurements when such measurements are clinically indicated. For those codes whose sole diagnostic goal is a biometric measure (**76514**, **76516**, and **76519**), permanently recorded images are not required. A final written report should be issued for inclusion in the patient's medical record. The prescription of the intraocular lens power satisfies the written report requirement for code **76519**. For those anatomic regions that have complete and limited ultrasound codes, note the elements that comprise a complete examination. The report should contain a description of these elements or the reason that an element could not be visualized (eg, obscured by bowel gas, surgically absent, etc).
- If less than the required elements for a complete examination are reported (eg, limited number of organs or limited portion of region evaluated), the limited code for that anatomic region should be used once per patient examination session. A limited examination of an anatomic region should not be reported for the same examination session as a complete examination of that same region.
- Doppler evaluation of vascular structures (other than color flow used only for anatomic structure identification) is separately reportable. To report, see Noninvasive Vascular Diagnostic Studies (**93875-93990**).
- Ultrasound guidance procedures also require permanently recorded images of the site to be localized as well as a documented description of the localization process, either separately or within the report of the procedure for which the guidance is used.
- Use of ultrasound, without thorough evaluation of organ(s) or anatomic region, image documentation, and final, written report, is not separately reportable.

**A-mode** implies a one-dimensional ultrasonic measurement procedure.

**M-mode** implies a one-dimensional ultrasonic measurement procedure with movement of the trace to record amplitude and velocity of moving echo-producing structures.

**B-scan** implies a two-dimensional ultrasonic scanning procedure with a two-dimensional display.

**Real-time** scan implies a two-dimensional ultrasonic scanning procedure with display of both two-dimensional structure and motion with time.

Within this series, one will find codes for reporting diagnostic ultrasound of the following anatomic sites:

| Code Ranges of Anatomic Sites | |
| --- | --- |
| Head and Neck | 76506-76536 |
| Chest | 76604-76645 |
| Abdomen and Retroperitoneum | 76700-76776 |
| Spinal Canal | 76800 |
| Pelvis (Obstetrical) | 76801-76828 |
| Pelvis (Non-Obstetrical) | 76830-76857 |
| Genitalia | 76870-76873 |
| Extremities | 76880-76886 |
| Ultrasonic Guidance Procedures | 76930-76965 |

## Obstetrical

The practice of obstetrical ultrasound has changed significantly. Advances in ultrasound technology allow evaluations and measurement of fetal characteristics and organ systems in much greater detail. Obstetric ultrasound services, reported with codes **76801-76817**, recognize these new advances in technology.

Codes **76801** and **76802** include determination of the number of gestational sacs and fetuses, gestational sac/fetal measurements appropriate for gestation (< 14 weeks 0 days), survey of visible fetal and placental anatomic structure, qualitative assessment of amniotic fluid volume/gestational sac shape, and examination of the maternal uterus and adnexa.

Codes **76805** and **76810** include determination of number of fetuses and amniotic/chorionic sacs, measurements appropriate for gestational age (≥ 14 weeks 0 days), survey of intracranial/spinal/abdominal anatomy, identification of four-chambered heart, umbilical cord insertion site, placenta location and amniotic fluid assessment, and, when visible, examination of maternal adnexa.

Codes **76811** and **76812** include determination of all elements of codes **76805** and **76810** plus detailed anatomic evaluation of the fetal brain/ventricles, face, heart/outflow tracts and chest anatomy, abdominal organ-specific anatomy, number/length/architecture of limbs, and detailed evaluation of the umbilical cord and placenta and other fetal anatomy, as clinically indicated.

Report should document the results of the evaluation of each element described previously or the reason for nonvisualization.

Codes **76813** and **76814** describe ultrasound measurement of nuchal translucency performed using either a transabdominal or transvaginal approach for the detection of chromosomal abnormalities such as Down syndrome. Performed in the first trimester of pregnancy, nuchal transparency measurement uses ultrasound to identify and measure fluid collections between the tissue covering the spine and the skin that covers it. This imaging procedure

> **CODING TIP**
>
> To report first trimester fetal nuchal translucency measurement, see **76813, 76814.**

takes advantage of the anechoic quality of this ultrasonographic anatomical feature. The calculation of chromosomal abnormality risk uses in the equation the measurements of maternal age, gestational age, and the deviation of the thickness of the nuchal translucency from the norm as compared to the crown-rump length of the fetus. Code **76815** represents a focused "quick look" examination limited to the assessment of one or more of the elements listed in code **76815**.

Code **76816** describes an examination designed to reassess fetal size and interval growth or reevaluate one or more anatomic abnormalities of a fetus previously demonstrated on ultrasound. This code should be used once for each fetus requiring reevaluation using modifier 59 for each fetus after the first.

Code **76817** describes a transvaginal obstetric ultrasound performed separately or in addition to one of the transabdominal examinations described previously. For transvaginal examinations performed for nonobstetrical purposes, use code **76830**.

Nonobstetrical ultrasound studies are reported using codes **76830**, **76831**, **76856**, and **76857**. The studies listed in the section include a transvaginal examination, a hysterosonography, and a transabdominal nonobstetrical ultrasound examination.

Codes for reporting noninvasive vascular diagnostic studies including vascular ultrasound are located in the Medicine section of the CPT codebook in the **93875-93990** series of codes. (The reporting of these codes is discussed in Chapter 9.)

Within the diagnostic ultrasound subsection of the CPT codebook, there are also listings for ultrasonic guidance procedures. Similar to the codes for CT guidance, codes for ultrasonic guidance (**76930-76965**) describe only the ultrasonographic portion of the specific procedure performed. Parenthetical notes appear after each code entry that direct the user to the appropriate code(s) for reporting the procedure. To completely describe the procedure performed, separate codes are reported for the imaging supervision and interpretation portion of the procedure and for the specific procedure performed. (Refer to the discussion of component coding found under the Interventional Radiology heading in this chapter.)

# Radiologic Guidance

Certain imaging modalities are used during many diagnostic and therapeutic radiologic procedures to observe the action of instruments being used. The following table lists the imaging modalities found in this subsection:

| Radiologic Guidance | |
| --- | --- |
| Fluoroscopy | 77001-77003 |
| Computed Tomography | 77011-77014 |
| Magnetic Resonance Guidance | 77021-77022 |
| Stereotactic | 77031 |
| Mammography | 77032 |

The ultrasound guidance procedures are listed in the Ultrasonic Guidance Procedures subsection and are reported using **76930, 76932, 76936, +76937, 76940, 76941, 76942, 76945, 76946, 76948, 76950, 76965, 76998**.

It is important to become familiar with the use of the fluoroscopy codes **77001-77003**. Fluoroscopic guidance can be performed as the sole imaging associated with a procedure (**77001-77003**) for which both the procedure and the fluoroscopic guidance are reported. Fluoroscopy may be performed in combination with other imaging during a procedure (eg, peripherally inserted central venous catheter using both ultrasound **76937** and fluoroscopic guidance **77001**) for which the procedure and both imaging codes are reported. For certain procedures, fluoroscopy is considered inclusive of the procedure (eg, **62263**) and not separately reportable. Fluoroscopic guidance is considered inclusive of certain organ/anatomic-specific radiological supervision and interpretation procedures **74320, 74355, 74445, 74470, 74475, 75809, 75810, 75885, 75887, 75980, 75982, 75989**. Since fluoroscopic imaging requires personal supervision, if the physician is not present in the operating room during a procedure that uses fluoroscopy or fluoroscopic guidance, that physician should not submit a code for fluoroscopy. However, the appropriate radiographic code to report the anatomy evaluated should be submitted in the event that (a) the radiologist's contract with the hospital requires that a radiologist issue a formal interpretation, or (b) the physician performing the study requests that a radiologist produce a formal report of the procedure from permanent images recorded.

**CODING TIP**

Fluoroscopic guidance is inclusive of organ/anatomic-specific radiological supervision and interpretation procedures **74320, 74355, 74445, 74470, 74475, 75809, 75810, 75885, 75887, 75980, 75982, 75989**.

# Breast, Mammography

For proper mammography coding, carefully consider the code descriptors and similarities that exist as well as the code's intended use. Furthermore, individual payer reporting and reimbursement policies may vary from CPT coding guidelines, so be certain to determine which are appropriate.

The CPT codes for reporting mammography include the following:

**77055**   Mammography; unilateral

**77056**   Mammography; bilateral

**77057**   Screening mammography, bilateral (2-view film study of each breast)

The key to the intended use of the codes can be found in the code descriptors. Code **77057** includes the word *screening* to indicate mammography performed on asymptomatic patients to detect unsuspected neoplasm. Codes **77055** and **77056** do not include this wording and therefore indicate a more definitive diagnostic procedure beyond that of a screening mammography.

Diagnostic mammography, represented by codes **77055** and **77056**, involves obtaining images of the breast to provide specific analytical information that will be used in problem solving for a patient with a significant clinical mammographic breast history, abnormal breast physical examination, or an abnormal screening mammogram. A diagnostic mammogram involves all of the interpretative skills included in a screening mammogram and in addition considerable physician supervision and more focused attention, often including multiple specialized views (eg, coned compression, magnification, special positioning). When documenting diagnostic mammography services, to clarify the use of the nonscreening code, include the clinical or historical information that necessitates a diagnostic mammogram.

Screening mammography, represented by code **77057**, is defined as images of each breast in two projections (eg, craniocaudal and mediolateral oblique). It is performed to detect unsuspected neoplasm in an early stage in asymptomatic women and is inherently bilateral. The bilateral modifiers are not used on this or any other code that contains the description "bilateral." (Refer to Chapter 10 for further discussion of the bilateral modifier.) Occasionally, supplemental views may be necessary to screen the entire breast (not specialized views). These additional views to ensure anatomic coverage are included in the screening examination when it is performed on an asymptomatic patient.

Codes **77051** and **77052** are add-on codes that describe computer-aided detection applied to either a diagnostic mammography or a screening mammography. As such, each of these add-on codes is intended to be reported exclusively with codes **77055**, **77056**, and **77057**. Special attention should be made to the cross-references following each of these codes that direct the user to the appropriate add-on code to report in conjunction with each mammography code. For example, code **77051** is reported for computer-aided detection applied to a diagnostic mammogram (**77055** or **77056**), while code **77052** is reported for computer-aided detection applied to a screening mammogram (**77057**). Computer-aided detection CAD codes **77051** and **77052** are also used on conjunction with HCPCS level II "G" codes used by Medicare to describe full field digital mammography procedures.

For patient convenience, many facilities screen mammographic images before the patient leaves the office. If it is determined that other specialized views are necessary and obtained (eg, magnification or compression spot views for calcification or a suspected abnormality), an additional diagnostic mammogram should be reported. A diagnostic mammogram may also be reported per Medicare guidelines. A "GG" modifier should be attached to the diagnostic study to designate the performance of a screening and a diagnostic mammogram on the same patient on the same day.

Since separate codes exist for both screening and diagnostic mammography, do not use code **76499**, Unlisted diagnostic radiologic procedure, to represent either of these procedures or any additional views taken during the examination.

# Radiation Oncology

Clinical radiation oncology is a highly complex medical specialty in which the actual course of therapy for individuals is customized for the disease parameters. Codes for reporting radiation oncology procedures and services can be found in the **77261-77799** series. These codes may be combined in various ways to accurately code and describe the entire course of treatment for a given disease entity. Each complete course of treatment is distinct. Should a patient return later with a new problem, this constitutes an entirely new course of radiation treatment.

Listings for radiation oncology provide for teletherapy and brachytherapy to include the following:

- Initial consultation
- Clinical treatment planning
- Simulation
- Medical radiation physics, dosimetry, treatment devices, special services clinical treatment management

Let us review the guidelines and notes available for the various subheadings in the Radiation Oncology section.

## Consultation: Clinical Management

When the radiation oncologist provides a preliminary consultation, with evaluation of the patient to determine the role of radiation therapy in the patient's care, an E/M code should be used.

Consultations performed by radiation oncologists do not differ from those conducted by other physicians. During consultations, physicians assess the health of a patient and determine whether to treat or which course of treatment will be most beneficial. To report an office consultation, use codes **99241-99245**; to report an inpatient consultation, use codes **99251-99255**, as appropriate.

If the radiation oncologist has determined that radiation therapy is appropriate, makes a recommendation to the requesting physician, and continues to provide E/M services, the patient is considered established. When E/M services are provided in this instance, codes from the office or other outpatient or hospital inpatient series are reported.

Codes from other sections of the CPT codebook are reported to describe additional services and procedures provided by the physician. These codes are reported separately in addition to the codes for the specific services and procedures provided from the Radiation Oncology subsection of the CPT codebook.

## Clinical Treatment Planning (External and Internal Sources)

Clinical treatment planning, described by codes **77261-77263**, is the cognitive process carried out by the physician to determine all of the parameters of a given course of radiation therapy. The clinical treatment planning process is a complex service including interpretation of special testing, tumor localization, treatment volume determination, treatment time/dosage determination, choice of treatment modality, determination of number and size of treatment ports, selection of appropriate treatment devices, and other procedures.

Treatment planning is usually reported only once for a given course of radiation therapy. If, however, a completely new area of disease develops during such a course, an additional treatment planning charge is justified. The three codes available for reporting treatment planning describe simple (**77261**), intermediate (**77262**), and complex (**77263**) therapeutic radiology treatment planning.

Simple planning requires a single treatment area of interest encompassed in a single port or simple parallel-opposed ports with simple or no blocking.

Intermediate planning requires three or more converging ports, two separate treatment areas, multiple blocks, or special time/dose constraints.

Complex planning requires highly complex blocking, custom shielding blocks, tangential ports, wedges or special compensators, three or more separate treatment areas, rotational or special beam considerations, brachytherapy, combination of therapeutic modalities, multileaf collimation, and intensity-modulated radiotherapy (IMRT).

## Simulation

Simulation, described by the codes in the **77280–77295** series, is the act of determining the configuration of the radiation treatment portals. Simulation is performed without actually delivering a treatment but uses all of the parameters of the treatment to be delivered.

Simulation is reported each time the procedure is performed. However, only one service is reported per day. These codes are defined as simple (**77280**), intermediate (**77285**), complex (**77290**), and three-dimensional (**77295**). Simulation may be carried out on a dedicated simulator, a virtual simulator using cross-sectional information from a diagnostic or therapy planning CT scan, a radiation therapy treatment unit, or a diagnostic X-ray machine.

The following definitions are provided for simple, intermediate, complex, and three-dimensional therapeutic radiology simulation-aided field setting:

**Simple** simulation of a single treatment area with either a single port or parallel opposed ports. Simple or no blocking. Block verification simulation.

**Intermediate** simulation of three or more converging ports, two separate treatment areas, multiple blocks.

**Complex** simulation of tangential portals, three or more treatment areas, rotation or arc therapy, complex blocking, custom shielding blocks, brachytherapy source verification, hyperthermia probe verification, any use of contrast materials.

**Three-dimensional** computer-generated three-dimensional reconstruction of tumor volume and surrounding critical normal tissue structures from direct CT scans and/or MRI data in preparation for noncoplanar or coplanar therapy. The simulation uses documented three-dimensional beam's eye view volume-dose displays of multiple or moving beams. Documentation with three-dimensional volume reconstruction and dose distribution is required.

The isodose plan, as described by codes **77305-77315**, is included in code **77295** and not separately reported.

## Medical Radiation Physics, Dosimetry, Treatment Devices, and Special Services

Medical radiation physics, dosimetry, treatment devices, and special services are reported with the codes in the **77300-77399** series. The appropriate radiation therapy planning code is reported according to the treatment delivery mode (eg, standard radiation delivery, intensity-modulated treatment delivery). Basic dosimetry (**77300**) is used in many different scenarios requiring delivery of a prescribed dose of radiation to a particular region. Multiple unique treatment ports to the same site or to different sites will each require separate calculations, as will off-axis or gap calculations. In brachytherapy, point doses and radioisotope decay may require multiple or repeated calculations.

The work described by CPT code **77300** is a distinct medical service separate from **77301**. Code **77300** is often used with complicated computer isodose planning for external beam radiation and implants. It is appropriately reported with all other planning codes, including **77305**, **77310**, and **77315** and is warranted with intensity modulated radiotherapy (IMRT) planning when medically necessary. To be clear, the calculations performed to determine treatment unit settings for IMRT planning are no different than for the previously mentioned isodose plan codes **77305**, **77310**, and **77315**; accordingly, code **77300** can be reported with **77301**. Code **77301** describes the particular type of planning required for intensity-modulated treatment delivery (**77418**). IMRT planning (**77301**) requires delineation of a tumor-bearing volume and a number of normal tissue volumes whose tolerance to radiation is less than that of the tumor. The radiation oncologist must specify the partial tolerances of the organs in continuity with the tumor by standard summation of modulated beams (forward planning) or by computer optimization after beam specification (inverse planning) or a combination of the two methods, so that dose to the tumor is maximized while dose to surrounding normal tissues is minimized. After creation of the plan, the radiation oncologist and physics staff must confirm the resultant dose distribution by means of both relative and absolute dosimetric methods (eg, diode, thermoluminescent dosimetry [TLD]). Only one IMRT plan may be reported for a given course of therapy to a specific treatment area. However, if there is clinical indication to change the treatment plan because of either changes in clinical condition or the need to change the parameters of treatment such as would be encountered in "boost" situations, the additional plan would be reported.

Codes **77305-77315** describe teletherapy isodose plans. As with the previous plan, only one teletherapy isodose plan may be reported for a given course of therapy to a specific treatment area. However, if there is clinical indication to change the treatment plan because of either changes in clinical condition or the need to change the parameters of treatment, such as would be encountered in boost situations, then the additional plan would be reported. An isodose plan is a plotting of lines of the same dosage within a given treatment field. An isodose plan is usually derived from a combination of treatment beams impinging upon a particular field of interest. The levels of doses delivered are expressed in percentages within this area of interest. More than one specific treatment area or treatment volume may be used during a single course of therapy (eg, a reduced volume boost as in treatment of cancer of the prostate).

Codes **77326-77328** are used to report a brachytherapy isodose plan. Refer to the discussion of clinical brachytherapy later in this chapter for explanation and discussion of these codes.

Special dosimetry, when prescribed by the treating physician, is reported with code **77331**. This code describes the use of special radiation measuring and monitoring devices (eg, solid-state diode probes, thermoluminescent dosimeters, microdosimetry).

Codes **77332-77334** are used to report the design and construction of treatment devices (eg, blocks, stents, wedges, molds or casts, compensators, and brachytherapy applicators).

Code **77336** is used to report continuing medical physics consultation. As indicated in the code descriptor, this code includes the assessment of treatment parameters, quality assurance of dose delivery, and review of patient treatment documentation in support of the radiation oncologist. This code is reported per week of therapy.

A special medical radiation physics consultation is reported with code **77370**. This code describes a consultation provided by the medical radiological physicist. A full consultative report is rendered by the medical radiological physicist. The procedure is ordered by the physician and the results are acknowledged by the physician, but the actual performance of this service is carried out exclusively by the physicist.

Stereotactic radiation therapy is the general term for stereotactic-based radiation treatment. This treatment usually consists of one to five high dose radiation treatments delivered by either a linear accelerator (**77372**) (sometimes called *linac radiosurgery* or *robotic-based radiosurgery*) or a Cobalt-60 unit (**77371**) (sometimes referred to as *radiosurgery* or by the proprietary name *GammaKnife®*). The linear accelerator can be contained in a traditional, rotational gantry, as in a typical course of radiation, or mounted on the end of an industrial robot, as in the CyberKnife®. Treatment delivery is achieved through rigid immobilization, such as with a head frame or frameless image-based immobilization and localization. For cranial lesions treated in a single fraction (ie, stereotactic radiosurgery), codes **77371** (Cobalt-60 unit based) and **77372** (linear accelerator based) are to be used. A team consisting of the radiation oncologist, neurosurgeon, and medical physicist is responsible for supervising the patient positioning and proper alignment of the treatment beams.

With the advent of new technologies for stereotactic treatments to noncranial areas, the term *stereotactic body radiation therapy* (SBRT) is used for designation of the extracranial targets (**77373**). Because of certain medical and tissue tolerance constraints, treatment may require single or multiple fractions. Code **77373**, Stereotactic body radiation therapy, treatment delivery, per fraction to 1 or more lesions, including image guidance, entire course not to exceed 5 fractions, should not be reported in conjunction with radiation treatment delivery codes

**CODING TIP**

When stereotactic radiation therapy is performed jointly by a surgeon and a radiation oncologist (eg, spinal or cranial), the surgeon reports radiosurgery with **61793**.

**77401-77416** or **77418**. For SBRT, radiation therapy management for the entire course of treatment is reported with CPT code **77435**, Stereotactic body radiation therapy treatment management, per treatment course to one or more lesions, including image guidance, entire course not to exceed 5 fractions.

## Radiation Treatment Delivery

Radiation treatment delivery, reported with the codes in the **77401-77416**, **77418** series, recognizes the technical component and the various energy levels of treatment delivery. Treatment is reported as each treatment is delivered. Radiation treatment delivery is reported for each single delivery given. Treatment delivery may occur less often than daily (eg, three times per week) or may even occur two to three times in the same day. This is frequently done in hyperfractionated radiotherapy for advanced tumors and in pediatrics.

Code **77418** is reported for intensity-modulated radiation treatment delivery. This mode of treatment is characterized by complex and conformal portal geometries. Modulated radiation treatment delivery results in the delivery of extreme patient-specific radiation treatment using binary or multileaf collimators to spatially and temporally modulate the radiation beams into a number of narrow "beamlets" that, when summated, generate the desired nonuniform intensity patterns. When all of the variously oriented beamlets are merged, this results in the delivery of a uniform dose fitted to the shape of the lesion while delivering a much lower dose to the sensitive normal tissues surrounding the tumor.

Code **77417** is used to report therapeutic radiology port film(s). Port films are X-rays taken during the delivery of radiation treatment using the treatment beam of the machine. Port films demonstrate the exact shape, size, and area covered by the treatment beam during an actual treatment. Port films are reported by the facility, once per five fractions or once per week of treatment management, per patient, regardless of the number of films required or portals evaluated. This is a technical-only code. The professional component or interpretation of these films is considered part of weekly treatment management. Alternatively, certain carriers request that port films be reported once per five fractions of therapy regardless of the number of films required.

## Radiation Treatment Management

Radiation treatment management is reported with the codes in the **77427-77499** series. Treatment management is the ongoing medical management of a patient receiving a course of radiation treatment. The professional services furnished during treatment management typically consist of the following:

- Review of port films
- Review of dosimetry, dose delivery, and treatment parameters
- Review of patient treatment set-up
- Examination of the patient for medical evaluation and management (eg, assessment of the patient's response to treatment, coordination of care and treatment, review of imaging, and/or laboratory test results)

Before the 2000 edition of the CPT codebook, radiation treatment management was reported with codes **77419**, **77420**, **77425**, and **77430**, which have been deleted from the CPT codebook. Radiation treatment management, as previously described by these codes, continues to be reported with code **77427**.

Radiation treatment management is reported per five fractions or treatment sessions, regardless of the actual time period in which the services are furnished. The services need not be furnished on consecutive days. A fraction is a single session of radiation treatment delivered to a specific area of interest at one setting.

Multiple fractions representing two or more treatment sessions furnished on the same day may be counted separately, as long as there has been a distinct break in therapy sessions and the fractions are of the character usually furnished on different days.

As indicated in the code descriptor, code **77427** is used to report radiation treatment management per five fractions or treatment sessions. This code is also reported if there are three or four fractions beyond a multiple of five at the end of a course of treatment. One or two fractions beyond a multiple of five at the end of a course of treatment are not separately reported. For example, radiation treatment management, eight treatments, would be reported with code **77427** times two. Radiation treatment management, seven treatments, would be reported with code **77427** only once.

Code **77431** is used to report radiation treatment management when the complete course of therapy consists of only one or two fractions. Note that this code is not used to "fill in" the last week of a long course of therapy.

Code **77432** describes stereotactic radiation treatment management of cerebral lesion(s). As indicated in the code descriptor, the complete course of treatment consists of only one session. If the course of treatment extends longer than one fraction, weekly treatment management (**77427**) may be used to report the remainder of the course of treatment.

Whenever any of the special procedures of radiation therapy are performed (eg, total body irradiation, hemibody irradiation, per oral cone irradiation, endocavitary or intraoperative cone irradiation, brachytherapy), IMRT, or combined radiochemotherapy, code **77470** will typically be used. This code is used to report the extra planning and effort required for the special procedure of hyperfractionation or other deviation from standard, total body irradiation, per oral or transvaginal cone irradiation, brachytherapy, concurrent hyperthermia, planned combination with chemotherapy or other combined modality therapy, and intraoperative radiation therapy in any other time-consuming treatment plan. This code may be reported in addition to conventional treatment planning.

### Proton Beam Treatment Delivery

Codes **77520–77525** are used to report proton beam treatment delivery. This is a radiation treatment modality using proton therapy as opposed to the more conventional photon radiation treatment delivery. These codes are classified by simple, intermediate, and complex delivery. *Simple* treatment is defined as delivery through a single port to a single treatment area and is further differentiated with separate codes by delivery with or without compensation. *Intermediate* treatment includes treatment to one or more treatment areas and is further distinguished from simple treatment by utilization of two or more delivery ports. *Complex* delivery is distinguished from intermediate delivery through the use of matching and patching centers and/or multiple isocenters. This series of codes includes treatment setup and verification images.

## Hyperthermia

Hyperthermia treatments are reported with the codes in the **77600-77620** series. The treatments listed in this section include external (superficial and deep), interstitial, and intracavitary hyperthermia.

Hyperthermia is the use of heat, generated either by microwave, ultrasound, or other heat-developing means, to raise the temperature of a specific area of the body in an attempt to increase cell metabolism, thereby increasing the potential for cell killing in a malignancy. Hyperthermia is used only as an adjunct to radiation therapy or chemotherapy. Radiation therapy when given concurrently is listed separately.

Codes **77600** and **77605** are used to report externally generated hyperthermia. They describe the use of an external heat-generating source such as ultrasound or microwave to produce localized heating to a specified depth. The appropriate code is reported based on whether the hyperthermia is superficial (heating to a depth of 4 cm or less) (**77600**) or deep (heating to depths greater than 4 cm) (**77605**).

Interstitial hyperthermia is reported with codes **77610** and **77615**. In this situation, probes act as small antennae or microwave radiators and are placed directly into the tumor-bearing area. The probes generate microwave fields within the tumor and thereby produce localized heating. The appropriate code is selected based on the number of interstitial applicators used. Code **77610** describes the use of five or fewer interstitial applicators. If more than five interstitial applicators are used, then code **77615** is reported. Interstitial hyperthermia may be used in combination with interstitial radiation treatments or external beam treatments.

Hyperthermia generated by intracavitary probe(s) is described by CPT code **77620**. A probe or applicator is inserted directly into a body cavity to produce hyperthermia of a localized area. Probes may be placed in the vagina, rectum, or esophagus to cause local heating in combination with external beam radiation therapy.

## Clinical Brachytherapy

Clinical brachytherapy is reported with the codes in the **77750-77799** series. The codes in this series include admission to the hospital and daily visits. Brachytherapy may be used as the sole form of radiation treatment but is often used with external beam radiation therapy to bring the total dose to the intended level.

Brachytherapy is the use of radioactive sources placed directly into a tumor-bearing area to generate well-defined regions of high intensity radiation. It requires the use of either natural or man-made radiation sources applied into or around a treatment field or volume of interest. The supervision of radiation sources and dose interpretation is performed solely by the therapeutic radiologist.

> **CODING TIP**
>
> Hyperthermia is used only as an adjunct to radiation therapy or chemotherapy and may be induced by a variety of sources (eg, microwave, ultrasound, low energy radiofrequency conduction, or by probes).

> **CODING TIP**
>
> The codes for reporting hyperthermia (**77600-77620**) include management during the course of therapy and follow-up care for three months after completion. Also included when reporting these codes are physics planning, interstitial insertion of temperature sensors, and use of external or interstitial heat-generating sources.

Brachytherapy may be categorized according to the relationship of the applicator to the body structures (ie, surface application vs intracavitary vs interstitial) and to the nature of the sources used in the process (ie, permanent or temporary brachytherapy). *Intracavitary* refers to placements directly into a body cavity and *interstitial* refers to the placements directly into the affected tissue.

A "source," a radioactive element that is used to deliver the radiation therapy, consists of various kinds of radioactive material completely sealed in small metal containers. Sources may be used to treat malignant or benign disease. They are available in several different formats including tubes or capsules, permanent seeds, and seeds embedded in ribbons and in various strengths or "activities." Tubes and capsules are commonly used for temporary intracavitary applications. Permanent seeds are very small (1 × 3 mm) sources of either low energy or short half-life. They are used for interstitial implantation, where they are left to decay completely over a period of months, thereby delivering a therapeutic amount of radiation. Code **77750** should be reported for infusion or installation of radioelement solutions, eg, strontium for bone metastases.

Seeds embedded in ribbons are usually referred to simply as "ribbons." Ribbons consist of very small sources embedded at specific intervals into thin plastic lines. They can be threaded into relatively thin needles or catheters and thus are used in the process of temporary interstitial brachytherapy. Ribbons may be cut or "edited" into specific lengths to control the distribution of the radiation treatment within the implant.

The complexity of a radiation source application is defined according to the number of sources or ribbons as simple, intermediate, or complex. A simple application has one to four sources/ribbons. An intermediate application has 5 to 10 sources/ribbons. A complex application has more than 10 sources/ribbons.

Within the **77750-77799** code series, there are specific codes for reporting intracavitary, interstitial, and remote afterloading high-intensity brachytherapy. A brief discussion of each of these types of brachytherapy follows.

### Intracavitary Brachytherapy

Intracavitary brachytherapy is reported with codes **77761-77763**. The codes are differentiated by the type of application performed (simple, intermediate, complex). Intracavitary brachytherapy is performed by the placement of an applicator into a body cavity. The most common intracavitary application is in the treatment of gynecologic malignancies such as carcinoma of the cervix or endometrium. A number of radiation sources are placed in the applicator (ie, the nonradioactive device or carrier that is placed first and serves as a receptacle for the radiation source) in a specific geometric configuration. It is designed to deliver a localized and concentrated dose of radiation. The applicator and sources are usually left in the patient for a period of one to three days.

### Interstitial Brachytherapy

Both permanent and temporary interstitial brachytherapy are reported with codes **77776-77778**. Again, the codes are differentiated according to the complexity of radioelement application that is defined by the number of sources or ribbons (ie, simple, intermediate, complex).

Interstitial brachytherapy is performed by the insertion of brachytherapy catheters or needles directly into and around tissue containing the cancer. These devices are subsequently loaded with the radiation source. Permanent seeds are inserted at the time of needle placement according to a previously calculated isodose plan. The permanent seeds remain in place and decay completely as they deliver the radiation dose. Temporary interstitial implants are afterloaded (ie, the radioelements in the form of ribbons are inserted some time during or after the isodose calculation is performed). Like temporary intracavitary implants, temporary interstitial applicators and sources are completely removed several days later when the desired dose of radiation has been administered.

Permanent seed interstitial, temporary intracavitary, and temporary interstitial brachytherapy deliver treatment relatively slowly over several days, so they are described as low dose rate brachytherapy.

### Remote Afterloading High-Intensity Brachytherapy

Remote afterloading high-intensity brachytherapy (RAHIB) is reported with codes **77781-77784**. Each code within this series is differentiated by the number of source positions or catheters used.

RAHIB is a technique that uses a special machine called a *remote afterloader*. It has a single, very small, high-intensity source of radioactive material located at the end of a long thin cable. It is capable of producing a very precise and controlled shape, volume, and intensity of radiation.

The brachytherapy applicators or catheters used in this form of brachytherapy are inserted in a manner similar to other temporary intracavitary or interstitial applications. Once the necessary therapeutic radiology simulation-aided field setting and the dosimetry and isodose plan calculations have been performed, the applicator or catheters are connected to the remote afterloader. The machine then inserts the high-intensity radiation source into the intracavitary applicator or into the complex array of interstitial catheters with millimeter precision. The source rests or "dwells" for specified periods of time at predetermined positions along each catheter to produce the desired radiation distribution pattern.

Because the source is of extremely high activity (thousands of times more powerful than a conventional brachytherapy source), the treatment is given in a matter of 5 to 30 minutes. Consequently, RAHIB is also known as high dose rate (HDR) brachytherapy. Because treatment is given in a shielded location, radiation safety is ensured. This form of brachytherapy, like external beam radiation therapy, is often given in a "fractionated" series of applications. Thus, a variety of treatment patterns and schemes are applicable, depending upon the clinical circumstances. The very short treatment time means that, unlike standard low dose rate brachytherapy, many of the HDR applications may be completed on an outpatient basis.

### Brachytherapy Therapeutic Radiology Simulation-Aided Field Setting

Simulation radiography for brachytherapy is a complex process. When using conventional or two-dimensional processes for simulation-aided field setting, this is reported with the code **77290**.

Brachytherapy may also be performed with three-dimensional reconstruction, in which case code **77295** is reported. When simulation radiography is necessary to check the implant position prior to succeeding HDR fractions (given in a series following an applicator placement procedure), the simple simulation code (**77280**) should be used.

### Brachytherapy Isodose Calculation

All forms of brachytherapy require the generation of brachytherapy isodose curves to accurately map the distribution of radiation over the treatment area or volume. Each brachytherapy procedure, whether it is preloaded, afterloading, or RAHIB, requires a brachytherapy isodose plan to be generated for each application. Brachytherapy isodose calculation is reported with the codes in the **77326-77328** series.

The isodose plan is necessary for the physician to determine the exact distribution of radiation around the brachytherapy radiation sources. In conventional brachytherapy, some adjustments may be made by changing the geometry of the sources to generate the desired plan.

With RAHIB, the isodose plan is predetermined and the machine and computer position the sources and set the dwell time for each position to generate a radiation distribution following the predetermined isodose plan. (Dwell time refers to the length of time that a RAHIB source will remain at any specific point along the catheter during treatment.) The complexity of the isodose plan is determined by the number of sources or dwell positions of the RAHIB source.

### Surgeon Services

The current clinical brachytherapy codes (**77750-77799**) describe the work of the therapeutic radiologist in placing the brachytherapy and do not describe the work provided by the surgeon in placing the radioelement(s). When a brachytherapy procedure requires the service of a surgeon in addition to the therapeutic radiologist, the specific CPT codes should be reported.

EXAMPLE 1: A 75-year-old patient with severe cardiac disease is diagnosed with uterine cancer. She is found not to be a candidate for surgery, and the decision is made to treat her cancer with radiation therapy including clinical brachytherapy. Insertion of Heyman capsules is performed. The therapeutic radiologist applies the radioactive element through these tubes into the capsules at the same session.

In this case, two physicians have worked together performing distinctly separate procedures. Code **58346**, Insertion of Heyman capsules for clinical brachytherapy, should be reported, without the use of a modifier, to describe the role of the surgeon in placing the capsules in the uterine cavity. The therapeutic radiologist should report code **77761**, Intracavitary radiation source application; simple, without the use of a modifier.

EXAMPLE 2: A patient undergoes intracavitary brachytherapy for treatment of carcinoma of the bronchus. A surgeon performs bronchoscopy with placement of catheter(s) for intracavitary radiation source application. The therapeutic radiologist then performs the radiation source application (an intermediate application with eight sources).

In this case, the bronchoscopy portion of the procedure is described by code **31643**, Bronchoscopy, (rigid or flexible); with placement of catheter(s) for intracavitary radiation source application. The surgeon will report this procedure code without the use of a modifier.

The intracavitary radiation source application is separately reported with code **77762**, Intracavitary radiation source application; intermediate. The therapeutic radiologist will report the intracavitary radiation source application with this code without the use of a modifier.

# EXERCISES

**1** What is the appropriate CPT code to report for supply of contrast materials?

**2** True or False: It is appropriate to separately report the intravascular administration of contrast when the phrase "with contrast" appears in the code descriptor.

**3** True or False: It is appropriate to separately report the supply of radio-pharmaceuticals with the appropriate CPT or HCPCS Level II codes.

**4** When a surgical procedure involving imaging is performed, the radiological portion of the procedure is designated as _____.

**5** Assign the appropriate code(s) for the following; code for the "complete procedure" where necessary:
   **a** CT scan of the cervical spine with and without contrast (intravenous injection of contrast)
   **b** Ultrasound guidance for percutaneous needle biopsy of the liver
   **c** MRA of the head performed both without and then with contrast injection
   **d** Bilateral mammography to detect unsuspected cancer in an early stage in an asymptomatic woman

**6** True or False: If the same vascular access is used for both a diagnostic and a therapeutic service on the same occasion, the access is only coded once.

**7** The cognitive process carried out by the physician to determine all of the parameters of a given course of radiation therapy is called _____.

**8** If a first-order and a second-order vessel within the same vascular family are selectively catheterized via the same access, how would the catheterization procedure be reported?

**9** True or False: Radiologists are restricted to reporting the codes in the **70000** series of the CPT Nomenclature.

**10** How should code **76816** be reported for a follow-up ultrasound of pregnant uterus for twins?

**11** What code should be used for nonobstetrical transvaginal ultrasound?

**12** Codes **76813** and **76814** describe fetal nuchal translucency measurement. What imaging modality is used to perform this procedure?

**13** True or False: The key distinction between CTA and CT is that CTA includes reconstruction postprocessing of angiographic images and interpretation.

**14** What basic dosimetry code is appropriately reported with all other planning codes, including **77305**, **77310**, and **77315**, and is warranted with IMRT planning when medically necessary?

**15** SBRT management for the entire course of treatment is reported with what code?

# CHAPTER 8

# Pathology and Laboratory

In this chapter, the Pathology and Laboratory section of the Current Procedural Terminology (CPT®) codebook is reviewed. Services in the Pathology and Laboratory section are provided by a physician, technologist, or other qualified laboratory personnel under the responsible supervision of a physician.

The following table provides a comprehensive listing of the subsections found in the Pathology and Laboratory section of the Current Procedural Terminology (CPT®) codebook.

## Pathology and Laboratory Subsections and Code Ranges

| Subsection | Code Range |
| --- | --- |
| Organ or Disease Oriented Panels | 80048-80076 |
| Drug Testing | 80100-80103 |
| Therapeutic Drug Assays | 80150-80299 |
| Evocative/Suppression Testing | 80400-80440 |
| Consultations (Clinical Pathology) | 80500-80502 |
| Urinalysis | 81000-81099 |
| Chemistry | 82000-84999 |
| Hematology and Coagulation | 85002-85999 |
| Immunology | 86000-86849 |
| Transfusion Medicine | 86850-86999 |
| Microbiology | 87001-87999 |
| Anatomic Pathology | 88000-88099 |
| Cytopathology | 88104-88199 |
| Cytogenetic Studies | 88230-88299 |
| Surgical Pathology | 88300-88399 |
| Transcutaneous Procedures | 88400 |
| Other Procedures | 89049-89240 |
| Reproductive Medicine Procedures | 89250-89356 |

This chapter, in addition to discussing appropriate coding for the collection of specimens, focuses on guidelines for codes in the following subsections:
- Organ or Disease Oriented Panels
- Drug Testing
- Therapeutic Drug Assays
- Evocative/Suppression Testing
- Clinical Pathology Consultations
- Urinalysis
- Chemistry
- Hematology and Coagulation
- Microbiology
- Cytopathology
- Fine Needle Aspiration
- Cytogenetic Studies
- Surgical Pathology
- Reproductive Medicine Procedures

# Collection of Specimen

The **80000** series of codes is for reporting the performance of the specific laboratory test only and does not include the collection of the specimen via venipuncture, arterial puncture, or other collection methodology (eg, lumbar puncture). The collection of the specimen by venipuncture or by arterial puncture is not considered an integral part of the laboratory procedure(s) performed.

Codes in the **36400-36425** series are used to report venipuncture for obtaining blood specimens. The collection of the specimen(s) by venipuncture is reported with code **36415**, Collection of venous blood by venipuncture. Collection of capillary blood specimen (eg, finger, heel, earlobe stick) is reported with code **36416**. Code **36415** should not be reported in conjunction with modifier 63. When venipuncture or finger/heel/earlobe stick is performed for collection of specimen(s), this code is reported in addition to the appropriate code(s) from the **80000** series for the laboratory procedure(s) performed.

CPT code **36600**, Arterial puncture, withdrawal of blood for diagnosis, is used to report the puncture of an artery for withdrawal of blood for diagnosis. If this procedure is performed, it would be appropriate to report code **36600** for the collection of the specimen. This code is reported in addition to the appropriate code(s) from the **80000** series for the laboratory procedure(s) performed.

# Organ or Disease Oriented Panels

Organ or disease oriented panels are reported with the codes from the **80048-80076** series. These panels were developed for coding purposes and should not be interpreted as clinical standards for testing.

Each panel includes a defined list of tests. The tests listed with each panel identify the defined components of that panel. To report a code for a panel, all of the tests listed in the panel definition must be performed, with no substitutions. If fewer tests are performed than those listed in the panel code, the individual code number(s) for each test should be listed rather than the panel code.

The panel components are not intended to limit the performance of other tests. If tests are performed in addition to those specifically listed for a particular panel, those tests would be reported separately in addition to the panel code.

The presence or absence of a specific code for a panel of tests in no way limits the physician's ability to order or perform a specific battery of tests. Whether a specific panel code exists or not affects only the method of reporting the tests performed.

Consider the following coding examples:

**EXAMPLE 1:** Dr Alder performs a lipid panel on automated equipment in his office. The battery of tests he uses include high-density lipoprotein cholesterol, total serum cholesterol, triglycerides, and a quantitative glucose. Dr Alder reports the following codes for the panel performed:

**80061**    Lipid panel

        This panel must include the following:

        Cholesterol, serum, total (**82465**)

        Lipoprotein, direct measurement, high-density cholesterol (HDL cholesterol) (**83718**)

        Triglycerides (**84478**)

**82947**    Glucose; quantitative, blood (except reagent strip)

**EXAMPLE 2:** Dr Bender performs a metabolic panel on automated equipment in her office. The tests she includes in her battery of tests are serum carbon dioxide, chloride, creatinine, glucose, potassium, sodium, and urea nitrogen (BUN).

The following two code listings are found in the CPT codebook for reporting metabolic panels:

**80048**    Basic metabolic panel

        This panel must include the following:

        Calcium, total (**82310**)

        Carbon dioxide (**82374**)

        Chloride (**82435**)

        Creatinine (**82565**)

        Glucose (**82947**)

        Potassium (**84132**)

        Sodium (**84295**)

        Urea nitrogen (BUN) (**84520**)

**80053**    Comprehensive metabolic panel

        This panel must include the following:

        Albumin (**82040**)

        Bilirubin, total (**82247**)

        Calcium (**82310**)

        Carbon dioxide (bicarbonate) (**82374**)

        Chloride (**82435**)

        Creatinine (**82565**)

        Glucose (**82947**)

Phosphatase, alkaline (**84075**)

Potassium (**84132**)

Protein, total (**84155**)

Sodium (**84295**)

Transferase, alanine amino (ALT) (SGPT) (**84460**)

Transferase, aspartate amino (AST) (SGOT) (**84450**)

Urea nitrogen (BUN) (**84520**)

Neither panel code **80048** nor **80053** accurately describes Dr Bender's metabolic panel. It would not be appropriate for Dr Bender to report code **80048**, since she does not include calcium (**82310**) as a component of her panel. It would also not be appropriate for Dr Bender to report code **80053**, as her panel does not include all of the test components listed in this code.

The appropriate way for Dr Bender to report her metabolic panel is to report the code for the electrolyte panel and separately report the creatinine, glucose, and BUN. The following codes would be reported:

Electrolyte panel (**80051**)

Creatinine (**82565**)

Glucose (**82947**)

BUN (**84520**)

# Drug Testing

The CPT codes used to report drug testing are located in three subsections of the Pathology and Laboratory section of the CPT codebook: Drug Testing (**80100-80103**), Therapeutic Drug Assays (**80150-80299**), and Chemistry (**82000-84999**). Qualitative assays (tests that detect whether a particular analyte, constituent, or condition is present) are reported with the drug testing codes; quantitative assays (tests that give results expressing the specific numerical amount of an analyte in a specimen) are reported with the therapeutic drug assay or chemistry codes.

The codes used to report qualitative drug testing distinguish between screening tests (**80100** and **80101**) and confirmatory testing (**80102**). The screening tests are further distinguished by the methods used to analyze multiple drug classes (**80100**) and those that test for a single drug class (**80101**). The codes are intended to distinguish among analytic methods rather than the platform or instrumentation on which any particular method is run.

For example, immunoassays, which are used to identify single drug classes, should be reported with code **80101** (when used in drug screening), whether the test is performed with a random access analyzer, a single-analyte test kit, or a multiple analyte test kit. Chromatography, which can identify multiple drug classes, is coded by means of code **80100** (when used in drug screening).

For code **80100**, each combination of stationary and mobile phase is to be counted as one procedure. For example, if screening for three drugs by chromatography requires one stationary phase with three mobile phases, report code **80100** three times. However, if multiple drugs can be detected with a single analysis (eg, one stationary phase with one mobile phase), report code **80100** only once.

**EXAMPLE 1:** A patient comes to the emergency department in a coma, and the treating physician orders a drug screen without identifying a specific drug class to be tested. The laboratory performs a multiple drug class screen by means of thin-layer chromatography with a single mobile and stationary phase.

For the pathology services provided, CPT code **80100** would be reported, because this code is used for qualitative drug screening by chromatographic methods. One unit would be coded for the single stationary and mobile phase combination.

For code **80101**, each single drug class method tested and reported is to be counted as one drug class. For example, if a sample is aliquotted to five wells and separate class-specific immunoassays are run on each of the five wells and reported separately, report code **80101** five times. Similarly, if a sample is run on a rapid assay kit composed of five class-specific immunoassays in a single kit and the five classes are reported separately, code **80101** should be reported five times.

**EXAMPLE 2:** A patient comes to the emergency department in a coma with a history of anxiety and depression under treatment with prescription medications. The physician orders a drug screen for alcohol, barbiturates, benzodiazepines, phenothiazines, and tricyclic antidepressants. The laboratory performs single drug class screening for each analyte by means of immunoassay methods in a random access analyzer.

Code **80101** would be reported five times, because this code is used to report immunoassay and enzyme assay, single drug class methods. Five units are reported as each single drug class is reported separately.

**EXAMPLE 3:** A patient comes to the emergency department in a coma with a history of illegal drug use. The treating physician orders a drug screen for amphetamines, barbiturates, benzodiazepines, cocaine and metabolites, opiates, phencyclidine, and tetrahydrocannabinoids. The laboratory performs single drug class screening for each analyte by means of a multiple-analyte rapid test immunoassay kit.

Code **80101** would be reported seven times, because immunoassay single drug class methods are reported with this code regardless of platform (random access analyzer or multiple-analyte test kit). Seven units are reported as each single drug class is reported separately.

For each procedure requiring confirmation, use code **80102**. As with the screening code (**80100**) for chromatography, each combination of stationary and mobile phase is to be counted as one procedure. For example, if confirmation of three drugs by chromatography requires one stationary phase with three mobile phases, report code **80102** three times. However, if multiple drugs can be confirmed with a single analysis (eg, one stationary phase with one mobile phase), report code **80102** only once.

> **EXAMPLE 4:** A patient comes to the emergency department in a coma with a history of illegal drug use. The treating physician orders a drug screen without necessarily identifying a specific drug class to be tested. The laboratory performs a multiple drug class screen and reports back positive results, consistent with opiates. The treating physician orders a confirmatory test, which the laboratory runs to confirm opiates by means of high-performance liquid chromatography (not quantitative).

To code the multiple drug class screen, use code **80100** (one unit would be coded). To code the confirmation test, use code **80102**, because this code is used to report confirmatory testing without quantification. One unit would be coded for the single stationary mobile phase.

Quantitative assays should be reported by means of the appropriate code in the Therapeutic Drug subsection (**80150-80299**) or Chemistry subsection (**82000-84999**). Quantitative chromatography for analytes not specified in those sections may be coded with code **82491** or **82492**.

## Table of Drugs and the Appropriate Qualitative Screening, Confirmatory, and Quantitative Codes

| Drug Qualitative | Multiple Drug Class Method | Single Drug Class Method | Confirmation | Quantitative |
|---|---|---|---|---|
| Alcohols | 80100[a] | 80101[b] | 80102[c] | 82055 or 82075[d] |
| Amphetamines | 80100[a] | 80101[b] | 80102[c] | 82145 |
| Barbiturates | 80100[a] | 80101[b] | 80102[c] | 80184 or 82205[e] |
| Benzodiazepines | 80100[a] | 80101[b] | 80102[c] | 80154 |
| Cocaine and metabolites | 80100[a] | 80101[b] | 80102[c] | 82520 |
| Methadone | 80100[a] | 80101[b] | 80102[c] | 83840 |
| Methaqualone | 80100[a] | 80101[b] | 80102[c] | 80299 or 82491[f] |
| Opiates | 80100[a] | 80101[b] | 80102[c] | 83925 |
| Phencyclidine | 80100[a] | 80101[b] | 80102[c] | 83992 |

| Drug Qualitative | Multiple Drug Class Method | Single Drug Class Method | Confirmation | Quantitative |
|---|---|---|---|---|
| Phenothiazines | 80100[a] | 80101[b] | 80102[c] | 84022 |
| Propoxyphene | 80100[a] | 80101[b] | 80102[c] | 80299 or 82491[f] |
| Tetrahydrocan-nabinoids | 80100[a] | 80101[b] | 80102[c] | 80299 or 82491[f] |
| Tricyclic antidepressants | 80100[a] | 80101[b] | 80102[c] | 80152, 80160, 80166, 80174, 80182[g]; 80299 or 82491[f] |

a Use code **80100** for each combination of mobile phase with stationary phase.

b Use code **80101** for each single drug class tested and reported.

c Use code **80102** for each combination of mobile phase with stationary phase used for drug confirmation.

d Code **82055** for "Alcohol (ethanol); any specimen except breath," and code **82075** for "Alcohol (ethanol); breath."

e Code **80184** for "Phenobarbital," **80188** for "Primidone," and **82205** for "Barbiturates, not elsewhere specified."

f If there is no appropriate quantitative code for the drug listed, use code **82491** for chromatographic determination or **80299** for other methods.

g Code **80152** "Amitriptyline," **80160** for "Desipramine," **80166** for "Doxepin," **80174** for "Imipramine," or **80182** for "Nortriptyline."

# Therapeutic Drug Assays

Therapeutic drug assays are reported with the codes in the **80150-80299** series. The material for examination may be from any source. The codes in this series represent quantitative examination (ie, the results will express the specific quantity of the drug present in the specimen, expressed as a numeric result). Nonquantitative or qualitative drug testing is reported with the codes in the **80100-80103** series. Qualitative tests detect only whether a particular analyte, constituent, or condition is present without expressing results as a numeric value.

The CPT Nomenclature lists the generic (nonproprietary) names of drugs whenever possible. If the specific drug for which the therapeutic drug assay is performed is not found in the **80150-80202** series, then code **80299**, Quantitation of drug, not elsewhere specified, is appropriately reported. When code **80299** is reported, it is necessary to identify the specific therapeutic drug assay performed.

The following table is provided to assist in cross-referencing commonly used trade names of drugs with their generic names. The trade names in this table are limited to those marketed in the United States. The table is not all-inclusive, and not every trade name in current use is listed for each drug. The inclusion or exclusion of a drug in this table does not indicate approval or disapproval of its use in any category, nor is any efficacy or safety implied.

| Crosswalk Table of Generic and Brand Name Drugs | |
|---|---|
| **Generic Name/Drug** | **Brand Name** |
| Amikacin | Amikin® |
| Amitriptyline | Elavil®, Endep® |
| Carbamazepine | Tegretol® |
| Desipramine | Norpramin® |
| Digoxin | Lanoxin® |
| Doxepin | Adapin® Sinequan® |
| Gentamicin | Garamycin® |
| Imipramine | Tofranil® |
| Lidocaine | Xylocaine® |
| Lithium | Eskalith®-Lithobid Lithoid® |
| Phenobarbital | Donnatal® |
| Phenytoin | Dilantin® |
| Primidone | Mysoline® |
| Procainamide | Pronestyl® |
| Quinidine | Quinaglute® Quinidex® |
| Theophylline | Respbid® Theo-Dur® Theo-24® |
| Tobramycin | Nebcin® |

# Evocative/Suppression Testing

Evocative/suppression testing is reported with the codes in the **80400-80440** series. In the code descriptors where reference is made to a particular analyte, for example, cortisol (**82533** × 2), the "× 2" refers to the number of times the test for that particular analyte is performed.

Some of the code descriptors indicate that the test is performed on pooled blood samples. When an analyte varies in the blood level from moment to moment, a more reliable value for baseline may be obtained by drawing several specimens several minutes apart, then pooling equal portions of each and obtaining one result (a pooled result).

The notes that appear at the beginning of this series of codes indicate how to code the additional physician services that may be a part of the complex series of events or actions carried out by the physician. Let us take a moment to review these notes.

Evocative/suppression test panels involve the administration of evocative or suppressive agents, and the baseline and subsequent measurement of their effects on chemical constituents. Codes **80400-80440** are used for the reporting of the laboratory component of the overall testing protocol. The panel itself may describe only a small portion of the protocol in some cases.

The physician's administration of the evocative or suppressive agents is reported separately with the codes in the **90760**, **90761**, **90765-90768** series describing hydration, therapeutic, prophylactic, and diagnostic injections and infusions. The supplies and drugs are separately reported with CPT code **99070**, or the appropriate Healthcare Common Procedure Coding System (HCPCS) Level II codes for supplies and drugs. (Refer to Chapter 9 for further discussion of codes **90760**, **90761**, and **90765-90768**.)

To report physician attendance and monitoring during the testing, use the appropriate evaluation and management (E/M) code, including the prolonged services codes if required. It is important to note that the prolonged services codes are not separately reported when the testing involves prolonged infusions reported with codes **90760**, **90761**, and **90765-90768**.

# Pathology Consultations

There are three different sets of codes in the Pathology and Laboratory section of the CPT codebook for reporting various types of consultative services. The three different types of consultative services include the following:
- Consultations (clinical pathology) (**80500-80502**)
- Consultation on referred material (**88321-88325**)
- Pathology consultation during surgery (**88329-88334**)

The various pathology consultation services codes are similar to the other CPT consultation codes found in the E/M section in that they describe physician pathology services provided at the request of another physician of the same or another facility or institution. In contrast to the E/M consultation services, pathology consultations do not require face-to-face encounter with the patient. If there is a face-to-face encounter, then the pathologist should use the appropriate E/M consult code(s).

The pathology consultation codes are reported if the services are performed as follows:
- At the request of the attending physician of the same or another institution relevant to test result(s) requiring further medical interpretation
- For consultation and report on material referred from another pathologist or facility
- For consultation provided to another pathologist in a different practice site or facility

> **CODING TIP**
>
> Codes **80500** and **80502** are used to report clinical pathology consultations.

- For consultation provided to another physician in the same facility/site on material from another institution (eg, review of slides before surgery or therapy at your facility)
- During surgery

Let us look next at the three sets of codes available and the guidelines for reporting these clinical pathology consultative services.

## Consultations (Clinical Pathology)

CPT codes **80500** and **80502** are used to report a clinical pathology consultation. The code descriptors appear in the CPT codebook as follows:

**80500**  Clinical pathology consultation; limited, without review of patient's history and medical records

**80502**  comprehensive, for a complex diagnostic problem, with review of patient's history and medical records

A clinical pathology consultation is a service including a written report rendered by the pathologist in response to a request from an attending physician in relation to test results requiring additional medical interpretive judgment. Code **80500** may also be used to report clinical correlation of gynecological cytology (ie, Pap test) and follow-up histology findings, as mandated by the Clinical Laboratory Improvement Act of 1988, when the clinical pathology consultations include a written report provided by the pathologist.

## Consultation on Referred Material

CPT codes **88321**, **88323**, and **88325** are used to report consultations and report on material referred from another source (ie, from another pathologist or facility). The code descriptors appear in the CPT code set as follows:

**88321**  Consultation and report on referred slides prepared elsewhere

**88323**  Consultation and report on referred material requiring preparation of slides

**88325**  Consultation, comprehensive, with review of records and specimens, with report on referred material

These codes are appropriate for use in reporting consultations provided to another physician in a different practice site or facility or in the same facility/site on material referred from an outside source (eg, review of slides from another institution before surgery or therapy at your facility).

As indicated in the code descriptors, code **88321** is used to report a consultation on referred material that does not require the preparation of routinely stained slides. Code **88323** describes consultation and report on referred material when the consultant prepares the slides for routine histologic staining.

When special stains or immunohistochemical stains are prepared in addition to the routine stain, they should be coded separately. Code **88325** is reported for a more comprehensive consultative service on referred material that involves review of records and specimens.

## Consultation During Surgery

Codes **88329**, **88331**, **88332**, **88333**, and **88334** are available for reporting a pathology consultation during surgery. The code descriptors appear in the CPT codebook as follows:

**88329**    Pathology consultation during surgery;

**88331**        first tissue block, with frozen section(s), single specimen

**88332**        each additional tissue block with frozen section(s)

**88333**        cytologic examination (eg, touch prep, squash prep), initial site

**88334**        cytologic examination (eg, touch prep, squash prep), each additional site

To appropriately report these codes, it is necessary to understand the definitions of *tissue blocks* and *sections*. A block is a portion of tissue from a specimen that is frozen or encased in a support medium such as paraffin or plastic, from which sections are prepared. A section is a thin slice of tissue from a block prepared for microscopic examination.

When the pathology consultation during surgery does not involve microscopic examination of tissue, the service is coded as **88329**, Pathology consultation during surgery. When a single frozen section (ie, the first tissue block) from a specimen is examined, the service is coded as **88331**, Pathology consultation during surgery; first tissue block, with frozen section(s), single specimen.

When frozen sections from more than one block from the same specimen are examined, the appropriate coding is one unit of service of code **88331** for the first tissue block and an additional unit of service of code **88332**, Pathology consultation during surgery; each additional tissue block with frozen section(s), for each block subsequent to the first.

Code **88332** is reported only when a single specimen requires multiple frozen section tissue blocks. CPT code **88332** cannot be reported for a specimen that has not already been examined, as indicated by code **88331**.

If more than one specimen is submitted for consultation, the services for each specimen would be coded, as appropriate.

Two intraoperative cytologic evaluation codes are also available: **88333** Pathology consultation during surgery; cytologic examination (eg, touch prep, squash prep), initial site, and **88334**, Pathology consultation during surgery; cytologic examination (eg, touch prep, squash prep), each additional site. These are structured similarly to the frozen section codes **88331** and **88332**. Codes **88333** and **88334** are reported for intraoperative cytologic examination (via touch or squash preparation) and consultation to provide immediate diagnoses during an intraoperative consultation without the involvement of frozen section. The important differentiation between the frozen section codes and the cytology codes is that where **88331** and **88332** are billed per block, **88333** and **88334** are billed per specimen site. An important list of parenthetical comments follows these codes defining the appropriate use of **88333** and **88334**. For example, when intraoperative cytology is performed in conjunction with frozen section analysis, the first frozen section per specimen is coded using **88331**, and all cytologic preparations performed on the same specimen are billed using one unit of **88334** per site. Also, for percutaneous needle biopsy requiring intraprocedural cytologic examination, use **88333**. However, if the frozen section and touch prep are performed simultaneously, complementarily aiding in the same specific diagnosis, only the frozen section code should be reported (eg, a squash preparation and a frozen section analyzed together on the same brain biopsy being assessed for glioma).

Following are a few examples of appropriate coding for pathology consultations during surgery.

**EXAMPLE 1:** A basal cell carcinoma is removed from a patient's forehead and submitted as a specimen for frozen section. Frozen section on one area is performed. The margin on one side is not adequate, so the surgeon has to resect more tissue from the same wound and submit this for frozen section. One frozen section is performed on this specimen.

For the pathology services provided, CPT code **88331** would be reported for the first specimen submitted. The margin on one side was not adequate and the surgeon had to resect more tissue from the same wound and submit this for frozen section. This second specimen submitted is reported as a "new" specimen and is reported as a separate frozen section examination with code **88331**. Therefore, to completely report the services described, code **88331** would be reported twice. The pathologist routinely also processes the tissue remaining after a frozen section. Those permanent sections also require analysis and, in the case described above, two units of **88305** (for the two tissue specimens) would be coded.

**EXAMPLE 2:** In the course of a radical prostatectomy, obturator lymph nodes from the right and left sides are submitted as separate specimens for immediate diagnosis with respect to involvement with metastatic disease. The pathologist examines each of these specimens and selects portions of lymph nodes resulting in two blocks on the right side and three blocks on the left side for frozen sections, which are examined microscopically.

In this example, for the specimen from the right side, the pathology services provided would be reported with codes **88331** and **88332** (two blocks on the right side—code **88331** for the first block and code **88332** for the second block).

For the separate specimen from the left side, the pathology services provided would be reported with code **88331** and code **88332** twice (three blocks on the left side—code **88331** for the first block and code **88332** twice, once for the second block and once for the third block).

Therefore, to code for the frozen section analyses in this example, code **88331** would be reported twice and code **88332** would be reported three times.

## Pathology Consultation Including Patient Examination

In instances when a clinical pathologist performs a pathology consultation including examination of the patient, the appropriate level of E/M code should be reported, provided the guidelines for reporting have been met and documented in the medical record.

# Urinalysis

Codes in the **81000-81099** series are used to report various types of urinalysis. The note at the beginning of this subsection indicates that many specific quantitative analyses are not reported with codes from this subsection; rather, the user is directed to see the appropriate section. For example, quantitative testing for chloride in the urine would be reported with code **82436**, Chloride; urine, from the Chemistry subsection. The codes available in this subsection include the following.

Codes **81000-81003** are used to report urinalysis by dip stick or tablet reagent. The following constituents are included when urinalysis by dip stick or tablet reagent is reported:

- Bilirubin
- Glucose
- Hemoglobin
- Ketones
- Leukocytes
- Nitrite
- pH
- Protein
- Specific gravity
- Urobilinogen

As indicated in the code descriptor, these codes are applicable when testing for any number of these constituents.

Appropriate code selection from the **81000-81003** series depends upon the type of test performed. To select the appropriate code, one must know whether the testing was automated or nonautomated and whether the testing was performed with or without microscopy.

When urinalysis is reported, multiple tests described in a single code should not be unbundled to produce multiple codes. For example, code **81000**, which describes urinalysis with microscopy, should not be coded as **81005** for the urinalysis and code **81015** for the microscopic examination.

Code **81005** is used to report qualitative or semiquantitative urinalysis, except for immunoassays. The parenthetical note following code **81005** directs the user to code **83518** for reporting a qualitative or semiquantitative immunoassay.

A urine pregnancy test performed by visual color comparison methods is reported with code **81025**. A visual color comparison involves a pad or stick that changes color dependent on the test results and is compared to a color chart that indicates positive or negative for pregnancy.

Code **81050** is reported for volume measurement for timed collection. A timed collection involves collection of all urine during a specific time period, such as 12 or 24 hours. As indicated in the code descriptor, this code is reported for each volume measurement.

This series of codes includes an unlisted urinalysis procedure (**81099**). This code is appropriately reported when a urinalysis is performed that is not more specifically identified with a code in the **81000-81050** series. (Refer to Chapter 2 for further discussion of unlisted codes.)

# Chemistry

When reviewing the codes in this subsection (**82000-84999**), one will notice that the code descriptors are primarily arranged alphabetically. The exception is the code series for molecular diagnostics (**83890-83914**). The note at the beginning of the molecular diagnostics procedures indicates that when these procedures are performed to test for oncology, hematology, neurology, or inherited disorder, the appropriate Genetic Testing Code modifier should be used to specify probe type or condition tested. Genetic Testing Code modifiers are intended for reporting with molecular laboratory procedures related to genetic testing. Genetic testing modifiers should be used in conjunction with CPT and HCPCS codes to provide diagnostic granularity of service to enable providers to submit complete and precise genetic testing information without altering test descriptors. These modifiers are categorized by mutation. The first (numeric) digit indicates the disease category, and the second (alphabetic) digit denotes gene type. Although this system does not allow complete capture of the human genome, it presents a viable solution to the expected growth of molecular genetic testing in clinical practice over the next decade while the technology and nomenclature systems mature. (For a complete listing of the Genetic Testing Code modifiers, see Appendix I of the CPT codebook. For more information on the appropriate applications of the Genetic Testing Code modifiers, see the Coding Commentary published in the July 2005 *CPT Assistant* newsletter.)

Here are some highlights of the guidelines that appear at the beginning of the Chemistry subsection.

The material for chemical analysis may be from any source. Exceptions to this guideline are evident when a code descriptor specifically lists the source of the specimen. A few examples include code **82480**, Cholinesterase; serum, in which the specimen is specifically identified as serum, and code **82436**, Chloride; urine, which specifies the specimen as urine. The results are quantitative unless otherwise specified. When an analyte is measured in multiple specimens from different sources or in specimens that are obtained at different times, the analyte is reported separately for each source and for each specimen. The listings in the Chemistry subsection represent quantitative examinations unless otherwise specified in the code descriptor. For multiple specimens or different sources, use modifier 59. For repeat laboratory tests performed on the same day, use modifier 91.

Mathematical calculations, that is, clinical information derived from the results of laboratory data that is mathematically calculated (eg, free thyroxine index or T7), are considered part of the test procedure and are not a separately reportable service.

When searching for the appropriate code(s) for a laboratory test, look first for a code that describes the specific analyte (substance analyzed). If no analyte-specific code is found, search for a code that describes the methodology used in the testing procedure. "Unlisted procedure" codes ending with 99 should be used only when the analyte or method code is not listed.

For example, when coding for prostate-specific antigen (PSA) testing, codes **84152**, **84153**, and **84154** specifically describe this testing procedure; these codes are analyte-specific. CPT code **86316**, Immunoassay for tumor antigen, quantitative (eg, CA 50, 72-4, 549), each, also describes tumor antigen testing but would not be appropriately reported because a specific code (PSA) exists. Code **86316** describes tumor antigen testing by the methodology (eg, immunoassay). This code is used to report tumor antigen testing when an analyte-specific listing is not available in the CPT codebook.

Although the cPSA (complexed PSA) result can be used much like the fPSA (free PSA), it should not be coded as such. The current code to report cPSA is code **84152**.

Codes in the series **84155**, **84156**, **84157**, and **84160** for measurement of total protein are intended to distinguish by specimen type. Protein electrophoresis methods are reported with codes in the **84165**, **84166** series.

**CODING TIP**

Code **83913** can be used to report any method of ribonucleic acid (RNA) stabilization.

# Hematology and Coagulation

Codes in the **85002-85999** series are used to report various hematology and coagulation procedures. Blood counts and clotting factor testing are some of the procedures described in this subsection.

The parenthetical note appearing at the beginning of this subsection indicates that blood banking procedures are not reported with codes in this subsection. Rather, codes in the Transfusion Medicine subsection of the CPT codebook are used to report blood banking procedures.

The hematology series of codes (**85002-85049**) contains variations of very specific component(s) and the specific methodology(s) used to obtain measurements of those components. The following components are typically included in a complete blood count (CBC):

- Red blood cell (RBC) count
- White blood cell (WBC) count

- Hemoglobin (Hgb)
- Hematocrit (Hct)
- Platelet count
- RBC indices—the calculation for determining the average size, hemoglobin content, and concentration of RBCs, including the following:
  - Mean cell volume
  - Mean cell hemoglobin
  - Mean cell hemoglobin concentrate
- Differential white blood cell count

Codes **85007-85009** describe current manual microscopic review of peripheral blood. Code **85007** describes microscopic examination of a blood smear with a manual differential leukocyte (WBC) count. Code **85008** describes a microscopic blood smear examination without a manual differential WBC count.

To report an automated CBC (**85027**) with a manual differential WBC count (**85007** or **85009**) or blood smear review (**85008**), code **85027** should be reported with **85007**, **85008**, or **85009**, as appropriate. If both an automated CBC and an automated differential WBC count are performed, code **85025** should be reported. Code **85032** describes each manual erythrocyte, leukocyte, or platelet count and is intended to allow for reporting of individual parts of the CBC. In the instance when a manual CBC (RBC, WBC, Hgb, Hct, differential, and indices) is performed, codes **85014** and **85018** should be reported one time, code **85032** should be reported two times and code **85007** or **85009** one time, as appropriate. Code **85041** describes an automated RBC count. This code should not be reported in conjunction with code **85025** or **85027**, as these codes already include an automated RBC count. It should be used to report automated RBC counts only. Code **85045** describes an automated reticulocyte count. Code **85048** is used to report an automated WBC count.

## Bone Marrow Aspiration, Bone Marrow Biopsy, Bone Biopsy

CPT code **85097** is used to report the interpretation of a smear resulting from the bone marrow aspiration procedure. The smears are stained in a hematology laboratory or a physician's office. Whether a differential cell count is performed or whether the findings are reported in a more descriptive fashion, the same code applies. If an aspirate clot is processed as a cell block in the histology laboratory, the additional code **88305** is also reported. When performed, codes **38220** and **38221** should be reported for the actual aspiration procedure and the actual bone marrow biopsy procedure, respectively.

The interpretation of the biopsy is reported with code **88305**. When performed, the decalcification procedure is separately reported with code **88311**.

The following codes are for pathologic examination:

- Code **85097** describes the examination of the bone marrow smear.
- Code **88305** describes the examination of the bone marrow cell block (also known as clot or particle section) prepared from the aspirate.

- Code **88305** describes the examination of the bone marrow biopsy.
- Code **88311** describes the decalcification of bone marrow biopsy or bone biopsy.
- Code **88313** describes the iron stain of bone marrow smear or clot section.

If additional testing is performed to establish the diagnosis (eg, additional special stains or immunohistochemical techniques), then other CPT codes may be reported as needed to describe the additional testing.

# Microbiology

Codes in the Microbiology subsection (**87001-87999**) include bacteriology, mycology, parasitology, and virology. When various microbiology testing procedures are reported, it is appropriate to designate multiple procedures that are rendered on the same date by separate entries.

The guidelines in the Microbiology subsection provide clear definitions of presumptive and definitive identification. Presumptive identification of microorganisms is defined as identification by colony morphology, growth on selective media, Gram stains, or up to three tests (eg, catalase, oxidase, indole, urease). *Definitive identification of microorganisms* is defined as an identification to the genus or species level that requires tests (eg, biochemical panels, slide cultures). If additional studies involve molecular probes, chromatography, or immunologic techniques, (**87140-87158**), they should be separately coded in addition to definitive identification codes. For multiple specimens/sites, use modifier 59. For repeat laboratory tests performed on the same day, use modifier 91.

The codes in the **87040-87077** series are intended to represent bacterial cultures. Specifically, codes **87040, 87045**, and **87046** are intended to be reported for aerobic bacterial culture of blood and stool. Code **87070** is reported for aerobic bacterial culture of any other source except urine, blood, or stool; eg, other body fluid or wound drainage. Codes **87071**, **87073**, **87075**, **87076**, and **87077** represent codes for aerobic and anaerobic techniques. These codes are also intended to be reported for presumptive and definitive identification of isolates.

Screening cultures are reported with codes **87081** and **87084**. Screening cultures are cultures used for the detection of a specific potential pathogenic organism. For example, a throat culture used to detect Group A Streptococcus only.

Codes **87086** and **87088** are intended to be used to report bacterial detection, quantitation, and presumptive identification of isolate(s) in urine specimens. Report **87086** for the initial urine culture and quantitation (if growth occurs) and **87088** for the presumptive identification of each potential pathogenic isolate. Urine cultures resulting in "no growth" are reported as **87086**.

Codes **87101-87107** describe fungal cultures. The appropriate code from this series is selected on the basis of the source of the specimen. Code **87101** describes fungal culture of the skin, hair, or nail. Code **87102** is intended to be reported for other source (except blood). Code **87103** describes a fungal culture of the blood.

Code **87106** is intended to be reported for definitive identification of each organism. This code is reported in addition to codes **87101**, **87102**, and **87103**, when appropriate. If definitive identification of more than one fungus is performed on a single specimen, it would be appropriate to report this code more than once per specimen. Again, code **87106** is intended to be reported for each organism definitively identified. Code **87107** is intended to be reported for mold cultures definitively identified.

Culture typing is reported with the codes in the **87140-87158** series. The appropriate code is selected on the basis of the method of testing used, eg, immunofluorescence, gas-liquid chromatography, or high-performance liquid chromatography.

Codes **87168**, **87169**, **87172**, **87177**, and **87209** are intended to report parasite testing. Code **87177** is not reported in conjunction with code **87015**.

Susceptibility studies are to be reported by means of codes **87181-87190**. The appropriate code is selected on the basis of the method of testing used (eg, disk method, enzyme detection). Code **87187** is reported in addition to code **87186** or **87188**.

Codes in the **87205-87210** series are used to report various smears with interpretation. CPT code **87205** is the appropriate code for reporting a Gram stain. Gram stain is a differential stain used to demonstrate the staining properties of bacteria of all types. The Gram stain confirms the presence of bacteria and their cell type.

As previously stated, it is appropriate to designate multiple procedures that are rendered on the same date by separate entries. Consider the following example:

**EXAMPLE:** A Gram stain is performed on the primary specimen in addition to an aerobic and anaerobic definitive bacterial wound culture. Additional identification methods are performed to determine the specific species within the organism group. Antibiotic sensitivity studies (minimum inhibitory concentration) are also performed.

In this case, one should separately report the Gram stain (**87205**), the aerobic bacterial wound culture (**87070**), the anaerobic wound culture (**87075**), the additional identification methods (**87076** and/or **87077**), and the antibiotic sensitivity studies (eg, **87186**).

Within the Microbiology subsection, codes **87260-87904** are specifically used for reporting infectious agent antigen detection. These codes are intended for primary source only. For similar studies on culture material, refer to codes **87140-87158**. The notes preceding the codes for infectious agent antigen detection direct the user to codes **86602-86804** for the detection of antibodies to infectious agents.

Included in codes **87260-87904** are separate code families based on the methodology used. Within each code family, the organisms listed represent those currently detectable by the specific methodology indicated.

General methodology codes are included in each family of codes and are to be reported when there is no agent-specific listing for the methodology used. For example, code **87299** is used to report detection of an infectious agent by immunofluorescent antibody technique when testing for an organism other than those specified in codes **87260-87290**.

The following table indicates the specific code families and methodologies available for reporting infectious agent antigen detection.

## Methodologies and Code Ranges

| Methodology Described | Code Range |
|---|---|
| Immunofluorescent technique | 87260-87300 |
| Enzyme immunoassay technique | 87301-87451 |
| Nucleic acid (DNA or RNA) | 87470-87801, 87901-87904 |
| Immunoassay with direct optical observation | 87802-87899 |

# Cytopathology

Codes **88104-88199** are used to report various cytopathology procedures. Separate code series are available for reporting the following:

- Cervical or vaginal cytopathology (**88141-88155**, **88164-88167**, **88174**, **88175**).
- Cytopathology of fluids, washings, or brushings (except cervical or vaginal) (**88104-88107**).
- Cytopathology smears from any other source (other than cervical or vaginal, or fluids, washings, or brushings) (**88160-88162**).
- Cytohistologic studies of fine needle aspirate (**88172**, **88173**). (Codes **10021** and **10022**, are discussed in the Surgery section under the heading of General.)

Cytopathology of fluids, washings, or brushings (except cervical or vaginal) are reported with the codes in the **88104-88107** series. Code **88104** is used to report cytopathology smears of fluids, washings, or brushings (except cervical or vaginal) with interpretation. Code **88106** is reported when only the filter method is used and includes interpretation. Code **88107** describes smears and filter preparation with interpretation.

Cytopathology smears of any other source (except cervical or vaginal; except fluids, washings, or brushings) are reported with codes **88160-88162**. Code **88160** is used to report cytopathology smears, screening, and interpretation. Code **88161** is reported for preparation, screening, and interpretation of cytopathology smears. Code **88162** describes an extended study involving more than five and/or multiple stains.

Codes for concentration (**88108**) as well as for concentration and enrichment techniques (**88112**) are not specimen source-specific except that they should not be used for cervicovaginal cytology. The primary uses for these codes currently are the cytocentrifuge techniques (**88108**), and the thin layer techniques (**88112**). Of note, one of the thin layer techniques currently uses a filter transfer technique. However, this does not suggest that this technique should be coded using **88106** or **88107**. Neither of these codes should be used for fine needle aspirate specimens, as this service is inclusive of the fine needle aspirate code **88173**.

An example for use of the **88160** series of codes is to report direct smear examinations for sputum, vesicle scrapings, nipple discharge smears, and other specimens not fulfilling the other cytologic code series (eg not a fine needle aspiration, fluid, brushing, or washing, and not analyzed using a concentration or concentration and enrichment techniques). Please note that although **88162** provides a code for extended cytologic study requiring the analysis of greater than five slides, again, this code is only applicable in studies that do not fulfill the criteria of the other cytologic code series.

## Pap Tests

Codes **88141-88155**, **88164-88167**, **88174-88175** are used to report cervical or vaginal screening by various methods and to report physician interpretation services. Codes **88150-88154** are used for manual screening of conventional Pap smears that are reported using the non-Bethesda system of reporting. Codes **88164-88167** are used for manual screening of conventional Pap smears that are reported using the Bethesda system of reporting. Codes **88142** and **88143** are used for manual screening of liquid-based specimens processed as thin-layer preparations that are reported using any system of reporting (Bethesda or non-Bethesda). Codes **88174** and **88175** are used for automated screening of liquid-based specimens that are reported using any system of reporting (Bethesda or non-Bethesda).

The four code families for reporting Pap smear services include the following:

- **88142**, **88143**, **88174**, **88175** (Thin Layer Preparation, Any System of Reporting, Manual or Automated Screening)
- **88147**, **88148** (Conventional Pap smears, Primary Screening by Automated System)
- **88150-88154** (Conventional Pap smears, Non-Bethesda Reporting, manual screening)
- **88164-88167** (Conventional Pap smears, Bethesda System of Reporting, manual screening)

When reporting Pap test procedures, within each of the code families listed above, choose the one code that describes the screening method(s) used. Codes **88141** and **88155** should be reported in addition to the screening code chosen when additional services are provided. Manual rescreening requires a complete visual reassessment of the entire slide initially screened by either an automated or manual process. A manual review represents an assessment of selected cells or regions of a slide identified by initial automated review.

Code **88141** should be used to report physician interpretation of a Pap test that is interpreted to be abnormal by personnel performing the initial screening, including those interpreted to be showing suspicious or malignant cells, those showing epithelial cell abnormality (eg, atypical cells of undetermined significance), or cellular changes simulating epithelial cell abnormality such as repair, radiation effect, and cellular changes associated with viral infection. Do not report this code for negative Pap tests that are reviewed solely for quality control purposes.

The following table is provided to summarize the Pap test code families.

## CPT Codes and Procedures for Pap Smear Procedures

| CPT Code | Service/Procedure Described |
|---|---|
| **88141** | Physician interpretation (used in conjunction with codes **88142-88154, 88164-88167, 88174, 88175**), any reporting system |
| **88142** **88143** | Automated thin layer preparation, manual screening, any reporting system |
| **88147** **88148** | Conventional Pap smears, Primary screening by automated system |
| **88150** **88152** **88153** **88154** | Conventional Pap smears, manual screening, Non-Bethesda reporting |
| **88155** | Add-on code definitive hormonal evaluation (used in conjunction with codes **88142-88154, 88164-88167, 88174** and **88175**) |
| **88164** **88165** **88166** **88167** | Conventional Pap smears, manual screening, Bethesda System of reporting |
| **88174** **88175** | Automated thin layer preparation, automated screening, any reporting system |

**CODING TIP**

Negative Pap smears (including smears reviewed for quality control purposes) that do not require physician interpretation should not be coded with the physician interpretation code **88141**. No separate listing in the CPT codebook exists to report Pap smears reviewed for quality control purposes.

### What Is the Bethesda System of Reporting?

The Bethesda System is a format for reporting cervical-vaginal cytologic diagnoses. This format for reporting provides uniform diagnostic terminology to facilitate unambiguous communication between the laboratory and the clinician.

The Bethesda System has the following four basic elements:

- Specimen type (conventional smear vs liquid-based preparation vs other).
- Statement of specimen adequacy—A statement of specimen adequacy is an integral part of the report. Specimens may be designated as satisfactory for evaluation or unsatisfactory for evaluation. (Specify reason and if the specimen was rejected and not processed or if it was processed and not able to be evaluated.)
- General categorization—The general categorization is included to aid clinicians in prioritizing cases for review or to assist laboratories in compiling statistical information. This should not be used as a substitute for a descriptive diagnosis. General categorizations include negative for intraepithelial lesion; epithelial cell abnormality, see interpretation/result; or other.
- Interpretation/Result—In the Bethesda System, descriptive diagnoses are grouped into categories: negative for intraepithelial lesion or malignancy (including organisms and other nonneoplastic findings); other malignant neoplasms; and epithelial cell abnormalities.

Ancillary testing and automated review, if performed, are also included in the Bethesda 2001 format.

## Fine Needle Aspiration

Codes **10021** and **10022** are used to report the technique of fine needle aspiration—the actual procedure performed by the clinical physician. Cross-references related to the use of these codes are found in the specific anatomic sections throughout the CPT codebook.

A fine needle aspiration is performed when material is aspirated with a long, slender needle and the cells are examined cytologically. This is in contrast to a biopsy, where a small piece of tissue is taken and examined for histologic architecture. Take a moment to review the code descriptors for fine needle aspiration procedures.

**10021**   Fine needle aspiration; without imaging guidance

**10022**      with imaging guidance

(For radiological supervision and interpretation, see **76942**, **77002, 77012, 77021**)

Code **10021** is reported if the fine needle aspiration is performed on superficial tissue. Code **10022** is reported for a fine needle aspiration of deep tissue under radiological guidance. As indicated by the parenthetical note following code **10021**, this code describes the needle aspiration procedure only; the radiologic guidance is reported separately by means of code **76942**, **77002**, **77012**, **77021**, depending on the type of guidance used. Codes **10021** and **10022** both include the preparation of smears, if smears are prepared. (Refer to Chapter 7 for further discussion of radiological guidance.) Retrieval and collection of ductal epithelial cells obtained through the ductal lavage procedure via insertion of microcatheters into the mammary ducts is reported with Category III codes **0046T** and **0047T**.

Codes **88172** and **88173** remain in the pathology and laboratory subsection and are used to report the evaluation of the fine needle aspirate specimen. These codes appear in the CPT codebook as follows:

**88172**   Cytopathology, evaluation of fine needle aspirate; immediate cytohistologic study to determine adequacy of specimen(s)

**88173**   interpretation and report

The material aspirated is frequently examined microscopically by a physician immediately to ensure that diagnostic material is present. Frequently this is done to render a preliminary diagnostic assessment so that a repeat operative procedure is not necessary. Code **88172** is used to report this service.

When a final definitive interpretation and written report are issued, the physician performing the definitive interpretation and written report should report code **88173**.

If the physician/pathologist performs both services (immediate evaluation to determine the adequacy of the specimen and the interpretation and report), it would be appropriate to report both codes, **88172** and **88173**, for the services provided.

As noted earlier, these codes are inclusive of other cytopathology codes (eg, for direct smears, cytocentrifuge, and thin layered preparations). Additional coding for an accompanying cell block preparation (**88305**), and any special studies, including special or other immunohistochemical stains, can also be appropriately reported.

# Cytogenetic Studies

The note at the beginning of the subsection indicates that when molecular diagnostic procedures are performed to test for oncologic or inherited disorder, use the appropriate Genetic Testing Code modifier to specify probe type or condition tested, when applicable. (See Appendix I of the CPT codebook for a complete listing of appropriate modifiers to report with molecular diagnostic and molecular cytogenetic procedures. For more information on the appropriate applications of the Genetic Testing Code modifiers, see the Coding Commentary published in the July 2005 *CPT Assistant* newsletter.)

# Surgical Pathology

Codes **88300-88309** are used to report surgical pathology. When these codes are reported, services include accession, examination, and reporting. They do not include the services designated in codes **88311-88399** or molecular pathology interpretations by pathologist, which are coded in addition when provided. Understanding the pathology service definition is necessary for proper use of the surgical pathology codes. The unit of service for codes **88300-88309** is the specimen. A *specimen* is defined as tissue or tissues submitted for individual and separate attention requiring individual examination and pathologic diagnosis. When material received for pathologic examination comprises multiple specimens, each specimen is considered a single unit of service and is to be reported using a single code.

Codes **88302-88309** should not be reported on the same specimen as part of Mohs surgery. The onus for correct coding lies with the Mohs surgeon. If a Mohs surgeon submits a specimen to a pathologist, the pathologist is then entitled to report the appropriate codes for the services rendered. The Mohs surgeon is proscribed from billing for the Mohs procedure under that circumstance. It would be inappropriate for the Mohs surgeon to report Mohs mircrographic surgery codes and submit tissue. However, it is appropriate for the pathologist to code for his or her services rendered.

More than 170 surgical pathology specimens are assigned individual CPT codes. Inevitably, some specimens will be encountered in practice that are not included in these lists. Unlisted specimens should be assigned the code that most closely reflects the physician work involved when the unlisted specimen is compared to other specimens assigned that code.

Since code selection for unlisted specimens is based on comparison of physician work to other listed specimens, those responsible for assigning the surgical pathology code to an unlisted specimen should communicate with the physician regarding appropriate code selection.

Now let us review appropriate coding for the following two examples:

**EXAMPLE 1:** Two separate skin lesions are submitted in a single container. One of these specimens is separately identified by a suture. Accompanying specimen information indicates "skin biopsy without suture from the left cheek; skin biopsy with suture from the right cheek." The physician work related to each of these separately identified specimens is coded as **88305** (two units of service).

**EXAMPLE 2:** Two separate skin lesions are submitted in a single container; however, they are not separately identified. This is a single specimen and coded as one unit of service with code **88305**.

Code **88300** is reported for any specimen that, in the opinion of the examining physician, can be accurately diagnosed without microscopic examination. Code **88302** is used when gross and microscopic examination is performed on a specimen to confirm identification of a presumptively normal specimen and absence of disease. Codes **88304-88309** describe all other specimens requiring gross and microscopic examination and represent additional ascending levels of physician work. Codes **88302-88309** are specifically defined by the assigned specimens.

As stated earlier, codes **88300-88309** do not include the services described by codes **88311-88372**. Codes in the **88311-88372** series represent additional surgical pathology services. The unit of service for codes in this section is the specimen, but unlike the tissue pathology section, the specimen submitted for special studies may be tissue or any body fluid or blood. These codes may be used alone or in addition to the code(s) reported for the primary surgical pathology services.

Additional services include:

- Decalcification procedure
- Special stains
- Determinative histochemistry or cytochemistry
- Frozen sections
- Immunohistochemistry
- Immunofluorescent studies, direct or indirect
- Electron microscopy
- Morphometric analysis
- Nerve-teasing preparations
- Tissue in situ hybridization
- Protein analysis of tissue by Western blot

As in coding for gross and microscopic examination of each specimen, a separate code should be used to report each additional service provided. For example, each antibody used in immunohistochemistry study of a specimen should be separately coded as **88342**.

The unit of service for special studies, like the basic gross and microscopic evaluation, is the specimen. As multiple special stains, immunohistochemical antibodies, and molecular probes are coded using the same CPT codes, the unit of service is further categorized appropriately. Hence, special (nonimmunohistochemical) stains are coded per special stain, per specimen; immunohistochemistry is coded per separately identifiable antibody, per specimen; and in situ hybridization is coded per separately identifiable molecular probe, per specimen.

Multiple molecular marker array-based evaluation codes series **88384-88386** is used to report array-based evaluation of multiple molecular probes. Specimens for these evaluations may be blood, fluid, or tissue. The code series encompasses both the professional component to capture the physician work and the technical component to capture the laboratory involvement of the array procedure. Laboratory preparation of the specimen for array-based evaluation should be additionally reported using codes **83890-83892, 83898-83901**. For preparation and analyses of arrays using less than 11 probes, codes **83890-83914** should be reported.

The following table is provided as an alphabetic reference for code assignment for surgical pathology specimens.

## Surgical Pathology Reference Table

| Specimen | Level | Code |
|---|---|---|
| **A** | | |
| Abortion, Induced | III | 88304 |
| Abortion—Spontaneous/Missed | IV | 88305 |
| Abscess | III | 88304 |
| Adrenal, Resection | V | 88307 |
| Aneurysm—Arterial/Ventricular | III | 88304 |
| Anus, Tag | III | 88304 |
| Appendix, Incidental | II | 88302 |
| Appendix, Other Than Incidental | III | 88304 |
| Artery, Atheromatous Plaque | III | 88304 |
| Artery, Biopsy | IV | 88305 |
| **B** | | |
| Bartholin's Gland Cyst | III | 88304 |
| Bone-Biopsy/Curettings | V | 88307 |
| Bone Exostosis | IV | 88305 |
| Bone Fragment(s), Other Than Pathologic Fracture | III | 88304 |
| Bone Fragment(s), Pathologic Fracture | V | 88307 |
| Bone Marrow, Biopsy | IV | 88305 |
| Bone Resection | VI | 88309 |
| Brain, Biopsy | V | 88307 |
| Brain/Meninges, Other Than for Tumor Resection | IV | 88305 |
| Brain/Meninges, Tumor Resection | V | 88307 |
| Breast, Biopsy, Not Requiring Microscopic Evaluation of Surgical Margins | IV | 88305 |
| Breast, Excision of Lesion, Requiring Microscopic Evaluation of Surgical Margins | V | 88307 |
| Breast, Mastectomy—Partial/Simple | V | 88307 |
| Breast, Mastectomy—With Regional Lymph Nodes | VI | 88309 |
| Breast, Reduction Mammoplasty | IV | 88305 |
| Bronchus, Biopsy | IV | 88305 |
| Bursa/Synovial Cyst | III | 88304 |

## Surgical Pathology Reference Table, *continued*

| Specimen | Level | Code |
|---|---|---|
| **C** | | |
| Carpal Tunnel Tissue | III | 88304 |
| Cartilage, Shavings | III | 88304 |
| Cell Block, Any Source | IV | 88305 |
| Cervix, Biopsy | IV | 88305 |
| Cervix, Conization | V | 88307 |
| Cholesteatoma | III | 88304 |
| Colon, Biopsy | IV | 88305 |
| Colon, Colostomy Stoma | III | 88304 |
| Colon, Segmental Resection, Other Than for Tumor | V | 88307 |
| Colon, Segmental Resection for Tumor | VI | 88309 |
| Colon, Total Resection | VI | 88309 |
| Conjunctiva-Biopsy/Pterygium | III | 88304 |
| Cornea | III | 88304 |
| **D** | | |
| Diverticulum-Esophagus/Small Intestine | III | 88304 |
| Duodenum, Biopsy | IV | 88305 |
| Dupuytren's Contracture Tissue | III | 88304 |
| **E** | | |
| Endocervix, Curettings/Biopsy | IV | 88305 |
| Endometrium, Curettings/Biopsy | IV | 88305 |
| Esophagus, Biopsy | IV | 88305 |
| Esophagus, Partial/Total Resection | VI | 88309 |
| Extremity, Amputation, Non-traumatic | V | 88307 |
| Extremity, Amputation, Traumatic | IV | 88305 |
| Extremity, Disarticulation | VI | 88309 |
| Eye, Enucleation | V | 88307 |

## Surgical Pathology Reference Table, *continued*

| Specimen | Level | Code |
|---|---|---|
| **F** | | |
| Fallopian Tube, Biopsy | IV | 88305 |
| Fallopian Tube, Ectopic Pregnancy | IV | 88305 |
| Fallopian Tube, Sterilization | II | 88302 |
| Fetus, With Dissection | VI | 88309 |
| Femoral Head, Fracture | IV | 88305 |
| Femoral Head, Other Than Fracture | III | 88304 |
| Fingers/Toes, Amputation, Non-traumatic | IV | 88305 |
| Fingers/Toes, Amputation, Traumatic | II | 88302 |
| Fissure/Fistula | III | 88304 |
| Foreskin, Newborn | II | 88302 |
| Foreskin, Other Than Newborn | III | 88304 |
| **G** | | |
| Gallbladder | III | 88304 |
| Ganglion Cyst | III | 88304 |
| Gross Examination Only | I | 88300 |
| Gingiva/Oral Mucosa, Biopsy | IV | 88305 |
| **H** | | |
| Heart Valve | IV | 88305 |
| Hematoma | III | 88304 |
| Hemorrhoids | III | 88304 |
| Hernia Sac, Any Location | II | 88302 |
| Hydatid of Morgagni | III | 88304 |
| Hydrocele Sac | II | 88302 |
| **I** | | |
| Intervertebral Disk | III | 88304 |
| **J** | | |
| Joint, Loose Body | III | 88304 |
| Joint, Resection | IV | 88305 |

## Surgical Pathology Reference Table, *continued*

| Specimen | Level | Code |
|---|---|---|
| **K** | | |
| Kidney, Biopsy | IV | 88305 |
| Kidney, Partial/Total Nephrectomy | V | 88307 |
| **L** | | |
| Larynx, Biopsy | IV | 88305 |
| Larynx, Partial/Total Resection | V | 88307 |
| Larynx, Partial/Total Resection—With Regional Lymph Nodes | VI | 88309 |
| Leiomyoma(s), Uterine Myomectomy—Without Uterus | IV | 88305 |
| Lip, Biopsy/Wedge Resection | IV | 88305 |
| Liver, Biopsy—Needle/Wedge | V | 88307 |
| Liver, Partial Resection | V | 88307 |
| Lung, Transbronchial Biopsy | IV | 88305 |
| Lung, Wedge Biopsy | V | 88307 |
| Lung—Total/Lobe/Segment Resection | VI | 88309 |
| Lymph Node, Biopsy | IV | 88305 |
| Lymph Nodes, Regional Resection | V | 88307 |
| **M** | | |
| Meniscus | III | 88304 |
| Mediastinum, Mass | V | 88307 |
| Mucocele, Salivary | III | 88304 |
| Muscle, Biopsy | IV | 88305 |
| Myocardium, Biopsy | V | 88307 |
| **N** | | |
| Nasal Mucosa, Biopsy | IV | 88305 |
| Nasopharynx/Oropharynx, Biopsy | IV | 88305 |
| Nerve | II | 88302 |
| Nerve, Biopsy | IV | 88305 |
| Neuroma—Morton's/Traumatic | III | 88304 |

## Surgical Pathology Reference Table, *continued*

| Specimen | Level | Code |
|---|---|---|
| **O** | | |
| Odontogenic/Dental Cyst | IV | 88305 |
| Odontogenic Tumor | V | 88307 |
| Omentum, Biopsy | IV | 88305 |
| Ovary, Biopsy/Wedge Resection | IV | 88305 |
| Ovary With or Without Tube, Neoplastic | V | 88307 |
| Ovary With or Without Tube, Non-neoplastic | IV | 88305 |
| **P** | | |
| Pancreas, Biopsy | V | 88307 |
| Pancreas, Total/Subtotal Resection | VI | 88309 |
| Parathyroid Gland | IV | 88305 |
| Peritoneum, Biopsy | IV | 88305 |
| Pilonidal Cyst/Sinus | III | 88304 |
| Pituitary Tumor | IV | 88305 |
| Placenta, Other Than Third Trimester | IV | 88305 |
| Placenta, Third Trimester | V | 88307 |
| Pleura/Pericardium-Biopsy/Tissue | IV | 88305 |
| Polyp, Cervical/Endometrial | IV | 88305 |
| Polyp, Colorectal | IV | 88305 |
| Polyp, Stomach/Small Intestine | IV | 88305 |
| Polyps, Inflammatory-Nasal/Sinusoidal | III | 88304 |
| Prostate, Except Radical Resection | V | 88307 |
| Prostate, Needle Biopsy | IV | 88305 |
| Prostate, Radical Resection | VI | 88309 |
| Prostate, Transurethral Resection (TUR) | IV | 88305 |
| **S** | | |
| Salivary Gland | V | 88307 |
| Salivary Gland, Biopsy | IV | 88305 |
| Sentinel Lymph Node | V | 88307 |
| Sinus, Paranasal Biopsy | IV | 88305 |

## Surgical Pathology Reference Table, *continued*

| Specimen | Level | Code |
|---|---|---|
| Skin—Cyst/Tag/Debridement | III | 88304 |
| Skin, Other Than Cyst/Tag/Debridement/Plastic Repair | IV | 88305 |
| Skin, Plastic Repair | II | 88302 |
| Small Intestine, Biopsy | IV | 88305 |
| Small Intestine, Resection, Other Than for Tumor | V | 88307 |
| Small Intestine, Resection for Tumor | VI | 88309 |
| Soft Tissue, Debridement | III | 88304 |
| Soft Tissue, Lipoma | III | 88304 |
| Soft Tissue Mass (Except Lipoma)—Biopsy/Simple Excision | V | 88307 |
| Soft Tissue, Other Than Tumor/Mass/Lipoma/Debridement | IV | 88305 |
| Soft Tissue Tumor, Extensive Resection | VI | 88309 |
| Spermatocele | III | 88304 |
| Spleen | IV | 88305 |
| Stomach, Biopsy | IV | 88305 |
| Stomach—Subtotal/Total Resection for Tumor | VI | 88309 |
| Stomach—Subtotal/Total Resection, Other Than for Tumor | V | 88307 |
| Sympathetic Ganglion | II | 88302 |
| Synovium | IV | 88305 |
| **T** | | |
| Tendon/Tendon Sheath | III | 88304 |
| Testicular Appendage | III | 88304 |
| Testis, Biopsy | V | 88307 |
| Testis, Castration | II | 88302 |
| Testis, Other Than Tumor/Biopsy/Castration | IV | 88305 |
| Testis, Tumor | VI | 88309 |
| Thrombus or Embolus | III | 88304 |
| Thymus, Tumor | V | 88307 |
| Thyroglossal Duct/Branchial Cleft Cyst | IV | 88305 |
| Thyroid, Total/Lobe | V | 88307 |
| Tongue, Biopsy | IV | 88305 |

## Surgical Pathology Reference Table, *continued*

| Specimen | Level | Code |
| --- | --- | --- |
| Tongue/Tonsil—Resection for Tumor | VI | 88309 |
| Tonsil, Biopsy | IV | 88305 |
| Tonsil and/or Adenoids | III | 88304 |
| Trachea, Biopsy | IV | 88305 |
| **U** | | |
| Ureter, Biopsy | IV | 88305 |
| Ureter, Resection | V | 88307 |
| Urethra, Biopsy | IV | 88305 |
| Urinary Bladder, Biopsy | IV | 88305 |
| Urinary Bladder, Partial/Total Resection | VI | 88309 |
| Urinary Bladder, Transurethral Resection (TUR) | V | 88307 |
| Uterus, With or Without Tubes and Ovaries, for Prolapse | IV | 88305 |
| Uterus, With or Without Tubes and Ovaries, Neoplastic | VI | 88309 |
| Uterus, With or Without Tubes and Ovaries, Other Than Neoplastic/Prolapse | V | 88307 |
| **V** | | |
| Vagina, Biopsy | IV | 88305 |
| Vaginal Mucosa, Incidental | II | 88302 |
| Varicocele | III | 88304 |
| Vas Deferens, Sterilization | II | 88302 |
| Vas Deferens, Other Than Sterilization | III | 88304 |
| Vein, Varicosity | III | 88304 |
| Vulva/Labia, Biopsy | IV | 88305 |
| Vulva, Total/Subtotal Resection | VI | 88309 |

## Reproductive Medicine Procedures

In vitro fertilization (IVF) involves a multitude of complex laboratory procedures performed over an interval of one to seven days. These procedures involve both the male and female gametes as well as the subsequent embryos that develop. The CPT code set initially had only one code to describe the laboratory procedures that took place from the time the oocyte was aspirated from the ovary until the embryo was transferred to the uterus or was cryopreserved. Codes in the subsection are intended to describe the many different components of work involved as the variety and complexity of assisted reproductive technology expanded.

Codes in the reproductive medicine subsection are intended to report oocyte/embryo culture and fertilization techniques (**89250**, **89251**, **89268**, **89272**, **89280**, and **89281**); oocyte/embryo biopsy techniques (**89290** and **89291**); and freezing, thawing, and storage techniques (**89258**, **89259**, **89335**, **89342**, **89343**, **89344**, **89346**, **89352**, **89353**, **89354**, and **89356**). These nonphysician procedures are performed in highly specialized clinical laboratories and should be reported separately from additional physician services. Codes **0058T** and **0059T** are intended to be used for reporting cryopreservation of ovarian tissue and oocytes and may apply to the IVF cycle.

## CHAPTER 8

# EXERCISES

**1** Dip stick urinalysis (nonautomated) with microscopy. Assign the appropriate code(s).

**2** Venipuncture. Quantitative therapeutic drugs assay to determine Lanoxin level. Assign the appropriate code(s).

**3** List the appropriate code(s) for reporting a laboratory panel that includes the following tests: carbon dioxide, chloride, potassium, and sodium.

**4** Collection of specimen by arterial puncture for blood gas determination (pH only). Assign the appropriate code(s).

**5** List the appropriate code(s) for reporting a laboratory panel that includes the following tests: calcium, carbon dioxide, chloride, creatinine, glucose potassium, sodium, and urea nitrogen (BUN).

**6** A segment of sigmoid colon is sent to the pathologist intraoperatively for immediate diagnosis. The pathologist examines the specimen and renders an intraoperative pathological diagnosis without subjecting any of the tissue to microscopic examination. How would the pathologist's intraoperative service be coded?

**7** A laryngectomy specimen is sent to the pathologist intraoperatively for immediate diagnosis with respect to involvement of resection margins by tumor. The pathologist examines the tissue and selects portions of the margins resulting in four blocks for frozen sections, which are then examined microscopically. How would the pathologist's intraoperative services be coded?

**8** True or False: If a specimen is submitted for frozen section and permanent sections are performed following frozen section examination, it would be appropriate to report both services separately.

**9** Three endoscopic biopsies are submitted from a colonoscopy. Each is in a separate container that is identified as to origin (hepatic flexure, descending colon, and rectum). Assign the appropriate surgical pathology code(s).

**10** A hysterectomy is performed for leiomyoma (benign neoplasm). The uterus containing leiomyomas is submitted in one container; for ease of resection only, the surgeon separately removes the ovaries and fallopian tubes. The right tube and ovary are separately identified in a second container; the left tube and ovary are separately identified in a third container. A fourth container is also received that contains the vermiform appendix. Assign the appropriate surgical pathology code(s).

**11**  What are the appropriate code(s) for reporting automated thin layer preparation techniques for cervical or vaginal smears?

**12**  True or False: It is appropriate to report code **80053**, even if all of the tests listed in the panel definition are not performed.

**13**  True or False: Codes **85025** and **85027** include an automated RBC count.

**14**  True or False: The CPT Nomenclature lists the generic (nonproprietary) names of drugs whenever possible.

**15**  To aid in clarifying a patient's prognosis and treatment options, the clinician orders comparative genomic hybridization array on the marrow for a patient diagnosed with multiple myeloma. Anticoagulated marrow aspirate is submitted to the laboratory for gene dosage testing at 300 different chromosomal loci using commercial reagents that have been previously analytically validated in the clinical laboratory. What is the correct code assignment (**88385** or **88386**) for the array-based evaluation of 300 different chromosomal loci using commercial reagents that have been previously analytically validated in the clinical laboratory?

# CHAPTER 9

# Medicine

The Medicine section of the Current Procedural Terminology (CPT®) codebook contains a variety of listings for reporting procedures and services provided by many different types of health care providers. In addition, many services and procedures provided by nonphysician practitioners can be found in the Medicine section. For example, codes in the Physical Medicine and Rehabilitation subsections are often used to report the services and procedures provided by physical and occupational therapists. Audiologists and speech-language pathologists find listings in the Special Otorhinolaryngologic Services subsection that describes some of the procedures and services they provide.

While the Medicine section is a single section, like the Surgery section, it contains many subsections to enable the user of CPT codes to more easily find the codes for the services that are to be described. Notice that there are two basic types of subsections: those that are procedure-oriented and those that refer to particular medical specialties. It is very important to remember that the codes in a "specialty" subsection, like gastroenterology, are not limited to use by gastroenterologists alone. Any qualified physician or, as appropriate, qualified health care professional may use any code in the CPT codebook. The performance of the services is regulated by state practice acts for the various professions and is not determined by the American Medical Association (AMA) or the CPT codebook.

The following table provides a summary of the subsections and associated code ranges available in the Medicine section of the CPT codebook.

## Medicine Subsections and Code Ranges

| Subsection | Code Range |
|---|---|
| Immune Globulins | 90281-90399 |
| Immunization Administration for Vaccines/Toxoids | 90465-90474 |
| Vaccines, Toxoids | 90476-90749 |
| Hydration | 90760-90779 |
| Therapeutic, Prophylactic, and Diagnostic Injections and Infusions | 90765-90779 |
| Injections, and Infusions (Excludes Chemotherapy) | 90760-90779 |
| Psychiatry | 90801-90899 |
| Biofeedback | 90901-90911 |
| Dialysis | 90918-90999 |
| Gastroenterology | 91000-91299 |
| Ophthalmology | 92002-92499 |
| Special Otorhinolaryngologic Services | 92502-92700 |
| Cardiovascular | 92950-93799 |
| Noninvasive Vascular Diagnostic Studies | 93875-93990 |
| Pulmonary | 94010-94799 |
| Allergy and Clinical Immunology | 95004-95199 |
| Endocrinology | 95250-95251 |
| Neurology and Neuromuscular Procedures | 95805-96004 |
| Medical Genetics and Genetic Counseling Services | 96040 |
| Central Nervous System Assessments/Tests (eg, Neuro-Cognitive, Mental Status, Speech Testing) | 96101-96120 |
| Health and Behavior Assessment/Intervention | 96150-96155 |
| Chemotherapy Administration | 96401-96549 |
| Photodynamic Therapy | 96567-96571 |
| Special Dermatological Procedures | 96900-96999 |
| Physical Medicine and Rehabilitation | 97001-97799 |
| Medical Nutrition Therapy | 97802-97804 |
| Acupuncture | 97810-97814 |
| Osteopathic Manipulative Treatment | 98925-98929 |
| Chiropractic Manipulative Treatment | 98940-98943 |
| Education and Training for Patient Self-Management | 98960-98962 |

| Medicine Subsections and Code Ranges, *continued* | |
| --- | --- |
| **Subsection** | **Code Range** |
| Special Services, Procedures, and Reports . . . . . . . . . . . . . . . . . . . . . . . | 99000-99091 |
| Qualifying Circumstances for Anesthesia . . . . . . . . . . . . . . . . . . . . . . . | 99100-99140 |
| Moderate (Conscious) Sedation . . . . . . . . . . . . . . . . . . . . . . . . . . . . . | 99143-99150 |
| Other Services and Procedures . . . . . . . . . . . . . . . . . . . . . . . . . . . . . | 99170-99199 |
| Home Health Procedures/Services . . . . . . . . . . . . . . . . . . . . . . . . . . . | 99500-99600 |

Like the other sections of the CPT codebook, the Medicine section contains specific guidelines that are necessary to appropriately interpret and report the procedures and services contained in that section. The text that follows will focus on various guidelines and codes for reporting the following services and procedures:

- Immunizations
- Hydration, therapeutic, prophylactic, and diagnostic injections and infusions
- Psychiatry
- Dialysis
- Gastroenterology
- Ophthalmology
- Special otorhinolaryngologic services
- Cardiovascular services
- Noninvasive vascular diagnostic studies
- Pulmonary
- Allergy and clinical immunology
- Endocrinology
- Neurology and neuromuscular procedures
- Medical genetics and genetic counseling services
- Health and behavior assessment/intervention
- Chemotherapy administration
- Photodynamic therapy
- Special dermatological procedures
- Physical medicine and rehabilitation
- Medical nutrition therapy
- Acupuncture
- Osteopathic manipulative treatment
- Chiropractic manipulative treatment
- Education and training for patient self-management
- Special services, procedures, and reports
- Moderate (conscious) sedation
- Home health procedures/services
- Home infusion procedures/services

# Immunizations

Immunizations are a major part of health care in the United States. It is recommended that all children receive routine immunizations according to the immunization schedule endorsed by the Advisory Committee on Immunization

Practices, the American Academy of Pediatrics (AAP), and the American Academy of Family Physicians. In addition, immunizations are advised for older adults and travelers.

In recent years, vaccine development has become very active, resulting in many new and combination vaccines, while various formulations and dosages of existing vaccines are also being made available. These changes and complexities are important considerations in immunization coding.

Certain carrier-specific policies may require reporting on a "per milliliter" (mL) basis, because currently the vaccine is produced in a specific formulation (ie, 20 $\mu$g/mL). Therefore, a 40-microgram ($\mu$g) dose requires 2 mL of vaccine to deliver the 40-$\mu$g dose. However, the administration of the 40-$\mu$g dose could be reported in different ways, depending on the carrier's claim reporting recognition of the units box. For example, a dialysis patient on a four-dose schedule is given 40 $\mu$g of hepatitis B vaccine, administered in a single intramuscular injection. In this instance, code **90471** is reported once and code **90747** is reported once.

As a further example, if the 40-$\mu$g dose was administered in two separate injections, code **90471** should be reported for the first injection and **90472** should be reported for the second injection. Code **90747** would be reported once, as stated previously.

To achieve the goal of uniformity and standardization in immunization reporting systems, the CPT codes have been restructured and expanded to be more usable and adaptable to today's changing environment. The AMA, in conjunction with the Centers for Disease Control and Prevention National Immunization Program and independent physicians in private practice, has worked to structure the CPT codes to support current and future reporting requirements for immunizations.

To assist users to report the most recent new or revised vaccine product codes, the AMA currently uses the CPT Web site, which features updates of CPT Editorial Panel actions regarding these products. Once approved by the CPT Editorial Panel, these codes will be made available for release on a semiannual (twice a year: July 1 and January 1) basis. As part of the electronic distribution there is a six-month implementation period from the initial release date (ie, codes released on January 1 are eligible for use on July 1, and codes released on July 1 are eligible for use January 1).

The CPT Editorial Panel, in recognition of the public health interest in vaccine products, has chosen to publish new vaccine product codes prior to Food and Drug Administration (FDA) approval. These codes are indicated with a $\nearrow$ symbol and will be tracked by the AMA to monitor FDA approval status. Once the FDA status changes to approved, the symbol will be removed. CPT users should refer to the AMA Internet site (www.ama-assn.org/ama/pub/category/ 10902.html) for the most up-to-date information on codes with the $\nearrow$ symbol.

## Immune Globulins

Codes **90281-90399** are used to report immune globulins. These codes identify the immune globulin product itself and the route of administration (eg, intramuscular, intravenous [IV]) and reflect dosage and formulation differences where applicable. An additional code from the Hydration, Therapeutic,

Prophylactic, and Diagnostic Injections, and Infusions subsection is required for reporting the administration of the immune globulin product. The appropriate administration code (**90765-90768**, **90772**, **90774**, **90775**) is reported separately in addition to the code for the immune globulin. The specific code selected should correspond with the route of administration.

## Immunization Administration for Vaccines/Toxoids

Codes **90465-90468** are reported for immunization administration and incorporate the work of physician immunization counseling for young children (under eight years of age). The majority of vaccines are mandated for early childhood when reactions can be both more frequent and more severe. Children react differently to vaccines because of the physiologic differences inherent in developing brains, with associated neurological events such as seizures and sequelae of an encephalopathic nature. The increased attention to claims of associated developmental problems and risks related to vaccines has increased families' concerns and the need for physician counseling prior to administration. Also, since many vaccines are mandated, physicians often spend additional time counseling those families who choose not to immunize their children.

Report codes **90465-90468** only when the physician provides face-to-face counseling of the patient and family during the administration of a vaccine. For immunization administration of any vaccine that is not accompanied by face-to-face physician counseling to the patient/family, report codes **90471-90474**.

Codes **90471-90474** are used to report the administration of vaccines/toxoids. These codes include percutaneous, intradermal, subcutaneous, and intramuscular injections and/or intranasal or oral administration. Code **90471** is reported for the percutaneous, intradermal, subcutaneous, or intramuscular immunization administration of one vaccine or toxoid (a single or combination vaccine/toxoid). Code **90472** is an add-on code, reported for the percutaneous, intradermal, subcutaneous, or intramuscular administration of each additional vaccine product (single or combination vaccine/toxoid). Code **90473** is reported for the intranasal or oral immunization administration of one vaccine or toxoid (a single or combination vaccine/toxoid). Code **90474** is an add-on code, reported for the intranasal or oral immunization administration of each additional vaccine product (single or combination vaccine/toxoid).

The codes for immunization administration (**90465-90474**) must be reported in addition to the vaccine and toxoid code(s) **90476-90749**. Separating the administration codes **90465-90474** from the vaccine product helps address the reporting of vaccines administered free of charge under state and national public health programs (eg, Vaccines for Children Program). When vaccines are provided free of charge, a zero dollar amount is indicated as the charge for the CPT vaccine/toxoid code, and the administration fees are reported separately with codes **90465-90474**. By using this method, important data collection is preserved by specifically identifying the vaccine administered, while distinguishing the service from those typically associated with the expense of purchasing and storing the vaccine. Codes **90476-90749** identify the vaccine/toxoid product only. These codes identify the complete generic vaccine name and recommended route(s) of administration. Only the generic names are used in CPT descriptor language. If you are unfamiliar with a specific manufacturer's vaccine trade name, a reference such as the *Physician's Desk Reference* that lists trade and generic vaccine names may prove invaluable.

There are often questions concerning the reporting of evaluation and management (E/M) services performed during the same visit when vaccines are administered in the office. The answer always depends on whether the provider performs a medically necessary and significant, separately identifiable E/M visit in addition to the immunization administration. If such a service is performed, an E/M code is reported, most likely from the **99201-99215** code family (office or other outpatient services), in addition to the appropriate code for immunization administration (**90465-90474**) plus the code for the vaccine product(s). In such cases, payers may require that modifier 25, Significant, Separately Identifiable Evaluation and Management Service by the Same Physician on the Same Day of the Procedure or Other Service, be appended to the E/M code to distinguish it from the actual administration of the vaccine.

The identification of a significant, separately identifiable service for E/M codes usually involves the performance and documentation of the "key components" (ie, history, physical examination, and medical decision making) or when time may be considered the key or controlling factor to qualify for a particular level of E/M service (ie, when counseling and/or coordination of care dominates more than 50% of the physician/patient and/or family encounter). However, the reporting of code **99211** is unique among E/M codes in having no key component requirements. The CPT descriptor for code **99211** states, "Office or other outpatient visit for the evaluation and management of an established patient, that may not require the presence of a physician. Usually, the presenting problem(s) are minimal. Typically, 5 minutes are spent performing or supervising these services." Therefore, how this concept is defined when the E/M code in question is **99211** needs further clarification.

To address this issue, it becomes important to determine:
- What services are included in the immunization administration codes?
- What additional services are required in order to appropriately report code **99211**?
- What are the documentation requirements for code **99211**?

## What Services are Included in the Immunization Administration Codes?

The following services are included in the immunization administration codes:
- Administrative staff services such as making the appointment, preparing the patient chart, billing for the service, and filing the chart
- Clinical staff services such as greeting the patient, taking routine vital signs, obtaining a vaccine history on past reactions and contraindications, presenting a Vaccine Information Sheet (VIS) and answering routine vaccine questions, preparing and administering the vaccine with chart documentation, and observing for any immediate reaction

The injectable immunization administration codes' relative value units (RVUs) were significantly increased in 2005. This increase accounted for the fact that many of the services noted earlier that were previously reported separately with code **99211** are now included in the immunization administration codes. For updated information on the new RVUs for the vaccine administration codes, please visit the Centers for Medicare and Medicaid Services (CMS) Web site at www.cms.hhs.gov.

### What Additional Services Are Required in Order to Appropriately Report Code 99211?

In addition to the fact that the E/M service must exceed those services included in the immunization administration codes, the service must be separate and significant from the immunization administration.

When the provider (typically a nurse) evaluates, manages, and documents the significant and separate complaint(s) or problem(s), the additional reporting of code **99211** is justified. In such circumstances, the nurse typically conducts a brief history and record review, along with a physical assessment (eg, indicated vital signs and observations) and provides patient education in helping the family or patient manage the problem encountered. These nursing activities are all directly related to the significant, separate complaint, and unrelated to the actual vaccine administration.

### What Are the Documentation Requirements for Code 99211?

All reported E/M codes must meet documentation requirements as outlined in CPT guidelines or in the CMS Documentation Guidelines. For most of the E/M services that physicians perform, this means that some designated combination of the key components of history, physical examination, and medical decision making must be met and clearly documented. Alternatively, if greater than 50% of the time spent during the E/M service is spent in counseling or coordinating care, time becomes the key, or controlling factor, in selecting a code.

Code **99211** is the one E/M service typically provided by the nurse and not the physician. As such, its documentation requirements differ. There are no required key components typical of the physician services noted previously. Further, the typical time published in the CPT codebook for code **99211** is five minutes. According to the AAP, it is beneficial to document the date of service and reason for the visit, a brief history of any significant problems evaluated or managed, any examination elements (eg, vital signs or appearance of a rash), a brief assessment and/or plan along with any counseling or patient education done, and signatures of the nurse and supervising physician.

While not required, it may help payers to better understand the medical necessity of the nurse E/M service if it is linked to a different (ICD-9-CM) code than the one used for the vaccine given, when appropriate. Further, encounter documentation should be a separate entry from the charting of the vaccine itself (product, lot number, site and method, VIS date, etc, which are all usually recorded on the immunization history sheet). Each practice should consider developing protocols and progress note templates for vaccine services.

Most "nurse" E/M services are carried out under a protocol of orders developed by the physician for the particular service and should be fully documented in the record. As always, the physician supervising the care should sign the chart entry.

Completion of a vaccination regimen is used to measure the clinic's performance for quality improvement, Health Plan Employer Data and Information Set, and other purposes. There are two schedules of administration of hepatitis B vaccine currently licensed in the United States for the dialysis or immunocompromised population: three-dose and four-dose. If only one code is used to report the administration of a dose, it would not be possible to tell whether a patient receiving three doses had completed a three-dose schedule or was incomplete for a four-dose schedule. Two codes specifying the dosing schedule will make the codes more useful for this purpose.

The codes for vaccines for hepatitis B are specific for the patient population and the schedule of administration. They do not specify the dose that must be given or the formulation. Those details are determined by the FDA license for the specific vaccine and are stated in the package insert. It is the physician's responsibility to follow the appropriate recommendations outlined. To determine which code to report, it is first necessary to determine which patient population the patient fits into (ie, child, adolescent, adult, or dialysis/ immunocompromised).

If the patient is in the category of dialysis or immunocompromised, the next question to answer is, "What is the schedule of administration for the specific vaccine given?" For example, certain dialysis formulations are administered on a three-dose schedule. The only code for the hepatitis B vaccine used in the dialysis or immunocompromised dosage on a three-dose schedule is code **90740**.

By comparison, the adult formulations are licensed to be given on a four-dose schedule for the dialysis or immunocompromised population, so it would be appropriate to report code **90747**, which specifies four-dose schedule and the administration code **90471**.

Consistent with the other vaccine codes, the administration code **90471**, Immunization administration (includes percutaneous, intradermal, subcutaneous, or intramuscular injections); one vaccine (single or combination vaccine/toxoid), is additionally reportable and not considered inclusive of either code **90740** or **90747**. Also consistent with the other vaccine codes, the descriptors of codes **90740** and **90747** do not indicate the micrograms/milliliters that must be given or the formulation. There has also been some confusion that codes **90747** and **90740** are reported one time to represent the total three/four-dose regimen. Codes **90747** and **90740** are reported for each dose administered according to the three- and four-dose regimen.

Multiple vaccine codes for the same vaccine were created to account for the following situations:

- When the schedule (number of doses or timing) differs for two or more products of the same vaccine type
- When one manufacturer makes more than one dosage or chemical formulation of the same vaccine type
- When both oral and parenteral (injectable) formulations of the same vaccine type are available

**CODING TIP**

A single-dose vial contains a single dose of antigen administered in one injection.

**CODING TIP**

What constitutes a dose? For allergy immunotherapy reporting, a dose is the amount of antigen(s) administered in a single injection from a multiple-dose vial.

When applicable, the common abbreviation, chemical formulation, and product dosage are reflected in the code descriptor. This degree of specificity in the vaccine/toxoid codes is intended to facilitate correct coding and enable physicians to comply with the various reporting requirements of immunization registries and programs.

Additionally, some of the language in the code descriptors serves as educational reminders. For example, the route of administration component of the vaccine codes could potentially prevent a patient from receiving an ineffective subcutaneous dose of hepatitis B vaccine. Also, the word "live" in the code descriptor (eg, poliovirus vaccine, live, oral) serves as a reminder of certain circumstances where live vaccines are contraindicated for patients.

Combination vaccines are also called *conjugate vaccines*. These vaccines combine two or more types of vaccine in one vial and are prepared by the manufacturer in this way. If a combination vaccine is provided (eg, diphtheria-tetanus-pertussis-Haemophilus influenza b [DTP-Hib]), it is not appropriate to report each component of the combination vaccine separately, as there are specific codes available for combination vaccines. For example, if the combination vaccine DTP-Hib was provided, then only CPT code **90720**, Diphtheria, tetanus toxoids, and whole cell pertussis vaccine and Haemophilus influenza B vaccine (DTP-Hib), for intramuscular use, would be reported. It would not be appropriate to report two separate codes, one for DTP and one for Hib, as there is a specific code that describes the combination vaccine. Sometimes, even though a combination vaccine may be commercially available, the physician or clinic may not have access to it or, for other clinical reasons, choose to administer the component vaccines as individual immunizations. In this instance, report each vaccine administered.

If there is no specific code that accurately describes the combination vaccine, the unlisted vaccine/toxoid code (**90749**) should be reported until a new code is available in the CPT codebook.

# Hydration, Therapeutic, Prophylactic, and Diagnostic Injections, and Infusions (Excludes Chemotherapy)

The drug administration codes are grouped into two categories: (1) hydration; and (2) therapeutic, prophylactic, and diagnostic injections and infusions.

The guidelines for the Hydration, Therapeutic, Prophylactic, and Diagnostic Injections and Infusions (Excludes Chemotherapy) subsection include definitions for the expected physician activity for reporting these codes and the requirements for reporting a separate E/M service. As indicated in the guidelines, "When administering multiple infusions, injections or combinations, only one 'initial' service code should be reported, unless protocol requires that two separate IV sites must be used. The 'initial' code that best describes the key or primary reason for the encounter should always be reported irrespective of the order in which the infusions or injections occur. If an injection or infusion is of a subsequent or concurrent nature, even if it is the first such service within that group of services, then a subsequent or concurrent code from the appropriate

**CODING TIP**

When fluids are used to administer the drug(s), the administration of the fluid is considered incidental hydration and is not reported separately.

**CODING TIP**

An initial service code is chosen irrespective of the order in which the infusions or injections occur. The primary service is key.

section should be reported (eg, the first IV push given subsequent to an initial one-hour infusion is reported using a subsequent IV push code)."

The guidelines for the Hydration, Therapeutic, Prophylactic, and Diagnostic Injections and Infusions (Excludes Chemotherapy) subsection define and list the services that are included, and therefore not separately reported, including the use of local anesthesia; IV start, access to indwelling IV, subcutaneous catheter or port; flush at conclusion of infusion, and standard tubing, syringes; and supplies. Users are instructed to report code **36550** for declotting a catheter or port.

Definition of the intent of the references to time (one hour, each additional hour) in the code descriptors is also provided in the guidelines. This definition indicates that when reporting codes for which infusion time is a factor, the actual time over which the infusion is administered should be used. This is because the time required for the infusion was used to define the range of services included in the infusion within the Hydration, Therapeutic, Prophylactic, and Diagnostic Injections and Infusions codes. Services leading up to the infusion and to conclude the infusion have been included in these services and are not separately reported. These services will include starting the IV and monitoring the patient postinfusion. Therefore, infusion time is calculated when administration commences (ie, the infusion starts dripping).

## Hydration Services

Hydration services are reported with codes **90760** and **90761**. As indicated in the Hydration guidelines, codes **90760** and **90761** are intended to report a hydration IV infusion to consist of a prepackaged fluid and electrolyte solutions (eg, normal saline, D5-1/2 normal saline + 30mEq KC1/L), but are not used to report infusion of drugs or other substances. Hydration IV infusions typically require direct physician supervision for purposes of consent, safety oversight, or intraservice supervision of staff. Typically, such infusions require little special handling to prepare or dispose of, and staff who administer these do not typically require advanced training. After initial setup, infusion typically entails little patient risk and thus little monitoring.

Codes **90760** and **90761** are intended to report IV infusions of prepackaged fluid and electrolytes but are not used to report infusion of drugs or other substances. Code **90760** is an initial service. Code **90761** is reported for hydration lasting beyond 1 hour and 30 minutes. Code **90761** is an add-on code that can be reported as a secondary service. More than 30 minutes of hydration in each subsequent hour must occur in order to report **90761** as a secondary or subsequent service. If hydration is an integral part of the drug administration, it should not be separately reported.

## Therapeutic, Prophylactic, and Diagnostic Injections and Infusions

The therapeutic, prophylactic, and diagnostic injections and infusions codes are used to report the administration of substances/drugs and are differentiated according to the route of administration (IV, intramuscular, intra-arterial,

**CODING TIP**

Only one "initial" drug administration code per encounter should be reported, unless the protocol requires that two separate IV sites must be used.

**CODING TIP**

Preparation of chemotherapy agent(s) is included in the service for administration of the agent. For example, mixing of chemotherapy drugs before administration is not separately reported, as this is included in the chemotherapy administration.

**CODING TIP**

Refilling and maintenance of portable pumps includes chemotherapy, narcotic pumps, and insulin pumps.

subcutaneous) and the injection status (initial, sequential, concurrent). When fluids are used to administer the drug(s), the administration of the fluid is considered incidental hydration and is not separately reported. These services typically require direct physician supervision for any or all purposes of patient assessment, provision of consent, safety oversight, and intraservice supervision of staff.

When administering multiple infusions, injections or combinations, only one initial service code should be reported, unless protocol requires that two separate IV sites must be used. The initial code that best describes the key or primary reason for the encounter should always be reported, irrespective of the order in which the infusions or injections occur. If an injection is of a subsequent or concurrent nature, even if it is the first such service within that group of services, a subsequent or concurrent code from the appropriate section should be reported (eg, the first IV push given subsequent to an initial one-hour infusion is reported using a subsequent IV push code).

A concurrent injection/infusion is the service in which multiple infusions are provided simultaneously through the same multiple-lumen catheter. Multiple substances mixed in one bag are considered to be one infusion and reported as a concurrent infusion. Each substance can be reported separately, but only one administration is reported.

A sequential infusion is considered to be an infusion of a different drug administered immediately following the initial infusion. Therefore, the sequential infusion within the category of infusions is appropriately reported in addition to any one of the initial infusion services reported with codes **90765**, **90775**, **96409**, and **96413**. Sequential infusion codes are reported one time only for the same infusate. Therefore, an infusion consisting of three substances in a single bag is not intended to be reported as three separate infusion services, as the parenteral administration codes are intended to report the separate work of administration access and not the inclusion of multiple agents in a bag prepared prior to access.

Different infusates can be reported with the same code as the original sequential code. However, additional hours required for infusion of the same infusate are reported with the add-on "each additional hour" infusion code of the same code series. In the instance where an anti-emetic drug was provided over a 1 hour and 15 minute IV infusion, following the initiation of a chemotherapy infusion over a 1 hour and 15 minute IV infusion, followed during the same treatment session by an IV push of the same anti-emetic drug, three codes would be reported. The initial chemotherapy drug infusion code **96413** would be reported, followed by the sequential IV infusion code **90767**, and the additional sequential IV push code **90775** for the new substance.

IV infusion therapy services are reported with codes **90765-90768**. Code **90765** is reported for an initial IV infusion up to one hour in duration for therapy (eg, pain management), prophylaxis (vaccine), or diagnosis (administration of the evocative or suppressive agents). Code **90767** is reported for an infusion of a second substance up to one hour in duration following the initial infusion in which the lines are flushed after the first infusion. An exclusionary cross-reference instructs that this code is reported only once for the same infusate mix and that code **90767** is reported for any infusion of a secondary or subsequent service or up to one hour in duration in addition to the initial infusion/injection codes **90765**, **90775**, **96409**, and **96413**.

Code **90768** is an add-on code reported for IV infusion into a multilumen catheter at the time of the initial infusion. As indicated in the exclusionary cross-reference, code **90768** is reported only once per encounter. Code **90768** is reported in addition to codes **90765**, **90766**, **96413**, **96415**, **96416**, **96422**, and **96423**.

Additional infusion hours are reported with add-on code **90766**. Code **90766** is reported one time for each one-hour IV infusion interval of greater than 30 minutes beyond a one-hour increment in addition to the base service codes **90765** and **90767** for initial and sequential IV infusion. As indicated in the guidelines, an IV push is defined as (1) an injection in which the health care professional who administers the substance/drug is continuously present to administer the injection and observe the patient or (2) an infusion of 15 minutes or less. It is not appropriate to report codes **90765-90779** with codes for which IV push or infusion is an inherent part of the procedure.

Short infusions that do not require continuous attendance should be reported as an injection. Code **90772** is reported for the performance of subcutaneous or intramuscular push injections. Cross-references for code **90772** indicate that (1) this code is reported for non-antineoplastic hormonal therapy injections and direct the user to code **96401** for antineoplastic hormonal therapy injections; (2) this code is reported for injections given with direct physician supervision, and code **99211** is reported for unsupervised injections; and (3) codes **90465-90466**, **90471-90472** are reported for administration of vaccines or toxoids.

Code **90773** is reported for the performance of intra-arterial push injections. Codes **90774** and **90775** are reported for the performance of IV push injections: code **90774** for the single or initial injection, and add-on code **90775** for each additional sequential IV push of a new substance/drug. A cross-reference instructs that code **90775** is reported in addition to any of the initial services described by codes **90765**, **90774**, **96409**, and **96413** and a second cross-reference supports the description of code **90775** as a subsequent service to these initial services. Code **90775** is not reported for IV push injection of additional agents in the same syringe. In the instance where the service consists of administration of only one syringe containing three nonchemotherapy drugs over 15 minutes, the single injection/substance IV push code **90774** would be reported one time only.

# Psychiatry

Codes in the **90801-90899** series are used to report various psychiatric services and procedures specifically related to medical management and are separate from the diagnostic, evaluative, and therapeutic procedures usually provided. Hospital care services involve a variety of responsibilities unique to the medical management of inpatients, such as physician hospital orders, interpretation of laboratory or other medical and psychological diagnostic studies, and observation.

Hospital care by the attending clinician in treating a mental health patient in an inpatient or partial hospital setting may be initial or subsequent in nature and may include exchanges with nursing and ancillary personnel. Partial hospitalization and intensive outpatient treatment involve services provided to patients who spend a portion or the majority of a day in a hospital setting but return to their homes or places of residence during the 24-hour day, returning to the hospital on the following day. Most of these settings operate on a five-day week, although there are settings that operate on a seven-day week. The partial hospital setting functions in the same fashion as a hospital in that the clinician is required to take a history and perform an examination, as well as write progress notes and a discharge summary. These services are similar to those a physician performs in a traditional hospital setting, where the patient remains throughout the 24-hour day.

The consultation codes from the E/M section of the CPT codebook may also be used to describe services provided. Consultations for evaluation of a patient include examination of the patient, exchange of information with the requesting physician and other informants such as nurses or family members, and preparation of a report. The consultation services codes are limited to initial or follow-up evaluation and do not involve psychiatric treatment. (Refer to Chapter 3 for further discussion of coding for consultative services.)

Some patients receive only hospital E/M services, while others receive E/M services and other procedures. If other procedures such as electroconvulsive therapy or psychotherapy are rendered in addition to hospital E/M services, these should be listed separately, eg, hospital care service plus electroconvulsive therapy or, when psychotherapy is done, an appropriate code defining psychotherapy with medical E/M services.

**CODING TIP**

For Mini-Mental Status Examination performed by a physician, see E/M service codes.

## Psychiatric Diagnostic or Evaluative Interview Procedures

Codes **90801** and **90802** are used to report psychiatric diagnostic interview examinations. A psychiatric diagnostic interview examination includes a history, mental status, and a disposition and may include communication with family or other sources. It may also include ordering and medical interpretation of laboratory or other medical diagnostic studies. In certain circumstances, other informants may be seen in lieu of the patient.

An interactive psychiatric diagnostic interview examination is typically furnished to children or other individuals with communication disorders. It involves the use of physical aids (eg, play materials) and nonverbal communication to overcome barriers to therapeutic interaction between the clinician and a patient who has not yet developed or has lost either the expressive language communication skills to explain his or her symptoms and response to treatment or the receptive communication skills to understand the clinician if he or she were to use ordinary adult language for communication. Physical aids used for interactive psychotherapy might include play materials such as puppets, dolls/dollhouse, animals, blocks, and vehicles, as well as other materials such as coloring materials, paper, and modeling clay. It could also include having an interpreter present to assist the clinician in communicating with a deaf patient.

The clinician elicits a complete medical and mental health history (from the patient and/or family), establishes a tentative diagnosis of the patient, and evaluates the patient's capacity to work psychotherapeutically.

The clinician also assesses the ability to establish a therapeutic alliance with the patient. This assessment allows the practitioner to evaluate the presenting problems/conditions to determine if psychopathology is present. The mental health history and general history may overlap. For example, the clinician may inquire about the chief complaint, history of present illness, family history, past personal history, sexual history, or medical history, depending on the informant (patient and/or family member).

The mental status examination focuses on the patient's condition during the interview. The psychiatric diagnostic interview examination includes a complete mental status examination and is not limited to problem areas. The clinician is looking for symptoms of psychopathology in the patient's general appearance, attitude toward the examiner, and overall behavior. In addition, the speech and stream of talk, emotional reaction and mood, perception, thought content, cognition, and potential for danger may be evaluated. The patient's condition determines the extent of this initial mental status examination.

The psychiatric diagnostic interview examination codes are used primarily during the initial phases of treatment. Frequently, in facility-based treatment, an E/M service or consultation code will be reported instead of the psychiatric diagnostic interview examination. If the clinician were unable to perform the psychiatric diagnostic interview examination at the initial encounter because of the patient's mental or physical condition, a code would be selected for the initial encounter specifically on the basis of what services/procedure the clinician provided.

## Psychiatric Therapeutic Procedures

Psychotherapy is the treatment for mental illness and behavioral disturbances in which the clinician establishes a professional contact with the patient related to resolution of the patient's problems and, through definitive therapeutic communication, attempts to alleviate the emotional disturbances, reverse or change maladaptive patterns of behavior, and support personality growth and development.

A patient receiving psychotherapy may also receive separate counseling related to areas such as laboratory findings, drug reactions, or treatment options. This counseling is separate and distinct from psychotherapy provided to treat mental illness. (Refer to Chapter 3 for further discussion of counseling as it pertains to E/M coding.)

Psychotherapy may be provided in many different settings. In the CPT codebook, two distinct categories are identified on the basis of the place of service: Office or Other Outpatient Facility (**90804-90815**) or Inpatient Hospital, Partial Hospital, or Residential Care Facility (**90816-90829**).

Outpatient settings include services provided in the clinician's office or in an outpatient or other ambulatory facility. In the residential care setting, the milieu is set up so that the patient lives in a more constructive and mentally healthy environment. The patient will usually attend school or obtain vocational training at the level that his or her abilities allow and will participate in group therapies, individual therapies, and adjunctive therapies (e.g., occupational therapy, specific behavioral therapies, movement therapies, music therapy, art therapy, etc.). As in the partial hospital setting and inpatient hospital setting, the physician in the residential care center is responsible for a psychiatric history, mental status examination, and the performance or supervision of a physical examination.

Within each setting category there are codes for insight-oriented, behavior-modifying, and/or supportive psychotherapy (**90804-90809**, **90816-90822**), and codes for interactive psychotherapy (**90810-90815**, **90823-90829**). Each family of codes is further divided according to the face-to-face time spent with the patient and whether E/M services are furnished in addition to psychotherapy: Insight-oriented, behavior-modifying, and/or supportive psychotherapy (**90804-90809**, **90816-90822**) and Interactive psychotherapy (**90810-90815**, **90823-90829**).

Insight-oriented, behavior-modifying, and/or supportive psychotherapy refers to the use of insight or affective understanding, behavior modification techniques, supportive interactions, or cognitive interventions or any combination of these to provide therapeutic change.

Some patients receive only psychotherapy, and others receive psychotherapy and medical E/M services. These E/M services involve a variety of responsibilities unique to the medical management of psychiatric patients. The medical management may include such services as a medical diagnostic evaluation (eg, evaluation of comorbid medical conditions, drug interactions, physical examinations), drug management when indicated, physician orders, interpretation of laboratory or other medical diagnostic studies, and observations. Each of the psychotherapy codes has an associated code to identify the provision of E/M services on the same day as psychotherapy.

If E/M services are provided on a day when psychotherapy is provided, the appropriate code for psychotherapy with medical E/M services should be reported. The following is an example of a psychotherapy-only code with its associated E/M services code. Each code describes the same type and length of psychotherapy. The difference between the two codes is the provision of E/M services in addition to the psychotherapy.

**90806**    Individual psychotherapy, insight oriented, behavior modifying and/or supportive, in an office or outpatient facility, approximately 45 to 50 minutes face-to-face with the patient;

**90807**    with medical evaluation and management services

With these codes, the appropriate code for psychotherapy with medical E/M services should be reported. Therefore, E/M services should not be reported separately when codes **90805-90829** are reported for services performed by the same provider on the same day.

If E/M services are provided on a day when psychotherapy is not provided, then the appropriate code from the E/M section of the CPT codebook should be reported. (Refer to Chapter 3 for further discussion of E/M coding.)

When reporting psychotherapy, select the appropriate code on the basis of the following:

- The place of service (office or other outpatient facility vs inpatient hospital, partial hospital, or residential care facility)
- The type of psychotherapy provided (insight-oriented, behavior-modifying, and/or supportive vs interactive)
- The face-to-face time spent with the patient during psychotherapy
- Whether E/M services are furnished on the same date of service as the psychotherapy

Traditionally, psychotherapy procedures have been reported in relation to the time spent providing the psychotherapy. Preservice and postservice work performed with a session of psychotherapy do not affect code selection, as these services are not performed during the face-to-face contact with the patient. Preservice work may include preparing to see the patient, reviewing records, or communicating with other health care professionals or the patient's family. Postservice work may include arranging for further services; communicating with other health care professionals, the patient's family, or the patient; and documenting the services provided.

Specific times are included in each of the psychotherapy code descriptors, indicating the approximate time spent face-to-face with the patient. If psychotherapy is provided for the time specified in the code, then the clinician reports that specific code. Modifiers 22, Unusual Procedural Service, and 52, Reduced Services, may be used to indicate that the time spent was greater or less than specified in the code. (Refer to Chapter 10 for further discussion of modifiers 22 and 52.) This includes time spent performing E/M services for the patient, which typically is an additional five to seven minutes of work either before or after the psychotherapy.

For example, 60 minutes (one hour) of individual insight-oriented, behavior-modifying, and/or supportive psychotherapy in an office or other outpatient facility may be reported with code **90806-22**.

## Other Psychotherapy

Code **90845** is used to report psychoanalysis. Psychoanalysis uses an investigative technique to gain insight into a person's unconscious motivations, conflicts, and symbols to effect a change in maladaptive behavior. Code **90845** refers to the practice of psychoanalysis and is not to be confused with psychotherapy codes. Reporting this code implies that the patient is being seen by a practitioner credentialed to practice analytic therapy and that psychoanalysis is the treatment being used with this patient. Psychoanalysis is reported on a 45–50 minute session basis.

**EXAMPLE:** A 37-year-old man with dysthymia and narcissistic personality disorder manifested by entitlement, inability to be intimate, and extreme variability of self-esteem is seen in the second year of psychoanalysis, just before going on a business trip. Argumentative and easily offended, he accuses the analyst of being insensitive and detached and angrily rejects any effort to explore the basis of his mood or behavior.

Codes **90846**, **90847**, and **90849** are used to report family psychotherapy. In family psychotherapy, the family is brought into the treatment process, and the dynamics within the family as they relate to the patient are the main theme of the psychotherapeutic sessions. These sessions may take place without the patient present (**90846**) or with the patient present (**90847**).

If multiple families are present in a group where similar issues for patients are being treated, code **90849** is used. This code is frequently used in hospitals and drug treatment centers, where psychotherapy with several different families occurs regarding issues surrounding hospitalization of the patient or the patient's abuse of substances. Code **90849** is reported for each family group present. For example, if three families are present, code **90849** would be reported three times, once for each identified patient within each family group.

Code **90853** is used to report group psychotherapy for other than a multiple family group. The psychotherapeutic process may be conducted with several patients in a group setting. The personal dynamics and behavior of an individual may be discussed. At times, the dynamics of the group are explored. Interpersonal interactions, support, emotional catharsis, problem solving, and reminiscing are other examples of the processes explored in group settings.

Code **90853** should be reported separately for each patient in the group.

Code **90857** is used to report interactive group psychotherapy. For example, this code may be used to report therapy for several children who are interacting with the clinician and each other through play equipment, physical devices, or an interpreter (deaf or language). When interactive group psychotherapy is reported, code **90857** is reported separately for each patient in the group.

## Other Psychiatric Services or Procedures

Code **90862** is reported in the following situations:
- When a physician manages medication for the patient who is in psychotherapy with a nonprescribing colleague
- When a patient's condition is being effectively treated with psychotropic drugs alone
- When a physician is primarily managing a patient who has an organic-type disorder (eg, senile dementia of the Alzheimer type) with the use of medication

The physician evaluates how the medication is affecting the patient, determines the proper dosage, and prescribes medication for the patient for the period of time before the patient is next seen.

Generally, the patient receives no other services from the physician at the encounter. If an E/M service is provided at that encounter, the pharmacologic management is included in the E/M service. In this case, the level of E/M service code reported should include the pharmacologic management as well as the other E/M services provided at that encounter. The psychotherapy provided in conjunction with code **90862** is very minimal and supportive.

Code **90865** is used to report narcosynthesis for psychiatric diagnostic and therapeutic purposes. Narcosynthesis is the administration of a medication to release inhibitions and allow a patient to discuss material that would otherwise be difficult for him or her to verbalize. In most instances, a barbiturate or benzodiazepine-type drug is administered intravenously in a very slow fashion to induce a state of drowsiness in the patient. During this time, an interview is conducted about the relevant material.

Code **90870** is used to report electroconvulsive therapy. Electroconvulsive therapy, usually used to treat depression or resistant life-threatening forms of psychosis, involves the application of electric current to the brain for a fraction of a second through scalp electrodes.

As indicated in the code descriptor, necessary monitoring is included when code **90870** is reported. In electroconvulsive therapy, it is necessary to monitor the patient. This includes the management of the seizure time by electroencephalographic tracing and observation. Decision making regarding further treatment is also considered part of the monitoring.

Codes **90875** and **90876** are used to report individual psychophysiological therapy incorporating biofeedback training. These codes include biofeedback training by any modality that the clinician chooses. Therefore, it is not appropriate to separately report codes **90901** and **90911** for the biofeedback provided.

Code **90880** describes hypnotherapy. Hypnotherapy is a treatment that makes use of an artificially induced alteration of consciousness characterized by increased suggestibility and receptivity to direction. It may be used for diagnostic or therapeutic purposes. If hypnotherapy is provided with psychotherapy, only code **90880** is reported for that session.

Code **90882** is used to report environmental intervention for medical management purposes on a patient's behalf with agencies, employers, or institutions. In certain circumstances, a clinician may be called upon to intervene on the patient's behalf. For example, in the case of certain situations for employers, a clinician may be called upon to present material to point out that shift work may be inappropriate for that patient to perform at his or her maximum. In that instance, the clinician actually goes into the employee's workplace to present the information and is in essence making an attempt to intervene in the environmental circumstances.

Code **90885** is used to report evaluation of psychiatric hospital records, other psychiatric reports, psychometric and/or projective tests, and other accumulated data for medical diagnostic purposes. This code is used when a clinician is asked to evaluate hospital records and develops a report for other agencies or individuals. It may also be used to report the evaluation of certain psychiatric reports, especially psychometric testing. Another use of this code is to report a records review requested by a peer review committee or for retrospective reviews requested by medical management companies.

Code **90887** is used to report interpretation or explanation of results of psychiatric or other medical examinations and procedures, or other accumulated data, to family or other responsible persons or to advise them how to assist the patient. The patient's treatment may require that certain aspects of his or her psychiatric care, which might include medical examinations, procedures, and accumulated data, be explained to family or to their employers to obtain their permission, participation, and/or support for the patient's treatment. In this

**CODING TIP**

Anesthesia administration for electroconvulsive therapy is separately reported with code **00104**.

**CODING TIP**

For home visit hemodialysis services performed by a non-physician health care professional, report code **99512**.

**CODING TIP**

For home infusion peritoneal dialysis performed by a nonphysician health care professional, report codes **99601-99602**.

instance, the clinician uses code **90887** to report the work performed in providing this service.

If this interpretation is provided on the day the clinician provides other services for the patient, it may be more appropriate to report an E/M code. Counseling and coordination of care (in the E/M code) could encompass code **90887**. When counseling and/or coordination of care dominates (more than 50%) the physician/patient face-to-face encounter, the E/M code is selected on the basis of the total time the physician spent with the patient and his or her family. (Refer to Chapter 3 for further discussion of E/M and counseling and coordination of care.)

Code **90889** is used to report preparation of a report of the patient's psychiatric status, history, treatment, or progress for other physicians, agencies, or insurance carriers.

The unlisted code, **90899**, is used to report a psychiatric procedure or service for which there is no specific code.

# Dialysis

Codes **90918-90921** are reported once per month to distinguish age-specific services related to the patient's end-stage renal disease (ESRD) performed in an outpatient setting. ESRD-related physician services include establishment of a dialyzing cycle, outpatient evaluation and management of the dialysis visits, telephone calls, and patient management during the dialysis, provided during a full month. These codes are not used if the physician also submits hospitalization codes during the month.

Codes **90918-90921** describe a full month of ESRD-related services provided in an outpatient setting. For ESRD and non-ESRD dialysis services performed in an inpatient setting and for non-ESRD dialysis services performed in an outpatient setting, see codes **90935-90937** and **90945-90947**.

E/M services unrelated to ESRD services that cannot be performed during the dialysis session may be reported separately.

Codes **90922-90925** are reported when outpatient ESRD-related services are not performed consecutively during an entire full month (eg, when the patient spends part of the month as a hospital inpatient or when the outpatient ESRD-related services are initiated after the first of the month). The appropriate age-related code from this series (**90922-90925**) is reported daily less the days of hospitalization. For reporting purposes, each month is considered to be 30 days.

**EXAMPLE:** Outpatient ESRD-related services are initiated on July 1 for a 57-year-old man. On July 11, he is admitted to the hospital as an inpatient and discharged on July 27.

In this example, code **90925** should be reported for each day outside of the inpatient hospitalization (30 days/month less 17 days/hospitalization = 13 days). Report inpatient E/M services as appropriate. Dialysis procedures rendered during the hospitalization (July 11–27) should be reported, as appropriate (**90935-90937**, **90945-90947**).

## Hemodialysis

Codes **90935** and **90937** are reported to describe the hemodialysis procedure with all E/M services related to the patient's renal disease on the day of the hemodialysis procedure. These codes are used for inpatient ESRD and non-ESRD procedures or for outpatient non-ESRD dialysis services.

Code **90935** is reported if only one evaluation of the patient is required related to that hemodialysis procedure.

Code **90937** is reported when patient re-evaluation(s) is required during a hemodialysis procedure. Use modifier 25 with E/M codes for services unrelated to the dialysis procedure or renal failure that cannot be rendered during the dialysis session.

Code **90940** is intended to report the technical component of hemodialysis access flow study by indicator method. This code includes indicator-based methods of hemodialysis access flow assessment including the conductivity dialysance method. Early detection and treatment of stenosis and access flow reduction of hemodialysis reduces the frequency of thrombosis and reduces access replacement rates. This study is not considered to be a part of routine dialysis.

## Miscellaneous Dialysis Procedures

Codes **90945** and **90947** describe dialysis procedures other than hemodialysis (eg, peritoneal dialysis, hemofiltration, or continuous renal replacement therapies) and all E/M services related to the patient's renal disease on the day of the procedure.

Code **90945** is reported if only one evaluation of the patient is required related to that procedure.

Code **90947** is reported when patient re-evaluation is required during a procedure. Use modifier 25 with E/M codes for services unrelated to the dialysis procedure or renal failure that cannot be rendered during the dialysis session.

# Gastroenterology

Code **91022** identifies duodenal motility studies, a technique used to evaluate the contractile activity of the proximal small bowel. Duodenal motility studies are indicated in pediatric and adult patients with unexplained nausea and vomiting, particularly when gastric emptying is normal, or equivocal, or when severe symptoms persist despite therapeutic trials. These studies are also indicated in patients with suspected pseudo-obstruction, systemic sclerosis, recurrent small bowel bacterial overgrowth, and to exclude diffuse gut motility prior to colectomy in a patient with constipation. If fluoroscopy is performed, report code **76000**. If a gastric motility (manometric) study is performed, report code **91020**.

Codes **91034** and **91035** identify nasal insertion of pH catheters (**91034**) or mucosal attachment of telemetry pH electrodes (**91035**) for detection of gastroesophageal reflux disease (GERD). These codes allow for testing of both acid and nonacidic reflux.

These codes describe important tests for the diagnosis of GERD. GERD results from the abnormal reflux of stomach contents into the esophagus. This can result in heartburn and other serious problems such as dysphagia, dysphonia, asthma, and Barrett's esophagus. Measuring the level of acid in the esophagus is an important step in the diagnosis of patients with symptomatic GERD and establishing treatment plans. Further, pH monitoring can be used to determine the effectiveness of treatment and the potential need for additional medical, pharmacologic, endoscopic, and/or surgical intervention.

Ambulatory pH monitoring can be accomplished by use of a catheter passed through the patient's nose and connected to a recording device (**91034**) performed for a 24-hour period or a telemetry-based system for measuring acid reflux (**91035**). The telemetry system involves the placement of a monitoring capsule that is temporarily inserted and attached to the patient's esophagus. The capsule monitors the presence of acid and transmits pH levels via radiofrequency telemetry to an external receiver worn by the patient. After a period of several days, the capsule is sloughed by the body and passes through the patient's digestive tract.

Codes **91037** and **91038** are used to describe esophageal impedance monitoring. Esophageal impedance testing measures all reflux, both acid and nonacid, over a period up to 1 hour (**91037**) or prolonged (**91038**) period. Code **91038** includes a specific time range in its descriptor to clearly define what constitutes a prolonged period for monitoring intraluminal impedance testing. Nonacid reflux may be associated with symptoms such as chest pain, regurgitation, cough, asthma, laryngitis, wheezing, and recurrent pneumonia in patients.

To perform esophageal motility testing (**91010**), a pressure-sensing catheter is inserted transnasally into the esophagus to measure sphincter function and esophageal muscular function. The motility (manometry) test quantifies sphincter location, length and closure pressure, function, and peristaltic muscular activity of the esophagus during swallow challenges of liquid material. During esophageal function testing, a bolus transit impedance catheter that includes incremental impedance sensors is inserted transnasally. The impedance test quantifies bolus transit dynamics and bolus transit effectiveness of the esophagus. Both liquid and viscous swallow challenges are used to optimally test the peristaltic process.

Code **91040** is used to report an esophageal balloon distention provocation study. For this procedure, serial insufflations of air or water are used to determine the threshold that reproduces symptomatic response in the patient. These insufflations are performed with the patient blind to the volume of substance infused to allow accurate results. The results are used by the physician to evaluate recurrent unexplained chest pain and dysphagia. Esophageal balloon provocation is used to evaluate for an esophageal source of chest pain in patients with or without GERD.

Noncardiac chest pain remains a common and vexing clinical problem. Provocative esophageal testing can help to identify an esophageal cause for the pain. Code **91065** is used to identify hydrogen breath testing, using the ability to determine malabsorption of dietary saccharides through use of a breath sample as opposed to an aspirate of gastric contents (sample of the contents of the stomach). Hydrogen breath testing for bacterial overgrowth requires different substrates and a different testing protocol than that used for lactose intolerance. The test is noninvasive and is therefore more readily tolerated by patients than alternative testing that requires jejunal intubation and aspiration of contents for detection of bacteria.

A parenthetical note follows code **91065** to direct users to the correct coding for *Helicobacter pylori* breath testing.

Hydrogen breath testing has been an established test for measuring gastrointestinal function for more than 20 years. It has been used to determine malabsorption of dietary saccharides such as lactose, the presence of bacterial overgrowth, and intestinal transit. Because of the type of sample used for this procedure, this code is used to report breath hydrogen testing for other disorders as well.

Fructose intolerance is a common and treatable condition in patients with unexplained chronic diarrhea, bloating due to gaseousness, and abdominal pain. It affects patients of all ages from infants to the elderly. The problem has become much more common since the food industry began to use high-fructose corn syrup as a sweetener in place of sucrose.

Bacterial overgrowth is particularly common and treatable in patients with unexplained chronic diarrhea and malabsorption, diabetics with chronic diarrhea, selected patients with refractory irritable bowel syndrome, and elderly patients with malabsorption. Since measurement of orocecal transit is useful in detecting motor disorders involving the stomach and small bowel such as diabetic gastroparesis, pseudo-obstruction secondary to scleroderma, diabetes, or dumping syndromes, it is of use in patients with symptoms of unexplained bloating and distention, diarrhea or constipation, nausea and vomiting, and abdominal pain. The test is useful in all age groups from infants to the elderly. Differentiation from small bowel bacterial overgrowth is important and can be difficult because overgrowth and delayed transit can coexist.

Codes **91110** and **91111** are specific to capsule endoscopy procedures, as wireless capsule endoscopy requires a fundamentally different approach to examining the gastrointestinal tract as compared with standard endoscopy procedures. Optical endoscopy methods use an endoscope that is inserted into an orifice of the body (oral or anal) and require specific manipulation of the device in order to view the appropriate predesignated areas of concern. To perform capsule endoscopy, the patient is required to swallow a capsule endoscope that generates numerous images as it passes through the gastrointestinal tract. Code **91110** describes capsule endoscopy from the esophagus to the ileum, performed over an eight- to nine-hour period. The images are recorded on a device worn by the patient as the patient goes through normal daily activities. At the conclusion of the recording period, the images are downloaded for subsequent review by the physician. The physician review necessary for these procedures can be quite extensive since the device captures 15 frames/second during the eight- to nine-hour period. The capsule is not retrieved and subsequently is eliminated.

Code **91111** identifies gastrointestinal tract imaging, intraluminal (eg, capsule endoscopy), of the esophagus, with physician interpretation and report. Because of the shorter duration for evaluation of the esophagus, the patient does not undergo prolonged monitoring. Do not report **91111** in conjunction with **91110**.

Code **91120** identifies measurement of rectal sensation, rectal tone, and compliance of the rectal wall as well as assessment of sensory properties of the rectal wall in response to controlled balloon distention of the rectum. Specifically, code **91120** describes a comprehensive assessment of sensory, motor, and biomechanical function of the rectum in patients with irritable bowel syndrome, constipation, and/or fecal incontinence. Testing is performed at rest and after provocative stimuli. The provocation stimuli include responses of the rectum to a graded balloon distention. The response provides data that the physician is able to analyze to determine information regarding rectal motility and function. For biofeedback training, use **90911**. For anorectal manometry, use **91122**.

# Ophthalmology

This section begins with definitions of intermediate and comprehensive ophthalmologic services. The codes that use these terms (**92002-92014**) are special codes that describe the unique nature of ophthalmologic examinations. These codes overlap with the general E/M codes described in Chapter 3. Either series may be used, though one may be more suitable depending on the specific services provided to the patient.

These codes share several definitions with the E/M codes, such as new and established patient. Differing from the E/M codes, the general ophthalmologic services describe the physician's activity as intermediate and comprehensive and do not follow the E/M framework of the three key components of history, examination, and medical decision making.

When coding ophthalmologic visits, be sure to confer with the physician to select either one of these codes or the appropriate E/M services codes, depending on the specific services provided to the patient at that visit.

As indicated in the definitions of ophthalmology services, the ophthalmology codes are more specific to the services and examination rendered during a visit related to the ocular system. However, E/M codes may be more appropriate when there are many eye problems, counseling and/or coordination of care dominates the visit, or an underlying medical condition of the patient is the primary reason for the visit. The code that most accurately describes the services performed should be the code reported, whether it is an E/M or an ophthalmology visit code.

Special ophthalmologic services include such procedures as determination of the refractive state (**92015**), ophthalmologic examinations under general anesthesia (**92018, 92019**), gonioscopy (**92020**), sensorimotor examinations (**92060**), orthoptic and/or pleoptic training (vision therapy) (**92065**), therapeutic contact lens fitting (**92070**), visual field examinations (**92081-92083**), tonometry and tonography (**92100-92130**), scanning computerized diagnostic imaging (**92135**), and provocative tests for glaucoma (**92140**).

Note that the determination of the refractive state of the eye (refraction) is listed as a separate code (**92015**), which is not included in the definition of an intermediate or comprehensive ophthalmologic service or E/M service. As noted previously, this code is one of the special ophthalmologic services codes. Special ophthalmologic services describes services in which a special evaluation of part of the visual system is made, which goes beyond the services included under general ophthalmologic services (or E/M services) or in which special treatment is given. Special ophthalmologic services are reported in addition to the general ophthalmologic services or E/M services.

If a refraction is performed in conjunction with an intermediate or comprehensive ophthalmologic service (**92002-92014**), it is appropriate to report code **92015** in addition to the appropriate code for the intermediate or comprehensive ophthalmologic service provided.

Also, if determination of the refractive state is performed in addition to an E/M service, it would be appropriate to report the determination of the refractive state separately and in addition to level of E/M service reported.

Refraction (**92015**) is intended to represent a bilateral procedure/service. It is not appropriate to report code **92015** per eye. It is also not appropriate to use modifier 50 when reporting this code (or the right or left Health Care Common Procedure Coding System [HCPCS] designation). Furthermore, if determination of refractive state is performed on one eye, modifier 52 should be appended to the code to indicate reduced services. (Refer to the table provided later in this chapter for further explanation of the use of modifiers 50 and 52 when reporting ophthalmologic services.)

Computerized corneal topography, unilateral or bilateral, with interpretation and report, is reported with code **92025**. Corneal topography is a computer-assisted test in which a special instrument projects a series of concentric light rings on the cornea, creating a color map of the corneal surface as well as a cross-section profile. This test is used to detect subtle corneal surface irregularity most often associated with a wide variety of corneal disease states. Computerized corneal topography is also known as computer-assisted video keratography, and corneal mapping. These data are compared to norms, and additional analyses are performed in addition to a visual inspection of the map. This code is intended to be reported when topography is not performed in conjunction with kerato-plasty procedures described by codes **65710**, **65730**, **65750**, and **65755**. Computerized corneal topography is considered to be integral to the postoperative management of these keratoplasty procedures. This code is not used for manual keratoscopy, often called *keratometry*, which is part of a single system E/M or general ophthalmological service.

Please notice throughout this section that several of the procedures are designated as "separate procedures." A separate procedure is one that is commonly carried out as an integral component of a more extensive service or procedure. The codes with the separate procedure designation should not be reported in addition to the code for the total procedure or service of which it is considered an integral component. (Refer to Chapter 4 for further discussion of the separate procedure designation.)

**CODING TIP**

Before coding for special ophthalmologic services, be sure to note whether the code is designated as a separate procedure. Consider whether the other services provided at that visit would include the separate procedure.

Ophthalmoscopy is the next section in the special ophthalmologic services section. A very important note prefaces these codes. The note under the ophthalmoscopy heading indicates that routine ophthalmoscopy is part of general and special ophthalmologic service and is not reported separately. When coding for eye-related services, ophthalmoscopy is part of the examination and the recorded findings. The codes in the series **92225-92260** are not to be used for routine ophthalmoscopy. The codes in this section describe extended types of ophthalmoscopic examinations, not routine ones, for relatively serious conditions and includes specific documentation. Be sure to read the medical record documentation carefully to avoid overcoding ophthalmoscopy services.

The final subsection under the special ophthalmologic services section is that of other specialized services. This section details special procedures, like electroretinography, external ocular photography, and other diagnostic procedures. In this section, there are specific references to other locations in CPT Nomenclature, such as other areas of the Medicine section and the Radiology section, where other diagnostic procedures related to the eye may be found. For those coding for services and procedures involving the eye and ocular adnexa, it is essential that these cross-references are considered.

A unique characteristic of this section is that many of the codes differentiate between the patient's condition, namely, aphakia and other than aphakia. Aphakia is defined as absence of the lens of the eye. The most common cause of this condition is surgical removal of the lens because of cataracts. Aphakia may also be because of absorption or degeneration of the lens or, very rarely, congenital absence of the lens.

When selecting codes for contact lens services, be sure to choose the code on the basis of whether the physician actually provides the lenses or supervises the fitting by an independent technician. For prescription, fitting, and/or medical supervision of ocular prosthetic adaptation by a physician, see E/M services or General Ophthalmological service codes **92002-92014**.

The supply of the contact lenses may be reported as part of the service of fitting. It may also be reported separately by using the appropriate supply code(s).

Following the codes for contact lens services are codes for ocular prosthetics or artificial eyes. These codes differentiate according to whether the physician actually fits and provides the prosthesis or only supervises the fitting by an independent technician.

If the supply of the prosthesis is not included in the service of prescription and fitting, modifier 26 should be used to indicate that only professional services were provided. On occasions when only the ocular prosthesis is supplied, it may be separately reported with the appropriate supply code.

The next section describes spectacle services excluding the refraction and prescription. The prescription of lenses for glasses is included in code **92015** and is not reported separately. The fitting of spectacles (glasses) is a separate service and may be reported by codes **92340-92371**. This series of codes uses special terms unique to spectacle services, including monofocal (single vision lenses), bifocal (two prescriptions in one lens), and multifocal (more than two prescriptions in one lens). Again, note that the fitting of spectacles is differentiated by aphakia and other than aphakia. Also note that in the codes referring to aphakia, the codes refer to the provision of prosthesis. This is because the lens of the glasses substitutes for the absent lens of the eye and is thus a prosthesis required to replace an absent body part.

Supply of spectacles is reported with the appropriate supply code.

As is common throughout the CPT Nomenclature, the section concludes with an "other procedures" category that contains an unlisted ophthalmologic service or procedure, code **92499**. This code should be used to report any service for which there is no specific CPT code.

## A Final Note

One of the most frequently asked questions deals with the use of the bilateral modifier when organs or body areas are paired, such as the eyes. This is particularly important in medical procedures (nonsurgical) in which a procedure is commonly performed on paired organs or body areas. The following table is essential to understanding the appropriate use of modifier 50 and modifier 52 in medical ophthalmology procedures. (Refer to Chapter 10 for further discussion of the use of modifiers 50 and 52.)

## Bilateral Modifier Usage for Medical Ophthalmology Procedures

| Code | Use bilateral modifier? | | Use reduced service modifier if performance is on one eye? | |
|------|:---:|:---:|:---:|:---:|
| | Yes | No | Yes | No |
| 92002 | | X | X | |
| 92004 | | X | X | |
| 92012 | | X | X | |
| 92014 | | X | X | |
| 92015 | | X | X | |
| 92018 | | X | X | |
| 92019 | | X | X | |
| 92020 | | X | X | |
| 92025 | | X | | X |
| 92060 | | X | X | |
| 92065 | | X | X | |
| 92070 | X | | | X |
| 92081 | | X | X | |
| 92082 | | X | X | |
| 92083 | | X | X | |
| 92100 | | X | X | |
| 92120 | X | | | X |
| 92130 | X | | | X |
| 92135 | X | | | X |
| 92136 | X | | | X |
| 92140 | X | | | X |
| 92225 | X | | | X |
| 92226 | X | | | X |
| 92230 | | X | X | |
| 92235 | X | | | X |
| 92250 | X | | | X |
| 92260 | | X | X | |
| 92265 | | X | X | |

## Bilateral Modifier Usage for Medical Ophthalmology Procedures, continued

| Code | Use bilateral modifier? | | Use reduced service modifier if performance is on one eye? | |
|------|:---:|:---:|:---:|:---:|
| | Yes | No | Yes | No |
| 92270 | X | | | X |
| 92275 | X | | | X |
| 92283 | | X | X | |
| 92284 | | X | X | |
| 92285 | X | | | X |
| 92286 | X | | | X |
| 92287 | X | | | X |
| 92310 | | X | X | |
| 92311 | | X | | X |
| 92312 | | X | | X |
| 92313 | X | | | X |
| 92314 | | X | | X |
| 92315 | | X | | X |
| 92316 | | X | | X |
| 92317 | X | | | X |
| 92325 | X | | | X |
| 92326 | X | | | X |
| 92340 | | X | X | |
| 92341 | | X | X | |
| 92342 | | X | X | |
| 92352 | | X | X | |
| 92353 | | X | X | |
| 92354 | | X | X | |
| 92355 | | X | X | |
| 92358 | | X | X | |
| 92370 | | X | X | |
| 92371 | | X | X | |
| 92499 | | X | | X |

# Special Otorhinolaryngologic Services

The function of the ears is to receive sound impulses and transmit them to the brain. The inner ear also houses the organs of balance. The nose allows air to enter the body and pass through the nasal cavity. After passing through the nasal cavity, the air reaches the pharynx, commonly known as the throat. The larynx, commonly known as the voice box, is the chamber located between the pharynx and the trachea. During the act of breathing, the vocal cords are separated to let air pass. During speech, they are closer together and sound is produced as air is expelled from the lungs, causing the cords to vibrate against each other.

These functions may not be performed properly because of disease or other conditions (eg, allergies, congenital disorders, ear or sinus infections, swallowing impairment because of stroke). These conditions can often be treated during a regular office visit; however, in some instances, additional assessments that are reported as special otorhinolaryngologic services should be performed. The special otorhinolaryngologic services relate to the ear (oto-), nose (rhino-), voice box (laryngo-), and throat (pharyngo-), as well as the neck and face. These services are often performed by otolaryngologists, audiologists, and speech-language pathologists (SLPs), or in collaboration with each other. The special otorhinolaryngologic services include those services performed by practitioners for the evaluation, analysis, treatment, and therapeutic services using various speech and hearing devices. This section focuses on CPT reporting for the evaluation and treatment of speech, language, voice, and other communication services as well as for swallowing function evaluation.

CPT codes **92506**, **92507**, and **92508** are specifically intended to identify the evaluation and treatment of speech, language, and voice communication disorder services. The code descriptors identify intent of use, as the code language indicates that the provider needs to be face-to-face with the patient when performing these services. These codes are intended to be reported one time per session and are not considered time-based codes. Specifically, code **92506** is intended to describe the basic assessment and evaluation of communication disorders. Professional intervention is based upon individual, ongoing assessment of a patient's communication skills. The professional starts by screening all areas of communication function and follows with an in-depth assessment of the particular areas that may be problematic. The assessment may include clinical observations and standardized and nonstandardized tests.

Codes **92507** (individual treatment) and **92508** (group treatment) are reported for the treatment of speech, language, voice, communication, and/or auditory processing disorders. These codes include most but not all aspects of treatment for a variety of communication disorders.

Since some of the special otorhinolaryngologic services include an assessment component as part of preservice work, use of these codes is dependent on whether the service being provided is a significant, separate service or simply a component of the more involved procedure. Since patient circumstances vary, choice of codes will depend on the specific patient encounter and the intent of the provider.

The determination of which areas to assess comprehensively is dependent upon the screening procedures suggested by the presenting problem. If the patient's language development appears to be delayed, then the assessment will focus on language areas. If language development is progressing well but fluency is an issue, then the clinician will evaluate fluency. Other patients will require voice assessment, assessment of semantic and pragmatic skills, etc. Some patients require detailed assessments across several areas that are performed by SLPs. For example, a child might have difficulties with speech, language, and fluency. The particular assessment and treatment approaches and procedures used by the professional will depend on the way the individual patient presents and his or her theories of development, disorders, and intervention.

CPT codes **92607** and **92608** represent evaluative services performed to provide prescription(s) for speech-generating augmentative and alternative communication (AAC) devices. These AAC devices are most commonly referred to as speech-generating devices (SGDs). The code descriptors identify intent of use, as the code language indicates that the provider needs to be face-to-face with the patient when performing these services. In addition, codes **92607** and **92608** are time-based, allowing for the use of code **92607** for the first hour of service and code **92608** for each additional 30-minute unit of service.

The AAC assessment is conducted to determine the appropriateness of aids, techniques, symbols, and/or strategies to augment or replace speech and enhance communication of patients with expressive and/or receptive communication disorders. Patients with severe expressive and/or receptive communication disorders who do not have a functional communication system to meet their needs are assisted in selecting and obtaining appropriate augmentative and/or alternative communication systems (eg, aids, techniques, symbols, strategies) to facilitate communication.

Patients of all ages are assessed as needed. The assessment is the result of a referral following a speech and language assessment (**92506**), or may follow unsuccessful speech and language treatment (**92507**). The patient who has been referred to an SLP for AAC assessment either currently does not have or is expected to lose the ability to communicate functional communication needs. The clinician must also be mindful that when the person's communication is impaired, other aspects of life (eg, health, education, vocation, socialization) are often negatively affected by lack of functional communication skills.

The tools of the SGD assessment (eg, tests, materials) vary depending on diagnosis, severity, age, age at onset, level of cognition, daily communication needs and abilities across environments and communication partners, and whether the expressive communication disorder is congenital, acquired, or progressive. Each assessment is unique and may include a wide range of formal and informal tests and observations. If the evaluating SLP cannot document functional ability in hearing, vision, cognition, seating and positioning, or motor abilities, appropriate referrals may be necessary. In addition, examination/observation of voice, speech, language, cognition, and communication systems including any existing adaptive AAC and/or orthotic devices currently used by the patient (eg, wheelchair, neck braces, communication boards, specialized electronic equipment) are included in the assessment process. The clinician must also evaluate the patient's ability to effectively use the SGD and required accessories. In addition to overall language skills and abilities, the method of access to the SGD (ie, direct or indirect) must be documented.

The assessment is conducted in a natural environment (eg, home or classroom) and/or in a clinical environment and includes a range of AAC aids, devices, and accessories to evaluate the patient's competencies. The assessment process considers the abilities, needs, and preferences of the patient and of the patient's communication partners (eg, family, caregivers, educators, service providers), history of substance abuse and/or mental illness, and the environment in which the AAC components will be used routinely. Documentation should include the following:

- Pertinent medical background information
- Communication diagnosis and severity
- Anticipated course (ie, degenerative, stable/chronic, improving) and results of device trials
- Rationale for devices and/or accessories as they relate to daily functional communication needs
- Measurable short- and long-term goals relating to functional communication needs
- A time frame for completing these goals

## Evaluative and Therapeutic Services

The codes included in this section identify services performed by practitioners for the evaluation, analysis, and, when appropriate, therapeutic services for various speech and hearing devices. In addition, codes have also been included that identify swallowing and laryngeal function. The strategic inclusion of parenthetical notes and guidelines helps instruct the user regarding the intent and use of the codes described in this section.

Codes **92601-92604** are used to report the postoperative analysis, fitting of the previously placed external learning device, connection of the external device to the cochlear implant, and programming of the stimulator. They are differentiated by the age of the patient (under seven years of age vs seven years and older) and by performance of programming or reprogramming of the device. Placement of the cochlear implant device is separately reported using code **69930** and does not include these services.

Diagnostic programming of the speech processor is a unique service that is critical to the safety and effectiveness of the cochlear implant system. This service is required after the initial fitting of the processor, usually four to six weeks after surgery and periodically for the first year. This programming includes adjustments to the stimulus parameters of the processor, which determine the signals delivered to the electrodes surgically implanted inside the cochlea. The connection of the external device and the fitting are also included as part of these services to ensure correct operation of the equipment used.

The cochlear implant periodic reprogramming is reported by codes **92602** and **92604** and includes any services performed after the first session.

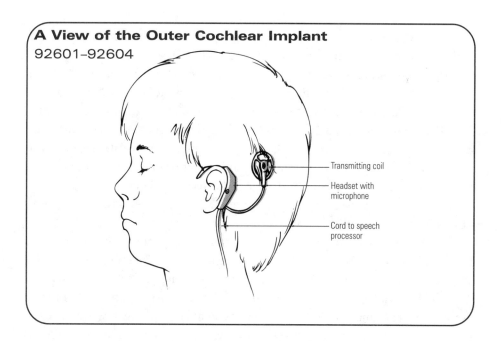

**A View of the Outer Cochlear Implant**
92601–92604

Transmitting coil

Headset with microphone

Cord to speech processor

Guidelines for codes **92601-92604** identify the complete services that are intended to be reported by these codes (postoperative analysis, fitting of previously placed external device, connection of the device to the cochlear implant, and programming of the stimulator). In addition, parenthetical notes have been placed within this series of codes to reference the correct codes to use for placement of the cochlear implant (**69930**), aural rehabilitation services following cochlear implant (**92626-92627**, **92630-92633**), and the intended method of reporting these codes (ie, exclusion of codes **92601** and **92603** when using codes **92602** and **92604**).

Codes **92605** and **92606** identify the evaluation for prescription and therapeutic services for the non-SGDs, respectively, and include low technology, non-SGDs such as Plexiglas devices, touch screen monitors, and communication boards. A parenthetical note has been placed after code **92597** to instruct the user of the appropriate codes to use to report AAC device services.

Codes **92607** and **92608** identify evaluation services performed to provide prescription(s) for speech-generating AAC devices. The code descriptors identify intent of use, as the code language indicates that the provider needs to be face-to-face with the patient when performing these services. In addition, the code **92607** and **92608** services are time based, allowing use of code **92607** for the first hour of service and code **92608** for each additional 30 minutes of service. Codes **92607-92609** differ from code **92597** because these codes identify evaluation for prescription of the device, while code **92597** identifies evaluation for use and/or fitting of a voice prosthetic such as a Passy Muir speaking valve. Only those codes that include time as part of the descriptor should be reported according to the time spent performing the service. Finally, code **92609** is used to report therapeutic services provided by the clinician for use of an SGD. Programming and modifications necessary for the device are included as part of the procedure and are therefore not separately reported.

Codes **92610** and **92611** are used to report a swallowing function evaluation. The structures of the larynx (eg, true and false vocal folds, arytenoid cartilages, epiglottis) move in a complicated and synchronized fashion to close, lift, and move forward during swallowing to divert food and liquids to the esophagus and down the digestive tract. When swallowing function is compromised, food and other materials can find their way into the bronchial tree and cause numerous problems such as aspiration pneumonia. Patients may also have difficulty with certain ingestants such as meat or pills or thin liquids. The procedure identified by code **92610** can be used to determine if problems exist, assessing whether airway protection exists. Code **92610** is a clinical, observational procedure typically performed by an SLP that assesses a patient's ability to chew food, form a bolus, and swallow different types of food and liquids. No instrumentation is involved. If the airway protective reflex is present, the patient will likely not choke, or aspirate, while he or she eats and swallows. If the reflex is diminished or absent, the risk of the patient choking or aspirating is extremely high, and dietary and behavioral changes will need to be recommended to prevent aspiration of secretions/ingestants into the tracheobronchial tree. Code **92611** is used to identify motion evaluation via use of fluoroscopy and incorporates the use of cine or video recording in order to accomplish the testing procedure. In many situations, an instrumental study such as code **92611** is indicated to more fully assess swallowing. Various consistencies of ingestants and maneuvers are tested to determine whether the patient can protect his or her airway and swallow adequately to maintain nutrition. Imaging for code **92611** is reported separately by using code **74230** to identify the radiologic supervision and interpretation. Code **92611** also differs from code **70371**, which is a videofluoroscopic study of the pharynx and speech evaluation that assesses movement and function of the soft palate as it closes during speech.

Another instrumental procedure for the assessment of the pharyngeal phase of the swallow is an endoscopic procedure. The code most frequently used is **92612**, Flexible fiberoptic endoscopic evaluation of swallowing by cine or video recording. These codes also differ from code **92520**, which applies to two different types of laryngeal function assays: acoustic testing of the voice and aerodynamic testing of voice function. Neither acoustic nor aerodynamic tests of voice have any direct relationship with the assessment of airway protection and swallowing. Therefore, separate codes are used to identify these very distinct services and generally should be reported with different diagnoses.

Codes **92612-92617** are used to report endoscopic performance of the same procedures identified previously. Each code includes language that differentiates its use from the other codes within the coding family according to the type of test performed (swallowing evaluation, laryngeal sensory testing, or both).

Code **92626** describes the first hour of evaluating auditory rehabilitation status in children and adults to determine current abilities to instruct the use of residual hearing provided by a cochlear implant or hearing aid. Code **92627** describes each additional 15 minutes of evaluation in conjunction with **92626**.

Code **92630** describes auditory rehabilitation; prelingual hearing loss. Prelingual denotes that the patient's hearing loss occurred prior to the development of speech. Code **92633** describes auditory rehabilitation; postlingual hearing loss. In this case the hearing loss was acquired following the development of speech and language. Code **92630** is reported to describe services performed primarily for pediatric patients who have no prior experience with hearing and are learning to hear through the use of hearing aids or cochlear implants. Code **92633** is reported for rehabilitation of adolescents and adults who had hearing and language, lost their hearing, and are receiving auditory assistance via a cochlear implant or hearing aid. Code **92633** represents the services that maximize use of residual hearing with a cochlear implant or hearing aid in a variety of listening situations.

Code **92640** is a special diagnostic procedure used to report diagnostic analysis with programming of auditory brainstem implant. An auditory brain stem implant is used in patients for whom a cochlear implant is not possible because of congenital absence, disease, or resection of the auditory nerve. This code is reported per hour.

Finally, code **92700** is used to report otorhinolaryngologic services that are not specifically identified within this code series.

# Cardiovascular

In the Cardiovascular subsection of the Medicine section of the CPT code set, there are specific categories of codes for reporting the following:
*   Therapeutic services (**92950-92998**)
*   Cardiography (**93000-93278**)
*   Echocardiography (**93303-93350**)
*   Cardiac catheterization (**93501-93581**)
*   Intracardiac electrophysiologic procedures/studies (**93600-93662**)
*   Peripheral arterial disease rehabilitation (**93668**)
*   Other vascular studies (**93701-93790**)
*   Other procedures (**93797-93799**)

Cardiovascular services in this section often involve complex anatomic and physiologic terms and concepts. It may be helpful to also refer to the Cardiovascular Surgery section of this text for additional heart illustrations.

## Therapeutic Services

The first code in this series is **92950** for reporting cardiopulmonary resuscitation (CPR). This code is intended to describe CPR to restore and maintain the patient's respiration and circulation after cessation of heartbeat and breathing. Basic CPR consists of assessing the victim, opening the airway, restoring breathing (eg, mouth-to-mouth, bag valve mask), then restoring circulation (eg, closed chest cardiac massage). In most instances, CPR is performed prior to, with continuation during, advanced life support interventions, eg, drug therapy and defibrillation, which would be included by reporting the appropriate critical care services code(s) from the E/M section of the CPT codebook.

CPR is not included in the reporting of critical care services. If CPR and critical care are both provided, it would be appropriate to separately report these services. Also, code **92950** includes no advanced life support interventions other than those described previously. Therefore, if endotracheal intubation is also performed, it would be appropriate to separately report code **31500** to describe the endotracheal intubation performed. (Refer to Chapter 3 for further discussion regarding coding for critical care services.)

Codes **92960** and **92961** are used to report cardioversion. Code **92960** specifically describes elective (nonemergency) external electrical cardioversion using an external electrical stimulator source, such as cardioversion paddles. Elective cardioversion may be used to treat atrial fibrillation and atrial flutter if antiarrhythmic drugs fail to convert the heart back to normal sinus rhythm or if the patient is hemodynamically unstable. The electric shock given in cardioversion is synchronized, ie, it is timed to occur during the R wave of the electrocardiogram. The patient will have his or her heart rhythm monitored for several hours after the procedure to ensure that the rhythm remains stable. Nonelective emergency defibrillation is discussed below.

Code **92961** is used to report internal cardioversion. This procedure is most commonly used to convert atrial fibrillation to normal sinus rhythm when external cardioversion is unsuccessful. Internal cardioversion requires vascular access, placement of catheters into the heart under fluoroscopy, and a much greater knowledge of electrophysiology procedures.

Code **92961** is designated as a separate procedure. Internal elective cardioversion is not separately reported when performed as an integral component of another procedure/service, as in an EP study or cardiac catheterization. However, if the internal elective cardioversion is performed independently, unrelated or distinct from other procedure(s)/service(s) provided at that time, it would be appropriate to separately report the internal cardioversion. The parenthetical note that follows this code indicates that it is not appropriate to report internal cardioversion in conjunction with codes **93618-93624**, **93631**, **93640-93642**, **93650-93652**, **93662**, and codes **93741-93744**. (Refer to Chapter 4 for further discussion of the *separate procedure* designation.)

Questions are often raised regarding use of the cardioversion codes to report defibrillation. Defibrillation is the delivery of an electrical impulse to the heart. This impulse is intended to interrupt abnormal rhythms (eg, ventricular fibrillation) and allow the normal sinus impulse and electrical conduction to resume. The electrical impulse must be strong enough to cause depolarization (neutralization of the positive and negative electrical charges) of a large percentage of the myocardium. The time of the defibrillation is not synchronized to the cardiac cycle.

No CPT code exists to report defibrillation as a procedure performed in isolation. Defibrillation may be performed as part of critical care services, at the end of open heart surgery, during cardiac catheterization, during cardioverter-defibrillator implantation, or during an electrophysiologic procedure. In all of these situations, defibrillation is not a separately reportable service.

Pharmacologic cardioversion (the use of drugs to convert the heart back to normal sinus rhythm) is reported on the basis of the specific services provided. For example, the use of prolonged services, critical care, E/M services, or codes describing therapeutic or diagnostic infusion or injection procedures may be appropriate, depending on the specific services provided.

## Angioplasty, Atherectomy, Stent Placement

Let us review the codes, specific reporting guidelines associated with their use, and some coding examples for angioplasty, atherectomy, and stent placement procedures and also when reported in addition to other add-on procedures (eg, coronary thrombectomy, coronary intravascular brachytherapy device placement).

Included in the therapeutic services series of codes are listings for reporting percutaneous transluminal coronary angioplasty (PTCA), percutaneous transluminal coronary atherectomy, and percutaneous transcatheter placement of intracoronary stents, with or without other therapeutic intervention. The exceptions are two therapeutic services codes, **92973** and **92974**, which are add-on codes, not performed as single procedures. Appropriate coding for therapeutic coronary procedures requires a thorough understanding of the codes and guidelines describing these procedures.

+**92973**    Percutaneous transluminal coronary thrombectomy
(List separately in addition to code for primary procedure)

(Use **92973** in conjunction with **92980, 92982**)

Code **92973** is an add-on code (meaning it is not performed in and of itself, but rather in conjunction with another procedure). As indicated in the cross-reference following code **92973**, this procedure may be reported for the removal of a thrombus from the lumen of a coronary artery by percutaneous technique when performed at the time of percutaneous intracoronary stent placement (**92980**) or percutaneous intracoronary balloon angioplasty (**92982**).

+**92974**    Transcatheter placement of radiation delivery device for
subsequent coronary intravascular brachytherapy (List separately
in addition to code for primary procedure)

(Use **92974** in conjunction with code(s) **92980, 92982, 92995, 93508**)

(For intravascular radioelement application, see **77781-77784**)

Similar to the reporting of code **92973**, the add-on code **92974** is also reported only in addition to certain other primary intracoronary procedures. Code **92974** is reported when transcatheter placement of a radiation delivery device is performed. This radiation delivery device will subsequently hold the brachytherapy seeds at the appropriate dose calculation. Code **92974** may be additionally reported when performed at the time of percutaneous intracoronary stent placement (**92980**), percutaneous intracoronary balloon angioplasty

(**92982**) or transluminal atherectomy procedures (**92995**), or when coronary arteriography, arterial coronary conduit or venous bypass graft angiography is performed without an associated left heart cardiac catheterization (**93508**).

**92980** Transcatheter placement of an intracoronary stent(s), percutaneous, with or without other therapeutic intervention, any method; single vessel

**+92981** each additional vessel (List separately in addition to code for primary procedure)

(Use **92981** in conjunction with code **92980**)

(To report additional vessels treated by angioplasty or atherectomy only during the same session, see **92984**, **92996**)

Codes **92980** and **92981** are used to report transcatheter placement of one or more intracoronary stents. Code **92980** is reported for placement of one or more stents into a single vessel. Each additional vessel with stent placement is reported with code **92981**. Code **92981** is an add-on code. The first parenthetical note following code **92981** indicates that code **92981** is reported in conjunction with **92980**.

**EXAMPLE:** Transcatheter placement of two stents in the right coronary artery is performed.

Code **92980** is reported one time.

**EXAMPLE:** One stent is placed in the right coronary artery and another stent in the left anterior descending coronary artery.

Codes **92980** and **92981** are both reported one time.

The code descriptor also describes "with or without other therapeutic intervention, any method." This language indicates that if PTCA or percutaneous transluminal coronary atherectomy is performed with subsequent stent placement, codes **92980** and **92981** are used to describe the angioplasty or atherectomy and the stent placement.

**EXAMPLE:** A PTCA of the right coronary artery with stent placement in the same vessel is performed.

Code **92980** is reported one time.

**EXAMPLE:** Percutaneous transluminal atherectomy with stent placement in the left anterior descending coronary artery is performed.

Code **92980** is reported one time.

The second parenthetical note following code **92981** provides further instruction regarding how to report additional vessels treated by angioplasty or atherectomy only during the same session. In those cases, use the add-on code(s) for the angioplasty and atherectomy procedures.

**EXAMPLE:** A PTCA with stent placement of the right coronary artery and PTCA only of the left anterior descending coronary artery are performed.

Code **92980** is reported for the PTCA and stent placement of the right coronary artery, and code **92984** is reported for the PTCA only of the left anterior descending coronary artery.

**EXAMPLE:** Percutaneous transluminal atherectomy with stent placement of the left circumflex artery and atherectomy only of the right coronary artery are performed.

Code **92980** is reported for the atherectomy and stent placement of the left circumflex artery, and code **92996** is reported for the atherectomy only of the right coronary artery.

**92982**     Percutaneous transluminal coronary balloon angioplasty; single vessel

**+92984**        each additional vessel (List separately in addition to code for primary procedure)

(Use **92984** in conjunction with code(s) **92980**, **92982**, **92995**)

(For stent placement following completion of angioplasty or atherectomy, see **92980**, **92981**)

Codes **92982** and **92984** are used to report PTCA. Code **92982** is reported for PTCA of a single vessel. Code **92984** is an add-on code reported for PTCA of each additional vessel. The first parenthetical note following code **92984** indicates that code **92984** is not reported without first reporting code **92980**, **92982**, or **92995**.

**EXAMPLE:** PTCA of the right coronary artery, the left anterior descending coronary artery, and the left main coronary artery is reported with codes **92982, 92984, 92984**.

Code **92984** is reported for each additional vessel treated by PTCA only. Therefore, in this example, **92984** is reported two times.

The second parenthetical note following code **92984** indicates that if stent placement is performed after completion of PTCA, codes **92980** and **92981** are to be reported.

**EXAMPLE:** PTCA of the left circumflex artery with stent placement is performed.

Code **92980** is reported to include the PTCA and the stent placement.

**92995** Percutaneous transluminal coronary atherectomy, by mechanical or other method, with or without balloon angioplasty; single vessel

**+92996** each additional vessel (List separately in addition to code for primary procedure)

(Use **92996** in conjunction with code(s) **92980**, **92982**, **92995**)

(For stent placement following completion of angioplasty or atherectomy, see **92980**, **92981**)

(To report additional vessels treated by angioplasty only during the same session, use **92984**)

Codes **92995** and **92996** are used to report percutaneous transluminal coronary atherectomy with or without balloon angioplasty. Code **92995** is reported for atherectomy (with or without balloon angioplasty) of a single vessel. Code **92996** is an add-on code reported for each additional vessel treated by atherectomy (with or without balloon angioplasty). The first parenthetical note following code **92996** indicates that code **92996** is reported in conjunction with codes **92980**, **92982**, or **92995**.

**EXAMPLE:** Percutaneous transluminal atherectomy of the left circumflex coronary artery and the left anterior descending coronary artery is performed.

Codes **92995** and **92996** are both reported one time.
The wording in the code descriptor indicates that if balloon angioplasty is performed in conjunction with the atherectomy, the angioplasty is included when codes **92995** and **92996** are reported.

**EXAMPLE:** Percutaneous transluminal atherectomy with balloon angioplasty of the left circumflex artery is performed.

Code **92995** is reported to include both the atherectomy and the angioplasty of the left circumflex artery.

**EXAMPLE:** Percutaneous transluminal atherectomy of the right coronary artery and atherectomy with balloon angioplasty of the left main coronary artery are performed.

Codes **92995** and **92996** are both reported one time.
The second parenthetical note following code **92996** indicates that for stent placement after completion of angioplasty or atherectomy, codes **92980** and **92981** are reported.

**EXAMPLE:** Percutaneous transluminal atherectomy of the left anterior descending coronary artery with stent placement is performed.

Code **92980** is reported to include both the atherectomy and the stent placement of the left main coronary artery.

The third parenthetical note following code **92996** instructs the user about how to report additional vessels treated by angioplasty only during the same session. In this case, code **92984** is reported.

**EXAMPLE:** Percutaneous transluminal atherectomy of the right coronary artery with PTCA of the left anterior descending coronary artery is performed.

Code **92995** is reported for the atherectomy of the right coronary artery, and code **92984** is reported for the PTCA of the left anterior descending coronary artery.

The therapeutic services of balloon angioplasty, atherectomy, and intracoronary stent placement procedures, represented by codes **92980**, **92981**, **92982**, **92984**, and **92995**, do not include diagnostic cardiac catheterization, nor do they describe any particular angiographic procedure. If a diagnostic cardiac catheterization and angiography are performed separately from the therapeutic service, it would be appropriate to separately report the services provided. However, angiography procedures performed during the course of a therapeutic coronary artery procedure (eg, injection of dye and imaging to determine catheter/balloon placement and postprocedural effectiveness) are considered an integral part of the therapeutic procedure and are not separately reported.

In coding for the therapeutic services of balloon angioplasty, atherectomy, and intracoronary stent placement, it may be noted that the physician performing the procedure indicates that the intervention was unsuccessful. Appropriate coding for unsuccessful procedures depends on the extent of the procedure performed. Consider the following examples.

**EXAMPLE 1:** A PTCA is unsuccessful in dilating a subtotal occlusion of the right coronary artery because of inability to cross the lesion with the balloon catheter. In this case, the code for the angioplasty is reported with modifier 52 appended.

**EXAMPLE 2:** A PTCA is unsuccessful in dilating a subtotal occlusion of the right coronary artery. However, the lesion was crossed and the angioplasty performed, but with an unacceptable outcome. In this case, the angioplasty would be coded without modifier 52 appended.

The codes included in the **93000-93278** series are used to report various methods of obtaining cardiographic readings for the heart. The correct code to use for the procedure is dependent on the capabilities of the equipment being used as well as the information that is obtained regarding heartbeat and any irregularities that may occur.

Codes **93000**, **93005**, and **93010** are used to report electrocardiographic services. The data itself can be obtained by a nonphysician provider, but the analysis and report require a physician's interpretation to perform. This procedure is carried out by attaching electrodes to the patient's limbs. Unipolar electrodes are then placed at appropriate locations on the chest to detect the depolarization and repolarization of the heart. The resultant information allows the physician to determine certain irregularities regarding the heartbeat and heart function. Since part of this service may be performed by either a physician or a nonphysician health professional, the codes included allow separate report of each of the components of this service. Code **93000** is intended to identify the complete service, which includes the reading (complete with hook-up, tracing, and monitoring), the interpretation of the procedure, and the report. If only the tracing or the interpretation and report are performed, separate codes should be used to identify the specific component provided (**93005** or **93010**).

As is implied by the parenthetical note included following code **93010**, if extended ECG monitoring is performed, the prolonged service codes should be appended to the appropriate E/M code (**99354-99360**) to identify the additional service provided.

Codes **93012** and **93014** are used to report ECG services that allow capture of postsymptomatic ECG readings via telephonic transmission. As indicated in the descriptor language, this code requires 24-hour attended monitoring for the patient and is performed over a 30-day period. Provision of this service requires participation on the patient's behalf, as the patient is required to take the device with him or her. When an episode occurs (arrhythmia), the patient attaches prefurnished electrodes and activates the device, which allows ECG monitoring during the event. The device also records some of the postsymptom ECG to allow additional information for analysis by the physician. After the episode, the patient transmits this information telephonically to the physician's office for interpretation. After a 30-day period, the device is returned to the physician's office for evaluation and interpretation of the data and for completion of the report. Similar to codes **93000-93012**, these codes are reported according to the specific component as indicated in the code descriptor, using code **93012** to identify tracing only or code **93014** for physician review with interpretation and report.

Codes **93015-93018** are used to report cardiovascular stress testing procedures. These procedures combine the use of a stressing agent or device (such as a treadmill, stationary cycle, or chemical stressor of the heart) with some type of ECG monitoring service. For this procedure, the physician places monitoring leads for information retrieval during the test. In addition to the ECG leads, the physician is also responsible for monitoring the heart rate, blood pressure, and any symptoms that may occur as a result of the testing. Once monitoring and data retrieval devices have been applied, the physician can apply stress to the heart in any of a number of methods including physical exercise by using a mechanical apparatus (exercise bike, treadmill, etc) or by administering a pharmacologic agent (eg, beta-1 agonist). At this point, the patient is monitored both for irregularity in heart function as well as for any other symptomatic responses to the stress (eg, labored breathing) to ensure the safety of the patient during the testing as well as to obtain pertinent information regarding possible pathology. Once the desired results are achieved, the patient is monitored to ensure safe return of the heart to a nonstressed state. The ECG recording and other information can then be analyzed by the physician.

Code **93015** is used to report the complete procedure, which includes physician supervision of the stressing of the patient, the ECG tracing procedure, and the interpretation and report provided following the administration of the test. (Note: Set-up of the equipment and application of the electrodes for monitoring are inherently included in the procedure.)

If the complete procedure is not performed, the provider should report codes **93016-93018** according to the specific procedures actually provided. Code **93016** is used to report physician supervision of the stress testing procedure itself and does not include the interpretation, report, or tracing. Code **93017** is used to report the tracing/recording procedure only, and code **93018** is used to report the physician interpretation and report only. If more than a single component is performed, it is appropriate to use multiple codes to identify the service(s) performed. (Note: Code **93015** should be used if all three components of this procedure are performed by a single physician.)

## Echocardiography

Codes in the **93303-93350** series are used to report echocardiography. Echocardiography includes obtaining ultrasonic signals (echoes) from the heart and great arteries, with two-dimensional image and/or Doppler ultrasonic signal documentation and interpretation and report. When the interpretation and report (professional component) are performed separately, the use of modifier 26 becomes necessary. (Refer to Chapter 10 for further discussion of the use of modifier 26.)

Transthoracic echocardiography, described by codes **93303-93308** and **93350**, is a noninvasive technique that involves the placement of an ultrasound transducer at various locations on the patient's chest and upper abdomen. Images obtained by ultrasonic transmission are recorded on videotape or stored in digital format into computer memory.

Transesophageal echocardiography (TEE), described by codes **93312-93318**, involves placement of an endoscopic ultrasound transducer through the mouth into the esophagus, during which two-dimensional images of internal structures of the heart (ie, cardiac chambers, valves, and great vessels) can be visualized and recorded.

The codes for reporting TEE allow for separate reporting of the placement of the transesophageal probe and the image acquisition, interpretation, and report when these services are provided separately. Code **93312** describes the complete service including probe placement, image acquisition, interpretation, and report. Code **93313** is used to report placement of the transesophageal probe only, and code **93314** is used to report the image acquisition, interpretation, and report only.

Consider the following examples:

**EXAMPLE 1:** Physician A places the transesophageal probe for TEE.
Physician B performs the image acquisition, interpretation, and report

> **CODING TIP**
>
> For transesophageal echocardiography (TEE) for intraoperative monitoring purposes only, use code **93318**. For transesophageal echocardiography (TEE) for diagnostic purposes, use code **93312-93317**. (Refer to Chapter 9 for further discussion.)

of the TEE. In this case, Physician A reports code **93313** to describe his services and Physician B reports code **93314**. Since code **93314** has a professional/technical component breakdown, Physician B will append modifier 26 if applicable (see Chapter 10).

**EXAMPLE 2:** Physician C performs TEE including probe placement, image acquisition, interpretation, and report. He performs the procedure in the hospital on hospital-owned equipment. In this case, Physician C reports code **93312** with modifier 26 appended to indicate that he is reporting for the professional component of the TEE (since the procedure is performed on hospital-owned equipment). (Refer to Chapter 10 for further discussion of the professional component and the use of modifier 26.)

When echocardiography is performed, it is often necessary to use pulsed wave and/or continuous wave Doppler with spectral display (**93320**, **93321**) and/or Doppler color flow-velocity mapping (**93325**). The codes used to describe these procedures are designated as add-on codes in CPT. Therefore, when these procedures are performed, appropriate add-on code(s) are listed separately, in addition to the code(s) for the echocardiography.

Codes **93303**, **93304**, and **93315-93317** are specifically used to report echocardiography for congenital cardiac anomalies. These codes are used to report echocardiographic examinations for suspected complex congenital heart disease. Or, in the case of follow-up or limited examinations, these codes are used to report a repeat echocardiographic study during or after a surgical or interventional repair procedure to verify or confirm the adequacy of the repair or function of the heart. However, these codes are not used when congenital heart disease is suspected but not found on echocardiographic evaluation. In this case, the noncongenital echocardiography codes should be used.

Code **93318** is a stand-alone code that differs from the previous TEE procedures in that it specifically describes TEE monitoring required to assess cardiovascular function and assist with therapeutic decisions (as opposed to diagnostic) performed intraoperatively. This code describes placement of a TEE probe and the use of TEE technology for continuous monitoring (not diagnostic) purposes during surgical operations and other types of interventions that produce acute and dynamic changes in cardiovascular function (eg, abdominal/thoracic aneurysm repair, open cardiac procedures).

To further differentiate usage, codes **93313** and **93316**, eg, are reported for placement of the transesophageal probe only and represent only the first step in the use of the TEE probe for monitoring. Codes **93314** and **93317**, which describe image acquisition, interpretation, and report, focus on a diagnostic assessment of cardiac anatomy and function at one point in time with the aim of specifying the disease process. These codes do not include continuous monitoring to detect acute and episodic changes occasioned by surgical manipulation and other interventions.

**EXAMPLE:** A patient is to undergo repair of an abdominal aortic aneurysm. As part of the surgical procedure, an aortic cross-clamp is applied during the operation while the surgeon excises the aneurysm and inserts a tube graft. TEE (code **93312**) images of left ventricular distention and impaired cardiac contractility would lead the anesthesiologist to (1) ask the surgeon to release the aortic cross-clamp at least partially, (2) administer a vasodilator, and (3) administer an inotrope (eg, digitalis, dopamine, dobutamine, amrinone). When the aortic cross-clamp is removed after the aortic graft is in place, hypotension usually ensues because of the sudden decrease in peripheral vascular resistance and reperfusion of tissues distal to the clamp. TEE images can guide the IV administration of fluid and blood products.

Code **93350** describes echocardiography during rest and cardiovascular stress test with the use of treadmill, bicycle exercise, and/or pharmacologically induced stress (stress echocardiography). The appropriate stress testing code from the **93015-93018** series should be reported in addition to code **93350** to describe the exercise stress portion of the study. Furthermore, if the stress is pharmacologically induced, it is appropriate to separately report the supply of the drug(s) used to induce the stress. The supply may be reported with CPT code **99070** or the appropriate HCPCS Level II code(s) for the specific drug(s) used. However, a separate code would not be reported for the administration of the drug(s). The administration procedure is considered an inclusive component of code **93350**.

## Cardiac Catheterizations

When coding for cardiac catheterization services, separate codes are reported to describe the following:

- The catheter placement
- Injection procedures performed in conjunction with the cardiac catheterization
- The imaging supervision, interpretation, and report for injection procedure(s) during cardiac catheterization

Codes **93501-93533** are intended to describe the insertion of catheters into the various chambers of the heart or arteries, veins, and great vessels. These codes include the introduction, positioning, and repositioning of catheter(s), when necessary; recording of intracardiac and intravascular pressure; and obtaining blood samples for measurement of blood gases or dilution curves and cardiac output measurements (Fick or other method, with or without rest and exercise and/or studies), with or without electrode catheter placement. They also include final evaluation and report of this portion of the cardiac catheterization procedure.

Coronary arteriography, arterial coronary conduit, or venous bypass graft angiography performed without an associated left heart cardiac catheterization is reported with code **93508**. It is appropriate to separately report injection procedures (**93539**, **93540**, **93544**, and **93545**) and imaging supervision, interpretation, and report (**93556**), when performed.

Codes **93530-93533** are specifically used to report cardiac catheterization for congenital cardiac anomalies. While it is true that the vast majority of patients undergoing congenital heart disease catheterization procedures are children (frequently newborns or infants younger than two years of age), more patients with congenital heart disease are surviving into adolescence and young adulthood. Therefore, there is no age limit included in the narrative description of these codes. As long as there is a congenital cardiac anomaly, it is appropriate to report these codes when cardiac catheterization is performed.

The codes in the **93501-93533** series do not include the injection procedure(s) performed in conjunction with cardiac catheterization. Codes **93539-93545** are reported for injection procedures for angiography performed in conjunction with cardiac catheterization. Injection procedures represent separately identifiable services and may be coded in conjunction with one another when appropriate. The technical details of angiography, supervision of filming and processing, and interpretation and report are not included in these codes. To report imaging supervision, interpretation, and report, use code **93555** and/or **93556**.

It is appropriate to report more than one code from the **93539-93545** series if multiple injection procedures are performed. For example, injection procedures for selective coronary angiography, left ventriculography, and pulmonary

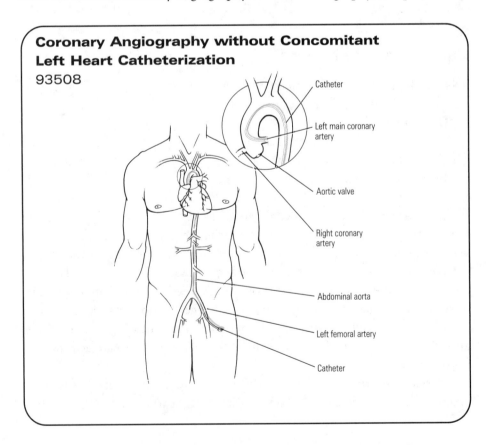

**Coronary Angiography without Concomitant Left Heart Catheterization**
93508

Catheter

Left main coronary artery

Aortic valve

Right coronary artery

Abdominal aorta

Left femoral artery

Catheter

angiography are separately reported with codes **93545**, **93543**, and **93541**, respectively. However, none of the codes in this series is reported more than once per cardiac catheterization session.

CPT codes **93555** and **93556** are intended to be used to report supervision of the angiographic imaging and interpretation and report for the injection procedure(s) during cardiac catheterization. Code **93555** describes imaging supervision, interpretation, and report for ventricular and/or atrial angiography. Code **93556** is used to report imaging supervision, interpretation, and report for pulmonary angiography, aortography, and/or selective coronary angiography (including venous bypass grafts and arterial conduits).

Codes **93555** and **93556** are designated as modifier 51-exempt, identified with the symbol placed before these codes. These codes appear in Appendix E of the CPT codebook and are exempt from the use of modifier 51 but have not been designated as CPT add-on codes. (Refer to Chapter 4 for further discussion of modifier 51-exempt codes.)

The use of the professional component modifier (modifier 26) is appropriate with codes **93501**, **93505-93533**, **93555**, and **93556** when only the professional component of cardiac catheterization procedures is provided (eg, when cardiac catheterization is performed on facility-owned equipment). However, it is not appropriate to append modifier 26 to the codes for injection procedure during cardiac catheterization (**93539-93545**), as these codes represent solely professional responsibilities. (Refer to Chapter 10 for further discussion regarding the use of modifier 26.)

Consider the following:

**EXAMPLE:** A combined right heart catheterization and retrograde left heart catheterization is performed with injection procedures for left ventricular angiography, aortography, and selective coronary angiography, including imaging supervision, interpretation, and report for the injection procedures.

In the previous example, it would be appropriate to report codes **93526**, **93543**, **93544**, **93545**, **93556**, and **93555** to completely describe the procedures performed.

## Repair of Septal Defects

Codes **93580** and **93581** are used to report repair of congenital atrial or ventricular septal defects via use of percutaneous transcatheter procedures. Since medicine has advanced to allow an alternative method for accomplishing this type of repair, these codes are used to identify this type of procedure, when performed. In addition, certain procedures are necessary when performing the repair, such as right heart catheterization and injection of contrast for atrial and/or ventricular angiograms. Therefore, parenthetical notes have been added to identify procedures that are inherently included as part of these percutaneous transcatheter septal defect repairs (ie, codes **93501**, **93529-93533**,

**93539**, **93543**, and **93555**). Notes have also been added that identify that echocardiographic services (codes **93303**, et al) should be separately reported if performed in addition to these transcatheter repair procedures.

## Intracardiac Electrophysiologic Procedures

Electrophysiology is a subspecialty of cardiology devoted to the diagnosis and treatment of heart rhythm disturbances. Because of the complex nature of electrophysiologic testing, it is necessary to understand the normal electrophysiology of the heart. The following illustration and flow chart on page 454 describe the normal electrical conduction of the heart.

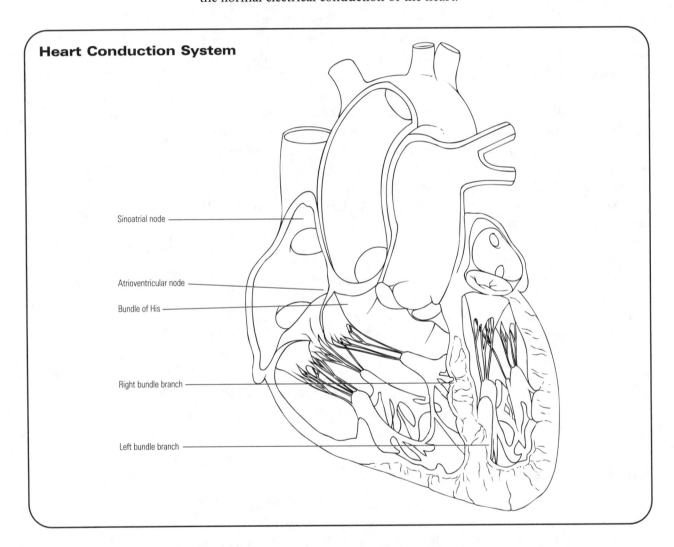

**Heart Conduction System**

Sinoatrial node

Atrioventricular node

Bundle of His

Right bundle branch

Left bundle branch

The sinoatrial (SA) node is the pacemaker of the heart; the cardiac cycle begins when this node fires. The impulse sent out by the SA node travels through the atrial tissue to the atrioventricular (AV) node. This same impulse causes the atria to contract. When the atria contract, blood is forced into the ventricles. Once the impulse reaches the AV node, it is rapidly transmitted to the AV bundle, or bundle of His. The bundle of His passes down the intraventricular septum before it divides into the left and right sides of the heart. From the bundle of His, the impulse is transmitted to the Purkinje fibers, which reach into the deeper muscle of the heart. Contraction of the ventricles occurs when the blood is forced out of the heart chambers into the lungs or body. The cardiac cycle is then complete, and the SA node is ready to fire again.

Codes **93600-93652** are used to report electrophysiologic (EP) procedures performed for diagnostic and/or therapeutic purposes. These codes include inserting and repositioning catheters. Intracardiac EP study(s) includes systematic intracardiac assessment of the heart's electrical event timing in various locations during rest and after a stimulated (induced) state. Recorded responses reveal the type, site, origin, and activity path of various cardiac conduction and rhythm disturbances.

During an EP study, an important element of the procedure is to attempt induction of an arrhythmia. This induction is done through the catheters that have already been placed in one or more of the heart chambers for recording and pacing. The electrophysiologist uses a programmable stimulator to deliver critically timed electrical impulses to the heart through any of the catheters that have been placed as part of the EP procedure. A specific protocol of stimulation is followed in the attempted induction of arrhythmia. In this process, stimulation may be performed in one or more sites in any cardiac chamber until the clinical arrhythmia has been induced or until the protocol has been completed. This process of programmed stimulation will initiate a cardiac arrhythmia (tachycardia) in most patients with tachycardia. Termination of arrhythmia by pacing methods or direct countershock during EP studies is considered an inclusive component of the EP study and not separately reported.

In addition to the induction of arrhythmias and their response to pharmacotherapy or device therapy, EP studies are used in the diagnosis and treatment of life-threatening and non-life-threatening cardiac arrhythmias. Therefore, EP studies offer a wealth of information about the heart's electrical activity in order to do the following:

- Investigate the patient's sinus node function and AV conduction
- Locate the origin of dangerous arrhythmias
- Assess supraventricular tachycardia and ventricular tachycardia
- Evaluate the effectiveness of drug therapy or an automatic implantable cardioverter-defibrillator
- Perform a radiofrequency ablation to destroy accessory conduction pathways or other sites of abnormal electrical activity that cause tachycardia

Intracardiac EP studies are invasive diagnostic medical procedures that include the insertion and repositioning of electrode catheters, recording of electrograms before and during pacing or programmed stimulation of multiple locations in the heart, analysis of recorded information, and report of the procedure.

EP studies are most often performed with two or more electrode catheters. In many circumstances, patients with arrhythmias are evaluated and treated at the same encounter. In this situation, a diagnostic EP study is performed, induced tachycardia(s) is mapped, and, on the basis of the diagnostic and mapping information, the tissue is ablated.

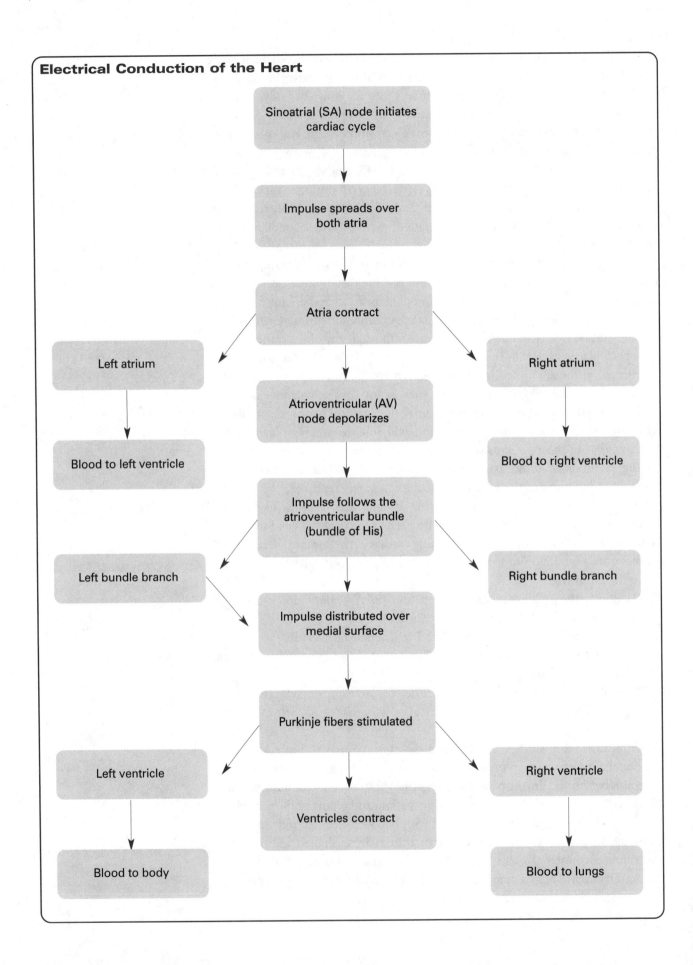

**Electrical Conduction of the Heart**

EP studies, mapping, and ablation represent distinctly different procedures, requiring individual reporting, whether performed on the same or subsequent dates.

**Arrhythmia Induction**—In most EP studies, an attempt is made to induce arrhythmia(s) from single or multiple sites within the heart. Arrhythmia induction is achieved by performing pacing at different rates, programmed stimulation (introduction of critically timed electrical impulses), and other techniques. Because arrhythmia induction occurs via the same catheter(s) inserted for the EP studies, catheter insertion and temporary pacemaker codes are not additionally reported. Codes **93600-93603**, **93610-93612**, and **93618** are used to describe unusual situations where there may be recording, pacing, or an attempt at arrhythmia induction from only one site in the heart. Code **93619** describes only evaluation of the sinus node, AV node, and His-Purkinje conduction system, without arrhythmia induction. Codes **93620-93624** and **93640-93642** all include recording, pacing, and attempted arrhythmia induction from one or more sites in the heart.

**Mapping**—Mapping is a distinct procedure performed in addition to a diagnostic EP procedure and should be separately reported by means of code **93609** or **93613**. Codes **93609** and **93613** identify different methods of mapping, using code **93509** to identify mapping performed for multiple sites within the atrium and/or ventricle and code **93613** to identify simultaneous computer-assisted, three-dimensional mapping from many electrodes. When a tachycardia is induced, the site of tachycardia origination or its electrical path through the heart is often defined by mapping. Mapping creates a multidimensional depiction of tachycardia by recording multiple electrograms obtained sequentially or simultaneously from multiple catheter sites in the heart. Depending on the technique, certain types of mapping catheters may be repositioned from point to point within the heart, allowing sequential recording from the various sites to construct maps. Other types of mapping catheters allow mapping without a point-to-point technique by allowing simultaneous recording from many electrodes on the same catheter and computer-assisted three-dimensional reconstruction of the tachycardia activation sequence (**93613**).

Parenthetical notes have been included with codes **93609** and **93613** to identify mutual exclusion when either service is performed.

**Ablation**—Once the part of the heart involved in the tachycardia is localized, the tachycardia may be treated by ablation (the delivery of radiofrequency energy to the area to selectively destroy cardiac tissue). Ablation procedures (**93651**, **93652**) may be performed independently on a date subsequent to a diagnostic EP study and mapping, or at the time a diagnostic EP study, tachycardia(s) induction, and mapping are performed. When an EP study, mapping, and ablation are performed on the same date, each procedure should be separately reported. In reporting catheter ablation, code **93651** and/or **93652** should be reported once to describe ablation of cardiac arrhythmias, regardless of the number of arrhythmias ablated.

Recording and pacing are described by codes **93600-93612**. In the early years of EP testing, it was fairly common to record and pace from only a single site. However, in most EP laboratories today, complex EP diagnostic procedures

---

**CODING TIP**

For three-dimensional intracardiac EP mapping, use code **93613**.

are performed according to a specific protocol that includes recording and pacing from multiple sites in a specific sequence to arrive at a precise diagnosis. Therefore, it is extremely unusual to record and pace from only one or two sites within the heart. Codes **93619-93622**, which describe these as combination procedures, will be used more often to describe EP evaluations. However, there are still occasional circumstances for which single catheter studies for either recording and/or pacing might be undertaken. That is, if recording electrograms alone are performed, codes **93600-93603** would be chosen either singly or in combination.

Code **93609** describes intraventricular and/or intra-atrial mapping of tachycardia site(s) with catheter manipulation to record from multiple sites to identify the origin of tachycardia. Code **93613** describes a mapping technique that allows simultaneous recording from many electrodes on the same catheter and computer-assisted three-dimensional reconstruction of the tachycardia activation sequence. If intracardiac mapping of tachycardia is performed with a comprehensive EP evaluation to localize the site of origin of the tachycardia, code **93609** or **93613** is reported in addition to code for the comprehensive evaluation. When an EP study, mapping, and ablation are performed on the same date, each procedure should be separately reported.

Pacing alone is coded with either **93610** or **93612**. Code **93610** describes intra-atrial pacing. Code **93612** is used to report intraventricular pacing. Either one of these codes is usually selected in circumstances where termination of an existing arrhythmia will be required as a separate procedure (not as part of a comprehensive study). It would not be appropriate to report code **93612** in addition to codes **93620-93622**.

Code **93618** describes the induction of arrhythmia by electrical pacing when this is performed without diagnostic mapping. Because codes **93619-93622** include arrhythmia induction (or attempted arrhythmia induction), it is not appropriate to additionally report code **93618**.

Most EP evaluations are comprehensive procedures, as described by codes **93619-93622**. In these comprehensive EP evaluations, three or more electrode catheters are inserted and positioned within the heart, usually in the right atrium, right ventricle, across the tricuspid valve, in the His bundle region, and sometimes in the coronary sinus or left ventricle. Because the combination codes for EP procedures include catheter insertion, recording, and stimulation, catheter insertion and temporary pacemaker codes are not reported in addition to codes **93619-93622**.

Selected electrodes are used for pacing, and endocardial electrograms are taken from the corresponding areas of the myocardium to evaluate conduction to localize the site of the arrhythmia. If the suspected arrhythmia is induced, the ectopic focus in the myocardium can be identified and treated. During the course of an evaluation, the catheters may be repositioned to provide better recording and/or pacing.

Occasionally during an EP study, it will be determined that permanent pacing should be performed in an urgent fashion for treatment of complete heart block or high grade second-degree heart block. In these circumstances, it is common practice to leave a pacing catheter in the right ventricle to provide backup pacing during insertion of a permanent pacemaker. Because the coding for the comprehensive EP procedure describes the original insertion of this catheter, an additional code for the insertion of a temporary pacing catheter is not reported.

Code **93619** describes a comprehensive EP evaluation with right atrial pacing and recording, right ventricular pacing and recording, and His bundle recording. This code is appropriate when a comprehensive evaluation with right atrial and ventricular pacing and recording and His bundle recording are performed without induction or attempted induction of an arrhythmia.

Code **93620** also describes a comprehensive EP evaluation, as in code **93619**. However, this code is reported when a comprehensive evaluation with right atrial and ventricular pacing and recording and His bundle recording is performed with induction or attempted induction of arrhythmia.

Add-on code **93621** describes a comprehensive EP evaluation with right atrial and ventricular pacing and recording and His bundle recording and also includes left atrial recordings from the coronary sinus or left atrium, with or without pacing. This code includes the induction or attempted induction of arrhythmia. Add-on code **93621** should be reported in addition to code **93620**. (Refer to Chapter 4 for further discussion of add-on codes.)

Add-on code **93622** describes a comprehensive EP evaluation with right atrial and ventricular pacing and recording, His bundle recording, and left ventricular recordings, with or without pacing. This code includes the induction or attempted induction of arrhythmia.

Add-on code(s) **93621** and/or **93622** may be reported in addition to code **93620** if a comprehensive EP study is performed as described by code **93620** with left atrial and/or left ventricular recordings. The appropriate codes are to be reported on the basis of the specific evaluation performed.

Code **93623** is an add-on code that describes programmed stimulation and pacing after IV drug infusion. This is an additional therapeutic assessment that involves IV drug infusion to suppress an inducible arrhythmia. This code is reported in addition to codes **93620**, **93621**, and **93622**, as appropriate.

Code **93624** describes an EP follow-up study with pacing and recording to test effectiveness of therapy. This code includes induction or attempted induction of arrhythmia. In some EP laboratories, serial drug testing for evaluation of therapeutic options for patients with tachycardia is performed by means of an indwelling catheter. This method of EP evaluation is not often performed, but when this approach is used, coding for subsequent studies is reported with code **93624**. Catheter insertion is not separately reported when an indwelling catheter has been used for an EP follow-up study.

Code **93631** describes intraoperative epicardial and endocardial pacing and mapping to localize the site of tachycardia or zone of slow conduction for surgical correction. This code is reported when the epicardial and endocardial pacing and mapping are performed via an open incision with the heart exposed. The surgeon exposes the heart, then the electrophysiologist performs the mapping. Once the arrhythmogenic focus (or foci) is determined, the surgeon ablates the specific focus (or foci). The ablation procedure is separately reported with codes from the **33250-33261** series of codes in the Surgery section of the CPT codebook.

Codes **93640-93642** describe the procedures undertaken by the electro-physiologist for evaluation of newly or chronically implanted single- or dual-chamber pacing cardioverter-defibrillators. These codes include defibrillation threshold testing that involves assessment of the device's sensing capability regarding the induction of ventricular arrhythmia(s) and the arrhythmia termination process.

Codes **93640** and **93641** are intended to be reported at the time of initial implantation or replacement of the pacing cardioverter-defibrillator. Code **93640** is reported when pacing cardioverter-defibrillator leads are implanted during insertion but are not connected to the pulse generator. When a pulse generator is connected and the entire system is tested, code **93641** is reported.

Codes **93640** and **93641** are reported in addition to the appropriate code(s) for the implantation or replacement of the pacing cardioverter-defibrillator from the cardiovascular system subsection of the Surgery section of the CPT codebook. (Refer to Chapter 5 for further discussion of the codes for implantation or replacement of a pacing cardioverter-defibrillator.)

Code **93642** is intended to describe subsequent or periodic EP evaluation of a previously implanted device (including induction of cardiac arrhythmias), performed in an EP laboratory.

Codes **93650-93652** describe intracardiac catheter ablation of arrhythmias. In catheter ablation coding, a single code is used to describe the ablation of cardiac arrhythmias, regardless of the number of arrhythmias ablated. If ablation is undertaken to cause complete heart block, code **93650** is reported. Because a temporary pacemaker is required, code **93650** includes the placement of a temporary backup pacemaker, but an additional and separate code is used to describe the insertion of the permanent pacemaker.

Catheter ablation undertaken for treatment of supraventricular tachycardia caused by dual AV nodal pathways or accessory AV connections or other atrial foci is reported with code **93651**. Code **93652** describes catheter ablation performed for treatment of ventricular tachycardia.

Code **93660** describes evaluation of cardiovascular function with tilt-table evaluation. Tilt-table testing involves the use of a motorized tilt table to provide passive upright posture for patients with a history of syncope. The procedure may be performed alone or with an EP study. Tilt-table testing often involves the use of IV infusion of drugs. As indicated in the code descriptor, when performed, pharmacological intervention is included in code **93660**.

**CODING TIP**

For thoracic electrical bioimpedance, use code **93701**.

## Other Vascular Studies

Code **93724** is used to report electronic analysis of an antitachycardia pacemaker system. In the procedure described by this code, an electrocardiogram is recorded. The device is programmed to allow induction of the tachycardia by noninvasive programmed stimulation, and the performance of the device is analyzed by interpreting recordings of electrograms and interrogation of the device. Such devices are now rarely used since catheter ablation of arrhythmias has become more common.

Codes **93731-93736** describe electronic analysis of single- and dual-chamber pacemaker systems obtained by direct recording or transtelephonic recording. Codes **93731** and **93734** describe analysis of single- and dual-chamber pacemaker systems in which direct patient contact occurs. Reprogramming is not a component of codes **93731** and **93734**. If there is a need to reprogram the device, code **93732** or **93735** should be reported.

If transtelephonic analysis of free-running and magnet strips is performed, codes **93733** and **93736** are used for dual- and single-chamber systems, respectively. Notice that the descriptors do not separate the technical from the professional components of this service. If only the professional component of these services is performed, modifier 26 is appended to the code. (Refer to Chapter 10 for further discussion of the use of modifier 26.)

Codes in the **93741-93744** series are used to report electronic analysis of pacing cardioverter-defibrillators. These codes are reported for postimplantation electronic analysis of an implantable cardioverter defibrillator or analysis of a wearable cardioverter defibrillator system performed in an office or outpatient setting. These services do not involve induction of arrhythmia.

Similar to the codes for electronic analysis of pacemaker systems, codes for the electronic analysis of pacing cardioverter-defibrillators differentiate services for single chamber/wearable devices without reprogramming (**93741**) and with reprogramming (**93742**) from those for dual-chamber analysis without reprogramming (**93743**) and with reprogramming (**93744**).

Code **93745** identifies the initial setup and programming provided by a physician for a wearable cardioverter-defibrillator device. Wearable cardioverter-defibrillator devices are worn outside of the body but still allow for the continuous monitoring of ECG information, including storage of pertinent data for later review by the treating physician and the capability of being programmed to deliver a shock protocol in the event of a life-threatening arrhythmia. This device also allows interaction by the user. Prior to delivery of a shock, the device issues several alerts that allow the wearer the opportunity to abort the shock sequence manually if the patient is conscious and not perceiving a threat that requires emergency defibrillation. In the event that the patient is unconscious and the device detects a heart rhythm that necessitates intervention, similar to other implanted defibrillator devices, the wearable cardioverter-defibrillator will deliver a life-saving shock in an attempt to re-establish the heart rhythm.

In addition to application/setup of the device, the physician provides a range of services prior to the initiation of patient use to ensure appropriate function of the device as well as to ensure the safety of the user and compliance with specifications regarding use. The procedure includes the efforts of the physician to program the device according to the patient's medical history, threshold for duration of occurrence, and threshold rate of ventricular tachycardia required to trigger the shock sequence.

The device also records the patient's ECG information regarding events that require defibrillation. This allows playback of arrhythmic events for physician review and downloading of ECG data for transmission to the health care facility for future analysis. The physician can view and print ECG events and generate reports related to patient wear-time compliance and overall monitoring performance.

# Noninvasive Vascular Diagnostic Studies

Noninvasive vascular diagnostic studies are reported with codes in the **93875-93990** series. Five series of codes exist for reporting these types of studies, including the following:

- Cerebrovascular arterial studies (**93875-93893**)
- Extremity arterial studies (including digits) (**93922-93931**)
- Extremity venous studies (including digits) (**93965-93971**)
- Visceral and penile vascular studies (**93975-93981**)
- Extremity arterial-venous hemodialysis access study (**93990**)

Vascular studies include patient care required to perform the studies, supervision of the studies, and interpretation of study results with written report for patient records including analysis of all data.

The codes in this series are not to be used to report the use of a simple handheld or other Doppler device that does not produce hard-copy output or that produces a record that does not permit analysis of bidirectional vascular flow. This type of evaluation is considered to be part of the physical examination of the vascular system performed as part of the E/M service provided and is not separately reported.

*Duplex scan* describes an ultrasonic scanning procedure with display of two-dimensional vascular structure, motion with time, and Doppler ultrasonic signal documentation with spectral analysis and/or color flow-velocity mapping or imaging. These are noninvasive tests that evaluate blood flow with the use of sound waves for imaging.

In Doppler ultrasonography, a graphic or audio recording (as opposed to imaging) is obtained by a handheld transducer that directs high frequency sound waves to the artery or vein being tested. The sound waves strike moving red blood cells and reflect back to the transducer, which then transforms the sound waves digital electronic signals to permit graphic recording of the blood flow motion including frequency shift and blood flow velocity measurements.

Noninvasive physiologic studies (**93875**, **93922-93924**, and **93965**) involve the use of nonimaging physiologic recordings of pressures (such as analysis of hard-copy bidirectional Doppler ultrasonic recordings of blood flow of eye or analysis of ocular blood pressure using oculoplethysmography—identified by code **93875**), Doppler analysis of bidirectional blood flow (such as those procedures identified by codes **93922-93924**, which provide analysis of upper or lower extremity arterial blood flow using methods such as Doppler waveform analysis, Doppler-derived ankle/brachial indices, volume plethysmography, or transcutaneous oxygen tension measurements), or plethysmography (such as that identified by code **93965**, which is an analysis of extremity venous blood flow using impedance plethysmography or air plethysmography).

If a duplex scan and Doppler ultrasonography are both performed, it is appropriate to separately report these procedures. They represent separately identifiable procedures that use different types of diagnostic instrumentation. However, Doppler spectral analysis and/or color flow Doppler recordings obtained on the same instrument at the same session as a duplex scan are considered to be an integral part of the duplex scan and are not separately reported.

For example, if a duplex scan of extracranial arteries is performed (a complete bilateral study as described by code **93880**) in conjunction with noninvasive physiologic studies of extracranial arteries, such as ocular plethysmography (as described by code **93875**), it would be appropriate to report both codes to completely describe the procedures performed. Code **93880** describes the duplex scan (imaging procedure), and code **93875** describes the noninvasive physiologic study.

The services described in each of these codes represent separately identifiable procedures that use different types of diagnostic instrumentation and should be reported separately.

In addition, codes **93890**, **93892**, and **93893** are cerebrovascular arterial studies codes used to report vasoreactivity studies and emboli detection when performed during transcranial Doppler examinations. These service codes go beyond the effort involved in a full or limited transcranial Doppler study of intracranial arteries, as performance of these procedures involves use of equipment, laboratory, and expertise not ordinarily included as part of the ordinary transcranial Doppler studies. This includes $CO_2$ reactivity measurement technique (used for vasoreactivity studies) as well as embolus detection monitoring of 30-60 (continuous monitoring of signals in cerebral vessels above that of a standard transcranial Doppler study). As is noted in the parenthetical note that follows the code listings, these codes should not be reported in addition to code **93888**.

# Pulmonary

## Ventilator Management

Codes **94002-94004** describe ventilation assist and management with initiation of pressure or volume preset ventilators for assisted or controlled breathing. Code **94005** is used to report home ventilator management care plan oversight of a patient (patient not present) in home, domiciliary, or rest home (eg, assisted living) requiring review of status, review of laboratories and other studies, and revision of orders and respiratory care plan (as appropriate) within a calendar month, 30 minutes or more. Code **94005** is not used in conjunction with **99339**, **99340**, or **99374-99378**.

Ventilatory management care plan oversight is reported separately from home or domiciliary, rest home (eg, assisted living) services. A physician may report **94005**, when performed, including when a different physician reports **99339**, **99340**, **99374-99378** for the same 30 days.

For those patients receiving ventilatory support, the management process involves the following key elements:

1  Initial establishment of the ventilator settings based on the patient's body size (ideal weight) and clinical condition

2  Assessment of the patient and the ventilator system to ensure that the patient is stabilized. This includes assurance of a patent airway and initial data gathered after stabilization.

3  Setting clinical goals for ventilatory support (plan of care)

4  Adjustments of support parameters as indicated by arterial blood gas or pulse oximetry results and the patient's clinical condition

5  Ongoing monitoring and assessment of the patient and ventilatory system, as often as indicated

6  Additional therapeutic intervention to treat the cause(s) and complications of respiratory failure when these are reversible

7  Definition of end-point goals to effect weaning from the ventilator once the problems resulting in respiratory failure have been corrected, where appropriate

Codes in the **94010-94799** series are used to report various pulmonary services and procedures. These codes include laboratory procedure(s) and interpretation of test results. The term *laboratory* does not refer to the services performed that are reported by codes from the Pathology and Laboratory section of the CPT codebook (**80002-89399** series). Rather, these codes describe diagnostic and therapeutic procedures performed in a pulmonary department or facility/pulmonary laboratory. If the services provided include services described by codes in the Pathology and Laboratory section of the CPT codebook, as well as pulmonary services from the **94010-94799** code series, then it is appropriate to report codes from both sections.

If a separately identifiable E/M service is performed, the appropriate E/M code should be reported in addition to code(s) from the **94010-94799** series. (Refer to Chapter 3 for further discussion of coding E/M services.)

The text that follows will discuss some of the specific codes for reporting pulmonary services and procedures.

Code **94010** is used to report spirometry, the measurement of the air entering and leaving the lungs, and is considered the basic foundation of pulmonary function testing. The patient performs a forced exhalation as the volume of air is plotted against time. This code includes a graphic record, total and timed vital capacity (the breathing capacity of the lungs, or the measurement of the amount of air that can be forcibly exhaled after a full inspiration/inhalation), and expiratory flow rate measurement(s). When performed, maximal voluntary ventilation is also included when code **94010** is reported. Spirometry provides a measurement of the air capacity of the lungs with a machine called a *spirometer* (a device that measures the volume or flow of air into and out of the lungs).

Codes **94014-94016** are used to report patient-initiated spirometric recording. This method of obtaining ongoing spirometric analysis of lung function is relatively new but is widely accepted in both the pulmonary medicine and transplant communities. Patient-initiated spirometric recording currently is being used after lung transplant and requires the patient to perform the spirometry at a predetermined time each day. The results are stored in a small computer that is part of the spirometer. At a scheduled time, the patient is contacted and the data are downloaded via modem from the spirometer's computer to another computer. The data is then trended and analyzed to identify problems such as rejection, infection, or bronchiolitis obliterans (obstruction of the bronchioles and alveolar ducts due to fibrous granulation tissue that forms as a result of ulcerations in the mucosal surface) after lung transplant.

Code **94014** is intended to describe a global service for patient-initiated spirometric recordings, ie, both the professional and technical components of the service. Code **94015** describes only the technical component of the service, including recording, hookup, reinforced education, data transmission, data capture, trend analysis, and periodic recalibration. Code **94016** is intended to represent only the physician (professional) component of the service.

Code **94060** is used to report bronchodilation responsiveness. This service and code includes spirometry as described by code **94010** before and after bronchodilator administration. In addition, the supply of the bronchodilator may be separately reported using code **99070** or an appropriate HCPCS supply code for the bronchodilator used. If a significant, separately identifiable E/M service is also provided, an appropriate code from the E/M section may be reported in addition to this procedure code.

Code **94070** is used to report prolonged postexposure evaluation of bronchospasm with multiple spirometric determinations after antigen, cold air, methacholine, or other chemical agent, with subsequent spirometrics. When code **94010** is used to report the initial spirogram, it is usually performed as a preliminary test, the results of which may lead to the performance of a provocative test with methacholine (**94070**). Under these circumstances, code **94010** is reported separately in addition to code **94070**, and modifier 59 may be appended to the secondary procedure to identify the distinctive nature of the procedure. However, the subsequent spirometrics are considered part of the procedure (**94070**) itself and should not be individually reported. Code **95070** is used by the laboratory or office administering the methacholine.

If a pulse oximetry (ie, the measure of the oxygen saturation of hemoglobin) procedure is performed in addition to spirometry testing (**94010**, **94060**, **94070**), both procedures may be separately reported (appending modifier 59 as necessary), since spirometry does not include pulse oximetry (**94760**).

Codes **94060** and **94070** both include administration of a bronchodilator. However, these services do not identify an inhalation treatment, since the bronchodilation administration performed for these procedures is administered to identify the patient's response to such treatments. Administering a bronchodilator for treatment requires separate effort by the physician. Therefore, when either procedure is performed, it would be appropriate to report inhalation treatment (ie, code **94640**) for the treatment administered for the acute airway obstruction.

As is indicated in the code **94640** descriptor, this procedure identifies a pressurized or nonpressurized inhalation treatment for acute airway obstruction or for sputum induction for diagnostic purposes. Namely, this means that the service is provided (1) as a treatment for the condition (as opposed to a "test" administration during analysis of the patient's breathing) and/or (2) for the procurement of a sputum sample for diagnostic purposes.

Code **94375** describes respiratory flow volume loop. This test consists of a forced expiratory maneuver followed by a forced inspiratory maneuver. Exhaled and inhaled air is collected or passed through a spirometer. The graphic presentation of the flow volume loop allows for inspection of the shape of the curve and its comparison with a normal loop.

Codes **94452** and **94453** are used to report high altitude simulation testing (HAST). This is a test that uses the administration of two (or more) hypoxic gas mixtures to identify patients who have a predisposition to high altitude sickness. The patient is usually predisposed to high altitude sickness because of chronic lung disease, but could also be vulnerable to this condition for other reasons, such as heart failure, neuromuscular disease, or other conditions.

Exposure to high altitude sickness can occur in circumstances such as commercial air travel, since commercial passenger aircraft usually fly at high altitudes. As a result of the high altitudes of flight, passenger cabins are typically pressurized to the equivalent of 5000 to 8000 feet of altitude. As a consequence of high altitude, the partial pressure of oxygen ($PO_2$) decreases and passengers receive less oxygen during their flight. The lower $PO_2$ experienced during air flight is well tolerated by most people, since hemoglobin dissociation for most people allows for some drop in arterial $PO_2$ without much reduction in blood oxygen content or delivery. However, patients with a reduced arterial $PO_2$ (typically from conditions such as chronic lung disease and other conditions previously mentioned) are at risk of significant hypoxia during air flight. Responsiveness to the administration of the hypoxic gases is an indication that the patient is a candidate for high altitude sickness, and that further evaluation and possibly treatment may be necessary for the patient regarding this situation.

To identify patients at risk of hypoxia during routine commercial flights, the HAST was developed almost 20 years ago. While individual tolerance of hypoxia is variable, high altitude-induced hypoxemia can induce significant clinical deterioration. As a result, HAST is now routinely performed in many hospital pulmonary function laboratories and in large group practices. In addition, all commercial airlines have policies and procedures for providing in-flight supplemental oxygen to patients based upon the results of HAST and a physician's prescription and completion of the appropriate airline forms.

These procedures do not include obtaining arterial blood gases. Therefore, blood gas procedures should be separately reported using code **36600** to identify the arterial puncture for obtaining the sample. Since this procedure includes pulse oximetry testing, codes **94760** and **94761** should not be reported separately.

Code **94610** is used to report intrapulmonary surfactant administration by a physician through an endotracheal tube. This code is not reported in conjunction with codes **99293-99296**. Additionally, this code is reported only once per dosing episode. For endotracheal intubation, report code **31500**.

Codes **94620** and **94621** are used to report simple and complex pulmonary stress testing. Simple and complex pulmonary stress testing methods are vastly different in the amount of resources required to perform the different tests. Simple pulmonary stress testing is typically performed as a six-minute hall walk or on a treadmill. Other types of exertional testing customized to specific patient needs could also be appropriately reported with this code. The purpose of a simple pulmonary stress test might include oxygen titration, exercise induced bronchospastic evaluation using pre- and postspirometry, or exercise prescription for pulmonary rehabilitation. Complex pulmonary stress testing is commonly performed on a treadmill or bicycle ergometer with cardiac monitoring and with a metabolic cart to measure $CO_2$ production and $O_2$ uptake. This test quantifies the aerobic work capacity as determined by peak oxygen uptake, and identifies the source(s) of a limited work capacity. Complex stress testing measures the integration of cardiac and pulmonary function and the status of physical fitness and includes measuring $CO_2$ production, $O_2$ uptake, and ECG recordings of the patient's response to the stress. The outputs of this panel of complex metabolic tests are analyzed and interpreted by the physician, and a report is generated.

Codes **94644** and **94655** describe continuous inhalation treatment with aerosol medication for acute airway obstruction.

Exercise with pulse oximetry to document desaturation or to determine oxygen flow to prevent desaturation is reported with code **94761**.

Code **94640** is reported for inhalation treatment for an acute airway obstruction such as asthma or croup and can represent an aerosol or nebulized administration of the appropriate medication as prescribed by the physician. If repeated treatments are required on the same date, code **94640** should be reported for each treatment performed, with modifier 76 appended to the additional code reported. (A parenthetical note has been included to describe the appropriate method to identify additional treatments performed on the same date.) For continuous inhalation treatment of one hour or more, use **94644, 94645**.

**EXAMPLE:** A 66-year-old patient with asthma is seen in the office with diffuse wheezing and bronchospasm. A nebulized bronchodilator is administered by means of a metered-dose inhaler and chamber. The treatment is repeated after 30 minutes with good clinical response.

In this case, code **94640** should be reported twice (**94640** and **94640-76**).

Code **94640** does not include the supply of the medication administered. The supply of the medication may be separately reported with CPT code **99070** or HCPCS Level II codes, as appropriate.

Code **94660** is used to report initiation and management of continuous positive airway pressure (CPAP) ventilation. CPAP is a technique of respiratory assistance that increases the functional residual capacity of the lung by expanding atelectatic (collapsed) areas within the lung and diminishing the tendency of alveoli to collapse on expiration. CPAP can be provided by mask or by endotracheal tube with or without a ventilator.

Code **94662** is used to report initiation and management of continuous negative-pressure ventilation. The primary use for negative-pressure ventilation is nighttime respiratory muscle rest for patients, eg, with chronic obstructive pulmonary disease or neuromuscular disorders. Negative-pressure ventilation is not usually used in the acute situation, but rather is used in chronic failure as a means of intermittent support.

Code **94664** is reported for the initial demonstration and/or evaluation of patient utilization of an aerosol generator, nebulizer, metered-dose inhaler, or intermittent positive-pressure breathing device. Code **94664** can be reported only once per date of service.

These codes do not include the supply of the medication administered. The supply of the medication may be separately reported with CPT code **99070** or HCPCS Level II codes, as appropriate.

Code **94664** does not include the services described by code **94640**. If the services described by code **94664** were performed in addition to the procedures performed in the preceding clinical scenario, codes **94640, 94640 76**, and **94664** should be reported.

> **EXAMPLE:** A 65-year-old man has chronic obstructive pulmonary disease and chronic bronchitis with thick secretions.

The patient is placed on a metered-dose inhaler with a chamber and is instructed in the appropriate use of the device and medication. The patient is observed using the medication and evaluated for its appropriate use and response.

In addition, code **94664** should be used to identify any number of demonstrations performed during the course of a day of treatment and should be reported only once, regardless of the number of demonstrations performed during that day. Code **97535** should not be reported for the patient instruction inherent in code **94664**.

As stated in the introductory notes of the Pulmonary subsection, if the physician meets the criteria for reporting an E/M code, an appropriate level E/M code should be reported in addition to the pulmonary procedure(s) performed. Modifier 25 should be appended to the appropriate level E/M code.

Codes **94680-94690** are used to report oxygen uptake, carbon dioxide production, and expired gas analysis. These codes are most commonly used to report indirect calorimetry performed to determine the nutritional needs of a patient in the intensive care unit. Code **94681** is used to report indirect calorimetry. These codes are used to describe the testing performed, regardless of the setting in which it is performed. These measurements are commonly performed as a component of complex pulmonary stress testing (represented by CPT code **94621**). When performed as part of complex pulmonary stress testing, it would not be appropriate to report codes **94680-94690** separately. Oxygen uptake and expired gas analysis may be done outside of pulmonary stress testing to evaluate oxygen uptake and $CO_2$ production directly.

Code **94774** describes pediatric home apnea monitoring event recording, including respiratory rate, pattern, and heart rate per 30-day period of time. This code includes monitor attachment, download of data, physician review, interpretation, and preparation of a report.

Code **94775** describes monitor attachment only, and includes hook-up, initiation of recording, and disconnection.

Code **94776** describes monitoring, download of information, receipt of transmission(s), and analyses by computer only.

Code **94777** describes physician review, interpretation, and preparation of report only.

# Allergy and Clinical Immunology

Codes in the **95004-95199** series are used to report allergy and clinical immunology procedures and services. There are separate categories of codes for reporting allergy testing (**95004-95075**) and allergen immunotherapy (**95115-95199**).

## Allergy Testing

Allergy sensitivity tests describe the performance and evaluation of selective cutaneous and mucous membrane tests in correlation with the history, physical examination, and other observations of the patient. The number of tests performed should be judicious and dependent on the history, physical findings, and clinical judgment of the practitioner. Not all patients should necessarily receive the same tests or the same number of sensitivity tests. For allergy laboratory tests, see **86000-86999**. For therapy for severe or intractable allergic disease, see **90765-90768, 90772, 90774, 90775**.

Codes **95004** and **95010** are used to report percutaneous tests (scratch, puncture, prick) for allergy testing. Code **95004** is used to report percutaneous tests with allergenic extracts. Code **95010** describes percutaneous tests with drugs, biologicals, or venoms. When reporting either of these codes, it is necessary to specify the number of tests performed.

Code **95012** describes nitric oxide expired gas determination. This test is performed before and after anti-inflammatory treatment is initiated to determine whether the anti-inflammatory treatment dosage is appropriate and to predict exacerbations. For nitric oxide determination by spectroscopy, use Category III code 0064T. Code **95012** differs from Category III code **0064T** in that it is not performed using spectroscopy. This procedure is performed using a nitric oxide monitoring system.

Codes **95015, 95024**, and **95027** describe intracutaneous (intradermal) tests that are evaluated immediately to determine if there is a reaction (immediate-type reaction). Each of these codes requires specifying the number of tests performed.

**CODING TIP**

Code **95027** is reported for dilution of each allergen tested.

Code **95015** is reported for intracutaneous (intradermal) tests with drugs, biologicals, or venoms. Code **95024** is used to report intracutaneous (intradermal) tests with allergenic extracts. Code **95027** is used to report sequential and incremental intracutaneous (intradermal) tests with allergenic extracts for airborne allergens.

Code **95028** is for intracutaneous tests with allergenic extracts that are evaluated in 24 to 72 hours to determine if there is a delayed reaction to the allergens (delayed-type reaction). Delayed reaction testing includes the intracutaneous administration of the allergenic extracts and the interpretation of the test results 24 to 72 hours later.

Code **95027** is used to report testing of airborne allergen(s) using various dilutional strengths. The dilutional strength is used to determine the appropriate concentration of allergen to use for immunotherapy. Code **95044** is used to report patch or application test(s). Patch or application tests involve topical application of the suspected allergen, which then may be covered with a bandage for a period of time. These services also include evaluation of the results. When this code is reported, it is necessary to specify the number of tests performed.

Code **95052** is used to report photo patch tests. When this code is reported, it is necessary to specify the number of tests performed.

Code **95056** is used to report photo tests. Some allergies are manifested upon exposure to sunlight and cause various kinds of skin eruptions. These photosensitivity reactions can be diagnosed by reproduction of the lesions with artificial or natural sunlight. The use of this code includes any number of reactions being tested at a single encounter.

Code **95060** is used to report ophthalmic mucous membrane tests. A small amount of antigen is applied to the lower conjunctival sac. This code includes evaluation of the results of the test(s). Any number of tests performed at the same encounter are included when this code is reported.

Code **95065** is used to report direct nasal mucous membrane tests. A number of methods exist for introducing the antigen into the nose. This code includes any number of tests performed at the same encounter and includes evaluation of the patient's response to the allergen.

Codes **95070** and **95071** describe inhalation bronchial challenge testing. Inhalation bronchial challenge testing involves the inhalation of agents that can trigger respiratory responses. The agents include drugs that cause airway constriction, antigens, and chemical sensitizers usually related to occupational breathing problems. These codes do not include the necessary pulmonary function tests. The parenthetical note following code **95071** directs the user to codes **94060** and **94070** to report the pulmonary function test(s).

Code **95075** is used to report ingestion challenge testing. This test involves the administration of sequentially or incrementally larger doses of the test item. Some examples of the test items that may be included are food, antibiotics, or other substances such as metabisulfite. This code is reported once per patient encounter, regardless of the number of items tested, and includes evaluation of the patient's response to the test items.

# Allergen Immunotherapy

Immunotherapy (desensitization, hyposensitization) is the parenteral administration of allergenic extracts as antigens at periodic intervals, usually on an increasing dosage scale, to a dose that is maintained as maintenance therapy.

Allergen immunotherapy is reported with codes **95115-95199**. The notes at the beginning of this series of codes indicate that an office or other outpatient visit may be reported in addition to allergen immunotherapy only when other identifiable services are provided with the immunotherapy. This may include services such as the examination of the patient, the interval history, and the evaluation of diagnostic studies. If allergen immunotherapy is the only service provided, it would not be appropriate to report an office visit code. (Refer to Chapter 3 for further discussion regarding coding for E/M services.)

Codes **95115** and **95117** reflect the administration (injection) of the allergenic extract when the extract is not included in the code descriptor. They do not include the provision or preparation of the extract. These codes are intended to be reported one time, regardless of the number of injections administered. Each injection should not be specified. Code **95115** is reported for a single injection, and code **95117** is reported if two or more injections are performed.

For example, an allergist provides a patient with an allergenic extract. The patient brings the extract to a family or primary care practitioner who administers the injection(s). In this case, either code **95115** or **95117** is reported to describe the services of the family or primary care practitioner. The appropriate code is selected on the basis of the number of injections performed.

Codes **95120-95134** describe the entire service of preparing, providing, and administering (injecting) the allergenic extract at a single patient encounter. Physicians who use a treatment board method, where small amounts of antigen are drawn from a number of separate vials containing different strengths of a particular antigen, accurately report their services with codes **95120-95134**. This type of treatment, referred to as "off the board," allows the physician to regulate and adjust the strength of the antigen at the encounter. Or this could be from a multiple-dose vial for which the patient had never been charged. This mixture is then injected into the patient. In this case it is not appropriate to use an injection code (**95115, 95117**) and a preparation code (**95144-95170**), since both are combined in codes **95120-95134**.

Code **95120** describes a single injection. Code **95125** is reported if two or more injections are administered. Codes **95130-95134** are intended to be reported on the basis of the total number of insect venom(s) injections administered. Each injection is not separately reported. For example, if the professional services for allergen immunotherapy are provided in the prescribing physician's office, including provision of the allergenic extract, and 1 mL of bee venom and 1 mL of wasp venom are given either by two separate injections or one injection, code **95131** is reported one time for the two stinging insect venoms.

Code **95144** represents the preparation and provision of extract furnished in single-dose vial(s) by the allergist for administration by another physician. Single-dose vials contain a single dose of antigen that is administered in one injection. The administering physician reports his or her services with the injection codes

**95115, 95117**. When code **95144** is reported, it is necessary to specify the number of vials (doses) provided.

Codes **95145-95170** describe the preparation of the antigen, the antigen extract itself, and the physician's assessment and determination of the concentration and volume to use, based on the patient's history and results of previous skin testing. These codes do not include the administration of the antigen. However, they do require that the number of doses be specified. It is immaterial whether the dose comes from a series of vials or from a single multiple-dose vial, because the code describes the dose, not the bottle from which it is drawn.

These codes enable physicians to equitably report the number of doses they prepare, whether they use a series of vials off a treatment board or a single multiple-dose vial to prepare the dosage. The code represents the type of preparation (ie, one, two, three, four, or five stinging insect venoms).

For example, code **95148** represents an extract containing four different stinging insect venoms.

Report the code that represents the total number of venoms. In the units box on the claim form, the total number of doses is specified. For example, the patient is provided with vials (the number of vials is irrelevant) containing four venoms, each with 10 doses. This is reported with code **95148** with a 10 in the units box.

When codes **95145-95170** are reported, the number of doses prospectively planned should be specified. This is the number of doses scheduled when the vial is provided. In most cases, that will be the number of doses administered. However, in some cases, because of reactions or other factors, the patient will not receive the number of doses intended.

The dosage depends on the amount of extract used in each preparation. One dose equals one administered injection of the venom. For example, if a patient is allergic to mixed vespid (yellow jacket and white- and yellow-faced hornet) and honeybee and gets 1 mL of each as maintenance immunotherapy, the correct code to use is **95148**, denoting four venoms.

## Coding Review

As a reminder, code **95165** describes the professional services for the supervision and provision of antigens for allergy immunotherapy, whether single or multiple antigens.

Code **95115** describes the single injection of an allergenic extract administered at a given patient encounter.

Code **95117** describes multiple (more than one) injections of an allergenic extract administered at a given patient encounter.

Code **95165** does not include the injection procedure(s) per se. Therefore, when a physician prepares allergenic extract(s) (same or different antigens), code **95165** should be reported in addition to either code **95115** or **95117**.

## Definition

For allergy immunotherapy reporting purposes, the definition of a *dose* is the amount of antigen administered in a single injection from a multiple-dose vial or drawn from a treatment board in one syringe.

## Examples

Let us consider a few coding examples for allergen immunotherapy.

**EXAMPLE:** A physician prepares a 10-dose multidose vial for a patient. At that same encounter, one dose from this vial is administered by one injection to the patient.

How to code?

**95165** × **10** in the units box + one injection code **95115**

In the previous example, code **95165** should be reported with the number 10 placed in the units box of the claim form. Code **95115** should be additionally reported, as one injection was performed.

**EXAMPLE:** A physician prepares two different multidose vials, each containing different antigens, and each vial containing 10 doses (total doses prepared: 2 × 10 = 20). At that same encounter, one dose from the first vial is administered in one injection and one dose from the second vial is administered in a second injection to the patient. Each injection contains one dose from each of the two multidose vials (two doses would be drawn from the treatment board in two syringes as noted previously).

The patient is also seen for an interval history and examination to assess the clinical status, as well as readjust the prescription drug treatment. The physician also questions the patient about reactions to injections from previously supplied vials.

The patient is then given the two vials to take to the primary care physician for administration of the remaining number of injections on the dosage schedule.

(Note: In this example, if the patient normally receives two doses and the two injections are performed on the same day, there should be 18 remaining doses in the vials given to the patient to then take to the primary care physician.)

How to code?

**95165** × **20** in the units box + one injection code **95117**, and the appropriate level E/M code with the modifier 25 appended

In the second example, code **95165** should be reported with the number 20 placed in the units box of the claim form. Code **95117** should be additionally reported, as two injections were performed. Also reported is an appropriate level E/M code with modifier 25 appended.

(Note: The previous example includes the scenario wherein subsequent immunotherapy administration will be performed by the primary care physician [eg, pediatrician, family physician, internist]. In this instance, code **95165** should not be reported by the primary care physician, since the allergy immunotherapy has already been determined and prepared and the vial[s] provided to the patient. For this specific coding example, the primary care physician would report code **95117** according to the prescribed dosage schedule. If the key components of an E/M service code have been met, the appropriate level E/M code should also be reported, with modifier 25 appended.)

# Endocrinology

Code **95250** has been included in the CPT code set to identify glucose monitoring procedures and includes all effort necessary to perform the service, including monitoring for up to 72 hours, setup of the equipment, training, and record. This procedure does not include the review, interpretation, reporting of the results, or actions taken in response to the findings. Therefore, an appropriate E/M service code may be used to identify the service. Since this procedure includes time as part of the descriptor for the service, this code should only be reported once to identify the specific effort provided when this procedure is performed for more than one day.

Code **95251** is reported for physician interpretation and report only.

# Neurology and Neuromuscular Procedures

Neurologic services are typically consultative, and any of the levels of consultation (**99241-99263**) services may be appropriate.

In addition, services and skills outlined under E/M levels of service appropriate to neurologic illnesses should be coded similarly.

For repetitive transcranial magnetic stimulation for treatment of clinical depression, see Category III codes **0160T, 0161T**.

The electroencephalography (EEG), autonomic function, evoked potential, reflex tests, electromyogram (EMG), nerve conduction velocity (NCV), and magnetoencephalography (MEG) services (**95812-95829**, **95920-95930**, and **95860-95967**) include recording, interpretation by a physician, and report. For interpretation only, use modifier 26.

## Sleep Testing

Codes **95805-95811** describe sleep studies and polysomnography, which refer to the continuous and simultaneous monitoring and recording of various physiologic and pathophysiologic parameters of sleep for six or more hours with physician review, interpretation, and report. The studies are performed to diagnose a variety of sleep disorders and to evaluate a patient's response to therapies such as nasal CPAP. Polysomnography is distinguished from sleep studies by the inclusion of sleep staging, which is defined to include a one- to four-lead EEG, an electro-oculogram, and a submental EMG. Additional parameters of sleep include the following, among others:

- ECG
- Airflow
- Ventilation and respiratory effort
- Gas exchange by oximetry, transcutaneous monitoring, or end-tidal gas analysis
- Extremity muscle activity, motor activity-movement
- Extended EEG monitoring
- Penile tumescence
- Gastroesophageal reflux
- Continuous blood pressure monitoring
- Snoring
- Body positions

The sleep services (**95805-95811**) include recording, interpretation, and report. For interpretation only, use modifier 26. Code **95805** describes the multiple sleep latency test or the maintenance of wakefulness test. The multiple sleep latency test measures a patient's ability to fall asleep, while the maintenance of wakefulness test measures a patient's ability to stay awake during the day.

For a study to be reported as polysomnography, sleep must be recorded and staged. Sessions in which less than six hours of recording are performed or other services are reduced should be reported with modifier 52. If nasal CPAP is initiated as part of polysomnography during a single sleep period, report code **95811** only. For example, if a patient arrives for a complex polysomnography on Wednesday night and nasal CPAP is initiated at any time during the patient's sleep period (Wednesday night to Thursday morning), only code **95811** would be reported.

## Routine Electroencephalography

Codes **95812-95830** are used to report various EEG procedures. These codes are distinguished according to the time noted in the code descriptor and specific circumstances involved in the testing (eg, coma/sleep testing EEG, cerebral death evaluation, etc). Parenthetical notes and guidelines have been included to identify (1) codes to use to identify routine and extended monitoring, (2) EEG codes used to identify 24-hour monitoring, (3) appropriate coding for the Wada test (**95958**), and (4) digital analysis of EEG (**95957**).

## Muscle and Range of Motion Testing

The codes included in this section (**95831-95857**) identify various muscle and range of motion testing procedures for various body areas and include provision of the report (when indicated in the descriptor). Codes **95831-95834** are specific to manual muscle testing procedures. Manual muscle testing findings can either be notated using a numerical scale (0–5) or equivalent language such as *zero, trace, fair, good,* or *normal.* These services may be reported in addition to the E/M service codes if the E/M service is performed as a significant, separately identifiable effort from the muscle and range of motion testing procedure performed. Computerized range of motion testing is also reported using these codes. However, computerized muscle testing should be reported using **97750**.

## Electromyography and Nerve Conduction Tests/Intraoperative Neurophysiology

EMG and nerve conduction studies codes (**95860-95904**) identify various aspects of testing for conduction of an electrical impulse from one anatomic location to another. The EMG testing professional component includes the needle examination and the formulation of an analysis of the test results. An E/M service may be performed on the same day and, in that case, it does not require the use of modifier 25. Needle electromyography procedures include the interpretation of electrical waveforms measured by equipment that produces both visible and audible components of electrical signals recorded from the muscle(s) studied by the needle electrode. EMG tests (**95860-95864**) should include five or more examined muscles in that extremity. If fewer are tested, use code **95870**. That code may be used more than once. For example, if three muscles are tested in each upper extremity, use code **95870** with two units of service, rather than code **95861**.

Code **95865** should be reported for needle electromyography of the larynx, which may be performed to identify laryngeal nerve and muscle disorders and facilitate intraoperative monitoring during laryngeal procedures and botulinum toxin injections in the laryngeal muscles. Needle EMG of the larynx is typically performed on both sides of the larynx; therefore, it is not appropriate to append the modifier 50 to **95865**. For a unilateral procedure, report **95865** with the modifier 52 appended.

Code **95866** should be reported for needle electromyography of the hemidiaphragm, which may be performed to identify respiratory muscle disorders and, less frequently, for intraoperative monitoring.

Prior to chemodenervation procedures, it may be necessary to perform a more precise localization for needle placement before the chemical is injected. Therefore, the physician may perform electrical stimulation or needle EMG to achieve this localization. Electrical stimulation for guidance in conjunction with chemodenervation is reported with code **95873**. Needle electromyography for guidance in conjunction with chemodenervation is reported with code **95874**.

Codes **95873** and **95874** are used in conjunction with chemodenervation codes **64612-64614**, but not in conjunction with needle electromyography procedure codes **95860-95870**. Code **95874** is not reported in conjunction with **95873**.

It has become standard to use EEG monitoring for certain surgical procedures (eg, clipping of some intracranial aneurysms). Add-on code **95920** describes ongoing EP testing and monitoring performed during surgical procedures. Code **95920** is reported per hour of service and includes only the ongoing EP monitoring time distinct from performance of specific type(s) of baseline EP study(ies) (**95860, 95861, 95867, 95868, 95870, 95900, 95904, 95928, 95929, 95933, 95934, 95936, 95937**) or interpretation of specific type(s) of baseline EP study(ies) (**92585, 95822, 95925, 95926, 95927, 95930**). The time spent performing or interpreting the baseline EP study(ies) should not be counted as intraoperative monitoring, but represents separately reportable procedures. Code **95920** should be used once per hour, even if multiple EP studies are performed. The baseline EP study(ies) should be used once per operative session.

Codes **95900**, **95903**, and **95904** identify nerve conduction studies (ie, to identify a specific nerve's ability to conduct electrical signals within the nervous system). The testing can be performed for different parts of a specific nerve (ie, different segments of a given nerve) to identify local pathological responses, if they exist. This could include information regarding the speed (latency and/or conduction velocity), size (amplitude), and shape of the response and therefore can reveal the status of myelin insulation of a particular nerve. (Note: A myelin sheath is the part of the nerve that insulates the nerve to protect, isolate, and expedite the signal being passed by a particular nerve.)

These codes are intended to be reported only once regardless of the number of sites tested on that specific nerve. (Parenthetical notes associated with these codes have been included to specify the intended use for these codes to the user.) For these studies, responses can be obtained from a nerve trunk (sensory nerve conduction study) or from a muscle innervated by that nerve trunk (motor nerve conduction study). The surface electrodes used can both stimulate and record information for that particular nerve.

Codes **95900** and **95903** involve the following nerves:

**I  Upper Extremity/Cervical Plexus/Brachial Plexus Motor Nerves**
  **A** Axillary motor nerve to the deltoid
  **B** Long thoracic motor nerve to the serratus anterior
  **C** Median nerve
    **1** Median motor nerve to the abductor pollicis brevis
    **2** Median motor nerve, anterior interosseous branch, to the flexor pollicis longus
    **3** Median motor nerve, anterior interosseous branch, to the pronator quadratus
    **4** Median motor nerve to the first lumbrical
    **5** Median motor nerve to the second lumbrical
  **D** Musculocutaneous motor nerve to the biceps brachia
  **E** Radial nerve
    **1** Radial motor nerve to the extensor carpi ulnaris
    **2** Radial motor nerve to the extensor digitorum communis

      **3** Radial motor nerve to the extensor indicis proprius

      **4** Radial motor nerve to the brachioradialis

   **F** Suprascapular nerve

      **1** Suprascapular motor nerve to the supraspinatus

      **2** Suprascapular motor nerve to the infraspinatus

   **G** Thoracodorsal motor nerve to the latissimus dorsi

   **H** Ulnar nerve

      **1** Ulnar motor nerve to the abductor digiti minimi

      **2** Ulnar motor nerve to the palmar interosseous

      **3** Ulnar motor nerve to the first dorsal interosseous

      **4** Ulnar motor nerve to the flexor carpi ulnaris

   **I** Other

**II Lower Extremity Motor Nerves**

   **A** Femoral motor nerve to the quadriceps

      **1** Femoral motor nerve to vastus medialis

      **2** Femoral motor nerve to vastus lateralis

      **3** Femoral motor nerve to vastus intermedialis

      **4** Femoral motor nerve to rectus femoris

   **B** Ilioinguinal motor nerve

   **C** Peroneal (fibular) nerve

      **1** Peroneal motor nerve to the extensor digitorum brevis

      **2** Peroneal motor nerve to the peroneus brevis

      **3** Peroneal motor nerve to the peroneus longus

      **4** Peroneal motor nerve to the tibialis anterior

   **D** Plantar motor nerve

   **E** Sciatic nerve

   **F** Tibial nerve

      **1** Tibial motor nerve, inferior calcaneal branch, to the abductor digiti minimi

      **2** Tibial motor nerve, medial plantar branch, to the abductor hallucis

      **3** Tibial motor nerve, lateral plantar branch, to the flexor digiti minimi brevis

   **G** Other

**III Cranial nerves**

   **A** Cranial nerve VII (facial motor nerve)

      **1** Facial nerve to the frontalis

      **2** Facial nerve to the nasalis

      **3** Facial nerve to the orbicularis oculi

      **4** Facial nerve to the orbicularis oris

   **B** Cranial nerve XI (spinal accessory motor nerve)

   **C** Cranial nerve XII (hypoglossal motor nerve)

   **D** Phrenic motor nerve to the diaphragm

   **E** Recurrent laryngeal nerve

   **F** Other

**IV Nerve Roots**

- **A** Cervical nerve root stimulation
    - **1** Cervical level 5 (C5)
    - **2** Cervical level 6 (C6)
    - **3** Cervical level 7 (C7)
    - **4** Cervical level 8 (C8)
- **B** Thoracic nerve root stimulation
    - **1** Thoracic level 1 (T1)
    - **2** Thoracic level 2 (T2)
    - **3** Thoracic level 3 (T3)
    - **4** Thoracic level 4 (T4)
    - **5** Thoracic level 5 (T5)
    - **6** Thoracic level 6 (T6)
    - **7** Thoracic level 7 (T7)
    - **8** Thoracic level 8 (T8)
    - **9** Thoracic level 9 (T9)
    - **10** Thoracic level 10 (T10)
    - **11** Thoracic level 11 (T11)
    - **12** Thoracic level 12 (T12)
- **C** Lumbar nerve root stimulation
    - **1** Lumbar level 1 (L1)
    - **2** Lumbar level 2 (L2)
    - **3** Lumbar level 3 (L3)
    - **4** Lumbar level 4 (L4)
    - **5** Lumbar level 5 (L5)
- **D** Sacral nerve root stimulation
    - **1** Sacral level 1 (S1)
    - **2** Sacral level 2 (S2)
    - **3** Sacral level 3 (S3)
    - **4** Sacral level 4 (S4)

Code **95904** involves the following nerves:

**I   Upper Extremity Sensory and Mixed Nerves**

- **A** Lateral antebrachial cutaneous sensory nerve
- **B** Medial antebrachial cutaneous sensory nerve
- **C** Medial brachial cutaneous sensory nerve
- **D** Median nerve
    - **1** Median sensory nerve to the first digit
    - **2** Median sensory nerve to the second digit
    - **3** Median sensory nerve to the third digit
    - **4** Median sensory nerve to the fourth digit
    - **5** Median palmar cutaneous sensory nerve
    - **6** Median palmar mixed nerve
- **E** Posterior antebrachial cutaneous sensory nerve

   **F** Radial sensory nerve
      **1** Radial sensory nerve to the base of the thumb
      **2** Radial sensory nerve to digit one
   **G** Ulnar nerve
      **1** Ulnar dorsal cutaneous sensory nerve
      **2** Ulnar sensory nerve to the fourth digit
      **3** Ulnar sensory nerve to the fifth digit
      **4** Ulnar palmar mixed nerve
   **H** Intercostal sensory nerve
   **I** Other

**II Lower Extremity Sensory and Mixed Nerves**
   **A** Lateral femoral cutaneous sensory nerve
   **B** Medial calcaneal sensory nerve
   **C** Medial femoral cutaneous sensory nerve
   **D** Peroneal nerve
      **1** Deep peroneal sensory nerve
      **2** Superficial peroneal sensory nerve, medial dorsal cutaneous branch
      **3** Superficial peroneal sensory nerve, intermediate dorsal cutaneous branch
   **E** Posterior femoral cutaneous sensory nerve
   **F** Saphenous nerve
      **1** Saphenous sensory nerve (distal technique)
      **2** Saphenous sensory nerve (proximal technique)
   **G** Sural nerve
      **1** Sural sensory nerve, lateral dorsal cutaneous branch
      **2** Sural sensory nerve
   **H** Tibial sensory nerve (digital nerve to toe one)
   **I** Tibial sensory nerve (medial plantar nerve)
   **J** Tibial sensory nerve (lateral plantar nerve)
   **K** Other

**III Head and Trunk Sensory Nerves**
   **A** Dorsal nerve of the penis
   **B** Greater auricular nerve
   **C** Ophthalmic branch of the trigeminal nerve
   **D** Pudendal sensory nerve
   **E** Suprascapular sensory nerves
   **F** Other

## Autonomic Function Tests

To regulate/maintain blood pressure and heart rate when an individual is in different positions (eg, standing up, lying down), the human body uses the autonomic nervous system. This system is controlled by the cerebrospinal nerve centers and allows control of certain body functions without requiring a deliberate, conscious effort by the individual to do so. In relation to heart function, the autonomic nervous system assesses changes in conditions that affect these functions and adjusts them according to the need.

The testing procedures identified by the codes in this section help identify problems that may exist for some. The language included in the codes in this section identifies the specific measures/components performed for the testing.

Definitions of some of the terms included in the descriptor language are as follows:

**Valsalva maneuver:** Any forced expiratory effort (strain) against a closed airway, whether at the nose and mouth or at the glottis. This causes high intrathoracic pressure that impedes venous return to the right atrium and therefore can be used to study cardiovascular effects of raised peripheral venous pressure and decrease cardiac filling and cardiac output, as well as poststrain responses. In the laboratory, this can be accomplished by allowing the patient to blow into a bugle with an expiratory pressure of 40 mm Hg and having the patient maintain the pressure for at least 10 seconds. The study is repeated to verify that the response is reproducible. A simple version would be to hold one's breath while maximally contracting the abdominal muscles.

**R-R interval:** Identifies the interval (in milliseconds) between the R wave of the QRS complex of two consecutive QRS complexes. The R-R interval is the reciprocal of the heart rate.

**Heart rate response to deep breathing:** A derived value from an analysis of the heart rate recordings with the subject breathing at a rate of five to six breaths per minute. All heart rate recordings are done with ECG monitoring of heart rate derived from R-R interval, displayed on a monitor and stored for off-line analysis.

**Valsalva ratio:** The maximum heart rate divided by the lowest heart rate. The subject performs a standardized Valsalva maneuver and the derived heart rate is analyzed.

**30:15 ratio:** The initial heart rate responses to standing consist of tachycardia at 3 seconds and then at 12 to 15 seconds followed by bradycardia at 20 seconds. The initial cardioacceleration is an exercise reflex, while the subsequent tachycardia and bradycardia are baroreflex mediated. The 30:15 ratio, (R-R interval at beat 30)/(R-R interval at beat 15) is widely used as an index of cardiovagal function.

**Passive tilt:** The act of placing a patient on a tilt table for the purpose of obtaining a baseline recording and later tilting the angle of the table to 60 to 80 degrees for at least five minutes (unless there is an excessive fall in blood pressure or other indicators of patient distress).

**Thermoregulatory sweat test:** A test of sympathetic nerves that supply the skin. For this procedure, the skin is dusted with an indicator powder that changes color when the patient sweats in response to raising the patient's temperature by raising ambient temperature in a heat cabinet.

**Quantitative sudomotor axon reflex test:** An evaluation that uses a quantitative noninvasive method to determine the integrity of the distal postganglionic sympathetic nerve fibers in diabetic and other neuropathies affecting autonomic nerves and in the progressive autonomic disorders. It uses the stimulation of sympathetic nerve fibers to the sweat glands at standard sites. The test is done optimally on one forearm site and three lower extremity sites in order to determine the severity and distribution of the sympathetic deficit.

## Evoked Potentials and Reflex Tests

The codes in this section are used to report somatosensory, reflex, and neuromuscular junction testing procedures. For those procedures that involve testing of specific nerves, the testing procedures included in this section include testing for any/all sites along that particular nerve. Parenthetical notes identify issues regarding laterality for these procedures as well as instructions regarding use of other related codes.

Codes **95928** and **95929** are used to report central motor-evoked potential studies (or transcranial motor stimulation) for the upper limbs (**95928**) and lower limbs (**95929**). As is indicated by the descriptor language, these codes are intended to monitor the motor tracts—separate codes are used to identify the monitoring of somatosensory evoked potentials (recordings typically done to monitor the sensory tracts during surgical procedures that involve exposure of the spinal cord [**95925-95927**]). The language for these codes differentiates the code that identifies upper limb monitoring (**95928**) from lower limb (**95929**).

Transcranial electrical motor stimulation is a method of testing that allows stimulation of the motor area of the cerebral cortex and recording from muscles over the upper and lower extremities. This method allows for a reliable assessment of motor pathway function and integrity. Any compromise of the pathways between these two locations would be detected via the stimulation testing and thus alert the physician and surgical staff of the problem. These changes most often indicate motor compromise from ischemia to the spinal cord.

## Special EEG Tests

Video EEG monitoring (**95951**) is used for prolonged monitoring of seizures. Usually, the coded procedure lasts 24 hours. Sometimes the monitoring is shorter, eg, because the patient was off monitoring to undergo magnetic resonance imaging (MRI). When monitoring is less than 12 hours but more than 6 hours, use modifier 52. When monitoring is less than 8 hours, use code **95813** instead of code **95951**.

Magnetoencephalography (MEG) is a noninvasive method for evaluating brain function. MEG is used for localizing areas of abnormal brain function, such as regions of epileptic activity, and for localizing areas important for normal function such as sensory and visual cortex. In an MEG procedure, magnetic fields of the brain associated with neuronal activity are measured with an array of very sensitive sensors positioned around the surface of the patient's scalp in a device known as a *biomagnetometer*.

Codes **95965-95967** are performed in the noninvasive localization of epileptic foci for planning of surgical treatment, including planning for implantation of invasive recording electrodes. Codes **95965-95967** are also performed for noninvasive localization of eloquent cortical areas (eg, sensory, motor, and language cortex) and for planning of surgical procedures (eg, tumor surgery, arteriovenous malformation surgery, or epilepsy surgery) in areas that might result in postsurgical functional deficits.

For EEG performed in addition to MEG, see codes **95812-95827**. For somatosensory-evoked potentials, auditory-evoked potentials, and visual-evoked potentials performed in addition to magnetic-evoked field responses, see codes **92585**, **95925**, **95926**, and/or **95930**. For computed tomography performed in addition to MEG, see codes **70450-70470** and **70496**. For magnetic resonance imaging (MRI) performed in addition to MEG, see codes **70551-70553**.

## Neurostimulators, Analysis—Programming

The codes included in this section are used to identify analysis (and, in some circumstances, programming) of previously implanted neurostimulator devices. The guidelines identify specifics regarding the intended use of these codes. For example, code **95970** is used to report electronic analysis of an implanted simple or complex brain, spinal cord, or peripheral (eg, peripheral nerve, autonomic nerve, neuromuscular) neurostimulator pulse generator system and excludes reprogramming. Codes **95972** and **95973** are used to describe intraoperative (ie, performed either at initial insertion or at revision) or subsequent electronic analysis of an implanted complex device. Each of the codes included in this section includes language that identifies the specific location of the device (and the testing performed) as well as whether or not programming is included as part of the procedure. In addition, the time necessary to perform the service is included as part of the descriptor if time is a factor for performance of the procedure. Time includes both the face-to-face time reprogramming as well as the in-office observation time between reprogramming cycles to evaluate the reprogramming efficacy.

## Other Procedures

Codes **95990** and **95991** are used to report refilling and maintenance of implantable delivery systems that include intrathecal, intraventricular, and epidural drug delivery. These codes allow a more granular (or service-specific) system that reflects the work, time, and intensity for the refill and maintenance of pumps providing spinal or brain infusion, as the refill and maintenance of these pumps is very different from that of systemic infusion. For refill and maintenance of implanted infusion pump or reservoir for systemic drug

**CODING TIP**

Use codes **96000-96003** to report comprehensive gait and motion-analysis procedures.

therapy (eg, chemotherapy or insulin), use **96522**. Codes **62367** and **62368** identify analysis and/or reprogramming of implantable infusion pumps. Refilling and maintenance of implanted infusion pumps or reservoirs for systemic drug therapy (eg, chemotherapy or insulin) is reported using **96522**.

# Motion Analysis

Codes **96000-96004** describe services performed as part of a major therapeutic or diagnostic decision making process. Motion analysis is performed in a dedicated motion analysis laboratory (ie, a facility capable of performing videotaping from the front, back, and both sides; computerized three-dimensional kinematics; three-dimensional kinetics; and dynamic EMG). Code **96000** may include three-dimensional kinetics and stride characteristics. Codes **96002** and **96003** describe dynamic EMG. Do not report codes **95860-95875** in addition to the motion-analysis codes. Code **96004** is reported once, regardless of the number of studies reviewed/interpreted.

## Functional Brain Mapping

Codes **96020** and **70555** were established to report neurofunctional brain mapping of blood flow changes in the brain by MRI in response to tests administered by physicians and psychologists correlating to specific brain functions (eg, motor skills, vision, language, and memory).

Functional brain mapping is a preoperative noninvasive test most commonly performed for patients with brain neoplasm (and metastases), arteriovenous malformations, intractable epilepsy, and any other brain lesion that may require invasive (eg, surgical excision) or focal treatment (eg, irradiation). The information derived from functional brain mapping is used to predict the potential for neurological deficits that may arise from tumor growths and surgical interventions, thus making it possible for the physician and patient to make informed decisions concerning the feasibility and risk of intervention, determine the extent of surgical intervention (eg, subtotal vs total resection), and identify expendable and nonexpendable cortical regions.

Preoperative noninvasive neurofunctional mapping is performed as an alternative to direct cortical stimulation or somatosensory evoked potentials performed intraoperatively, which may be unsuccessful and associated with visual distortion, seizure, and increased surgical time.

Code **96020** is used to report neurofunctional testing selection and administration during noninvasive imaging functional brain mapping, with test administration entirely by a physician psychologist, with review of tests results and report. Code **96020** includes selection and administration of testing of language, memory, cognition, movement, sensation, and other neurological function when conducted in association with functional neuroimaging, monitoring of performance of this testing, and determination of validity of neurofunctional testing relative to separately interpreted functional magnetic resonance images. E/M services should not be reported on the same day as **96020**.

# Medical Genetics and Genetic Counseling Services

Genetic counseling is a communication process that deals with the human problems associated with the occurrence, or the risk of an occurrence, of a genetic disorder in the family. This process involves an attempt by appropriately trained persons to help the individual or family to

- comprehend the medical facts, including the diagnosis, probable course of the disorder, and the available management;
- appreciate the way heredity contributes to the disorder, and the risk of recurrence in specified relatives;
- understand the alternatives for dealing with the risk of occurrence;
- choose the course of action that seems to them appropriate in view of their risk, family goals, and ethical and religious standards, and to act in accordance with that decision; and
- make the best possible adjustment to the disorder in an affected family member and/or the risk of recurrence of that disorder.

This process is most often performed after a thorough collection and interpretation of the genetic family history; a pedigree analysis and assessment of the risk of disease occurrence or recurrence; and the identification of interventions to manage and, in many cases, ameliorate disease risk.

Code **96040** is used to report medical genetics and genetic counseling services, each 30 minutes face-to-face with patient/family. These services are provided by trained genetic counselors and may include obtaining a structured family genetic history, pedigree construction, analysis for genetic risk assessment, and counseling of the patient and family. These activities may be provided during one or more sessions and may include review of medical data and family information, face-to-face interviews, and counseling services. For genetic counseling and education provided by a physician to an individual, see the appropriate E/M codes.

# Health and Behavior Assessment/Intervention

Health and behavior assessment procedures are used to identify the psychological, behavioral, emotional, cognitive, and social factors important to the prevention, treatment, or management of physical health problems. The focus of the assessment is not on mental health but on the biopsychosocial factors important to physical health problems and treatments.

Health and behavior intervention procedures are used to modify the psychological, behavioral, emotional, cognitive, and social factors identified as important to or directly affecting the patient's physiologic functioning, disease status, health, and well-being. The focus of the intervention is to improve the patient's health and well-being by means of cognitive, behavioral, social, and/or psychophysiologic procedures designed to ameliorate specific disease-related problems.

Codes **96150-96155** describe services offered to patients who present with established illnesses or symptoms, are not diagnosed with mental illness, and may benefit from evaluations that focus on the biopsychosocial factors related to the patient's physical health status. These services do not represent preventive medicine counseling and risk factor reduction interventions.

For patients who require psychiatric services (**90801-90899**) as well as health and behavior assessment/intervention (**96150-96155**), report the predominant service performed. Do not report codes **96150-96155** in addition to codes **90801-90899** on the same date. E/M service codes should not be reported on the same day as health and behavior assessment/intervention services codes **96150-96155**.

These codes are not intended to represent preventive medicine services, as these services do not identify the comprehensive evaluation services as identified in the **99381-99397** series. If comprehensive evaluation services are performed, these codes (**99381-99397**) should be used to identify those specific services.

These codes should not be reported on the same day, in addition to preventive medicine counseling and/or risk factor reduction services (**99401-99412**).

## Chemotherapy Administration

While the chemotherapy administration codes continue to be reported for parenteral administration of nonradionuclide antineoplastic drugs, these codes are also reported for antineoplastic agents provided for the treatment of noncancer diagnoses or for substances such as monoclonal antibody agents and other biologic response modifiers.

The secondary service categories of codes are intended to report additional sequential infusions, sequential IV pushes, and IV chemotherapy pushes for additional drugs for hydration and therapeutic, prophylactic, or diagnostic IV infusions or injections.

Three subheadings distinguish the codes in this section according to access, specifying IV, intra-arterial, and other chemotherapy administration.

The Chemotherapy Administration guidelines direct the appropriate reporting for these services. The guidelines indicate the drug agents with which the drug administration codes are appropriately reported. These agents are based upon the inherent risk of the agent administration and are linked to the management of the possible toxic effects of the drug rather than upon the cancer diagnosis most commonly associated with chemotherapy treatment. These procedures therefore include parenteral administration of nonradionuclide antineoplastic drugs and antineoplastic agents provided for treatment of noncancer diagnoses (eg, cyclophosphamide for autoimmune conditions) or to substances such as monoclonal antibody agents and other biologic response modifiers. The guidelines further define the efforts required of the provider in order to report these codes and define those elements, which are included and not separately reported.

The chemotherapy administration codes include confirmation or recalculation of doses based upon the condition of the patient on the day of chemotherapy administration.

The Chemotherapy Administration guidelines reinforce the instruction that these codes are not limited for reporting by any specialty. The guidelines define the level of difficulty expected for provision of these services including direct physician supervision for patient assessment, provision of consent, safety oversight, and intraservice staff supervision. Typically, such chemotherapy services require advanced practice training and competency for staff providing the services; special consideration in preparation, dosage, or disposal; and in the potential patient risk and requirements for frequent monitoring.

Similar to the Hydration, Therapeutic, Prophylactic, and Diagnostic Injections, and Infusions guidelines, the Chemotherapy Administration guidelines define and list the services that are included and therefore are not separately reported, including local anesthesia; the IV start, establishment of access to, and indwelling IV, subcutaneous catheter, or port; the flush at conclusion of infusion; administration supplies including standard tubing and syringes; and the preparation of chemotherapy agents.

The guidelines also instruct separate reporting for each method and technique of chemotherapy administration. These instructions support the intent of the codes to reflect the additional effort required for each technique of administration. An infusion consisting of three substances in a single bag is not intended to be reported as three separate infusion services, as the parenteral administration codes are intended to report the separate work of administration access and not the inclusion of multiple agents in a bag prepared prior to access. Further instructions direct the user to report administration of all other hydration, therapeutic, prophylactic, and/or diagnostic injections, and infusions with the appropriate codes from the **90760-90779** series. The user is cautioned, however, that fluid used to administer the drug(s) is considered to be incidental hydration and is not separately reportable.

Guidelines define the initial service to distinguish the initial service code from the subsequent or concurrent injection and infusion and to instruct reporting for initial, subsequent, concurrent, and multiple infusions, injections, or combination of services. These instructions clarify that the definition of the service is based less upon the chronological order of the services than it is upon the primary reason for the encounter. The definitions of *subsequent* and *initial* also indicate that an initial service code is reported only one time per encounter and that subsequent, sequential, and concurrent codes are reported regardless of the subsection (Hydration, Therapeutic, Prophylactic, and Diagnostic Injections, and Infusions; Chemotherapy Administration) in which the initial service code appears.

Definition of the intent of the references to time (one hour, each additional hour) in the code descriptors is provided in the guidelines. This definition indicates that reporting the time of the service should be based only upon the administration time for the infusion. This is because the time required for the infusion was used to define the range of services included in the infusion within the Chemotherapy Administration codes. Services leading up to the infusion and to conclude the infusion have been included in the infusion service and are not separately reported. These services will include starting the IV and monitoring the patient postinfusion.

If a significant, separately identifiable E/M service is performed, the appropriate E/M service code should be reported using modifier 25 in addition to codes **96401-96549**.

Chemotherapy services are typically highly complex and require direct physician supervision for any or all purposes of patient assessment, provision of consent, safety oversight, and intra-service supervision of staff. An exclusionary cross-reference directs the user to codes **99601** and **99602** for home infusion services.

Injection and Intravenous Infusion Chemotherapy is the first subsection of the Chemotherapy Administration codes. Guidelines specific to this subsection provide the definition of IV or intra-arterial push to distinguish these services from the infusion codes.

Code **96401** is intended to report subcutaneous or intramuscular nonhormonal antineoplastic administration services. Antineoplastic hormonal therapy injections are reported with code **96402**.

Code **96405** is reported for the injection of chemotherapeutic substances into one to seven lesions. This code describes the number of lesions treated, not the number of injections and should be reported once, when one to seven lesions are treated, even if a particular lesion is injected more than once. Intralesional chemotherapy for more than seven lesions is reported with code **96406**.

Codes **96409** and **96411** are reported for IV push chemotherapy administration services. These codes are distinguished by the administration of the single or initial substance and administration for additional substances. Because add-on code **96411** is reported for the administration of a sequential substance, a cross-reference directs that this code is appropriately reported with initial IV chemotherapy service codes **96409** and **96413**, as provided for in the Chemotherapy Administration guidelines.

Codes **96413** and **96417** are reported for IV infusion chemotherapy administration services. These codes are distinguished by the administration of the single or initial substance and administration for additional substances. Code **96413** is reported for the IV infusion administration of a single or initial chemotherapeutic drug. Add-on code **96417** is reported for the infusion of a sequential substance. A cross-reference following code **96417** directs the user (1) that this code is appropriately reported with code **96413**, (2) that this code should be reported only once per sequential infusion, and (3) that additional hour(s) of sequential infusion are reported with code **96415**.

Code **96415** is intended to be reported one time for each additional hour of IV infusion chemotherapy administration services. The add-on cross-reference directs that this code is appropriately reported only with the initial IV infusion chemotherapy service code **96413**. An exclusionary cross-reference defines the length of infusion required to be performed in order to report each additional hour of infusion. Because code **96415** is not intended to be reported for nonchemotherapeutic subsequent IV services, a cross-reference directs the user to the appropriate nonchemotherapeutic secondary or subsequent services **90761**, **90766**, **90767**, and **90776**, which should be reported with code **96413** when these services are provided. For instance, drugs that are incidental to chemotherapy are not reported with the chemotherapy services codes. Therefore, administration of an antiemetic drug, while often performed at the same session as chemotherapy administration, would be reported with the secondary or therapeutic prophylactic subsequent services codes **90761**, **90766**, **90767**, and **90776**, based upon the route of administration.

Code **96416** is reported for initiation of prolonged IV infusion chemotherapy administration services defined as a service greater than eight hours and requiring use of a portable or implantable pump. A directional cross-reference instructs the user to refer to codes **96521-96523** to report services for refilling and maintenance of a portable pump or an implantable infusion pump or reservoir for drug delivery.

The family of IV infusion codes is not completely synchronous with the nonchemotherapy series **90765-90768**. There is no code for concurrent administration of chemotherapeutic drugs. Multiple drugs given at the same session are considered to be sequential injections rather than concurrent and are reported with code **96411** to report IV push administration of additional drugs/substances at the same session and **96417** to report IV infusion administration of additional drugs/substances at the same session.

Code **96423** is reported for each additional hour of up to eight hours of intra-arterial infusion and is used in conjunction with code **96422**. An exclusionary cross-reference instructs that this code is reported for infusion intervals of greater than 30 minutes beyond one-hour increments.

The guidelines in the final subsection of the Chemotherapy Administration codes are specific to the portable pump and implantable infusion pump or reservoir services. Codes **96521-96523** may be reported when these devices are used for therapeutic drugs other than chemotherapy. Code **96523** does not require direct physician supervision.

Chemotherapy supplies should be reported with the most specific supply code.

**CODING TIP**

Be sure to find out whether HCPCS Level II codes are required by a third-party payer to report chemotherapy supplies.

## Special Dermatological Procedures

Codes **96900-96999** are used to report various dermatologic procedures that use both diagnostic and therapeutic services. As indicated in the guidelines for these services, these diagnostic and therapeutic services may be reported in addition to E/M services including but not limited to consultations (appending modifier 25, as appropriate, to the E/M code used).

Code **96902** is a diagnostic service, as this procedure is used to identify hair growth pathology. As noted in the descriptor, this procedure requires that the hair specimen be obtained by the provider.

Code **96904** is used to report whole body photography. This service is used to monitor high risk patients with dysplastic nevus syndrome or a history of dysplastic nevi, or patients with a personal or familial history of melanoma. This code is intended to report the use of photography as a benchmark for skin cancer identification and is meant to be used no more than once per year for retention in the patient's record.

Codes **96900**, **96910**, **96912**, **96913**, and **96920-96922** identify various skin treatment methods and are differentiated according to the type of method (eg, photochemotherapy, laser, etc) used for the procedure. Those procedures that are used for certain specific conditions include language within the descriptor that indicates the condition treated and, when necessary, the amount of time necessary to provide the treatment. In addition, laser treatment codes **96920-96922** included in this section differ from destruction services reported in the **17000**s series, as these services are intended to report treatment of inflammatory skin conditions and not to identify destruction of skin lesions.

# Physical Medicine and Rehabilitation

Codes in the **97001-97799** series are used to report various physical medicine and rehabilitation procedures and services. Within this subsection of codes, separate series of codes are available for reporting as follows:
- Evaluations and re-evaluations
- Modalities (supervised and constant attendance)
- Therapeutic procedures
- Tests and measurements
- Active wound care management
- Orthotic management and prosthetic management
- Other procedures

These codes are not restricted to use by a specific specialty group. Instead, they may be used by any qualified health care provider whose scope of practice as defined by regulation permits them to perform the service represented by the specific code. Licensure and credentialing vary on a state-by-state and institutional basis. Relevant state and institutional authorities should be consulted regarding the appropriate provision of these services by qualified health care professionals.

Codes **97001-97004** are used to report physical and occupational therapy evaluation and re-evaluation. These codes identify a dynamic process in which clinical judgments are made on the basis of data gathered. These evaluations result in the development of a plan for management of a patient's problems as they relate to his or her disease or disability. Codes **97005** and **97006** describe athletic training evaluation and re-evaluation, respectively.

Since some of the physical medicine services include an assessment component as part of preservice work, use of the evaluation (**97001**, **97003**) and re-evaluation (**97002**, **97004**) codes is dependent on whether the service being provided is a significant, separate service or if it is simply a component of the more involved procedure. Since patient circumstances vary, deciding when to use these codes depends on the specific patient encounter and identification of what has been actually done. Evaluations (**97001**, **97003**) signal the beginning of the episode of care. State practice acts require that evaluation services be performed at the beginning of the episode. Re-evaluations (**97002**, **97004**) are performed at appropriate intervals during the episode to reflect the gathering of new data that will impact the future management of patient care.

Two series of codes exist for reporting modalities. Codes **97010-97028** are used to report supervised modalities, and codes **97032-97039** are used to report constant attendance modalities.

These codes are used according to whether direct (one-on-one) patient contact is provided (constant attendance) or whether the application of the modality does not require direct patient contact by the provider (supervised modalities).

Both the supervised modality codes (**97010-97028**) and the constant attendance codes (**97032-97039**) include language in the descriptor that indicates "application of a modality to one or more areas." The number of areas of application is not a consideration in the reporting of these codes. For example, if hot packs are placed on the knee and cervical spine, code **97010** is reported once for that patient encounter, despite the fact that two hot packs were placed.

The constant attendance modality codes, however, also include a time component. The descriptor language for the constant attendance codes indicates that these codes are reported for each 15 minutes.

The time frames indicated in the descriptor language of the constant attendance modality codes describe the total time, ie, preservice, intraservice, and postservice time spent in performing the modality being reported. Codes that do not include an increment of time in the descriptor do not use time as a component for determining the use of the code. One unit of the supervised modalities code is reported without regard to the length of time spent performing the service or the number of body parts treated with that particular modality. When more than one modality is used during an encounter, whether supervised or constant attendance or any combination, each modality provided should be separately reported.

The therapeutic procedure codes, **97110-97546**, identify procedures that effect change through the application of clinical skills and reflect services that attempt to improve the patient's function. When reporting these codes, the provider is required to have direct (one-to-one) patient contact.

Common components of preservice work include chart reviews for treatment, set-up of activities and the equipment area, and review of previous documentation as needed. Also included is communication with other health care professionals (such as the physician, social worker, and/or nurse) and discussions with the family. After the therapeutic service is provided, the treatment is recorded, and typically the progress is documented.

Other services may also be required to effectively administer the various treatments involved. Therefore, as was previously indicated, the use of the physical therapy or occupational therapy evaluation and re-evaluation codes with a particular therapeutic procedure may be used when a significant, separately identifiable service is performed in addition to the therapeutic service being provided.

Many of the therapeutic procedure codes have narrative language that describes the desired outcome of care (eg, strengthening, posture, balance), and this helps the provider select the most appropriate code to represent the services provided. It is very typical for more than one procedure and/or modality to be provided on the same date of service. It is also typical that in the early stages of treatment, the patient is seen multiple times per week.

Code **97140** is to be reported for manual therapy techniques, several examples of which are listed in the descriptor nomenclature. The manual therapy code is based on each 15 minutes of manual therapy provided to one or more regions, and more than one manual therapy technique can be provided to the patient on the same date of service. If this happens, the provider should total the minutes associated with the delivery of manual therapy techniques and report the appropriate number of timed units for that session. Code **97140** is not intended to include chiropractic manipulation techniques (CMT). The appropriate CMT procedure code(s) should be reported for those manipulation techniques.

Since it is possible that manual therapy technique(s) may be required in addition to CMT procedure(s), it may be appropriate to additionally report the manual therapy technique(s) (based on 15-minute intervals of service). For example, manual traction is performed to treat a cervical spine injury and on the same day the chiropractor also performs chiropractic manipulation to the lumbar region. Therefore, codes **97140 59** and **98940** should be reported and the documentation should support the claim.

Within this series of codes, code **97150** is available for reporting therapeutic procedure(s) provided to patients in a group setting. If any combination of the therapeutic procedures in the Physical Medicine and Rehabilitation subsection are performed simultaneously with two or more individuals, only code **97150** is reported. This code is reported separately for each member of the group. Do not code the specific type of therapy in addition to the group therapy code. Group therapy procedures involve constant attendance by the provider but by definition do not require one-to-one patient contact by the provider.

Code **97532** is intended to report the provision of 15 minutes of care intended to facilitate the patient who may have been diagnosed with a cognitive deficit (eg, psychiatric disorder, brain injury, or cerebrovascular accident) to resume independent living, return to work, or function safely in his or her living environment.

Code **97533** should be used to report the provision of sensory integrative techniques intended to improve the patient's ability to process input from a deficient sensory system (ie, vestibular, proprioceptive, tactile, visual, or auditory), enhance the patient's sensory processing, and promote appropriate adaptive responses (eg, balance, task completion) of the patient to environmental demands.

Codes **97535-97537** are used to report rehabilitative training provided to an individual who has experienced a loss in functional ability to perform certain common tasks independently in the home environment. As indicated in the code descriptor language, this service may include use of assistive technology devices/adaptive equipment. Code **97537** is used to represent the provision of similar services in the community environment.

Code **97542**, Wheelchair management and training, is intended to represent services including assessing the patient for a wheelchair, determining the appropriate wheelchair model, measurement of the patient, fitting of the wheelchair, making necessary adjustments, and training the patient and/or caregiver in the use of the wheelchair. This is a timed code and each unit represents 15 minutes. This code is usually reported in multiple units and will be reported on more than one date of service. The determination of the need for a wheelchair and the measurement for the chair are usually performed on one date of service.

The receipt of the chair and fitting and adjustments as well as training in the use of the chair are performed on subsequent visits.

Two codes are available in the tests and measurements series. Code **97750**, Physical Performance Test or Measurement, represents a separate service from those occurring during an evaluation (**97001**, **97003**) or re-evaluation (**97002**, **97004**). Code **97750** is used to report testing/measurement of physical performance of a select area or number of areas. This code could represent testing such as functional capacity, isokinetic measurements, timed walking tests, computerized muscle testing, and other tests that measure physical performance. As indicated in the descriptor language, use of this code is based on time of performance and therefore should be used according to the time spent providing the service, analyzing the data, and providing instruction to the patient. In addition, it varies from the use of codes **97001-97004** in that it requires a separate written report from other evaluations that may be done.

Code **97755** is used to report an assessment of a person with severe disabilities to use assistive technological devices intended to help the person interface with his or her environment. Assistive technology facilitates a higher level of functional independence in areas such as wheeled mobility, activities of daily living, and written and verbal communication. This type of assessment may provide opportunities for people with disabilities to fully participate in all aspects of life. The provider must have knowledge of available assistive technology components and how that technology has the potential to facilitate improved function based on the patient's level of disability. This knowledge and skill allow the provider to assess the functional capacity of the individual and match the functional need to a technology option—whether off-the-shelf, modified, or via a custom solution. The assessment requires knowledge of disability, including prognosis regarding functional issues, and knowledge of technology options designed to assist the person in meeting functional needs. This code is not intended for a routine assessment for a standard or powered wheelchair absent this higher level technology component.

## Active Wound Care Management

Active wound care interventions, as performed by physical therapists, occupational therapists, and enterostomal nurses, are reported using codes **97597-97606**. These codes describe active wound care procedures, which are intended to remove devitalized (dead) tissue and remove tissue exudates that inhibit wound healing. These procedures use both selective and nonselective debridement techniques without the use of anesthesia and are not reported in addition to codes **11040-11044**. For wound debridement performed by physicians, see codes **11040-11044**.

### Definitions

Selective debridement as described by codes **97597** and **97598** is the removal of specific areas of devitalized tissue from a wound. Sharp selective debridement techniques include the use of scalpels or scissors to cut along a line of demarcation, separating viable tissue from that which is devitalized (necrotic tissue).

When selective debridement techniques are performed, no prior preparation of tissue is required.

Selective debridement includes use of the following:

*   Autolysis or other selected agents
*   Sharp instruments such as scissors, scalpel, and forceps
*   High-pressure water jet

If whirlpool (**97022**) is performed in conjunction with this procedure, it is not separately reportable.

Nonselective debridement, as described by code **97602**, includes the gradual removal of loosely adherent devitalized tissue, usually over more than one patient visit. This technique will include preparation to soften and loosen the involved tissue through the use of pulsed lavage, irrigation, or hydrotherapy techniques. Nonselective debridement may be performed with instruments such as forceps and, on occasion, scissors to remove loosely adherent necrotic tissue. Nonselective debridement includes the following types of debridement/ dressings:

*   Enzymatic agents
*   Wet
*   Wet to dry
*   Wet to moist

Code **97602** includes the application and removal of any protective or bulk dressings. Performance of a dressing change only, or in the absence of wound care, is not separately reported and is included within the E/M service.

Negative pressure wound therapy identifies any wound care management method that requires a vacuum (or suctioned pulling force) to remove excessive tissue exudates (fluidic discharge that usually results in scab formation) within the wound that inhibit wound healing. It is intended to facilitate wound healing with minimal scar formation. The vacuum cleanses the wound and stimulates the wound bed, reduces localized edema, and improves local oxygen supply. This procedure places mechanical stress on the tissue and thereby increases rates of cellular proliferation in the wound site as well as granular tissue formation and new vessel growth.

Codes **97597**, **97598**, **97605**, and **97606**, for selective debridement and negative pressure wound care management, should be reported according to the size of the area treated, as these codes include language in the descriptor that notate use in this manner. In addition, since "wound(s)" is stated in the code descriptor language (indicating a single wound site or multiple wound sites), codes **97597**, **97598**, **97605**, and **97606** are intended to describe an entire debridement session, regardless of the number of wounds or areas debrided at that specific session. Therefore, these codes should not be reported for each anatomic site debrided, nor should modifier 59, Distinct Procedural Service, be appended to depict the additional debridement performed at more than one anatomic site at that session. However, if selective debridement is performed on one site and nonselective debridement is performed at another site during the same visit, a modifier 59 would be appropriate.

Another exceptional use of modifier 59 would be in the instance when active wound care management is provided at two distinctly separate sessions on the same date. For example, pressure sores of the right ankle and right hip are debrided in the morning, but because of the patient's condition, the selective debridement of the sacral pressure sore is performed at a separate session in the afternoon on that same date by the same provider. In this specific example, codes **97597** and **97602 59** should be reported to identify procedures that are not normally reported together but are appropriate under the circumstance and represent a different session or patient encounter, different procedure, and different site. Because carrier-specific reimbursement policy may not recognize the use of modifier 59 in this circumstance, one should provide documentation to substantiate use of this modifier and the multiple reporting of debridement codes on the same date of service.

Codes **97597**, **97598**, and **97602** include the application and removal of any protective or bulk dressings. These procedures also include any assessment regarding the active wound care management that is necessary. Therefore, assessment to determine the type of wound care treatment required is not separately reported.

## Orthotic Management and Prosthetic Management

Code **97760**, Orthotic management and training, is a timed code intended to represent services associated with the provision and training of orthotics. If an HCPCS Level II "L" code is reported, the L code includes the evaluation and fitting of the orthotic. Any minutes associated with training in the use of the orthotic can be reported using **97760**. However, if an L code is not reported, then the total number of minutes associated with assessment, fitting, and training for an orthotic can be reported using **97760**. This code can be reported on more than one date of service. For example, if a patient was provided a dynamic, custom-made hand orthotic to use following surgery for flexor tendon repair, it would be expected that the orthotic would be modified and refitted during the healing of the tendon, allowing for progressively more tendon excursion in a protected range of motion. The appropriate number of units of **97760** can be reported each time the orthotic is remolded, the tension of the elastic bands are revised, and the patient is instructed in the proper use of the orthotic. Fabrication time is included in the definition of code **97760**. This code includes both static and dynamic orthotics. Materials and supplies may be separately reported with a supply/material code (eg, CPT code **99070** or HCPCS Level II code). Code **97760** should not be reported with **97116** for the same extremity.

Code **97761** is a timed code meant to identify services related to prosthetic training.

Code **97762** is intended to identify the practitioner's checkout/review of an orthotic or prosthetic to facilitate the patient's ability to use the device. As is indicated in the descriptor, both procedures are provided for established patient checkout, such as readjustments of a prosthetic as a result of surgical revisions to the application site or changes made to an orthotic because of physical

**CODING TIP**

For gait training including stair climbing, use code **97116**.

changes at the orthotic site (eg, a decrease in edema resulting in poor conformity of the orthotic to the limb or an increase in edema causing patient discomfort and breakdown in skin integrity). Any adjustments or repairs may be made to ensure alignment, and reinstruction may be given at this time as well.

Code **97762** differs from code **97760**, which describes orthotics fitting and training. Code **97760** identifies the initial fitting as well as the patient training required to properly use orthotic devices.

Application of a cast or strapping device is used when the desired effect is to provide total immobilization or restriction of movement. *Strapping* refers to the application of overlapping strips of adhesive plaster or tape to a body part to exert pressure on it and hold a structure in place. Strapping may be used to treat strains, sprains, dislocations, and some fractures. These services are reported using codes in the **29000** series.

Orthosis application differs from the purpose of an application of a cast or strapping device. Orthotics are used to support a weak or ineffective joint or muscle. They are used to provide support while the patient transitions through treatment (ie, provides mobility with support) as well as to permanently support a part (eg, ankle-foot orthotic used to prevent foot drop during gait). Some examples of orthotic devices include wrist-hand-finger splints, spinal orthotics, shoe inserts, and ankle-foot orthotics.

A cross-reference also appears at the end of the Application of Casts and Strapping subsection notes to refer the reader to code **97760** to report orthotics fitting and training. This cross-reference is to make it clear that casting and strapping codes should not be reported for orthotics fitting and training.

Also, the cross-reference is intended to make clear that the casting and strapping codes should not be reported in addition to code **97760** unless it is for a different body part. When describing orthotic procedures, dynamic splints are considered orthotics and therefore the dynamic splint application service should be identified by code **97760**.

# Medical Nutrition Therapy

Medical nutrition therapy (MNT) includes nutritional diagnostic therapy and counseling services provided by a registered dietician (RD) or licensed nutrition professional for the purpose of managing disease. MNT is provided to patients of all age groups from extremely low birth-weight preterm infants to the elderly. RDs and licensed nutrition professionals provide MNT to individuals with acute and chronic diseases or conditions where malnutrition, including overnutrition and undernutrition, may be evidenced. Malnutrition leads to poor outcomes and should be avoided or treated if present.

MNT is an essential component of any system designed to provide quality, cost-effective care throughout the life cycle. The level of safety, timeliness, responsiveness, and cost are all qualities of a system. Following valid and reliable nutrition screening, MNT provided by RDs has the potential to significantly reduce several clinically relevant endpoints (eg, infectious complications, hospital stay, and mortality).

MNT occurs over multiple encounters. The typical MNT service includes an initial assessment and intervention followed by multiple reassessment and intervention encounters. In addition, for chronic disease states, annual follow-up MNT encounters are scheduled.

RDs and licensed nutrition professionals who provide MNT use codes **97802**, **97803**, and **97804**, as well as **G0270** and **G0271**. Some insurance plans use these codes for RDs and licensed nutrition professionals who provide preventive nutrition services and nutrition services within complementary alternative medicine programs. RDs and licensed nutrition professionals provide MNT in all care settings, including physicians' offices, outpatient clinics, cardiac rehabilitation units, intensive care units, acute care hospitals, skilled nursing units, rehabilitation facilities, long-term care units, home care settings, and RD private practices. Physicians who provide nutrition services use E/M or preventive medicine services codes for reporting this service. Frequently, a physician referral is needed for RDs or licensed nutrition professionals to provide MNT.

The MNT code **97802** includes MNT assessment and intervention services for the individual patient for the first visit (new patient). Code **97803** includes MNT reassessment and intervention for the individual patient and is used for all subsequent follow-up MNT services with individual patients. MNT code **97804** is used for group MNT services. The codes for individual MNT services are reported for each 15 minutes of service. Group MNT is reported for each 30 minutes of service. RDs should use MNT code **97804** (for groups) after an individual assessment and evaluation and MNT code **97802**, where the RD determines that group MNT therapy is appropriate for the patient. The American Dietetic Association evidence-based MNT guides for practice/protocols indicate that a typical, individual, initial visit is 60 to 90 minutes and typical, follow-up, individual visits are 30 to 45 minutes. MNT codes **97803** and **97804** may be used in the initial calendar year when reassessment and intervention are provided and also in subsequent follow-up years.

Two additional codes are used by RDs and licensed nutrition professionals with qualifying Medicare patients for reassessment and subsequent MNT intervention following a second referral in the same calendar year for a change in diagnosis, medical condition, or treatment regimen. The two G codes, **G0270** for reassessment and intervention for individual MNT services, and **G0271** for reassessment and intervention for group MNT services, are used when additional hours of MNT services are performed beyond the hours typically covered by Medicare. MNT code **G0270** is reported for each 15 minutes, and code **G0271** is reported for each 30 minutes.

# Acupuncture

Codes **97810-97814** describe acupuncture and electroacupuncture services and capture the varying times required to perform these services. Codes **97810** and **97811** describe acupuncture services without electrical stimulation. Similarly, codes **97813** and **97814** describe acupuncture services with electrical stimulation.

A critical element necessary to understand and appropriately apply the intent of the acupuncture code family pertains to the 15-minute increment. Acupuncture is reported based on 15-minute increments of personal (face-to-face) contact with the patient and not the duration of acupuncture needle(s) placement.

If no electrical stimulation is used during a 15-minute increment, codes **97810** and **97811** should be reported, as appropriate. If electrical stimulation of any needle is used during a 15-minute increment, codes **97813** and **97814** should be reported, as appropriate.

Only one code may be reported for each 15-minute increment. Code **97810** or code **97813** should be reported for the initial 15-minute increment. In addition, only one initial code is reported per date of service. The acupuncture codes may be reported by any qualified provider according to any state and licensure requirements.

If the patient's condition requires a significant, separately identifiable E/M service above and beyond the usual preservice and postservice work associated with the acupuncture services, E/M services may be reported separately using modifier 25.

## Osteopathic Manipulative Treatment

Osteopathic manipulative treatment (OMT) is reported with codes in the **98925-98929** series. OMT is a form of manual treatment applied by a physician to eliminate or alleviate somatic dysfunction and related disorders. This treatment may be accomplished by a variety of techniques. OMT refers to more than 20 different manual treatment techniques. The procedures may be reported by DOs and MDs.

E/M services may be separately reported if and only if the patient's condition requires a significant, separately identifiable E/M service above and beyond the usual preservice and postservice work associated with the procedure. In this case, modifier 25 would be appended to the E/M code reported. It is important to note that the E/M service may be caused or prompted by the same symptoms or condition for which the OMT service was provided. Therefore, different diagnoses are not required for the reporting of OMT and E/M on the same date.

The codes for OMT are reported on the basis of the number of body regions involved. The body regions referred to are as follows:

- Head region
- Cervical region
- Thoracic region
- Lumbar region
- Sacral region
- Pelvic region
- Lower extremities
- Upper extremities
- Rib cage region
- Abdomen
- Viscera region

# Chiropractic Manipulative Treatment

Codes **98940-98943** are used to report chiropractic manipulative treatment (CMT). CMT is a form of manual treatment to influence joint and neurophysiologic function and can be accomplished using of a variety of techniques.

Chiropractic adjustment is a therapeutic procedure that uses (1) controlled force, (2) leverage, (3) direction, (4) amplitude, and (5) velocity, which are directed at specific joints or anatomic regions. Chiropractors commonly use such procedures to influence joint and neurophysiologic function.

CMT takes into account a variety of factors including subluxation. A subluxation is a motion segment in which the alignment, movement integrity, and/or physiologic function are altered, although contact between joint surfaces remains intact.

Chiropractic is a health care discipline that emphasizes the inherent recuperative power of the body without the use of drugs or surgery. This is accomplished by focusing on the relationship between structure, primarily the spine, and function, as coordinated by the nervous system, as that relationship may affect the preservation and restoration of health.

As is true with all of the codes in the CPT Nomenclature, the CMT codes are not limited to use by a specific specialty group. Any procedure or service in any section of the CPT codebook may be used to designate the services rendered by any qualified physician. It would also be reasonable to check with your third-party payer for reimbursement policy and payment issues.

The CMT codes include a premanipulation patient assessment. Additional E/M services may be reported separately by means of modifier 25 if and only if the patient's condition requires a significant, separately identifiable E/M service above and beyond the usual preservice and postservice work associated with the procedure.

For purposes of CMT, there are spinal regions and extraspinal regions to consider. The five spinal regions referred to are as follows:
· Cervical region (includes atlanto-occipital joint)
· Thoracic region (includes costovertebral and costotransverse joints)
· Lumbar region
· Sacral region
· Pelvic (sacroiliac joint) region

The five extraspinal regions referred to are as follows:
· Head (including temporomandibular joint, excluding the atlanto-occipital) region
· Lower extremities
· Upper extremities
· Rib cage (excluding costotransverse and costovertebral joints)
· Abdomen

# Education and Training for Patient Self-Management

Code **98960** is reported for education and training for patient self-management by a qualified, nonphysician health care professional using a standardized curriculum, face-to-face with the patient (could include caregiver/family) each 30 minutes, individual patient. Code **98961** is reported for two to four patients. Code **98962** is reported for five to eight patients.

# Special Services, Procedures, and Reports

The codes in the **99000-99091** series provide the reporting physician or other qualified health care professional with the means of identifying the completion of special reports and services that are an adjunct to the basic services rendered. These codes describe special circumstances under which practitioner services are performed. None of the codes in this series can be reported separately. These codes are reported in addition to the basic service(s) provided. Let us review the codes available for reporting special services and reports.

Code **99000** is used to report the handling and/or conveyance of a specimen for transfer from the physician's office to a laboratory. For example, a patient collects a 24-hour urine specimen and brings it to the physician's office. The conveyance of the specimen to the laboratory is reported in addition to the office visit code in which the need for the test was identified. Code **99000** is appropriately reported when the physician incurs costs for the handling and/or transportation of a specimen to the laboratory.

Another typical use of code **99000** is when a venipuncture is performed in the office to obtain a blood specimen (reported with code **36415**) and in addition, the physician's office performs the work involved in the preparation of the specimen before sending it to the laboratory. Since code **99000** is also intended to reflect this work, it would be appropriate to report code **99000** to describe the typical work involved in this preparation. This work may include centrifuging a specimen, separating serum, labeling tubes, packing the specimens for transport, filling out laboratory forms, and supplying necessary insurance information and other documentation.

Code **99000** is not intended to be used to report obtaining a specimen (eg, Pap smear, throat culture). The services to obtain the Pap smear specimen or throat culture are inherent in the procedure being performed and are not reported separately.

Code **99001** describes handling and/or conveyance of a specimen for transfer from the patient in other than a physician's office to a laboratory. This could include specimens obtained in the patient's home or in a nursing facility that does not have laboratory facilities in which to provide the services requested for that specimen.

Code **99002** describes handling, conveyance, and/or any other service in connection with the implementation of an order involving devices. This code is applicable when devices such as orthotics, protectives, and prosthetics are fabricated by an outside laboratory or shop but have been designed by and are to be fitted and adjusted by the attending physician.

Code **99024** is used to report postoperative follow-up visits included in the surgical package. Normally, a follow-up visit during the normal, uncomplicated follow-up care of a surgical procedure is not separately reported. Sometimes, however, providers wish to track these follow-up visits that are part of the surgical package for administrative reporting. This code provides a means of tracking those follow-up visits. (Refer to Chapter 4 for further discussion of this code and follow-up care.)

Codes **99026** and **99027** are used to report physician hospital-mandated on-call services. To assist the user, a cross-reference was added following **99360** to instruct that hospital-mandated on-call services are reported with codes **99026** and **99027**.

Code **99050** is used to report services provided in the office at times other than regularly scheduled office hours or on days when the office is normally closed (eg, Saturdays, Sundays, and holidays) in addition to the basic service.

Code **99051** is used to report services provided in the office during regularly scheduled evening, weekend, or holiday office hours in addition to the basic service.

Code **99053** is used to report service(s) provided between 10 PM and 8 AM at a 24-hour facility in addition to the basic service.

Code **99056** describes the provision of services that are provided in a location other than the physician's office when the services would normally be provided in the office. This code is used to indicate that the patient requested the location where the service was provided. For example, a patient who has a sore throat and high fever requests that her attending physician provide an E/M service in the emergency department rather than in the physician's office.

Code **99058** is used to report office services provided on an emergency basis that disrupt other scheduled office services in addition to the basic service. If a patient presents to the physician's office and requires unscheduled emergency care, code **99058** may be reported in addition to the other service(s) provided. This code is reported for those office patients whose condition, in the clinical judgment of the physician, warrants the physician's interrupting his or her care of another patient to deal with the emergency. This code is not reported when the physician's usual practice is to have time slots available in the schedule and patients are fit into that schedule.

Code **99060** is reported for service(s) provided on an emergency basis out of the physician's office that disrupt other scheduled office services. Code **99060** is also reported in addition to the basic service.

Code **99070** is used to report supplies and materials (except spectacles) provided by the physician over and above those usually included with the office visit or other services rendered. Code **99070** is also not to be used to report educational supplies such as books, tapes, and pamphlets. Educational supplies are reported by means of code **99071**.

Code **99071** is used to report educational supplies provided for the patient's education at cost to the physician. For example, a patient may be taught to give his own insulin. A videotape that emphasizes the various steps in the administration of insulin may be sent home with the patient to watch and gain proficiency in the technique.

Code **99075** is reported when the practitioner provides medical testimony, for example, in a court or arbitration hearing.

Code **99078** describes physician educational services rendered to patients in a group setting. Examples of the use of this code include prenatal, obesity, or diabetic education. This is not a time based code. It is appropriate to report the code once for each patient in the group, regardless of the time spent providing the service. Individual counseling of patients with established illness is included in the counseling component of the E/M services codes. (Refer to Chapter 3 for further discussion of counseling and E/M coding.)

Code **99080** describes the completion of special reports, such as insurance forms, that include more than the information conveyed in the usual medical communications or standard reporting form. There are occasions when a practitioner must complete other than a standard reporting form (eg, detailed forms related to accidents, injuries). This code may be used to report the completion of these special reports. However, physicians are often asked to complete brief standard reports (eg, return-to-work forms, hospital discharge summaries). Completion of these routine forms is not reported separately. To assist the user, a cross-reference was added following code **99080** to instruct that this code should not be reported in conjunction with codes **99455** and **99456** for the completion of workers' compensation forms.

Code **99082** is used to report unusual travel, such as travel and escort of a patient. Codes **99289** and **99290** are used to report the physical attendance and direct face-to-face care by a physician during the interfacility transport of a critically ill or injured patient. For the purpose of reporting codes **99289** and **99290**, face-to-face care begins when the physician assumes primary responsibility of the patient at the referring hospital/facility and ends when the receiving hospital/facility accepts responsibility for the patient's care. Only the time the physician spends in direct face-to-face contact with the patient during the transport should be reported. Patient transport services involving less than 30 minutes of face-to-face physician care should not be reported with codes **99289** and **99290**.

Code **99090** describes analysis of clinical data stored in computers (eg, ECGs, blood pressures, hematologic data). Often, data is stored on computers and made available in another format for the physician to review. Reporting this code requires that the physician write a formal report on the analysis of the information stored in the computer. This code is not intended to be used to report, eg, the brief analysis of an ECG rhythm strip that has been recorded with a presymptom or postsymptom memory loop.

Code **99091** should be reported no more than once in a 30-day period to include the physician or health care provider time involved with data accession and review, data interpretation, modification of care plan as necessary (including communication to patient and/or caregiver), and associated documentation. If the services described by code **99091** are provided on the same day the patient presents for an E/M service, these services should be considered part of the E/M service and not separately reported. Code **99091** is not intended to be separately reported for the collection and interpretation of data that occurs in the same 30 days of provision of care plan oversight services (**99374-99380**);

for the transfer or interpretation of data from hospital or clinical laboratory computers; or if more specific CPT codes exist to describe the service (eg, codes **93014**, **93227**, **93233**, and **93272** for cardiographic services; code **95250** for continuous glucose monitoring).

## Moderate (Conscious) Sedation

Moderate (conscious) sedation is a drug-induced depression of consciousness during which patients respond purposefully to verbal commands, either alone or accompanied by light tactile stimulation. No interventions are required to maintain a patent airway, and spontaneous ventilation is adequate. Cardiovascular function is usually maintained. It is also important to note that moderate sedation does not include minimal sedation (anxiolysis), deep sedation, or monitored anesthesia care (**00100-01999**).

Codes **99143-99150** are used to report moderate sedation services and are distinguished by provider, patient age, and additional time.

Codes **99143** and **99144** are used to report moderate sedation services provided by the same physician who also performs the diagnostic or therapeutic service that the sedation supports. Code **99143** is reported for patients under five years of age for the first 30 minutes of intraservice time. Conversely, code **99144** is reported for patients age five years or older for the first 30 minutes of intraservice time.

Codes **99143-99145** require the presence of an independent trained observer to assist in the monitoring of the patient's level of consciousness and physiological status.

The following information from the American Society of Anesthesiologists (ASA) and the American Academy of Pediatrics (AAP) is provided to help clarify the definition of an independent trained observer.

The ASA guidelines for sedation and analgesia by nonanesthesiologists indicate that a designated individual, other than the practitioner performing the procedure, should be present to monitor the patient throughout procedures performed with sedation/analgesia. The individual responsible for monitoring the patient should be trained in the recognition of complications associated with sedation/analgesia. In addition, at least one qualified individual capable of establishing a patent airway and positive pressure ventilation, as well as a means to summon additional assistance, should be present whenever sedation/analgesia is administered. It is recommended that an individual with advanced life support skills be immediately available.

The AAP guidelines for monitoring and management of pediatric patients during and after sedation for diagnostic and therapeutic procedures indicate that the practitioner responsible for the treatment of the patient and/or the administration of drugs for sedation must be trained in and capable of providing, at the minimum, pediatric basic life support; training in pediatric advanced life support is strongly encouraged.

In the AAP's guidelines, it is also encouraged that the independent trained observer be trained in pediatric basic life support. This individual shall have specific assignments in the event of an emergency and thus, current knowledge of the emergency cart inventory.

Both codes **99143** and **99144** are reported for the first 30 minutes of intraservice time. Code **99145** is an add-on code that is reported in addition to codes **99143** and **99144** for each additional 15 minutes of intraservice time.

Intraservice time starts with the administration of the sedation agent(s), requires continuous face-to-face attendance, and ends at the conclusion of personal contact by the physician providing the sedation.

Contrary to codes **99143** and **99144**, codes **99148** and **99149** are reported when a second physician other than the health care professional performing the diagnostic or therapeutic services provides moderate (conscious) sedation in the facility setting. Code **99148** is reported for patients under age five, while code **99149** is reported for patients age five and older. Both codes are reported for the first 30 minutes of intraservice time. Code **99150** is an add-on code that is reported in addition to codes **99148** and **99149** for each additional 15 minutes of intraservice time.

The following services are included as part of the moderate sedation and are not reported separately:

- Assessment of the patient (not included in intraservice time)
- Establishment of IV access and fluids to maintain patency, when performed
- Administration of agent(s)
- Maintenance of sedation
- Monitoring of oxygen saturation, heart rate, and blood pressure
- Recovery (not included in intraservice time)

Codes for pulse oximetry (**94760-94762**) are not to be reported in addition to the codes for moderate (conscious) sedation services **99143-99150**, as these services are considered an inclusive component.

If catheter placement is performed in conjunction with moderate (conscious) sedation, it would be appropriate to report this procedure separately with a code from the **36000** series. While both the ASA and the AAP guidelines suggest the presence of an IV line for all patients who receive sedation/analgesia, they are not mandatory for patients who receive their medications through non-IV routes. The current practice standard for sedation/analgesia does not result in the routine placement of an IV catheter. Therefore, it would be appropriate to separately report catheter placement when performed.

Appendix G provides a list of procedures that include conscious sedation as an inherent component of providing the procedure. It is not appropriate for the same physician to report both the procedure and the sedation codes **99143-99145**, as the services listed in Appendix G include moderate sedation. There may be some unusual circumstances when a second physician other than the health care professional performing the diagnostic or therapeutic services provides moderate sedation in the facility setting for the procedures listed in Appendix G. In this instance, it would be appropriate for the second physician to report codes **99148-99150** in conjunction with codes listed in Appendix G. However, when these services are performed by the second physician in the nonfacility setting, codes **99148-99150** would not be reported.

# Home Health Procedures/Services—Including Home Infusion Procedures/Services

The codes included in this section (**99500-99512** and **99601-99602**) are intended to identify services provided by nonphysician health care professionals for various health and maintenance issues necessary for a patient's continued recovery, health improvement, and general welfare. These services include such activities as maintenance for stoma care (following colostomy or cystostomy) and home visits for mechanical ventilation care.

Physicians performing services of this nature should not report these codes. Instead, physicians should use the home visit codes **99341-99350** and CPT codes other than **99500-99602** for any additional procedure(s) or service(s) provided to a patient living in a residence. If a health care professional who is authorized to use E/M home visit codes (**99341-99350** according to state licensure requirements) performs these services in addition to a significant, separately identifiable E/M service, both services may be reported, appending modifier 25 to the home visit code to identify this service as significant enough to report and as a separate effort from the home health procedure that was provided.

CHAPTER 9

# EXERCISES

Assign the appropriate code(s) for the following procedures/services.

1 Subcutaneous administration of the conjugate measles, mumps, and rubella virus vaccine, live.

2 A dialysis patient on a four-dose schedule is given 40 mcg of hepatitis B vaccine, administered in a single intramuscular injection.

3 Five-hour hydration IV infusion administered by the physician.

4 Interactive group psychotherapy for a five-patient group.

5 Forty minutes of individual psychotherapy, insight-oriented, behavior-modifying, and/or supportive, in the clinician's office.

6 Mini-mental state examination performed by a physician.

7 Sixty minutes (one hour) of individual insight-oriented, behavior-modifying, and/or supportive psychotherapy in an office or other outpatient facility.

8 End-stage renal disease services consecutively provided over a full month, in outpatient setting.

9 ESRD-related services not performed consecutively during an entire full month for a four-year-old receiving continuous peritoneal dialysis during 16 days of daily outpatient care, preceding or following a period of hospitalization.

10 Comprehensive ophthalmological services, established patient visit, with determination of refractive state.

11 Gonioscopy under general anesthesia.

12 Fitting of monofocal spectacles.

13 Percutaneous transluminal atherectomy and balloon angioplasty of the left anterior descending coronary artery. Percutaneous transluminal atherectomy only of the right coronary artery.

14 Percutaneous transluminal coronary thrombectomy and percutaneous intracoronary stent placement.

15 Percutaneous transcatheter placement of a radiation delivery device for subsequent coronary intravascular brachytherapy performed at the time of coronary arteriography (without associated left heart catheterization).

16 PTCA with stent placement of the left anterior descending coronary artery. PTCA only, left circumflex.

**17** Complete transthoracic echocardiography with Doppler echocardiography and color flow-velocity mapping.

**18** Placement of a transesophageal echocardiography (TEE) probe and use of transesophageal echocardiography (TEE) for continuous monitoring during a surgical operation.

**19** Echocardiography (ECG) during rest and cardiovascular stress test.

**20** Left heart catheterization with injection procedures for coronary angiography and left ventriculography, including imaging supervision, interpretation, and report.

**21** Comprehensive EP evaluation with right atrial and ventricular pacing and recording, His bundle recording, with induction of arrhythmia and intracardiac mapping of tachycardia to localize the site of origin of the tachycardia.

**22** Intracardiac EP three-dimensional mapping.

**23** One session of peripheral arterial disease rehabilitation performed on a group of four patients.

**24** A physician prepares a 10-dose multivial for a patient. At that same encounter, one dose from this vial is administered by one injection to the patient.

**25** A patient is known to be allergic to three different insect venoms (honeybees, hornets, and yellow jackets). The allergist prepares a dosage schedule for treatment, which includes venom for all three of the stinging insects combined into two multiple-dose vials containing five doses. The patient on subsequent visits receives a weekly injection consisting of one dose drawn from the prepared multiple-dose vials.

**26** A physician prepares two different multidose vials, each containing different antigens and each vial containing 10 doses (total doses prepared: $2 \times 10 = 20$). At that same encounter, one dose from the first vial is administered in one injection and one dose from the second vial is administered in a second injection to the patient. Each injection contains one dose from each of the two multidose vials (two doses would be drawn from the treatment board in two syringes as noted previously). The patient is also seen for an interval history and examination to assess the clinical status, as well as to readjust the prescription drug treatment. The physician also questions the patient about reactions to injections from previously supplied vials.

**27** Noninvasive method for evaluating brain function using magnetic fields.

**28** Assessment/interventions to modify the psychological, behavioral, emotional, cognitive, and social factors identified or affecting patient physiologic functioning, disease status, health, and well-being (without psychiatric diagnosis).

**29** Application of a hot pack to the neck and knee. Manual electrical stimulation, 15 minutes.

**30** Sharp selective debridement of a sacral pressure ulcer having black eschar surrounded by chronic inflammation with dark pigmentation. The total wound surface area selectively debrided is 18 sq cm.

**31** Individual patient medical nutrition therapy (MNT) reassessment and intervention, of 30 minutes' duration.

**32** OMT cervical region, lumbar region, and pelvic region.

**33** CMT lumbar region and myofascial release of the cervical region.

**34** CMT cervical region and lower extremities.

**35** Application of paraffin bath to left hand. Orthotics fitting and training, 15 minutes.

**36** Handling and/or conveyance of a specimen for transfer from the patient in other than a physician's office to a laboratory.

**37** A postoperative follow-up visit included in a global service.

**38** Office services provided to a patient presenting and requiring unscheduled emergency care.

**39** Collection and interpretation of physiologic data (eg, ECG, glucose monitoring) digitally stored and/or transmitted.

**40** True or False: Pulse oximetry may be reported in addition to conscious sedation.

**41** True or False: Subsequent reprogramming of a cochlear implant on a different day is included as part of the diagnostic analysis procedure.

**42** True or False: The home visit codes (**99500-99512**) included as part of the Home Health Procedures subsection are intended to be used only by physicians.

**43** True or False: Codes ESRD **90918-90921** do not include the dialysis treatment.

**44** True or False: Stress testing codes **93015-93018** should be reported in addition to code **93350** to describe the exercise stress portion of the study.

# CHAPTER 10

# Modifiers

The Current Procedural Terminology (CPT®) Nomenclature uses modifiers as an integral part of its structure. A modifier provides the means to indicate that a service or procedure that has been performed has been altered by some specific circumstance but not changed in its definition or code. Modifiers also enable health care professionals to effectively respond to payment policy requirements established by other entities. This chapter reviews the two-digit numeric modifiers found in the CPT code set and in Appendix A of the CPT codebook.

In the CPT Nomenclature, modifiers may be used in many instances. Some examples include the following:

- To report only the professional component of a procedure or service
- To report a service mandated by a third-party payer
- To indicate that a procedure was performed bilaterally
- To report that multiple procedures were performed at the same session by the same provider
- To report that a portion of a service or procedure is reduced or eliminated at the physician's discretion
- To report assistant surgeon services

To report a modifier:

Append the modifier to the procedure code usually reported. If the computer system being used allows eight or more digits to report a service on one line, the two-digit modifier may be appended as follows:

Example:    **49500 50**

In addition to the CPT (Health Care Common Procedure Coding System [HCPCS] Level I) modifiers, there are a number of HCPCS Level II (national) modifiers available for reporting purposes. HCPCS Level II modifiers are updated by the Centers for Medicare and Medicaid Services (CMS). (Refer to Chapter 1 for further discussion of the HCPCS Level II codes.) Information regarding HCPCS Level II national modifiers can be obtained from one's CMS regional office. Information can also be found in the American Medical Association's (AMA's) HCPCS Level II codebook, available by contacting the AMA Customer Service Department at 800-621-8335. Be sure to become familiar with these modifiers and the specific requirements for their use.

## Review of All CPT Modifiers

CPT modifiers are two-digit numeric indicators—except for the physical status modifiers also found in the guidelines of the Anesthesia section of the CPT Nomenclature. (Refer to Chapter 6 for further discussion of the physical status modifiers.)

This chapter focuses on the two-digit numeric modifiers found in the CPT code set. Appendix A of the CPT codebook contains a complete listing of these modifiers and their definitions. In the text that follows, the definitions are reviewed and the use of each modifier is illustrated.

## Modifier 21, Prolonged Evaluation and Management Services

When the face-to-face or floor/unit service(s) provided is prolonged or otherwise greater than that usually required for the highest level of evaluation and management (E/M) service within a given category, it may be identified by adding modifier 21 to the E/M code number. A report may also be appropriate.

### Illustration of Modifier 21

A physician assesses an established patient in the office who has multiple, concurrent diseases requiring more than the highest level of office and other outpatient services (eg, the physician examines the patient for osteoarthritis, gout, emphysema, and advanced diabetes with a stasis ulcer). After assessing the patient, the physician counsels the patient and his family, adding time to the visit. The decision making and examination, plus the time spent with the patient (90 minutes), all exceed the highest level of E/M service in that category.

In this case, the physician provided all of these services continuously and directly to the patient and did not leave the patient during the 90-minute visit. Since the physician's service exceeds the highest level of E/M service, modifier 21 is appended to code **99215**.

In this scenario, the important difference between modifier 21 and prolonged physician service with direct (face-to-face) patient contact is that the time spent with the patient is continuous and the services exceed the highest level of service in that category. The prolonged physician services with direct (face-to-face) patient contact can be intermittent and reported with any level of E/M service. For further discussion of the prolonged physician services codes, refer to Chapter 3 of this text and the guidelines in the CPT codebook.

## Modifier 22, Unusual Procedural Services

When the service(s) provided is greater than that usually required for the listed procedure, it may be identified by adding modifier 22 to the usual procedure number. Documentation must support the substantial additional work and the reason for the additional work (ie, increased intensity, time, technical difficulty of procedure, severity of patient's condition, physical and mental effort required). Note: This modifier should not be appended to an E/M service.

The word *procedural* in the descriptor of modifier 22 is intended to indicate that modifier 22 may be used with any procedure but is not used with the E/M codes. Modifier 21, Prolonged Evaluation and Management Services, the nonprocedural counterpart of modifier 22, may be reported "when the service(s) provided is prolonged or otherwise greater than that usually required for the highest level of E/M service within a given category."

### Illustration of Modifier 22

A physician excises a lesion located in a crease of the neck of a very obese person. The obesity makes the excision more difficult. The physician indicates the complexity of the removal of the lesion by appending modifier 22 to the code used to report the removal of the lesion. When reporting this service to a third-party payer, it may be helpful to include a copy of the operative report to demonstrate the increased services provided.

## Modifier 23, Unusual Anesthesia

Occasionally, a procedure that usually requires either no anesthesia or local anesthesia because of unusual circumstances must be done under general anesthesia. This circumstance may be reported by adding modifier 23 to the procedure code of the basic service.

The guidelines in the Surgery section of the CPT codebook for the CPT Surgical Package Definition indicate that a given CPT surgical code includes, on a procedure-by-procedure basis, a variety of services. In addition to the operation per se, one of the services included is local infiltration, metacarpal/metatarsal/digital block, or topical anesthesia, when used. Certain codes in the CPT Nomenclature represent services performed under anesthesia (eg, **57410**, Pelvic examination under anesthesia); for these codes, modifier 23 would not be appended.

Procedures that generally do not require general anesthesia may, in some cases, require general anesthesia because of the extent of the service or other circumstances. In these cases, modifier 23 is appended to the procedure code reported.

### Illustration of Modifier 23

The physical condition of some patients, such as patients who are mentally retarded, extremely apprehensive, or have particular physical conditions (eg, tremors, spasticity), may require the use of general anesthesia to perform certain procedures that would normally not require anesthesia. To report these cases, append modifier 23 to the procedure code.

## Modifier 24, Unrelated Evaluation and Management Service by the Same Physician During a Postoperative Period

The physician may need to indicate that an E/M service was performed during a postoperative period for reasons unrelated to the original procedure. This circumstance may be reported by adding modifier 24 to the appropriate level of E/M service.

Modifier 24 is used when a physician provides a surgical service related to one problem and then, during the period of follow-up care for the surgery, provides an E/M service unrelated to the problem requiring the surgery. In this circumstance, diagnosis code selection is particularly critical to indicate the reason for the additional E/M service.

### Illustration of Modifier 24

An orthopedic surgeon performs a hip replacement on Mrs Jones. During the normal, uncomplicated postoperative period related to the hip surgery, she falls and sprains her wrist.

**CODING TIP**

Append modifier 24 to the appropriate skilled nursing facility admission code, should the admission be due to an unrelated condition during the postoperative period. Modifier 24 should not be appended to the subsequent hospital care codes (**99231-99233**), unless a different diagnosis is reported, identifying the service as unrelated to the original procedure.

The orthopedic surgeon reports the E/M service (related to the sprained wrist) performed in the office using the established patient, office or other outpatient service codes. The level of E/M service reported is based on the services provided related to the sprained wrist. Appending modifier 24 to the E/M service indicates to the third-party payer that the E/M service provided is related to the sprained wrist, and not to the hip replacement.

## Modifier 25, Significant, Separately Identifiable Evaluation and Management Service by the Same Physician on the Same Day of the Procedure or Other Service

It may be necessary to indicate that on the day a procedure or service identified by a CPT code was performed, the patient's condition required a significant, separately identifiable E/M service above and beyond the usual preoperative and postoperative care associated with the procedure that was performed. A significant, separately identifiable E/M service is defined or substantiated by documentation that satisfies the relevant criteria for the respective E/M service to be reported (see Evaluation and Management Services Guidelines for instructions on determining level of E/M service). The E/M service may be prompted by the symptom or condition for which the procedure and/or service was provided. As such, different diagnoses are not required for reporting an E/M service on the same date. This circumstance may be reported by adding modifier 25 to the appropriate level of E/M service. Note: This modifier is not used to report an E/M service that resulted in a decision to perform surgery. See modifier 57. For significant, separately identifiable non-E/M services, see modifier 59.

Modifier 25 is not restricted to a specific level of E/M service and may be reported with the appropriate code for the level of service supported by documentation in the medical record.

Modifier 25 is used to indicate that a significant, separately identifiable E/M service is performed by the same physician on the day of a procedure. As stated in the definition, the E/M service must be "above and beyond" the other service or "beyond" the usual preoperative and postoperative care associated with the procedure. CPT guidelines do not require different diagnoses for an E/M service and the procedure/service performed to be separately reported. However, the E/M service must either meet the key components (ie, history, examination, medical decision making) or be selected based on time when counseling and/or coordination of care dominates (more than 50%) the physician/patient and/or family encounter (face-to-face time in the office or other outpatient setting or floor/unit time in the hospital or nursing facility), of that level of E/M, including medical record documentation.

### Illustration of Modifier 25

A physician examines a patient exhibiting a fever, headache, vomiting, and stiff neck and performs a spinal tap, as well as the services described in code **99214**. To report this patient encounter, the physician appends modifier 25 to code **99214**, and separately reports code **62270**, Spinal puncture, lumbar, diagnostic, to indicate that both a significant E/M service and a procedure were performed on a given day.

Do not use modifier 25 to report an E/M service that results in a decision to perform surgery; for this circumstance, use modifier 57.

## Modifier 26, Professional Component

Certain procedures are a combination of a physician component and a technical component. When the physician component is reported separately, the service may be identified by adding modifier 26 to the usual procedure number.

Properly reporting the technical and professional components for procedures is a complex process. Since CPT codes are intended to represent physician and other health care practitioner services, the CPT Nomenclature does not contain a coding convention to designate the technical component for a procedure or service. CPT coding guidelines do not specifically address billing for the technical component of a procedure or service.

However, many third-party payers have established modifiers and/or specific reporting policies for reporting the technical component. For example, Medicare established the TC modifier for reporting the technical component. Other insurance companies may also require the use of the TC modifier, or they may have developed their own method for such reporting. When reporting the technical component of a procedure or service, become familiar with the various reporting requirements of individual insurance companies in one's area, because reporting and reimbursement policies vary among insurance companies.

CPT coding does provide modifier 26 for separately reporting the professional (or physician) component of a procedure or service. Certain procedures are a combination of a physician professional component and a technical component. For procedures with both a technical and professional component, modifier 26 is used to indicate that the professional component of the procedure is being reported separately.

In general, if a procedure is composed of both a technical and a professional component and is performed on facility-owned equipment, it may be necessary for the physician to indicate that he or she is reporting only the professional component by appending modifier 26 to the procedure code(s) reported. This is because a hospital or other facility may be reporting the technical component of the procedure.

Unmodified CPT codes are intended to describe both the technical and professional components of a service. The professional and technical components together are referred to as the "global service." If the technical and professional components of the service are performed by the same provider, it is not appropriate or necessary to report the components of the service separately.

### Illustration of Modifier 26

Sometimes a physician performs a complex cystometrogram in his or her office, while other times he or she may only interpret the results of a complex cystometrogram. When the physician only interprets the results and/or operates the equipment, the professional component modifier 26 is appended.

> **CODING TIP**
>
> Modifier 26 is not appended to the cardiac catheterization injection procedure codes **93539-93545**, as these are solely performed by the physician.

The guidelines for reporting urodynamic studies, found preceding code **51725**, indicate that all procedures in that section imply that these services are performed by or under the direct supervision of a physician and that all instruments, equipment, fluids, gases, probes, catheters, technician's fees, medications, gloves, trays, tubing, and other sterile supplies are provided by the physician. Thus, when the physician only interprets the results and/or operates the equipment and does not provide the equipment, supplies, technicians, etc, modifier 26 is used to identify the physician's services.

## Modifier 32, Mandated Services

Services related to mandated consultation and/or related services (eg, third-party payer, governmental, legislative, or regulatory requirement) may be identified by adding modifier 32 to the basic procedure.

### Illustration of Modifier 32

Occasionally, some third-party payers require the patient to undergo certain mandated services, such as a second or third opinion on a surgical procedure. In these instances, when the physician is aware that the patient is scheduled for an appointment for these types of services, the code for the service provided is reported with modifier 32 appended.

## Modifier 47, Anesthesia by Surgeon

Regional or general anesthesia provided by the surgeon may be reported by adding modifier 47 to the basic service. (This does not include local anesthesia.) Note: Modifier 47 would not be used as a modifier for the anesthesia procedures.

If a physician personally performs the regional or general anesthesia for a surgical procedure he or she also performs, modifier 47 would be appended to the surgical code, and no codes from the Anesthesia section would be used.

### Illustration of Modifier 47

A surgeon performs a regional nerve block prior to performing surgery to decompress the nerve at the carpal tunnel. To report this, the physician uses code **64721**, Neuroplasty and/or transposition; median nerve at carpal tunnel, with modifier 47 appended. Code **64415**, Injection, anesthetic agent; brachial plexus, would also be reported to describe the regional nerve block performed.

Use of modifier 47 alerts the third-party payer that the surgeon personally performed the anesthesia. Listing the code for the anesthesia (in this case a nerve block) indicates specifically which nerve was blocked. Under no circumstance should modifier 47 be appended to the anesthesia procedure codes **00100-01999**.

## Modifier 50, Bilateral Procedure

Unless otherwise identified in the listings, bilateral procedures that are performed at the same operative session should be identified by adding modifier 50 to the appropriate five-digit code.

This modifier is used to report bilateral procedures that are performed at the same operative session. The use of this modifier is applicable only to services/procedures performed on identical anatomical sites, aspects, or organs (eg, arms, legs, eyes). The intent is for the modifier to be appended to the appropriate unilateral code as a one-line entry on the claim form to indicate that the procedure was performed bilaterally.

Furthermore, when a procedure is reported with modifier 50 appended to the code, the units box on the claim form should indicate that "1" unit of service was provided since one procedure is being performed bilaterally.

Although the intended reporting of modifier 50 is that the code be listed only once, one's local third-party payer reporting guidelines may require that the code be listed twice, with modifier 50 appended to the second line entry. One may want to contact the various payers regarding their preferred method of reporting bilateral procedures.

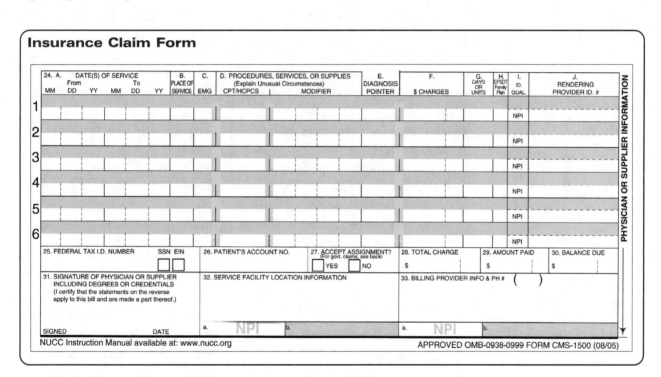

### Illustration of Modifier 50

A physician repairs bilateral reducible inguinal hernias on a two-year-old. The physician reports code **49500**, Repair initial inguinal hernia, age 6 months to younger than 5 years, with or without hydrocelectomy; reducible, with modifier 50 appended (**49500 50**).

Note that although the text of this modifier refers to "operative session," these words are used in a broad context. Diagnostic as well as therapeutic procedures may require the use of the bilateral modifier if the anatomical structures are found bilaterally and the identical procedure is performed on both sides.

## Modifier 51, Multiple Procedures

When multiple procedures, other than E/M services, Physical Medicine and Rehabilitation services or provision of supplies (eg, vaccines), are performed at the same session by the same provider, the primary procedure or service may be reported as listed. The additional procedure(s) or service(s) may be identified by appending modifier 51 to the additional procedure or service code(s). Note: This modifier should not be appended to designated "add-on" codes (see Appendix D).

Historically, payers and providers have used modifier 51, Multiple Procedures, in varying ways. To alleviate confusion about the intent of the modifier, the definition includes language to indicate that it is not appended to "add-on" codes, as listed in Appendix D of the CPT codebook, E/M codes, or codes designated as modifier 51-exempt, as listed in Appendix E of the CPT codebook. (Refer to Chapter 4 for further discussion of add-on codes and codes designated as modifier 51-exempt.)

Also, the language, "by the same provider," is included in the definition to indicate that this modifier is not to be appended to procedures performed and reported by another physician at the same session.

Modifier 51 has four applications, namely, to identify the following:

- Multiple medical procedures performed at the same session by the same provider
- Multiple, related operative procedures performed at the same session by the same provider
- Operative procedures performed in combination at the same operative session by the same provider, whether through the same or another incision or involving the same or different anatomy
- A combination of medical and operative procedures performed at the same session by the same provider

## Modifier 52, Reduced Services

Under certain circumstances, a service or procedure is partially reduced or eliminated at the physician's discretion. Under these circumstances, the service provided can be identified by its usual procedure number and the addition of modifier 52, signifying that the service is reduced. This provides a means of reporting reduced services without disturbing the identification of the basic service. Note: For hospital outpatient reporting of a previously scheduled procedure/service that is partially reduced or cancelled as a result of extenuating circumstances or those that threaten the well-being of the patient prior to or after administration of anesthesia, see modifiers 73 and 74 (see modifiers approved for ambulatory service center [ASC] hospital outpatient use).

> **CODING TIP**
>
> Modifier 51 may be appended to the same related family of codes when repairing multiple surgical endoscopic/laparoscopic/arthroscopic procedures.

Illustration of Modifier 52

Some codes, such as those below, indicate that the associated services performed are inherently bilateral. However, sometimes a procedure cannot be performed as described in the CPT code set. For example, if an extremity arterial study is performed on a patient who previously had an above-the-knee amputation, modifier 52 would be appended to code **93923** to indicate that this test was not performed in its entirety.

**93923**   Noninvasive physiologic studies of upper or lower extremity arteries, multiple levels or with provocative functional maneuvers, complete bilateral study (eg, segmental blood pressure measurements, segmental Doppler waveform analysis, segmental volume plethysmography, segmental transcutaneous oxygen tension measurements, measurements with postural provocative tests, measurements with reactive hyperemia)

## Modifier 53, Discontinued Procedure

Under certain circumstances, the physician may elect to terminate a surgical or diagnostic procedure. Due to extenuating circumstances or those that threaten the well-being of the patient, it may be necessary to indicate that a surgical or diagnostic procedure was started but discontinued. This circumstance may be reported by adding modifier 53 to the code reported by the physician for the discontinued procedure. Note: This modifier is not used to report the elective cancellation of a procedure prior to the patient's anesthesia induction and/or surgical preparation in the operating suite. For outpatient hospital/ASC reporting of a previously scheduled procedure/service that is partially reduced or cancelled as a result of extenuating circumstances or those that threaten the well-being of the patient prior to or after administration of anesthesia, see modifiers 73 and 74 (see modifiers approved for ASC hospital outpatient use).

Modifier 53 is used for physician reporting purposes. It is used to report circumstances when patients experience unexpected responses (eg, arrhythmia, hypotensive/hypertensive crisis) that cause the procedure to be terminated. Modifier 53 differs from 52 (which describes a procedure that was reduced at the physician's discretion) in that a patient's life-threatening condition precipitates the terminated procedure. Modifier 53 is not used to report elective cancellation of procedures prior to anesthesia induction or surgical preparation in the surgical suite, including situations where cancellation is due to patient instability.

Illustration of Modifier 53

Following anesthesia induction, the patient experiences an arrhythmia that causes the procedure to be terminated. The physician reports the code for the planned procedure with modifier 53 appended.

## Modifiers 54, 55, 56

### Modifier 54, Surgical Care Only

When one physician performed a surgical procedure and another provided preoperative and/or postoperative management, surgical services may be identified by adding modifier 54 to the usual procedure number.

### Modifier 55, Postoperative Management Only

When one physician performed the postoperative management and another physician performed the surgical procedure, the postoperative component may be identified by adding modifier 55 to the usual procedure number.

### Modifier 56, Preoperative Management Only

When one physician performed the preoperative care and evaluation and another physician performed the surgical procedure, the preoperative component may be identified by adding modifier 56 to the usual procedure number.

### Illustration of Modifiers 54, 55, 56

In certain locations or types of practice, a surgeon may be asked to perform a surgical procedure while another physician(s) performs the preoperative and postoperative services associated with a particular service. The operating surgeon reports the surgical procedure performed and appends modifier 54 to the surgical procedure code. The physician who provides the preoperative and postoperative management appends modifiers 55 and 56 to the surgical procedure code.

For example, a patient travels to a famous medical center for specialized surgery and subsequently receives postoperative care from his or her local physician. The surgeon, in this case, reports the preoperative management and the surgical procedure code (ie, report the surgical procedure with modifiers 54 and 56). The physician who performed the postoperative management reports the operative procedure code with modifier 55 appended. Reporting the postoperative management indicates that the physician performed all of the postoperative care.

In some specialties, the internal medicine physician (eg, a cardiologist) provides the preoperative and postoperative management related to the medical component of the patient's care. In this case, one should check with the third-party payer(s) for the preferred method of reporting.

## Modifier 57, Decision for Surgery

An E/M service that resulted in the initial decision to perform the surgery may be identified by adding modifier 57 to the appropriate level of E/M service.

Modifier 57 provides a means of identifying the E/M service that results in the initial decision to perform the surgery. The modifier, supported by documentation that the decision for surgery was made at the time of the visit, may allow separate payment for the E/M service if covered by the payer. Many variations and coverage interpretations can exist among payers regarding this modifier.

## Illustration of Modifier 57

A physician is consulted to determine whether surgery is necessary for a patient with abdominal pain. The physician's services meet the criteria necessary to report a consultation (ie, documents findings, communicates by written report to the requesting physician). The requesting physician agrees with the consultant's findings and requests that the consultant assume the case and discuss his findings with the patient.

The patient consents to undergo surgery to repair a perforated ulcer; the operation is performed later that same day. To code this, the surgeon reports the E/M services (consultation) using the appropriate consultation code and appends modifier 57. The surgeon also reports the appropriate code for the specific surgery (without a modifier) in addition to the E/M service.

It is incorrect to append modifier 25 to the consultation code for the decision to perform surgery. Appending modifier 57 to the consultation described previously indicates to the third-party payer that the consultation is not part of the global surgical procedure.

## Modifier 58, Staged or Related Procedure or Service by the Same Physician During the Postoperative Period

It may be necessary to indicate that the performance of a procedure or service during the postoperative period was: (a) planned or anticipated (staged), (b) more extensive than the original procedure, or (c) for therapy following a surgical procedure. This circumstance may be reported by adding modifier 58 to the staged or related procedure. Note: For treatment of a problem that requires a return to the operating/procedure room (eg, unanticipated clinical condition), see modifier 78.

At times it is necessary for a surgeon to perform one operation and then during the postoperative period associated with that surgery, perform a staged or related procedure. Modifier 58 should be appended for surgeries performed by the original surgeon or provider during the postoperative period of the original procedure that were planned prospectively, at the time of the original procedure; for follow-up surgeries that are more extensive than the original procedure; or for therapy following a surgical procedure.

## Illustration of Modifier 58

A surgeon performs a mastectomy on a patient. During the postoperative global period, the surgeon inserts a permanent prosthesis (**11970**). The surgeon reports the code for the permanent prosthesis insertion with modifier 58, to indicate that the service was related to the mastectomy (staged to occur at a time after the initial surgery). If the physician did not append modifier 58, a third-party payer could reject the claim because the surgery occurred during the postoperative period associated with the mastectomy.

In a second case, a diabetic patient with advanced circulatory problems has three gangrenous toes removed from her left foot (**28820, 28820 51, 28820 51**). During the postoperative period, it becomes necessary to amputate the patient's left foot. To report this, modifier 58 would be appended to the code for the amputation of the foot (**28805 58**).

Since the amputation is related to the reason for the previous amputation of the toes (diabetic gangrene), modifier 58 is used (rather than modifier 78) even though the use of an operating room is necessary. The amputation of the foot was not due to a complication of the first surgery but was due to the underlying disease process.

## Modifier 59, Distinct Procedural Service

Under certain circumstances, it may be necessary to indicate that a procedure or service was distinct or independent from other non-E/M services performed on the same day. Modifier 59 is used to identify procedures/services, other than E/M services, that are not normally reported together but are appropriate under the circumstances. Documentation may support a different session, different procedure or surgery, different site or organ system, separate incision/excision, separate lesion, or separate injury (or area of injury in extensive injuries) not ordinarily encountered or performed on the same day by the same individual. However, when another already-established modifier is appropriate, it should be used rather than modifier 59. Only if no more descriptive modifier is available and the use of modifier 59 best explains the circumstances, should modifier 59 be used. Note: Modifier 59 should not be appended to an E/M service. To report a separate and distinct E/M service with a non-E/M service performed on the same date, see modifier 25.

### Separate Procedure

Modifier 59 is also intended to assist in the reporting of codes with the "separate procedure" designation. Some of the codes listed in the CPT Nomenclature have been identified with the term *separate procedure* in the code descriptor. (Refer to Chapter 4 for further discussion of separate procedure.)

When a procedure or service that is designated as a separate procedure is carried out independently or considered unrelated or distinct from other procedures/services provided at that time, it may be reported by itself or in addition to other procedures/services by appending modifier 59 to the specific separate procedure code reported. This indicates that the procedure is not considered a component of another procedure but is a distinct, independent procedure, such as a different session, different site or organ system, separate incision/excision, separate lesion, or treatment of a separate injury (or area of injury in extensive injuries).

Codes designated as separate procedures may not be additionally reported when the procedure/service is performed as an integral component of another procedure/service.

## Modifier 62, Two Surgeons

When two surgeons work together as primary surgeons performing distinct parts of a procedure, each surgeon should report his or her distinct operative work by adding modifier 62 to the procedure code and any associated add-on code(s) for that procedure as long as both surgeons continue to work together as primary surgeons. Each surgeon should report the cosurgery once using the same procedure code. If additional procedure(s) (including add-on procedure [s]) are performed during the same surgical session, separate code(s) may also be reported with modifier 62 added.

Note: If a cosurgeon acts as an assistant in the performance of additional procedure(s) during the same surgical session, those services may be reported using separate procedure code(s) with modifier 80 or modifier 82 added, as appropriate.

### Co-Surgeon Modifier

Co-surgery may be required because of the complexity of the procedure(s), the patient's condition, or both. The additional surgeon is not acting as an assistant at surgery in these circumstances but is performing a distinct portion of the procedure.

### General Guidelines for Spine Surgery

Modifier 62 is not to be used with instrumentation or bone graft codes. Documentation to establish medical necessity for both surgeons is required for some services.

The approach surgeon and the spine surgeon must discuss, before a scheduled surgery, what portion of the operation each is expected to perform based on the case's complexity. If because of the complexity of the procedure the approach surgeon is needed as a co-surgeon (both the spine and approach surgeon serve as primary surgeons) to also perform additional procedures, modifier 62 may be appended to these agreed-upon procedures.

When an approach surgeon opens and closes only, modifier 62 is appended to the distinct principal procedure along with any additional levels that require approach work by only the approach surgeon.

Modifier 62 may be added to additional procedural codes only if both surgeons agree to continue to work together as primary surgeons based on complexity of the case.

Modifier 80 may be appended to additional procedural code(s) by the approach surgeon, provided both surgeons agree the approach surgeon is needed to continue to work as an assistant to the spine surgeon.

Following is an example:

**PROCEDURE:** Anterior Thoracic Two-Level Arthrodesis, Anterior Single-Level Discectomy, Anterior Plate Instrumentation, Structural, Autograft Iliac Crest Bone Graft

**EXAMPLE 1:** Approach Surgeon Performs Approach and Closure Only

*Surgeon Performing Approach Only*

**22556 62**

**22585 62**

---

> ### CODING TIP
>
> Modifier 62 should not be appended to the bone graft codes **20900-20938** and spinal instrumentation codes **22040-22855**.

*Surgeon Performing the Spine Procedure*

**22556 62**

**22585 62**

**63077 51**

**22845**

**20938**

**EXAMPLE 2:** Approach Surgeon Performs as Co-surgeon with Spine Surgeon for Entire Case

*Surgeon Performing Approach and Serving as Co-surgeon for Entire Case*

**22556 62**

**22585 62**

**63077 62 51**

*Surgeon Performing the Spine Procedure*

**22556 62**

**22585 62**

**63077 62 51**

**22845**

**20938**

**EXAMPLE 3:** Approach Surgeon Performs Approach and Closure and Performs Rest of Case as Assistant to Spine Surgeon

*Surgeon Performing Approach and Serving as an Assistant for Entire Case*

**22556 62**

**22585 62**

**63077 80 51**

*Surgeon Performing the Spine Procedure*

**22556 62**

**22585 62**

**63077 51**

**22845**

**20938**

## Modifier 63, Procedure Performed on Infants Less Than 4 kg

Procedures performed on neonates and infants up to a present body weight of 4 kg may involve significantly increased complexity and physician work commonly associated with these patients. This circumstance may be reported by adding modifier 63 to the procedure number. Note: Unless otherwise designated, this modifier may only be appended to procedures/services listed in the **20000-69979** code series. Modifier 63 should not be appended to CPT codes listed in the Evaluation and Management Services, Anesthesia, Radiology, Pathology/Laboratory, or Medicine sections.

Modifier 63 is intended to be appended only to invasive surgical procedures and reported only for those invasive procedures performed on neonates/infants up to the 4-kg cutoff. Modifier 63 is intended to represent the significant increase in work intensity required in this population of patients. The factors related to this increase in work intensity include difficulties in maintenance of temperature control, obtaining intravenous access (which may require upwards of 45 minutes), and in the performance of the procedure itself, which is technically more difficult, especially with regard to maintenance of homeostasis.

There are many procedures with which it would be inappropriate to report modifier 63. These procedures are those performed solely on the very young patient, for which the difficulty of the procedure has already been considered in the establishment of the code. Procedures that include the work inherent in modifier 63 and that would not be reported in addition to this modifier are denoted with a parenthetical statement. The following is an example:

**44055**   Correction of malrotation by lysis of duodenal bands and/or reduction of midgut volvulus (eg, Ladd procedure)

(Do not report modifier 63 in conjunction with **44055**)

CPT procedure codes to which modifier 63 would be appropriately appended include code **44120**, Enterectomy, resection of small intestine; single resection and anastomosis; code **44140**, Colectomy, partial; with anastomosis; and code **33820**, Repair of patent ductus arteriosus; by ligation.

### Illustration of Modifier 63

A physician performs a patent ductus arteriosus repair on a three-week-old, 800 g, 28-week premature neonate patient. Special services required in performing this procedure include maintenance of the operating suite temperature at an appropriately hot level, establishment of adequate venous access, careful positioning of the patient on the Bovie grounding plate, and placement of appropriate barriers for prevention of heat loss. The patent ductus arteriosus repair is subsequently completed. The patient is placed into the isolate and transferred to the neonatal intensive care unit (NICU), still on the ventilator. This surgery is often further complicated by the fact that the procedure is performed in the NICU, relocating the operating team and equipment to the

NICU to lessen the risk of the transfer to the operating suite in these delicate neonates.

**33820 63**    Surgeon Performing the Cardiac Procedure

## Modifier 66, Surgical Team

Under some circumstances, highly complex procedures (requiring the concomitant services of several physicians, often of different specialties, plus other highly skilled, specially trained personnel, various types of complex equipment) are carried out under the "surgical team" concept. Such circumstances may be identified by each participating physician with the addition of modifier 66 to the basic procedure number used for reporting services.

In certain CPT codes, one major procedure is listed without indicating the various components of that service (eg, code **33945**, Heart transplant, with or without recipient cardiectomy). This code lists one major service that combines the work of several physicians and other specially trained personnel.

### Illustration of Modifier 66
Generally, each physician on a heart transplant team performs the same portion of the surgery each time. Perhaps one surgeon opens the chest and inserts the chest tubes while another surgeon prepares the great vessels for anastomosis to the donor heart. Each surgeon reports the same code with the same modifier, in this case code **33945 66**. It is important that all of the physicians on the surgical team jointly provide a description of each physician's general role on the heart transplant team and send the report to each third-party payer, to indicate each physician's role in the performance of the surgery.

If one surgeon assists another surgeon with a procedure, modifiers 80, Assistant Surgeon; 81, Minimum Assistant Surgeon; or 82, Assistant Surgeon (when qualified resident surgeon not available) may be more appropriate to report than modifier 66.

## Modifiers 76, 77, 78, 79

### Modifier 76, Repeat Procedure or Service by Same Physician
It may be necessary to indicate that a procedure or service was repeated subsequent to the original procedure or service. This circumstance may be reported by adding modifier 76 to the repeated procedure/service.

### Modifier 77, Repeat Procedure by Another Physician
It may be necessary to indicate that a basic procedure or service performed by another physician had to be repeated. This situation may be reported by adding modifier 77 to the repeated procedure/service.

Modifier 78, Unplanned Return to the Operating/Procedure
Room by the Same Physician Following Initial Procedure
for a Related Procedure During the Postoperative Period
It may be necessary to indicate that another procedure was performed during
the postoperative period of the initial procedure (unplanned procedure following initial procedure). When this procedure is related to the first and requires
the use of an operating/procedure room, it may be reported by adding modifier
78 to the related procedure. (For repeat procedures, see modifier 76.)

Modifier 79, Unrelated Procedure or Service by the Same
Physician During the Postoperative Period
It may be necessary to indicate that the performance of a procedure or service
during the postoperative period was unrelated to the original procedure. This
circumstance may be reported by using modifier 79. (For repeat procedures on
the same day, see modifier 76.)

Illustration of Modifiers 76, 77, 78, 79
A physician performs a femoral-popliteal bypass graft in the morning. Later that
day, the graft clots and the entire procedure is repeated by the same physician.
The initial procedure is reported with code **35556**, Bypass graft, with vein;
femoral-popliteal. The repeat procedure is reported as code **35556 76**.
Appending modifier 76 alerts the third-party payer that code **35556** has not
accidentally been reported twice. Documentation supporting the reoperation
should be provided to the third-party payer when reporting these services.

Now consider the same example with two different surgeons involved. The
patient has a femoral-popliteal graft in the morning and it clots later that day.
However, Physician A performs the surgery in the morning but is not available
to perform the repeat operation later that day. A second surgeon, Physician B,
performs the same procedure later that night. Physician A reports code **35556**,
and Physician B reports code **35556 77**.

Physician B is not affected by Physician A's global service. Physician B's performance of a surgical service (**35556**) will begin a global package related to the
repeat surgical procedure. Again, documentation should be provided to the third-
party payer to clarify that a repeat procedure was performed by another surgeon.

Let us expand on this coding example. The patient who had the repeat
femoral-popliteal graft (**35556**) goes home and the incision and graft heal well.
However, the patient develops acute renal failure a week after returning home
and is hospitalized within the postoperative period of the bypass procedure. The
patient does not respond to medical treatment of the renal failure. Hemodialysis
is indicated, and Physician B inserts a cannula for hemodialysis: code **36810**,
Insertion of cannula for hemodialysis, other purpose (separate procedure); arteriovenous, external (Scribner type).

Physician B's services for the insertion of the cannula for hemodialysis are
reported as code **36810 79**, because this service (**36810**) is unrelated to the
femoral-popliteal bypass graft (**35556**) performed during the previous hospitalization. If modifier 79 is not appended to this procedure, the third-party
payer may not know that this service is unrelated to the femoral-popliteal graft

(ie, the computer program used by the third-party payer may not be able to distinguish that this service is not related to the previous surgery and may automatically reject this claim). One must provide documentation to the third-party payer to indicate that this service is unrelated to the first procedure.

In another case, if a patient's operative site bleeds after an initial surgery and requires a return to the operating room to stop the bleeding, the same procedure is not repeated. Thus, a different code, **35860**, Exploration for postoperative hemorrhage, thrombosis or infection; extremity, would be reported with modifier 78 appended. Since the same procedure is not repeated, modifier 76 would not be appropriate to use.

Modifier 78 is appended to procedures that are performed during the postoperative period that require a patient to return to the operating/procedure room and are directly associated with the performance of the initial operation.

## Modifiers 80, 81, 82

> **CODING TIP**
>
> The assistant surgeon reports the same CPT code as the operating surgeon, with modifier 80 appended.

Although the intent of the assistant surgeon modifiers is to report physician services, many users report these modifiers for a variety of nonphysician surgical assistant services. The most common misinterpretation of the assistant surgeon modifiers is to report physician assistant (PA) or nurse practitioner (NP) assistant surgical services. Although from a CPT Nomenclature perspective, the assistant surgeon modifiers are not intended to be reported for PA or NP assistant surgical services, some third-party payers consider this an acceptable means of reporting these services during surgery. Many have established their own guidelines for reporting assistant surgeon services.

Modifier 80, Assistant Surgeon
Surgical assistant services may be identified by adding modifier 80 to the usual procedure number(s).

*Illustration of Modifier 80*

**PROCEDURE:** Closure of Intestinal Cutaneous Fistula

**EXAMPLE:** Primary Operating Surgeon Performs Approach and Closure and Assistant Surgeon assists during entire surgical case

*Surgeon Performing Approach and Closure*

**44640**

*Assistant Surgeon*

**44640 80**

One physician may assist another physician in performing a procedure. If an assistant surgeon assists a primary surgeon and is present for the entire operation or a substantial portion of the operation, the assisting physician reports the same surgical procedure code as the operating surgeon. The operating surgeon does not append a modifier to the procedure code that he or she reports. The assistant surgeon reports the same CPT code as the operating physician, with modifier 80 appended. The individual operative report submitted by each surgeon should indicate the distinct service(s) provided by each surgeon.

### Modifier 81, Minimum Assistant Surgeon

Minimum surgical assistant services are identified by adding modifier 81 to the usual procedure number.

*Illustration of Modifier 81*

While a primary operating physician may plan to perform a surgical procedure alone, during an operation circumstances may arise that require the services of an assistant surgeon for a relatively short time. In this instance, the second surgeon provides minimal assistance for which he or she reports the surgical procedure code with modifier 81 appended.

### Modifier 82, Assistant Surgeon (When Qualified Resident Surgeon Not Available)

The unavailability of a qualified resident surgeon is a prerequisite for use of modifier 82 appended to the usual procedure code number(s).

*Illustration of Modifier 82*

In certain programs (eg, teaching hospitals), the physician acting as the assistant surgeon is usually a qualified resident surgeon. However, there may be times (eg, during rotational changes) when a qualified resident surgeon is not available and instead another surgeon assists in the operation. In these instances, report the services of the nonresident assistant surgeon with modifier 82 appended to the appropriate code. This indicates that another surgeon is assisting the operating surgeon instead of a qualified resident surgeon.

## Modifier 90, Reference (Outside) Laboratory

When laboratory procedures are performed by a party other than the treating or reporting physician, the procedure may be identified by adding modifier 90 to the usual procedure number.

This modifier is used by a physician or clinic when the laboratory tests performed for a patient are performed by an outside or reference laboratory. This modifier is used to indicate that although the physician is reporting the performance of a laboratory test, the actual testing component was a service from a laboratory.

### Illustration of Modifier 90

Dr Jones, an internist, performs an examination of a patient and as part of the examination orders a complete blood count. Dr Jones does not perform in-office laboratory testing. He has an arrangement with a laboratory to bill him for the testing procedure, and in turn he bills the patient. Dr Jones' staff performs the venipuncture. Dr Jones may report an appropriate E/M code as well as code **36415**, Collection of venous blood by venipuncture, and also reports that the laboratory analysis of the specimen was performed by an outside laboratory, for example, code **85025 90**, Blood count; complete (CBC), automated (Hgb, Hct, RBC, WBC and platelet count) and automated differential WBC count.

## Modifier 91, Repeat Clinical Diagnostic Laboratory Test

In the course of treatment of the patient, it may be necessary to repeat the same laboratory test on the same day to obtain subsequent (multiple) test results. Under these circumstances, the laboratory test performed can be identified by its usual procedure number and the addition of modifier 91. Note: This modifier may not be used when tests are rerun to confirm initial results, because of testing problems with specimens or equipment, or for any other reason when a normal, one-time, reportable result is all that is required. This modifier may not be used when other codes describe a series of test results (eg, glucose tolerance tests, evocative/suppression testing). This modifier may be used only for laboratory test(s) performed more than once on the same day on the same patient.

### Illustration of Modifier 91
This modifier is used to report that the same laboratory test was performed more than once on the same day for the same patient to obtain subsequent (multiple) test results. If it is necessary in the course of treatment of the patient to repeat the same laboratory test on that patient on the same day to obtain subsequent test results, modifier 91 is appended to the laboratory code reported to indicate this circumstance.

## Modifier 92, Alternate Laboratory Platform Testing

When laboratory testing is being performed using a kit or transportable instrument that wholly or in part consists of a single-use, disposable analytical chamber, the service may be identified by adding modifier 92 to the usual laboratory procedure code (for example, HIV testing, reported with the code series **86701-86703**). The test does not require permanent dedicated space, hence by its design may be hand carried or transported to the vicinity of the patient for immediate testing at that site, although location of the testing is not in itself a determining factor in the use of this modifier.

### Illustration of Modifier 92
This modifier is used to report laboratory testing performed using a kit or transportable instrument that wholly or in part consists of a single-use, disposable analytical chamber.

## Modifier 99, Multiple Modifiers

Under certain circumstances two or more modifiers may be necessary to completely delineate a service. In such situations, modifier 99 should be added to the basic procedure, and other applicable modifiers may be listed as part of the description of the service.

This modifier is used to alert third-party payers that several modifiers are being used to report a service.

### Illustration of Modifier 99

This modifier would be used to report a situation in which a surgical procedure is performed using an assistant surgeon (modifier 80), and at the physician's discretion, a portion of the procedure is reduced or eliminated (modifier 52). The service provided by the assistant surgeon would be reported as follows:

**43510 99** or

**43510 99 80 52**

# CHAPTER 10

# EXERCISES

**1** Match the modifier number in column one with the description found in column two.

| Modifier Number | | Description | |
|---|---|---|---|
| **22** | Increased Procedural Services | **a** | A patient is seen in consultation for a second opinion for a surgical procedure, as required by the third-party payer. |
| **23** | Unusual Anesthesia | **b** | A procedure/service is performed on facility-owned equipment and the physician is reporting for only his or her portion of the procedure/service. |
| **24** | Unrelated E/M Service by the Same Physician During a Postoperative Period | **c** | A patient with severe tremors undergoes an upper gastrointestinal endoscopy under general anesthesia. |
| **26** | Professional Component | **d** | A cholecystectomy is made more difficult because of a patient's severe obesity. |
| **32** | Mandated Services | **e** | The services of an assistant surgeon are required for a relatively short time. |
| **47** | Anesthesia by Surgeon | **f** | A physician provides an office visit during which a decision is made to perform surgery two weeks later. |
| **52** | Reduced Services | **g** | An orthopedic surgeon performs a total knee replacement. During the postoperative period of the knee replacement, the patient returns for a sprain of the opposite knee. The E/M service for the sprained knee is reported with this modifier appended. |
| **57** | Decision for Surgery | **h** | This modifier may be used to represent procedures not ordinarily encountered or performed on the same day by the same physician. |

| Modifier Number | | Description |
| --- | --- | --- |
| **58** Staged or Related Procedure | **i** | A surgeon places a self-retaining, indwelling ureteral stent following a cystourethroscopic procedure. During the postoperative period, the patient returns to the operating room for removal of the stent by the same operating surgeon. |
| **59** Distinct Procedural Service | **j** | A surgeon provides the regional or general anesthesia for a surgical procedure that he or she performs. This modifier is appended to the surgical procedure code reported. |
| **81** Minimum Assistant Surgeon | **k** | At the physician's discretion, a portion of a procedure is eliminated. |

**2** True or False: Modifier 21, Prolonged Evaluation and Management Services, may be appended only to the highest level of E/M service in a given category.

**3** True or False: Modifier 57, Decision for Surgery, is used only with the consultation categories of E/M codes.

**4** When the same laboratory test is repeated to obtain subsequent (multiple) test results, which modifier is appended to the laboratory code reported?

**5** Indicate the appropriate code(s) for reporting a bilateral frontal sinusotomy performed with a trephine.

**6** Multiple, related operative procedures performed at the same session by the same provider are identified using which CPT modifier?

**7** True or False: Modifier 53, Discontinued Procedure, is reported by the physician to report the elective cancellation of a procedure prior to the patient's anesthesia induction and/or surgical preparation in the operating suite.

**8** The unavailability of a qualified resident surgeon is a prerequisite for the use of which CPT modifier?

**9** True or False: The CPT Nomenclature does not contain a coding convention to designate the technical component of a procedure or service.

**10** Which modifier is used to indicate that an E/M service was performed during a postoperative period for reason(s) unrelated to the original procedure?

**11** True or False: Modifier 47 should be used with the anesthesia codes (**01000-01996**).

**12** Which modifier indicates alternate laboratory platform testing?

**13** True or False: Modifier 51 may be appended to multiple endoscopic/laparoscopic/arthroscopic procedures in the same related series.

**14** A surgeon performs only open incisional anterior access and closure to the cervical/thoracic vertebrae for another surgeon to perform spine procedures; which modifier is used?

# CHAPTER 11

# Correct Coding Initiative Edits

On January 1, 1996, the Medicare program implemented its National Correct Coding Initiative comprising nearly 83,000 code edits in an attempt to eliminate unbundling or other inappropriate reporting of Current Procedural Terminology (CPT®) codes. The purpose of this initiative is to reduce program expenditures by detecting inappropriate coding on Medicare claims and denying payment for them. This chapter is a review of what the National Correct Coding Initiative (NCCI) is and the American Medical Association's response to the NCCI.

# What Is the National Correct Coding Initiative (NCCI)?

The Centers for Medicare and Medicaid Services (CMS), formerly named the Health Care Financing Administration, contracts with Correct Coding Solutions, LLC (CCS LLC) to develop and refine a system of Healthcare Common Procedure Coding System (HCPCS/CPT) code (procedure-to-procedure) edits and correct coding policies that are used nationally by all Medicare Part B carriers. These coding edits and policies are known as the NCCI. The NCCI edits are released on a quarterly basis into the Medicare Part B claims processing system. The NCCI correct coding policies are updated on an annual basis effective October 1 of each year.

According to CMS, the HCPCS/CPT code edits are developed based on an annual and/or ongoing review of changes in HCPCS/CPT code descriptors, HCPCS/CPT coding instructions and guidelines, local Medicare carrier and national Medicare edits and policy initiatives, and Medicare billing history. The correct coding edits that result from this process are incorporated into claims processing systems used by Medicare carriers to determine payments to physicians. As of April 1, 2007, there will be approximately 289,002 active coding edits in the NCCI. CMS has identified approximately 13,197 of these edits as "correct coding edits for mutually exclusive codes," ie, those codes that represent services that cannot reasonably be performed in the same session. The remaining 275,805 edits are classified as "correct coding edits for column one/column two codes" that represent various coding and payment policies where the column one code will be paid and the column two code disallowed for two procedures performed on the same patient, on the same date of service, by the same provider. Following are examples of each type of edit.

## A Correct Coding Edit for Column One/Column Two Codes

### Column One Code

**36216**   Selective catheter placement, arterial system; initial second order thoracic or brachiocephalic branch, within a vascular family

### Column Two Code

**36215**   Selective catheter placement, arterial system; each first order thoracic or brachiocephalic branch, within a vascular family

In this example, the Column One code will be paid and the Column Two code will be denied, unless an appropriate modifier is appended to one of the codes on the claim.

## A Correct Coding Edit for Mutually Exclusive Codes

### Column One Code

**63045**   Laminectomy, facetectomy and foraminotomy (unilateral or bilateral with decompression of spinal cord, cauda equina, and/or nerve root(s), (eg, spinal or lateral recess stenosis)), single vertebral segment; cervical

## Column Two Code

**63040**    Laminotomy (hemilaminectomy), with decompression of nerve root(s), including partial facetectomy, foraminotomy, and/or excision of herniated intervertebral disk, reexploration, single interspace; cervical

In this example, the Column One code will be paid and the Column Two code will be denied, unless an appropriate modifier is appended to one of the codes on the claim.

## Modifier 59

In each of the previous examples, and in most of the NCCI edits, a CPT modifier may be appropriate and necessary to indicate that distinct or independent services were performed and that the inclusion of both codes on the same claim form reflects appropriate coding. The modifier that is most used to attest to distinct services performed on the same date is modifier 59, defined as follows: Modifier 59, Distinct Procedural Service. Under certain circumstances, the physician may need to indicate that a procedure or service was distinct or independent from other services performed on the same day. Modifier 59 is used to identify procedures/services that are not normally reported together but are appropriate under the circumstances. This may represent a different session or patient encounter, different procedure or surgery, different site or organ system, separate incision/excision, separate lesion, or separate injury (or area of injury in extensive injuries) not ordinarily encountered or performed on the same day by the same physician. However, when another already established modifier is appropriate, it should be used rather than modifier 59. Only if no more descriptive modifier is available, and the use of modifier 59 best explains the circumstances, should modifier 59 be used.

Modifier 59 allows physicians to indicate that two codes, which would otherwise be subject to a code edit (meaning that one of the two codes in the pair would not be payable), were actually provided as distinct procedures to the same patient on the same day. (Refer to Chapter 10 for further discussion of modifier 59.)

# The AMA's Correct Coding Policy Committee (CCPC)

In response to the CMS proposal to implement the NCCI, the AMA insisted that practicing physicians be allowed to review the proposed coding edits prior to implementation each year. CMS agreed to the AMA's proposal to establish a process that would allow formal input from the AMA and organized medicine to the NCCI. The AMA believes such a process is essential to preserve the AMA's leadership in maintaining the CPT coding system and determining what constitutes correct or incorrect coding.

In 1995, the CCPC was formed and included 14 physicians from various specialties, as well as one non-MD/DO health professional who represented the interests of those non-MD/DOs who use the CPT code set to report their services. The CCPC has coordinated a process to allow for comment on edits proposed by CMS prior to implementation by all Medicare carriers. These proposed edits are primarily based on the annual changes to the CPT codebook. Those involved in this comment process include the following:

- Physician advisors from the CPT Advisory Committee
- Specialty society coding and reimbursement staff
- The members of the Healthcare Professional Advisory Committee, to allow greater input from non-MD/DO health care professionals

These various specialty societies may also share the proposed edits with coding committees and others within their specialty to receive input prior to submitting comments. As a result, many individuals have the opportunity to submit comments to CMS on several proposed additions to the NCCI. Input provided to CMS from carrier medical directors or individual physician offices also leads to changes in the quarterly updates of the NCCI.

## Phase I

The first phase of the NCCI included the 83,000 code edits first implemented on January 1, 1996. More than 50 individual specialty societies commented on these initial edits, stating that 951 of these edits were inappropriate. CMS later asked the CCPC to review these edits. In April of 1996, the CCPC met to review these problematic edits and agreed that 469 of the edits should be removed completely from the NCCI. CMS subsequently accepted the committee's recommendations on all but 325 of the 951 edits. The CCPC has asked CMS to justify retaining the 325 edits.

## Phase II and Phase III

In 1996 and 1997, the national medical specialty societies and the CCPC reviewed more than 30,000 proposed coding edits. These edits were primarily related to coding changes for CPT 1996 and CPT 1997. The majority of these proposed edits were implemented by CMS, with little opposition by the AMA, specialty societies, or the CCPC, as they represented correct use of the codes in question.

## Phase IV

AdminaStar proposed more than 300,000 additional edits to CMS in July 1998. CMS subsequently compared these proposed code pairs against their January through June 1998 Medicare claims data on the same date of service, for the same beneficiary, and by the same provider. As a result, only 12,754 proposed code pairs were found to ever be reported together. These edits were reviewed by the national medical specialty societies and the CCPC from August 1998 to March 1999. Of the 12,754 proposed edits, specialty societies agreed that only 1744 were appropriate. The majority of those that were problematic were related to E/M services performed on the same date as minor services or diagnostic tests. As a result of the objections from the AMA, specialty societies, and the CCPC, CMS did not implement the edits related to E/M services at that time. There are 515 edits that were implemented despite objections. These edits were implemented on April 1, 1999, (329 edits) and July 1, 1999 (186 edits). The April 1, 1999, (Version 5.1) update included edits resulting from a review of deleted codes for CPT 1999.

## Phase V

CMS and CCS LLC continue to review all CPT coding changes for the CPT nomenclature and propose new coding edits for each CPT cycle. CMS reviews the reporting of the code pairs against their claims data and forwards these edits, which are based on the annual changes to the CPT codebook, to the AMA for specialty society comment.

Although the AMA would not concede that the NCCI system is perfect, it appears that of all the edits implemented by CMS, no more than 1% to 2% are considered inappropriate by those who have been involved in their review. The NCCI editing system has allowed physicians and other health care professionals to participate in the process prior to implementation. The NCCI edits for physicians are available on the CMS Web site at www.cms.hhs.gov.

## Medically Unlikely Edits (MUEs)

On January 1, 2007, CMS implemented a new program of edits called the Medically Unlikely Edits (MUEs). The MUEs, previously known as the Medically Unbelievable Edits, are units of service edits that reflect the maximum number of units of service that a provider might report for the same HCPCS/CPT codes for the same beneficiary on the same date of service. According to CMS, the purpose of the MUE project is to detect and deny unlikely claims on a prepayment basis to prevent inappropriate payments.

CMS will be implementing the MUEs in multiple quarterly phases. Phase I, which was implemented on January 1, 2007, consists of edits based on anatomical considerations that are determined by limitations based on anatomical structures. For example, the MUE for cataract surgical procedures would be two, since there are two eyes. Phase II will be implemented April 1, 2007, and will include edits based on anatomical considerations, CPT code descriptors/CPT coding instructions, CMS policies, nature of procedure/ service, nature of analyte, or nature or equipment. Future phases will be based on criteria other than claims data analysis. As with NCCI edits, proposed MUEs are sent to the AMA for distribution to the national medical specialty societies for review and comment.

# Chapter Exercise Answers

# Chapter 1

**1**  The American Medical Association (AMA)

**2**  Level I, CPT; Level II, HCPCS national codes

**3**  CMS (formerly HCFA)

**4**  Category I codes are implemented January 1 of each year. Category II and III codes are early released biannually for implementation either January 1 or July 1 of a CPT cycle.

**5**  Category I codes

**6**  False

**7**  False. The first character of HCPCS Level II codes is alpha.

**8**  From the HCPCS/Medicare Web site, http://www.cms.hhs.gov/medicare/hcpcs

**9**  A listing of descriptive terms and identifying codes for reporting medical services and procedures

**10**  False. Category II codes may not be used as a substitute for Category I codes.

**11**  False. The alphabetical listing allows the user the ability to locate a particular measurement code according to a disease or condition for which it may apply.

**12**  Composite Measures codes

**13**  Semiannual

# Chapter 2

**1**  Eight. The six sections pertain to the following Category I codes:

Section 1    Evaluation and Management
Section 2    Anesthesia
Section 3    Surgery
Section 4    Radiology
Section 5    Pathology and Laboratory
Section 6    Medicine

The seventh section includes the Category II codes. Category III codes comprise the eighth section.

**2**  The E/M section, for ease of reference because these codes are used most by physicians in reporting their services.

**3**  **71060**  Radiology
**49060**  Surgery
**99241**  Evaluation and Management

**01440** Anesthesia

**99058** Medicine

**84443** Pathology and Laboratory

**64831** Surgery

4 **31625** Bronchoscopy, rigid or flexible, with or without fluoroscopic guidance; with bronchial or endobronchial biopsy(s), single or multiple sites.

**73202** Computed tomography, upper extremity; without contrast material, followed by contrast material(s) and further sections

**42415** Excision of parotid tumor or parotid gland; lateral lobe, with dissection and preservation of facial nerve

**28805** Amputation, foot; transmetatarsal

**64704** Neuroplasty; nerve of hand or foot

5 **97028** **97010**

**87530** **87470**

**59515** **59514**

**40844** **40840**

**99292** **99291**

6 True

7 True

8 1 D

2 A

3 E

4 B

5 C

6 J

7 L

8 G

9 H

10 K

11 F

12 I

13 M

9 False. Any procedure or service in any section of the CPT codebook may be used to designate the services rendered by any qualified physician or other qualified health care professional.

10 The bullet symbol

11 1. Procedure or service, eg, Allergen Immunotherapy

2. Organ or other anatomic site, eg, abdomen, bladder

3. Condition, eg, abscess, blepharoptosis

4. Synonyms, eponyms, and abbreviations, eg, Anderson tibial lengthening, CBC

# Chapter 3

**1** History, Examination, Medical Decision Making

**2** A new patient is one who has not received any professional services from the physician, or another physician of the same specialty who belongs to the same group practice, within the past 3 years.

**3** **99347**

**4** **99396** for the preventive service, **99213 25** for the problem-oriented E/M service

**5** Office or Other Outpatient Services—New Patient, level of service **99203**

**6** **99214**

More than 50% of the encounter was spent providing counseling and/or coordination of care. Therefore, the level of service may be selected using time as the key or controlling factor for this encounter. The level is selected based upon the total time of the face-to-face physician/patient encounter.

**7** All three key components must meet or exceed the stated requirements to qualify for a particular level of service.

**8** True

**9** False. The emergency department services codes are not limited to use by the emergency department physicians.

**10** Location: Right forearm. Duration: A week.

**11** **99289, 99290**

**12** Yes; however, the initial date neonatal critical care code (**99295**) may be reported only after the patient has been admitted to the neonatal intensive care unit.

**13** The consulting physician may perform the evaluation of the patient, initiate diagnostic services, and initiate therapy at the same encounter. This activity assumes that the consultation has been requested and that the consulting physician provides and documents it and communicates his or her consulting opinion and any services provided in a written report to the requesting physician. The service may be coded as a consultation.

**14** Any period less than 60 continuous outpatient days is not reported. If less than the specified minimum number of services per period are performed, it would not be appropriate to report the anticoagulant management service codes **99363-99364**.

**15** True. When immunizations are performed at the same visit as preventive medicine services, the immunizations and the associated administration code are always coded separately.

**16** Consultations provided in the emergency department are reported with the Office or Other Outpatient Consultations codes **99241-99245**.

**17** **99238**, Hospital discharge day management, would be reported for this service.

# Chapter 4

**1** True

**2** **99024**

**3** In defining the specific services included in a given CPT surgical code, the following services are always included in addition to the operation per se:
- Local infiltration, metacarpal/metatarsal/digital block or topical anesthesia
- Subsequent to the decision for surgery, one related E/M encounter on the date immediately prior to or on the date of procedure (including history and physical)
- Immediate postoperative care, including dictating operative notes, talking with family and other physicians
- Writing orders
- Evaluating the patient in the postanesthesia recovery area
- Typical postoperative follow-up care

**4** The ✚ symbol

**5** **99070**, Supplies and materials (except spectacles), or the specific supply code provided by the physician over and above those usually included with the office visit or other services rendered (list drugs, trays, supplies, or materials provided)

**6** True. These codes are exempt from the multiple procedure concept.

**7** True. Add-on codes describe procedures or services that are always performed in addition to the primary procedure or service.

**8** **64831**, **64832**

**9** **43202**, Esophagoscopy, rigid or flexible; with biopsy, single or multiple

**10** True.

**11** False. When procedures for reporting, reimbursement, or other purposes are evaluated, it is essential that each procedure be considered on its own merits, not simply based on the location or placement of the code in the CPT codebook.

**12** False. Codes designated as separate procedures may not be additionally reported when the procedure or service is performed as an integral component of another procedure or service.

13 False. CPT coding guidelines do not include listings of codes or procedures for which it is appropriate to separately report supply items (eg, surgical trays). Reimbursement of supplies and materials provided by the physician may vary from carrier to carrier.

# Chapter 5

1  **a 10021 b 10022, 77012**

2  False

3  False

4  Only one code is selected based on the classification of the repair performed, the size of the repair, and the location of the repair. The method of the repair plays a factor only if adhesive strips are used.

5  False. When lesion excisions are coded, each lesion excised through a separate excision is reported separately. The codes reported for this example should be **11420** for the 0.5-cm lesion on the hand and **11420 59** for the 0.5-cm lesion on the foot. Only the repair codes are based on the sum of lengths of repairs. As stated in the repair guidelines, "When multiple wounds are repaired, the lengths of those wounds in the same classification (eg, simple, intermediate and complex) and from all anatomic sites that are grouped together into the same code descriptor should be added together and reported as a single item."

6  **16035, 16035 59**

7  Code **17000** for the first lesion and code **17003** with a "13" in the units column for the remaining 13 lesions.

8  Code **15100** for the first 100 sq cm, code **15101** for the additional 100 sq cm, code **15101** for the additional 30 sq cm, as code **15101** includes grafts up to and including 100 sq cm.

9  **19102, 76095**

10  **19103, 77031**

11  **22558, 22585, 20937, 22845**

12  **22521, 22522**

13  **63042**

14  **31628 × 1**

15  **31624**

16  **32442**

17  **32486**

18  **31526**

19  **31505**

20  **33141**

21  **33208, 33235, 33233**

22  **35600**

23  **33533, 33517, 33530**

24  **34812-50**

25  a **36831, 36833**  b **36870**  c **36860** or **36861**

26  **37204** and **75894**

27  **33226**

28  **36578** × **2**

29  **44127**

30  **43239** × **1**

31  **43750, 74350**

32  **45315**

33  **45384, 45385**

34  **49561, 49568**

35  **52290**

36  **53853**

37  **52647**

38  **57023**

39  **58346**

40  **58353**

41  **56630**

42  **58150**

43  **57160, 99070** or **A4561** or **A4562**

44  **59414** for the delivery of the placenta and code **59430** for the provision of postpartum care

45  **61618**

46  **64483 50, 64484 50, 77003 26**

47  **64475, 64476, 77003 26**

48  **66984**

**49** **65235**

**50** **67311 50**

**51** **69436 50**

**52** **69718**

**53** It would not be appropriate to report two excision of lesion codes if an additional excision is performed for complete tumor removal. Instead, only one code should be reported based on the final widest excised diameter.

**54** True

**55** Both the spine surgeon (ie, primary surgeon) and the approach surgeon would append modifier 62 to the primary procedure and any associated add-on codes. The additional surgeon is not acting as an assistant at surgery in these circumstances but is performing a distinct portion of the procedure. As stated in the modifier 62 language, when two surgeons work together as primary surgeons performing distinct part(s) of a procedure, each surgeon should report his or her distinct operative work by adding modifier 62 to the procedure code. If a co-surgeon acts as an assistant in the performance of additional procedure(s) during the same surgical session, those services may also be reported using separate procedure code(s) with modifier 80 or modifier 82 added, as appropriate.

**56** True

**57** False. Synovial biopsy, when performed at the first MTP joint in conjunction with a bunion correction procedure, is considered an integral component of the bunion procedure and not reported separately.

**58** **29075**, for the cast application, and the appropriate level of emergency department services E/M code (**99281-99285**) based on key components that have been met, with modifier 25 appended.

**59** **24516**

**60** Code **20550** should be reported only once when multiple injections are administered to the same tendon.

**61** True

**62** True

**63** True

**64** False. Separately report **35500**.

**65** False

**66** False

**67** True

**68** True

**69** False

**70** True

**71** a **49507 50**    b **49521**    c **49520**    d **55040**

**72** a **50590 50**    b **51701**

**73** a **52320**    b **52332**

**74** a **59610**    b **58605**

**75** True

**76** True

**77** **61609, 61610, 61611, 61612**

**78** False. Code **20660** is designated as a "separate procedure." Therefore, when the application of a stereotactic frame is performed as a component of a larger procedure (eg, stereotactic biopsy of an intracranial lesion), it would not be reported separately.

**79** **70450, 70460, 70470,** MRI codes **70551, 70552, 70553**

**80** True, use **95974** and **95975**

**81** a **62350**    b **62351**

**82** True

**83** **96522**

**84** **63030**

**85** False

**86** Chemodenervation

**87** True

**88** Unilateral

**89** a **67221**    b **67221, 67225**

**90** True

**91** **58544**

**92** True.

**93** Yes. Although **61623** departs from traditional interventional radiology component coding convention, codes **61624** and **61626** follow the component coding usage. Therefore, code **75894** should be reported in addition to codes **61624**. Code **75898** should also be reported for postembolization arteriography.

**94** False. Codes **62200** and **62201** may be used to describe third ventricle ventriculocisternostomy performed by stereotactic method only, combined stereotactic and endoscopic methods, or endoscopic method only (with an endoscope but without the use of stereotactic method).

95  False. Codes **62263** and **62264** include the procedure of injections of contrast for epidurography (**72275**) and fluoroscopic guidance and localization (**77003**) during initial or subsequent sessions.

96  Epidurography at the cervical and lumbar region would be reported by means of codes **62310** and **72275** (cervical) plus **62311** and **72275 59** (lumbar). If injections are performed at different spinal levels, the spinal injection codes should be reported for each level of the involved spinal region.

97  **66984**

98  **65235**

99  **67311 50**

100  The terms *simple*, *intermediate*, and *complex* are not used in the Eye section, whereas they are used in the Integumentary System section. Therefore, the repair of an ocular laceration is described by location of the laceration and not the type of repair performed. The sum of the lengths of the lacerations is also not a feature of this coding structure in the eye section, although these lengths may sometimes be found in the operative report.

101  False

102  True

# Chapter 6

1  P4

2  True

3  The anesthesia code representing the most complex procedure is reported. The time reported is the combined total for all procedures. Add-on codes are an exception. They are reported in addition to the code for the primary anesthesia service.

4  False. More than one qualifying circumstances code may be selected and reported, as appropriate.

5  The American Society of Anesthesiologists

6  **99143-99145**

7  Modifier 47, Anesthesia by Surgeon

8 Anesthesia time begins when the anesthesia provider starts preparing the patient for anesthesia in the operating room or an equivalent area. Anesthesia time ends when the patient is safely placed under postoperative supervision.

9 **01462-01522**

10 **01760**

11 **01953, 01968, 01969**

12 **01924-01933**

13 **01958-01969**

14 False. Invasive forms of monitoring (eg, intra-arterial, central venous, and pulmonary artery catheters and transesophageal echocardiography) are not included in basic anesthesia administration services.

15 False. The anesthesia codes for hernia repairs **00834-00836** include the skill and effort required to provide anesthesia services to young infants.

16 True.

17 True.

18 False. Moderate (conscious) sedation is not an anesthesia service.

# Chapter 7

1 **99070**

2 False. The contrast administration procedure, when performed intravascularly, is not separately reported when the phrase "with contrast" appears in the code descriptor.

3 True

4 Radiological supervision and interpretation

5 a. **72127** Computed tomography, cervical spine; without contrast material, followed by contrast material(s) and further sections
  b. **76942** Ultrasonic guidance for needle placement (eg, biopsy, aspiration, injection, localization device), imaging supervision and interpretation
    **47000** Biopsy of liver, needle; percutaneous
  c. **70546** Magnetic resonance angiography, head; without contrast material(s) followed by contrast material(s) and further sequences.
  d. **77057** Screening mammography, bilateral (2-view film study of each breast)

6 True

7 Clinical treatment planning

8 With the code for the second order catheterization only

9 False. Any procedure or service in any section of the CPT codebook may be used to designate the services rendered by any qualified physician.

10 Code **76816** should be reported once for each fetus requiring follow-up ultrasound, with modifier 59 appended for each additional fetus.

11 **76830**

12 Ultrasound

13 True

14 **77300**

15 **77435**

# Chapter 8

1 **81000**

2 **36415, 80162**

3 **80051**

4 **36600, 82800**

5 **80048, 80053, 80069**

6 **88329**

7 **88331** × **1** and **88332** × **3**

8 True

9 **88305** (three units of service)

10 **88302, 88307**

Rationale: The uterus and the right and left tubes and ovaries constitute a single specimen, even though they are separately identified and submitted in separate containers. The physician's work related to the uterus, tubes, and ovaries is coded as one unit of service of code **88307**. The vermiform appendix does constitute a separate specimen, and the physician effort related to this specimen is reported with code **88302**.

11 **88174, 88175**

12 False. Each panel includes a defined list of tests. The tests listed with each panel identify the defined components of that panel. To report a code for a panel, all of the tests listed in the panel definition must be performed, with no substitutions. If fewer tests are performed than those listed in the panel code, then the individual code number(s) for each test should be listed rather than the panel code.

**13** True

**14** True

**15** **88386.** If additional steps are required to prepare a sample for microarray analysis, then these codes may be reported in addition to the appropriate microarray code.

# Chapter 9

**1** **90471, 90707**

**2** **90471 × 1, 90747 × 2**

**3** **90760, 90761 × 4**

**4** **90857** (report once for each patient in the group)

**5** **90806**

**6** Not separately reportable. Included in an appropriate level E/M service code, when performed.

**7** **90806 22**

**8** Appropriate code from **90918-90921** series

**9** **90923**

**10** **92014, 92015**

**11** **92018**

**12** **92340**

**13** **92995, 92996**

**14** **92973, 92981**

**15** **92974, 93508**

**16** **92980, 92984**

**17** **93307, 93320, 93325**

**18** **93318**

**19** **93350**

**20** **93510, 93543, 93545, 93555, 93556**

**21** **93609, 93620**

**22** **93613**

**23** **93668**

**24** **95165 × 10** in the units box and code **95115**

25 **95147** × **5** in the units box to indicate the number of doses prepared

26 **95165** × **20** in the units box and code **95117** and the appropriate E/M code with modifier 25 appended

27 Appropriate code from **95965-95967** series

28 Appropriate code from **96150-96155** series

29 **97010, 97032**

30 **97597**

31 **97803** × 2 in the units box or **97803** × 2

32 **98926**

33 **98940, 97140**

34 **98940, 98943**

35 **97018, 97760**

36 **99001**

37 **99024**

38 **99058**

39 **99091**

40 False

41 False. Code **92602** identifies subsequent reprogramming performed for cochlear implantations.

42 False. These codes are intended to be used by nonphysician health care professionals. Physicians should use the home visit codes **99341-99350** and **99500-99600** for any additional procedures/services provided to patients living in a residence.

43 True

44 True

# Chapter 10

1 a. 32
  b. 26
  c. 23
  d. 22
  e. 81
  f. 57
  g. 24

      h. 59

      i. 58

      j. 47

      k. 52

**2** True

**3** False. Modifier 57 may be appended to any E/M service that results in the initial decision to perform surgery.

**4** Modifier 91, Repeat Clinical Diagnostic Laboratory Test

**5** **31070 50**; or **31070, 09950**

**6** Modifier 51, Multiple Procedures

**7** False

**8** Modifier 82, Assistant Surgeon (When Qualified Resident Surgeon Not Available)

**9** True

**10** Modifier 24

**11** False

**12** Modifier 59

**13** True

**14** Modifier 62

# APPENDIX B

# Resources

# Resource Materials for the Physician Office

Every physician's office needs comprehensive medical reference material to code diagnoses and procedures appropriately. Many of the questions answered at the American Medical Association (AMA) can be researched in common reference books that are easy to use and provide additional information on choosing correct code(s). While each physician office requires specific reference tools, the following is a suggested list of coding resources for the medical office.

All references listed here are distributed or published by the AMA. To order, please call the AMA at 800 621-8335. (Please note: The AMA does not endorse any specific non-AMA reference book. The books listed are examples of commonly used reference materials and guidebooks.)

1  *Current Procedural Terminology (CPT®)*—stay in compliance with code changes each year with AMA's official coding resource for procedural codes, rules, and guidelines.

2  *CPT® Changes: An Insider's View*—serves as the definitive text on additions, revisions, and deletions to the CPT code set. To assist CPT users in applying new and revised CPT codes, this book includes clinical examples that describe typical patients who might receive the procedure and detailed descriptions of the procedure.

3  *CPT Reference of Clinical Examples*—this is the only reference organized by CPT codebook section that provides more than 475 detailed case studies of reported codes pulled from the proprietary CPT information database and Medicare claims data.

4  *Healthcare Common Procedure Coding System (HCPCS)*—lists Medicare's national Level II codes used to bill Medicare and other third-party payers for various medical supplies, devices, and services.

5  *ICD-9-CM, Volumes 1 and 2*—lists diagnosis codes and descriptions. The ICD-9-CM diagnoses must be reported on the insurance claim form for Medicare and most other third-party payers.

6  *Medicare RBRVS: The Physicians' Guide*—an easy-to-use guide to understanding Medicare's resource-based relative value scale (RBRVS) payment system and calculate payment schedules.

7  *CPT® Assistant*—the official monthly newsletter for CPT coding issues, with guidance from the AMA.

8  *Clinical Examples in Radiology: A Practical Guide to Correct Coding*—a quarterly newsletter from the AMA and the American College of Radiology that is designed to provide up-to-date coding information.

9  *CPT Network*—an Internet-based inquiry system that allows one to search an online knowledge base of CPT code information filled with frequently asked questions and clinical examples (vignettes). This service is provided to AMA members as a benefit of membership and is also available as a subscription fee-based service for nonmembers and subscribers. Log on to www.cptnetwork.com to view the different packages available.

10  *Physician's Desk Reference (PDR)*—provides the latest and most accurate data on more than 4000 prescription drugs, including product overviews of the most commonly prescribed drugs.

11  *Medical dictionaries*—provide definitions of procedures and diagnoses. Stedman's Medical Dictionary and Dorland's Illustrated Medical Dictionary are two frequently used medical dictionaries. If a description is not found in the CPT codebook index, often there may be another word to describe the procedure that can be located in the dictionary.

12  *Netter's Atlas of Human Anatomy for CPT® Coding*—a reference for CPT codebook users who want to understand anatomic structures described within CPT code descriptions.

13  *Merck Manual*—provides detailed information on specific diagnoses including etiology, symptoms, treatment, and clinical features.

The following reference materials are generally available at a local medical bookstore:

1  *Laboratory Test Handbook*—a useful guide in assigning CPT codes for laboratory tests. This book explains the laboratory tests, gives definitions and CPT codes, and provides hints for terms you can look up in the CPT index to obtain the appropriate code.

2  *Medical acronyms and abbreviations*—useful in transcription and interpreting operative and other reports.

The following additional references may prove useful:

1  Hospital medical staff directories—these will enable one to look up referring and consulting physician information for submission of claims.

2  Third-party payer guidebooks—useful in filing claims with specific third-party payers. These guidebooks can also give additional information on the levels of HCPCS codes they accept. These manuals are usually provided to the office when a physician submits claims to a particular insurer.

# Electronic Health Records Implementation Resources (Available From the AMA)

1  *HIPAA Plain and Simple*—provides an overview of the legislation and regulations in detailed yet simplified terms. Includes sample forms and agreements, staff training, and other critical points regarding compliance.

2  *EHR Implementation: A Step-by-Step Guide for the Medical Practice*—this is an invaluable resource that guides physicians and administrators through the evaluation, selection, negotiation, and culture management transition to an electronic environment.

In addition to these reference tools, there are also many clinical specialty books available. Some are listed here; however, for those specialties not listed, office staff may confer with their physicians to determine other reference books that may be helpful.

1   *Ultrasound Coding User's Guide.* American College of Radiology, 703 648-8900.

2   *User's Guide for the Radiation Oncology Related CPT Codes.* American College of Radiology, 703 648-8900.

3   *Interventional Radiology Coding User's Guide.* Society of Cardiovascular and Interventional Radiology, 703 691-1805.

4   *The American College of Cardiology Guide to CPT-4.* American College of Cardiology, 202 375-6000.

5   *Global Service Data for Orthopaedic Surgery.* American Academy of Orthopaedic Surgeons, 800 346-2267.

6   *Pediatric Procedural Terminology.* American Academy of Pediatrics, Publications Department, 847 434-4000.

7   *CPT Coding in Obstetrics and Gynecology.* American College of Obstetricians and Gynecologists, 800 762-2264.

8   *Frequently Asked Questions in Obstetric and Gynecologic Coding.* American College of Obstetricians and Gynecologists, 800 762-2264.

9   *Coding in Rheumatology.* American College of Rheumatology, 404 633-3777.

10  *Using CPT for Cardiothoracic Reimbursement: A Manual for Surgeons and Insurance Billing Specialists.* Society of Thoracic Surgeons, 312 202-5800.

11  *Report of the Task Force on Global Surgical Services Intraoperative Services.* American Podiatric Medical Association, Inc, Health Affairs Department, 301 571-9200.

12  *Coding Tips for the Urologist's Office.* American Urological Association, 410 689-3700.

13  *Current Dental Terminology.* American Dental Association, 312 440-2500.

14  *NASS Common Coding Scenarios.* North American Spine Society, 708 588-8080.

15  *AANS Guide to Coding: Mastering the Global Service Package for Neurological Surgery Services.* American Association of Neurological Surgeons, 888 566-2267 or www.AANS.org.

16  *Practical Tips for the Practicing Oncologist.* American Society of Clinical Oncology, 703 299-0150.

# Other Resources

**1** *The National Correct Coding Manual* is available by contacting NTIS at 800 553-6847. The Correct Coding Initiative edits are also available on CD-ROM.

**2** Information about the AMA/Specialty Society RVS Update Committee (RUC) and Resource-Based Relative Value Scale (RBRVS) is available by contacting the Department of Physician Payment Policy and Systems at the AMA, 312 464-4736.

# Index

# A

Abdomen, peritoneum, and omentum, 234–235
    introduction, revision, and/or removal of cannula or
        catheter in, 234–235
Abdominal aortic aneurysm, endovascular repair of, 208
Abortions
    coding for treatment of, 258
    complete, 259, 260
    incomplete, 259, 260
    induced, 258, 260–261
    missed, 259, 260
    septic, 259
    spontaneous, 258, 259, 260
    threatened, 258
Acellular dermal replacements, 148, 149
Active wound care management, 134, 491–493
Acupuncture, 495–496
Acute airway obstruction, 465
Add-on codes, 115–117
    ✚ to identify, 30, 115
    criteria to identify, 115–116
    as not reported alone, 128
Additional lesion add-on code, 116
Additional procedures, addendum to operative report
        describing, 126
Additional time add-on code, 117
Adenoidectomy, 220
Adjacent tissue transfer or rearrangement, 145–146
Advisory Committee on Immunization Practices,
        408–409
Agency for Healthcare Research and quality (AHRQ), 12
Allergen immunotherapy, 469–470
    administration of allergenic extract for, 469, 470
    antigen extract for, 470
    coding review for, 470
    definition of dose for, 471
    entire service for allergenic extract for, 469
    examples for, 471–472
    multiple injections for, 470
    single-dose vials for, 469–470
    single injection, 469
Allergy and clinical immunology, 467–472
Allergy testing, 467–468
    airborne allergen, 468
    ingestion challenge, 468
    intracutaneous (intradermal), 467–468
    nasal mucous membrane, 468
    nitric oxide expired gas determination for, 467
    ophthalmic mucous membrane, 468
    percutaneous, 467
    photo patch, 468
Allograft, 147, 148, 149
Allotransplantation/transplantation, 218–219
Alphabetic index in CPT codebook, 35
Ambulatory Quality alliance (AQA), 12

American Academy of Family Physicians, 409
American Academy of Pediatrics (AAP), 409, 501
American Hospital Association, official coding
        guidelines for ICD-9-CM from, 126
American Medical Association (AMA)
    appealing decision of CPT Editorial Panel to staff of, 7
    Board of Trustees of, CPT Editorial Panel members
        appointed by, 4
    Board of Trustees of, Performance Measures Advisory
        Group appointed by, 13
    Correct Coding Policy Committee for proposed edits
        to NCCI of, 537–539
    CPT Editorial Panel of, 4, 6–7, 8, 12, 13, 20–21, 409
    CPT Web site of, 20, 409
    Executive committee of CPT Editorial Panel of, 4, 7
    Health Care Professionals Advisory Committee
        (HCPAC) of, 5–6
    immunization code structure by, 409
    product order information for, 559
    reference tools available from, descriptions of,
        559–562
    Web site of, 13, 19
American Society of Anesthesiologists (ASA), 501
Amniocentesis, 253
Anesthesia, 315–325
    administration services for, 318–319
    for electroconvulsive therapy, 423
    exercise answers for, 551–552
    exercises for, 324–325
    modifiers for, 320
    multiple surgical procedures during, reporting,
        320–322
    paracervical uterine nerve injection as, 285
    for patient of extreme age, 323
    qualifying circumstances for, 322–323
    regional or general, 319
    separately reportable services for, 321
    subsections and code ranges for, 317
    by surgeon, 514
    time reporting for, 320
    unusual, 511
Anesthesia administration services, basic, 318–319
Aneurysm, arteriovenous malformation, or vascular
        disease, surgery for, 270
Angiogram, diagnostic, 216
Angiographic imaging, supervision of, 451
Angiography
    carotid, cerebral, bilateral, radiological supervision
        and interpretation, 346
    diagnostic, 269, 347–348
    pulmonary, 450–451
    selective coronary, 450–451
    venous bypass graft, 449–450
Angioplasty or stenting, intracranial, 270
Annual nursing facility assessment, 86–87

Coronary artery bypass procedures, 203–204
  harvesting radial artery for, 203
  redo, 205–206
Corpus uteri code series, 249, 250
Correct Coding Initiative edits, 533–539
  for column one/column two codes, 535
  modifier for distinct procedures to avoid, 536
  for mutually exclusive codes, 535–536
Correct Coding Solutions, LLC (CCS LLC),
  HCPCS/CPT code edits developed and
  refined by, 535
Co-surgeon modifier for spine surgery, 163,
  174–175, 521
Counseling
  constituting more than 50% of physician-patient
    and/or family encounter, 45, 56
  as contributory factor for E/M services, 42, 44
  definition for E/M services of, 47
  genetic, 483
  for groups of patients with symptoms or established
    illness, 98
  immunization, 410
  for interpretation of psychiatric examinations and
    procedures, 424
  preventive medicine, 98
  types of discussions included in E/M services for, 47
CPT Advisory Committee
  coding change request forms referred to, 7
  members and objectives of, 5
  review of proposed coding changes by, 6, 13
*CPT Assistant*
  Genetic Testing code modifiers in, 382, 391
  green ⊃ to denote articles in, 31
  ordering information for, 559
CPT classification of procedures vs nomenclature, 28–29
CPT codebook
  ►◄ for new and revised text in, 30
  alphabetic index in, 35
  appendixes to, 17–19, 33–35
  basics of, 25–37
  code symbols used in, 30–31
  guidelines at beginning of each section of, 31
  index of, to locate type of procedure performed, 126,
    127, 128
  ordering information for, 559
  section numbers and sequences in, 27
CPT codes
  annual updates to, 21
  appeals process for rejected requests for new,
    flowchart of, 9
  categories of, 9–21
  deleted, crosswalk to, 35
  effective date of, 21
  for E/M services, payer policies on who may report, 104
  exempt from modifier 51, ⊘ symbol for, 30, 117–118
  new procedure, ● symbol for, 30

  process for adding new, diagram of, 8
  requests for new, 13
  schematic diagram of, 41
  separate procedure, 118–119
  with substantially altered descriptions, ▲ symbol
    for, 30
  for unlisted procedure or service, 32
CPT codeset
  as national standard under HIPAA, 4
  placement of code in, 28–29
CPT code symbols in codebook, 30–31
CPT coding terminology, 29–30
CPT-5 project workgroup, 9–10
CPT nomenclature, 1–23
  AMA organizations maintaining, 4–6
  attributes developed or evolving for, 10
  basics of, 25–37
  classification vs, 28–29
  core elements defining, 9–10
  definition of, 3
  development of, 3–4
  exercise answers for, 543, 543–544
  exercises for, 23, 36–37
  function of, 3
  instructions for using, 27–28
  as Level I of HCPCS coding system, 4, 21
  modifiers in structure of, 32
  review of suggested changes to, 6–9
  submitting changes to, 6
  surgical package definition in, 113–114
Cranial Neurostimulator subsection, 272
Craniectomy or craniotomy, 265–267, 273
Critical Care Services E/M category, 75–79
  additional time for, 117
  first day of services in, 78, 117
  for inpatient pediatric critical care, 78–79
  reported with other E/M services to same patient on
    same date by same physician, 75, 81–82
  reporting codes for, 77–78
  reporting conventional E/M services with, 81–82
  services included in reporting, 76
Critical care time reporting, 77–78
  additional, 76, 117
Cryosurgical ablation of prostate, 245
*Current Procedural Terminology*, history of, 3–4
Custodial Care Services, Established Patient, 65
Cystourethroscopy
  laterality of codes for, 241–242
  separate reporting for, 240–241
  stent insertion and removal during, 242–243
  steroid injection into stricture for, 242
Cytogenetic studies, 391
Cytologic evaluation codes, intraoperative, 379
Cytology codes distinguished from frozen section
  codes, 380
Cytopathology, 387–390

# D

# E

Fructose intolerance, 427
Functional brain mapping, 482
Fungal cultures, 385–386

# G

Gait and motion-analysis procedures, 482
Gastric restrictive procedures, 229–230
Gastric stimulation for gastroparesis and morbid
　　obesity, 230–231
Gastroenteral stent placement, 229
Gastroenterology, 425–428
Gastroesophageal reflux disease (GERD), 425–426
Gastrointestinal tract imaging, intraluminal, of the
　　esophagus, 427–428
Gastroparesis, gastric neurostimulator electrodes to
　　treat, 230
Genetic counseling services, 483
Genetic Testing Code modifier, 382, 391
Global services for routine obstetric care, 255–257
　　for twins, 258
Global surgical package, evaluations included in, 61
Glucose monitoring procedures, 472
Graft material
　　arterial, 203
　　arterial-venous, 203–204
　　fat, for excision of acoustic neuroma, 266
　　open procurement of, 204
　　venous, 203, 204
Gynecologic surgery, 246

# H

Hair growth pathology, 487
Hallux valgus, 176–180
　　Akin procedure phalanx osteotomy for, 179
　　double osteotomy for, 179
　　Joplin procedure for, 177
　　Keller type procedure for, 177
　　Lapidus-type procedure for, 178
　　Mitchell procedure for, 178
　　Silver-type simple resection procedure for, 176
Hammertoe operation, 176
Hand, diagram of bones, muscles, and tendons of, 158
Harvesting of upper extremity artery for coronary artery
　　bypass, 204
HCPCS (Healthcare Common Procedure Coding
　　System) (CMS), 21–22
　　CPT nomenclature as Level I of, 4, 21
　　national codes as Level II of, 22
　　ordering information for, 559
Health and behavior assessment/intervention, 483–484

Health Care Professionals Advisory Committee
　　(HCPAC), 4
Health Employer Data Information Set (HEDIS)
　　(NCQA), 12
Health Insurance Association of America, I codes
　　reserved for, 22
Health Insurance Portability and Accountability Act of
　　1996 (HIPAA)
　　elimination of local codes under, 20
　　standard code sets under, 5
Heart
　　conduction system of, diagram of, 452
　　diagram of electrical conduction of, 454
Heart rate response to deep breathing, 479
Hematology and coagulation, 383–385
　　interpretation of smear from bone marrow
　　　aspiration, bone marrow biopsy, or bone
　　　biopsy, 384–385
Hemodialysis, 425
　　access creation for, 214–215
Hepatitis B vaccine, 413
Hernia repair, 235–237
　　anesthesia for, 323
　　implantation of mesh or other prosthesis for,
　　　236–237
　　initial inguinal, performed on preterm infants, 235
　　medical, 235
　　open surgical, 235
　　reducible, incarcerated, or strangulated, 235, 236
　　vaginal, 248
High altitude simulation testing (HAST), 464
Histologic staining, 378
History for E/M services, 48, 49–53
　　definitions of types of, 53
　　interval, 64–65, 85
　　items included in, 49
　　as key component for level of E/M services, 42, 44
　　of normal newborn infant, 100, 101
　　for preventive services visits, comprehensive, 96, 97
　　required by life insurance company, 102
History of present illness (HPI), 49, 50
Home apnea monitoring event recording, pediatric, 467
Home health procedures/services—including home
　　infusion procedures/services, 503
Homeostasis, maintaining, 264
Home Services E/M category, 89–91
　　for established patient, 65, 89, 91
　　for new patient, 89, 90
Home visits by physicians, 503
Hospital Discharge Services E/M category, 66
　　for newborn, 100
Hospital Inpatient Services E/M category, 62–65
　　initial hospital care for new or established
　　　patient in, 64
　　subsequent hospital care for new or established
　　　patient in, 65

Tubal ligation or transaction procedures
abdominal or vaginal approach for, 251
done at time of cesarean delivery or intra-abdominal surgery, 251
as inherently unilateral or bilateral, 251
Tumor antigen testing, 27–28
Twins, coding for delivery of, 258
Tympanostomy
diagram of, 308
insertion of ventilating tube in, 307

## U

Ulnar styloid fracture, closed treatment of, 175
Ultrasonic guidance for cryosurgical ablation
of fibroadenoma, 155
of prostate, 245
Ultrasound, diagnostic, 348–350
code ranges of anatomic sites for, 349
obstetrical, 349–350
vascular, 350
Ultrasound guidance for intrauterine fetal surgical procedures, 253
Unlisted procedure
anterior segment of eye, 298
esophagus, 225
of external ear, 306
intestine except rectum, 221
laparoscopy or hysteroscopy, 251
nervous system, 280
nonobstetrical procedures of female genital system, 246
radiological, 332
rectum, 221
urinalysis, 382
Unlisted procedure or service, reporting, 32
Unlisted service or procedure, reporting, 332
Unlisted specimens, 392
Unplanned return to operating/procedure room by same physician, 525
Unrelated E/M service by same physician during postoperative period, 511–512
Unrelated procedure or service by same physician, 525
Unusual procedural services, 510–511
Ureteral strictures, endoscopic treatment of, 243
Urgent care setting for Office or Other Outpatient Services, 58
Urinalysis, 381–382
by dip stick or tablet reagent, 381
multiple tests for, 381
qualitative or semiquantitative, 382
Urinary System surgery subsection, 237–245
diagram of, 238

Uterine artery embolization, 216
Uterine fibroids, excision of, 249

## V

Vaccine development, 409
Vaccine, hepatitis B, 413
Vaccines, conjugate (combination), 414
Vaccines pending FDA approval, ✗ for, 30, 409
Vaccines/toxoids, immunizations for, 410–414
E/M services performed during same visit as, 411
Vacuum extraction during vaginal delivery, 254
Vagina, dilation of, 248
Vaginal hematoma, 247
Vagina repair, 248, 254
Valsalva maneuver, 479
Valsalva ratio, 479
Vascular access (catheterization procedures), 344
noncoronary, 344–345
nonselective, 345
selective, 345
Vascular disease, surgery for, 270
Vascular injection procedures, 211–215
Vascular interventional radiology, 342–348
arterial system anatomy for, 342–343
coding conventions for, 343–348
Vascular studies
Doppler ultrasonography, 460, 461
duplex scan, 460, 461
noninvasive physiologic, 460, 461
vasoreactivity, 461
Vascular ultrasound, 350
Venoarterial cannulation for chemotherapy perfusion, 213
Venogram, diagnostic, 216
Venography, diagnostic, 347–348
Venous conduit harvest, 204
Venous grafting or arterial grafting, 203
Venipuncture to obtain blood specimen, 498
Ventilating tube for ear
insertion of, 307
removal of, 308
Ventilator management, 461–467
Ventricular catheter placement or replacement and attachment to shunt system, 277–278
Ventriculography, left, 450–451
Vertebrae, types of, 162
Vertebral body, embolization or injection for, 165
Vertebroplasty of each vertebral body, 165
Vessel branches off arch of aorta, diagram of, 343
Video-assisted thoracic surgery (VATS), 190

Code ranges (eg, **00100–01999**) indicate reference to the entire code range, not to individual codes within that range.

64479-64484; 287, 289, 290
64480; 286, 287, 288, 289, 290
64483; 290
64484; 286, 287, 289, 290
64517; 290
64553; 275
64553-64581; 277
64553-64595; 272
64573; 274
64585; 277
64590; 230, 231
64595; 230, 277
64600-64640; 290
64600-64681; 290
64612-64614; 290, 474
64622; 291
64622-64627; 289, 291
64623; 291
64626; 291
64627; 291
64721; 514
64831; 116
64832; 116
64999; 280, 290
65091-65114; 295
65091-68899; 111
65093; 296
65125-65175; 295
65205-65265; 296
65270-65286; 296
65400-65426; 296
65430-65600; 297
65710; 429
65710-65755; 297
65730; 429
65750; 429
65755; 429
65800-66030; 297
65860; 297
66130-66250; 297
66500-66770; 297
66680; 296
66820-66986; 298
66990; 298
66999; 298
67005-67040; 298
67005-67299; 298
67101-67228; 298
67105; 299
67107; 299
67141; 304
67145; 304
67208-67220; 304
67220; 300
67221; 299, 300

67225; 299, 300
67227; 304
67228; 304
67229; 304
67311; 301
67311-67318; 301
67311-67999; 300
67318; 301
67400-67599; 300
67413; 296
67430; 296
67434; 296
67700-67999; 300
67810; 135, 300
67930; 296
67935; 296
67938; 296
68020-68399; 302
68399; 302
68400-68899; 303
68530; 296
68760; 303
68761; 303, 304
68810; 303
68811; 303
68815; 303
69000-69399; 305
69000-69979; 111
69150; 306
69155; 306
69200-69222; 306
69210; 306
69399; 306
69400-69799; 305, 306
69424; 308
69433; 307
69433-69436; 308
69436; 307
69535; 307
69610; 308
69714; 306
69714-69718; 306
69715; 306
69717; 306
69718; 306
69799; 306
69801-69949; 305, 307
69930; 307, 436, 437
69949; 307
69950-69979; 305, 307
69990; 111, 168, 169, 185, 266, 270, 282, 295, 306
70000; 225, 253, 329, 331, 332, 340, 346
70010-79999; 27

70015; 265
70030-70160; 335
70030-70330; 329
70190-70328; 335
70332; 339, 340
70333; 339
70336; 337
70360-70370; 335
70371; 438
70380; 335
70450; 271, 273, 332
70450-70470; 337, 481
70450-70498; 329
70460; 271, 332
70470; 271, 332
70480-70482; 337
70486-70488; 337
70490-70492; 337
70496; 335, 338, 481
70498; 335, 338
70540-70543; 337
70544; 336
70544-70546; 337
70544-70549; 335
70547-70549; 337
70551; 271, 273
70551-70553; 337, 481
70552; 271
70553; 271
70554; 335, 337
70555; 335, 337, 482
70557-70559; 337
71010; 75, 76
71010-71035; 335
71015; 75
71020; 75, 76
71040; 189
71060; 189
71075; 76
71090; 198
71100-71130; 335
71250-71270; 337
71275; 335, 338
71550-71552; 337
71555; 335, 337
72010; 330
72010-72120; 335
72125-72127; 337
72128-72130; 337
72131-72133; 337
72141; 337
72142; 337
72146; 337
72147; 337
72148; 337

**90768;** 417
**90772;** 410, 417, 467
**90773;** 417
**90774;** 410, 417, 467
**90775;** 410, 416, 417, 467
**90776;** 486, 487
**90801;** 418
**90801-90899;** 407, 417, 484
**90802;** 418
**90804-90809;** 420
**90804-90815;** 419
**90805-90829;** 420
**90806;** 420, 421
**90807;** 420
**90810-90815;** 420
**90816-90822;** 420
**90816-90829;** 419
**90823-90829;** 420
**90845;** 421
**90846;** 422
**90847;** 422
**90849;** 422
**90853;** 422
**90857;** 422
**90862;** 422
**90865;** 422
**90870;** 423
**90875;** 423
**90876;** 423
**90880;** 423
**90882;** 423
**90885;** 423
**90887;** 423, 424
**90989;** 424
**90901;** 423
**90901-90911;** 407
**90911;** 423, 428
**90918-90921;** 424
**90918-90999;** 407
**90922-90925;** 424
**90925;** 424
**90935;** 425
**90935-90937;** 424
**90937;** 425
**90940;** 425
**90945;** 425
**90945-90947;** 424
**90947;** 425
**91000-91299;** 407
**91010;** 426
**91020;** 425
**91022;** 425
**91034;** 425, 426
**91035;** 425, 426
**91037;** 426

**91038;** 426
**91040;** 426
**91065;** 426, 427
**91105;** 75, 76
**91110;** 427, 428
**91111;** 427, 428
**91120;** 428
**91122;** 428
**92002;** 432
**92002-92014;** 428, 429, 430
**92002-92499;** 407
**92004;** 432
**92012;** 432
**92014;** 432
**92015;** 428, 429, 430, 432
**92018;** 428, 432
**92019;** 428, 432
**92020;** 428, 432
**92025;** 429, 432
**92060;** 428, 432
**92065;** 428, 432
**92070;** 428, 432
**92081;** 432
**92081-92083;** 428
**92082;** 432
**92083;** 432
**92100;** 432
**92100-92130;** 428
**92120;** 432
**92130;** 432
**92135;** 428, 432
**92136;** 432
**92140;** 428, 432
**92225;** 432
**92225-92260;** 430
**92226;** 432
**92230;** 432
**92235;** 432
**92250;** 432
**92260;** 432
**92265;** 432
**92270;** 433
**92275;** 433
**92283;** 433
**92284;** 433
**92285;** 433
**92286;** 433
**92287;** 433
**92310;** 433
**92311;** 433
**92312;** 433
**92313;** 433
**92314;** 433
**92315;** 433
**92316;** 433

**92317;** 433
**92325;** 433
**92326;** 433
**92340;** 433
**92340-92371;** 430
**92341;** 433
**92342;** 433
**92352;** 433
**92353;** 433
**92354;** 433
**92355;** 433
**92358;** 433
**92370;** 433
**92371;** 433
**92499;** 431, 433
**92502;** 305
**92502-92700;** 407
**92506;** 434, 435
**92507;** 434, 435
**92508;** 434, 435
**92520;** 438
**92585;** 475, 481
**92597;** 437
**92601;** 437
**92601-92604;** 436, 437
**92602;** 436, 437
**92603;** 437
**92604;** 436, 437
**92605;** 437
**92606;** 437
**92607;** 437
**92607-92609;** 437
**92608;** 437
**92609;** 437
**92610;** 438
**92611;** 438
**92612;** 438
**92612-92617;** 186, 438
**92626;** 438
**92626-92627;** 437
**92627;** 438
**92630;** 438, 439
**92630-92633;** 437
**92633;** 439
**92640;** 439
**92700;** 439
**92950;** 76, 439, 440
**92950-93799;** 407
**92950-92998;** 439
**92951;** 76
**92952;** 76
**92953;** 75, 76
**92960;** 440
**92961;** 440
**92973;** 441

# The perfect companion to
# Principles of CPT® Coding, fifth edition

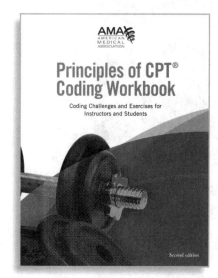

## Principles of CPT® Coding Workbook, second edition
### (formerly CPT® Coding Workbook)

Revised and expanded by more than 150 pages, the second edition lays a foundation for understanding CPT coding by providing detailed examples designed to strengthen coding skills. In-depth instruction on key coding concepts is provided by CPT code section, with extensive coding scenarios and operative procedure exercises given at the end of each chapter to test knowledge. A detailed answer key with comprehensive rationales walks the reader through the process of code assignment.

Written by the AMA's CPT coding experts and specialty society advisers, this resource was developed as a companion to the best-seller *Principles of CPT Coding* to provide additional code instruction and exercises, and can also be used as a stand-alone teaching tool. Features and tools in this new edition include:

- **Two new chapters** explain Category II codes and the CPT codebook appendixes
- **New illustrations** enable readers to visualize the area being discussed
- **Decision tree flowcharts for selected specialties** demonstrate correct code selection
- **Expanded chapters** on E/M, medicine, surgery, anesthesiology and radiology now include updated coding information and instruction

Softbound, 8-1/2"x11", 300 pages
ISBN: 978-1-57947-883-4   Order #: OP570407
Price: $59.95   AMA member price: $44.95

---

## New coding and documentation resources from "The Source of CPT"—the AMA

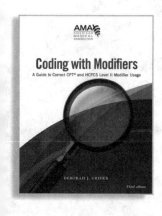

### Coding with Modifiers, third edition

The new, third edition of *Coding with Modifiers* explains revisions made to modifiers in CPT® 2008, along with new tools to aid in modifier instruction. This edition contains updated CMS, third party payer and AMA modifier guidelines to assist in coding accurately and avoiding payment delays. Coding tips and decision tree flow charts help clear up confusion surround modifier usage. A new test-taking tool is provided on CD-ROM, giving users a stimulated test taking environment. New clinical examples and additional test-your-knowledge questions are also included.

Available December 2007
Softbound, 8-1/2"x11", 500 pages
ISBN: 978-1-57947-889-6   Order #: OP322007
Price: $92.95   AMA member price: $69.95

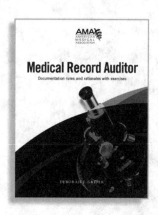

### Medical Record Auditor, second edition

The new, second edition of *Medical Record Auditor* expands on the principles of medical record documentation and provides instructions on how to perform a medical record audit in the physician's or outpatient office. This edition contains extensive coverage of E/M documentation and chart audits, guidelines for auditing radiology and operating room records, information on how to ensure medical records are compliant with current regulation and more than 110 auditing case examples and report templates. PowerPoint® presentations outlining each chapter and answer keys are included on CD-ROM.

Softbound, 8-1/2"x11", 458 pages
ISBN: 978-1-57947-884-1   Order #: OP301007
Price: $74.95   AMA member price: $54.95

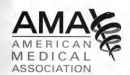

AMERICAN
MEDICAL
ASSOCIATION

**Order Today! Call toll-free (800) 621-8335 or order online at *www.amabookstore.com***

# Stedman's CPT® Dictionary

## End the guesswork of code assignment by expanding your understanding of CPT® code descriptions

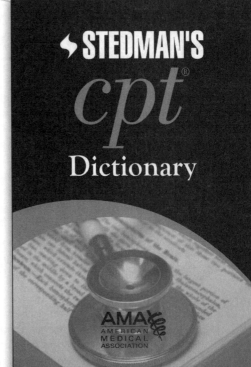

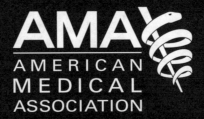

AMA
AMERICAN
MEDICAL
ASSOCIATION

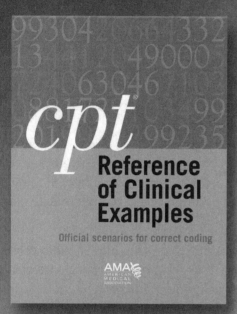
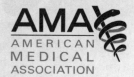

# CPT® coding answers—
## *straight from the source!*

## With the *AMA's CPT® Network*, get expert answers and data fast, all from your desktop.

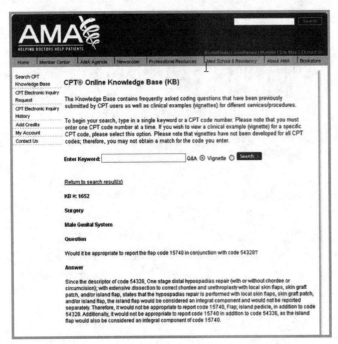

Brought to you by the American Medical Association (AMA) coding professionals who develop the Current Procedural Terminology (CPT®) code system, CPT® Network is a subscription-based online inquiry system that helps you find fast, accurate answers to all of your coding questions.

CPT® Network allows you to quickly research the network's Knowledge Base of commonly asked coding questions and clinical examples as well as:

- Submit electronic inquiries directly to a CPT expert for timely, accurate results
- Track inquiry history
- Add credits to your account toward additional electronic inquiries (special pricing available)

■ Easily update customer profile information, and more

**Choose the subscription package that best meets your needs.**

| CPT® Network | Description | Price | AMA member price | Users |
|---|---|---|---|---|
| Package A | 50 electronic inquiries + Knowledge Base | $2,600 | $2,250 | 2–5 |
| Package B | 25 electronic inquiries + Knowledge Base | $1,500 | $1,200 | 2–5 |
| Package C | 5 electronic inquiries + Knowledge Base | $480 | $255 | Single |
| Package D | 2 electronic inquiries + Knowledge Base | $320 | $108 | Single |
| Package E | Knowledge Base access only | $200 | FREE | Single |

**Subscribe today! Visit *www.cptnetwork.com* for details.**

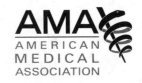

AMERICAN MEDICAL ASSOCIATION

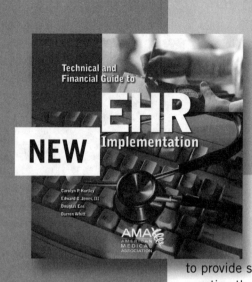
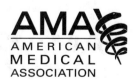

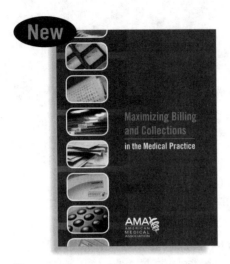
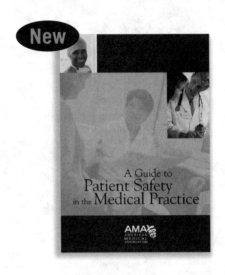
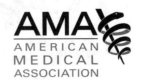

## Principles of CPT® Coding, Fifth Edition

CD-ROM Installation Instructions

This *Principles of CPT Coding* CD-ROM is a cross platform CD-ROM that will run on both Windows-based and Macintosh PCs.
To install the CD-ROM, follow these steps:

### Users

1. Insert the CD into your CD-ROM drive.
2. If Autoplay is enabled, the CD will open automatically to reveal two files labeled Principles PowerPoint® Presentation and Facilitator's Discussion. Click either of the two files that appear in the CD window to begin using the files on the CD-ROM.
3. If AutoPlay is *not* enabled and the CD-ROM does not open automatically, follow these steps:
   a. Select Start > My Computer and double click the CD-ROM icon to display its contents. You should see the two files on the CD-ROM.
   b. To begin, click any of them.

### Minimum System Requirements

### Windows

- CD-ROM drive
- Microsoft® Windows® NT, 2000, XP, Vista
- 64 MB RAM
- Microsoft® PowerPoint® 2002 or later

### Macintosh

- CD-ROM Drive
- Apple Mac OS 9.0 or higher
- 64 MB RAM
- Microsoft® PowerPoint® 2002 or later